# AGE ERASERS *for* Women

## Actions You Can Take Right Now to Look Younger and Feel Great

By the Editors of **PREVENTION** Magazine Health Books
and the Rodale Center for Women's Health

Doug Dollemore, Mark Giuliucci, Sid Kirchheimer,
Ellen Michaud, Elisabeth Torg, Laura Wallace-Smith, Mark D. Wisniewski

Edited by Patricia Fisher

Rodale Press, Emmaus, Pennsylvania

Copyright © 1994 by Rodale Press, Inc.
Cover photograph copyright © 1994 by James McLoughlin
Illustrations copyright © 1994 by Susan Rosenberger

**Library of Congress Cataloging-in-Publication Data**

Age erasers for women : actions you can take right now to look younger and feel great / by the editors of Prevention Magazine Health Books and the Rodale Center for Women's Health.
    p.  cm.
  Includes index.
  ISBN 0–87596–214–9 (acid-free paper) hardcover
    1. Middle aged women—Health and hygiene.   2. Aged women—Health and hygiene. 3. Middle aged women—Mental health.   4. Aged women—Mental health.   5. Longevity. I. Prevention Magazine Health Books.   II. Rodale Center for Women's Health.
RA778.A34   1994
613′.04244—dc20                                    94–28251
                                                  CIP

**Distributed in the book trade by St. Martin's Press**

  4  6  8  10  9  7  5  3      hardcover

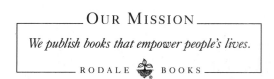

OUR MISSION

*We publish books that empower people's lives.*

RODALE ❦ BOOKS

# *AGE ERASERS FOR WOMEN* EDITORIAL AND DESIGN STAFF

SENIOR MANAGING EDITOR: PATRICIA FISHER

SENIOR EDITOR: RUSSELL WILD

STAFF WRITERS: DOUG DOLLEMORE, MARK GIULIUCCI, SID KIRCHHEIMER, ELLEN MICHAUD, ELISABETH TORG, LAURA WALLACE-SMITH, MARK D. WISNIEWSKI

CONTRIBUTING WRITERS: STEFAN BECHTEL, JEFF CSATARI, LISA DELANEY, TIM FRIEND, MARK GOLIN, MARCIA HOLMAN, CLAIRE KOWALCHIK, RICHARD LALIBERTE, JEFF MEADE, MELISSA MEYERS, RICHARD TRUBO, JOSEPH M. WARGO, STEPHEN WILLIAMS

ART DIRECTOR: STAN GREEN
INTERIOR AND COVER DESIGNER: ACEY LEE
STUDIO MANAGER: JOE GOLDEN
LAYOUT DESIGNER: LYNN N. GANO
TECHNICAL ARTISTS: KRISTEN PAGE MORGAN, DAVID Q. PRYOR, COLIN SHERMAN
COVER PHOTOGRAPHER: JAMES MCLOUGHLIN
ILLUSTRATOR: SUSAN ROSENBERGER

RESEARCHERS AND FACT-CHECKERS: SUSAN E. BURDICK, HILTON CASTON, CHRISTINE DREISBACH, VALERIE EDWARDS-PAULIK, JAN EICKMEIER, THERESA FOGARTY, CAROL J. GILMORE, DEBORAH PEDRON, SALLY A. REITH, SANDRA SALERA-LLOYD, ANITA SMALL, CAROL SVEC, MICHELLE M. SZULBORSKI, JOHN WALDRON

COPY EDITORS: SUSAN G. BERG, KATHY DIEHL

OFFICE STAFF: ROBERTA MULLINER, MARY LOU STEPHEN, JULIE KEHS

## *PREVENTION* MAGAZINE HEALTH BOOKS

EDITOR-IN-CHIEF, RODALE BOOKS: BILL GOTTLIEB
EXECUTIVE EDITOR: DEBORA A. TKAC
ART DIRECTOR: JANE COLBY KNUTILA
RESEARCH MANAGER: ANN GOSSY YERMISH
COPY MANAGER: LISA D. ANDRUSCAVAGE

# CONTENTS

# Part III: Boost Your Youthfulness

# INTRODUCTION

## It's Earlier Than You Think

**M**aybe death and taxes are inevitable, but for most of us, those two aren't nearly as fearsome as the prospect of getting older. Getting older. *Aaarrrgghh!* The words alone are enough to chill the heart of any red-blooded American woman. And we cringe at the timeworn images that accompany those words—of gray hair, deep wrinkles, flaccid arms, saggy thighs, the end of attraction and romance and possibility.

It was fine for Gloria Steinem to say proudly, during one of her milestone decades, "This is what 40 looks like." She said it again on her 50th birthday—cheerfully adding on another ten years, of course.

But most of us aren't so cavalier and confident. And we're certainly not laughing in public as the birthdays roll by. We stopped admitting our ages after 29, and we change the subject when anybody younger says "So when did you graduate from college?"

That's why we wrote *Age Erasers for Women.*

After a year of talking to experts and doing extensive research on how to stem the tide of time, our team of writers found that it is indeed possible for any woman to turn back the clock—or at least to freeze it in place. At the very least, this book will help you redefine your image of aging, so you can move into tomorrow with energy and anticipation.

We embarked on this project after you told us that aging was one of your biggest worries. It's a concern that we share—and why not? In America, youth is king, especially for women.

When a man gets gray around the temples, he's distinguished. When he develops a paunch, he's cute. When he starts playing golf instead of pickup games with 18-year-old guys at the local basketball court, he's settling down.

When that happens to a woman, she's getting older.

But it doesn't have to be that way. The hundreds of simple strategies in this book will help you feel and look younger, no matter what your age.

We also wrote a book for men, who, despite society's tolerance for their pot-bellies and thinning hair, told us that they're uneasy about aging, too. *Age Erasers for Men* speaks to their concerns; *Age Erasers for Women* speaks to ours.

So take this book—please. And have some fun with it. The future is better than you think.

*Patricia Fisher*

Patricia Fisher
Senior Managing Editor
Rodale Books

# Part I

## How a Woman Ages

# Stop the Clock

## And Make the Years Treat You Right

Pepper Herman plays killer golf, drives a sports car and zips back and forth between her home in Charlottesville, Virginia, and voice-over jobs for ad agencies in Wilmington, Delaware, and Philadelphia.

Her hair is long and dark. Her skin is smooth. People tell her that she looks a lot like Cher.

Oh, and one other thing: Pepper Herman is 60.

Back in her thirties and forties, Pepper started to create the vibrant, energetic woman she is today. You can do that, too.

## The Real Age Makers

Aging today is not like it was for our mothers.

Lots of us had mothers who put on an extra ten pounds at age 30. They got wrinkles at 35, dry skin at 40, joint stiffness at 45, high cholesterol at 50, heart disease at 55, memory loss at 57 and osteoporosis at 60.

We don't.

We don't because today we know that a low-fat diet prevents the weight gains and increases in cholesterol associated with aging.

We know that staying out of the sun and using sunscreens prevent the proliferation of wrinkles.

We know that alpha-hydroxy acids—acids found in fruit and milk—prevent the dry, patchy skin that comes with age spots and baggy skin.

We know that exercise—particularly water aerobics and swimming—delays the onset of arthritis.

We know that aerobic exercise, a low-fat diet, aspirin and relaxation exercises prevent the progression of clogged arteries to heart disease.

We know that working crossword puzzles and reading the op-ed section of a newspaper can counteract the memory loss that results from an aging brain.

And we know that weight-bearing exercise and getting enough calcium can prevent the thinning of a woman's bones that leads to osteoporosis.

In other words, we know that although overweight, wrinkles, dry skin, arthritis, high cholesterol, heart disease, memory loss, osteoporosis and a whole host of other things could rob us of our youth, the real age maker is not physical: It's the mind-set that allows us to veg out in front of the television, eat high-fat foods, smoke, skip vegetables, bake in the sun and forget to play and challenge ourselves.

Aging, for the most part, is what we do to ourselves.

# The Biology of Aging

"The human body is designed to last 110 years," says Ben Douglas, Ph.D., professor of anatomy at the University of Mississippi Medical Center in Jackson and author of *AgeLess: Living Younger Longer*. "Just like other members of the animal kingdom, our bodies are designed to last roughly five times the age of when we reach our sexual maturity. And with proper care, we should."

So what is it about aging that stops us? Let's take a part-by-part look, keeping in mind that much of what we call aging can be overcome.

*Skin.* In your twenties, accumulated sun damage may cause skin across your forehead to wrinkle. In your thirties it may wrinkle between your eyes. By age 40, crow's-feet appear and by age 50, wrinkles will have started at the corners of your mouth. Your skin will grow thinner, drier and less elastic with time—mostly due to a dwindling supply of connective tissue and estrogen that begins in the forties.

*Cardiovascular System.* After age 25, there's a small but steady decline in your cardiovascular system's ability to deliver oxygenated blood throughout your body during exercise. Typically, a woman's aerobic capacity drops 5 to 10 percent a decade between the ages of 25 and 75, which, as a practical matter, means that you get winded easier as you get older. The heart itself shrinks and beats at a slower rate. Blood vessels narrow and become less flexible. Systolic blood pressure—the top number on a blood pressure reading—increases about 20 to 30 percent between the ages of 30 and 70.

*Muscles.* After the age of 45 or so, your muscles begin to shrink as fat deposits expand. Muscle strength declines approximately 30 percent between the twenties and seventies, while muscle mass declines up to 40 percent.

*Bones.* Minerals—particularly calcium—are constantly being added and withdrawn from your bones throughout life. Deposits exceed withdrawals until around age 35. After that, there's a steady decline in bone strength and density. Partly because women's skeletons are smaller than men's to begin with, and partly because hormonal changes after menopause accelerate bone loss, osteoporosis tends to be more of a problem for women than it is for men. The risk of hip fractures starts to increase in the forties, then doubles every six years thereafter. In fact, researchers estimate that a woman is likely to have lost 30 percent of her peak bone mass by the time she's 70—making her increasingly prone to breaks.

*Joints.* A little stiffness in the knees, hips and neck begins somewhere in the forties. It gradually gets worse until your doctor diagnoses it as arthritis somewhere in your sixties. The disks between your vertebrae begin to degenerate and your spine stiffens somewhere in your seventies.

*Metabolism.* Starting around age 20, the number of calories your body needs gradually declines. By the time you're 70, you need 500 fewer calories a day.

*Brain.* We start life with a fixed number of neurons designed to provide a lifetime of service. Although we lose some nerve cells throughout life, in the absence of any disease, nerve cells function, repair, regenerate and make new connections during our entire lives. So what causes senility? Most of what we think of as senile behavior in older folks is caused by disease—not the loss of neurons.

*Immune System.* After age 60, the gradual decline in your immune system makes you more vulnerable to infection. If there's a bug around, you're more likely to get it.

*Cholesterol.* The amount of cholesterol in your blood—which is generated by the liver from saturated fats and cholesterol in your diet—tends to increase with age. It generally reaches a peak between the ages of 60 and 70, about a decade later than a man's peak.

*Hair.* Graying can start at any time. By age 50, half of us will have gray hair. By age 80, 40 percent of us will have more facial hair than we want.

*Bladder.* As estrogen begins to decline in the late forties, you may lose urine when you exercise. After menopause, you may be more prone to bladder infections.

*Reproduction.* The ovaries may produce less estrogen and progesterone after age 35. Fertility gradually ends and menopause begins.

*Eyes.* When you start holding the newspaper at arm's length somewhere in your early forties, the lens in your eye is losing its elasticity, making it less able to focus on close objects or shift from near to far. By age 65, you may begin to develop cataracts and by age 80, you may need three times as much light to see as clearly as you do now.

*Ears.* Your ability to hear begins to decline in your sixties. It declines in men as well, but at a faster pace.

*Nose.* Your ability to smell declines gradually after age 45.

*Mouth.* Your ability to sense subtle distinctions between flavors is reduced as the number of taste buds on your tongue declines.

# The Age Erasers

Despite what you've just read, very little of what we call aging has to happen. Somewhere around the age of 40, for instance, Pepper Herman realized that if she wanted to maintain her youthful body and energetic personality into her sixties and

*(continued on page 8)*

# Before the Looking Glass

Most of us keep track of the aging process with our mirrors. Here's what a woman can and can't see as she watches her face and body throughout the adult years.

*Twenties. She looks good and feels great. But by her early twenties, the first faint signs of aging begin to show. Her muscles begin losing fullness and firmness due to the loss of muscle fibers. The rate at which her body burns calories begins to slow, dropping off by 2 percent a decade from now on. Her high-pitched hearing also begins to fade.*

*Thirties. Laugh lines and fine furrows appear around her eyes and mouth, and if she's overly fond of a California tan, she may have other wrinkles, too, along with age spots. That's because her skin is gradually slowing production of pigment-producing melanocytes, tiny cells that help protect against ultraviolet radiation. In her early thirties, crow's-feet may appear. She also has to stay active to slow the decline in cardiovascular fitness, which begins now and may drop 30 to 40 percent by age 65. The gradual loss of bone strength begins around age 35.*

*Forties. As the sebaceous glands in her skin cut back production and supportive fibers grow less elastic, primarily as a result of sun damage, she notices that her skin is becoming drier, thinner and more inclined to wrinkle. She may notice bags under her eyes. To her sur-*

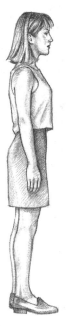 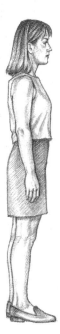 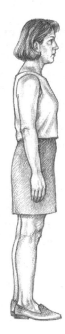

Twenties               Thirties              Forties

prise, she finds that she needs reading glasses—the lenses in her eyes began to stiffen at around age 40 and now she has difficulty focusing on close objects. She may also begin to see a slight weight gain.

**Fifties.** Most women's ovaries stop producing estrogen and progesterone at approximately age 50. The change accelerates bone loss, reduces vaginal lubrication and raises cholesterol levels—increasing the risk of osteoporosis, heart attack and stroke. Her skin will loosen and sag in the middle of her cheeks, jowls and neck. Skin tone becomes more irregular.

**Sixties.** She begins asking people to repeat what they said because her hearing has begun to fade. She may also discover she's actually begun to lose weight—mostly because she's lost muscle mass and gained fat. Since fat weighs less than muscle, she's now a size or so smaller. She also begins to grow ever-so-slightly shorter, losing half an inch over the next twenty years. Her skin is rougher and loses its uniform color, resulting in more splotches. She may also notice that she's more likely to pick up any bug that might come around, since a gradual decline in her immune system makes her more vulnerable to infections.

**Seventies.** She takes life just a bit easier now. Her muscle strength has declined from its peak in her thirties, and reduced muscle tone means that she may have difficulty holding her urine or having food move through her digestive tract. She also needs twice as much light to see as clearly as she once did, but the odds are ten to one that she's still as sharp mentally as she ever was.

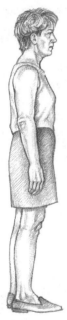 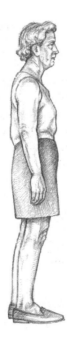 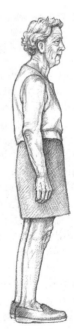

| Fifties | Sixties | Seventies |

## Our Longevity Bonus

Women may be tougher than men from the moment of conception.

The reason remains a mystery, scientists say. But they note that although 170 male embryos develop for every 100 female embryos, only 106 boys are actually born for every 100 girls.

More baby boys also die during infancy and childhood, so that by the time reproductive hormones start to flow during adolescence, the ratio of boys to girls is roughly one to one.

After that, the guys seem intent on leaving the planet. They are twice as likely to die from an unintentional injury as women and nearly three times as likely to die from suicide or murder.

Part of the reason for the early demise of so many men are the social expectations that encourage men to perform hazardous jobs, experts say. That's why men are 29 times more likely than women to fall to their deaths from a ladder, 23 times more likely to get killed by machinery or nearly 20 times more likely to be electrocuted.

Of course, as women gain more opportunities in the workplace, they'll probably also have an equal opportunity to be smashed, mangled and

seventies, she'd better develop a battle plan to fight off the encroachment of age.

Pepper approached it in her usual way: She talked to her friends, visited doctors and read everything she could get her hands on about maintaining a healthy body. Then she experimented to find what was right for her.

She started on an eating regimen that included beans, brown rice, broccoli, miso soup and rice cakes along with tomatoes, green peppers and chicken.

The diet was so successful that it made her look and feel about ten years younger. "My cholesterol dropped from 300 to 167 and I lost weight," she admits. "But I didn't exercise, so my build still wasn't good."

Finally a friend dragged her to an aerobics class that was simultaneously trying to build "buns of steel," "super abs" and "power pecs." "It was awful," says Pepper. "They all looked like movie stars, and I couldn't keep up. I could only do a quarter of what they did."

Exhausted, Pepper decided that she might need exercise, but not to that degree of intensity. "I found a local exercise class in which I felt more comfortable and went twice a week," she says. "I also started walking with my sister-in-law and playing golf.

"I started losing more weight, and toned and tightened myself up," she adds. "My body became better than it had been in my twenties and thirties."

zapped, so it's a good bet, experts say, that the discrepancies in death rates between men and women that are related to occupation will vanish.

In the meantime, statistics indicate that three things seem to increase longevity in women: education, work and an above-average income.

A 25-year-old American woman who did postgraduate work can look forward to living another 59 years, while a woman the same age who didn't get any further than fourth grade will probably live only another 54 years, reports the U.S. Census Bureau.

A 25-year-old woman who works outside the home can look forward to living another 61 years, while a woman the same age who works at home will probably live only another 56 years. And a white woman with family income over $50,000 annually can look forward to living another 58 more years, while a woman the same age whose family income is $5,000 or so will probably live only 54 more years.

But however women achieve extra years, the fact is that by the time men and women reach age 65, there are going to be eight women for every seven guys.

Eventually, Pepper says, she added a relaxation technique, popped some vitamins—especially vitamins C and E plus beta-carotene—chewed a calcium-enriched gum, earned her master's degree, hung out with creative people who stimulated her mind, got involved with political action groups and seduced her husband on energizing trips to Sante Fe, Anguilla, Vermont and anywhere else that took her fancy.

The result? The Pepper we have today: the prototype of an exciting, seemingly ageless woman—a woman who smashes every previous generation's concept of "old."

Not everyone can become a Pepper, of course. But everyone can hold aging at bay by changing the way they think about getting old.

To stay young, says Mary M. Gergin, Ph.D., associate professor of psychology at Pennsylvania State University's Delaware County campus, "We need to liberate ourselves from outdated notions of aging. We need to be unafraid and daring and willing to take risks. And we need to be willing to break the mold of aging."

Once we do, says Dr. Gergin, we need to use the age erasers that most suit our own individual needs just as Pepper Herman did.

Which ones? Here's a sample of strategies you might want to consider.

# Get Out and Sweat

If there's anything close to a genuine youth drug, it's sweat.

"There's nothing science can do for you that could be of more benefit than exercise," says William Evans, Ph.D, director of the Noell Laboratory for Human Performance Research at Pennsylvania State University in University Park and co-author of *Biomarkers: The Ten Determinants of Aging You Can Control.*

A single classic experiment vividly illustrates his point. In the late 1960s, a Swedish physiologist named Bengt Saltin asked five young men, two of them athletes, to lie in bed for three weeks while he monitored their bodies' physiological response to prolonged disuse.

The result? In the space of 21 days, doing nothing reduced the men's aerobic capacity so dramatically that Saltin concluded it was equivalent to almost 20 years of aging.

Fortunately, subsequent research found that exercise could not only reverse Saltin's results, it could actually reverse the results of age. In one study, for example, 11 healthy men and women from 62 to 68 years old were put on a moderately strenuous walking program for six months, and it boosted their aerobic capacity an average of 12 percent. When they continued the program for another six months, at double the intensity, their aerobic capacity climbed an additional 18 percent.

Many other physiological changes that were normally associated with aging can also be prevented or delayed with moderate exercise. What does "moderate" mean? About 20 minutes of aerobic activity, three times a week, should do the trick.

Researchers at Tufts University put a group of elderly volunteers on an eight-week strength training program and found that women as old as age 96 were able to increase their muscle size and strength by more than 200 percent.

Other researchers have found that weight-bearing exercises such as walking, jogging and dancing can keep bones strong and help prevent osteoporosis.

And still other researchers have found that exercise can prevent the age-related increases in weight, triglycerides, cholesterol and diastolic blood pressure—the bottom number in a blood pressure reading.

In a study at the University of Pittsburgh School of Medicine, researchers recorded weight, triglycerides, cholesterol and blood pressure for 500 women between the ages of 42 and 50 both at the beginning of the study and then again three years later. In the years between measurements, diastolic blood pressure, weight, triglycerides and total cholesterol levels went up for everyone. But the women who exercised the most gained the least weight and had healthier blood cholesterol levels.

How much exercise is necessary to keep your body youthful into your sixties and seventies?

"For years, exercise zealots kept saying that you had to work out for 30 to

40 minutes, three times a week, in order to get any benefit," says Dr. Evans. "But there's now good evidence that fairly low-level activity is also beneficial."

Low level means taking the stairs when you could take the escalator, he adds. It means parking the car far from the entrances of malls, supermarkets, work-places—in short, anywhere you go. It also means walking ten minutes in the morning or at lunch and another ten minutes around dinnertime or before bed.

"It all adds up," says Dr. Evans. And the bottom line is that it will erase many of the problems that make you old before your time.

## Eat Veggies for Longevity

Florets of broccoli, a heap of steamed carrots or a few ruffled leaves of kale may not seem important in the larger scheme of life. But these unassuming vegetables are actually "longevity foods"—clean-burning, high-octane fuels that can prevent many causes of premature aging.

Broccoli, brussels sprouts, carrots and most leafy green vegetables are packed with beta-carotene, the vitamin A–producing substance that has been shown to block cancer and prevent heart attacks.

Kale and other green vegetables are loaded with calcium, the mineral your body needs most to maintain its youthful bone strength.

And all vegetables have almost no fat or cholesterol, which will help keep age-related weight gains, high blood pressure readings and clogged arteries at bay.

## Feast on Fruit

Nutrients called antioxidants—vitamins C and E and beta-carotene—turn out to be key players in what could be described as an "anti-aging diet." Contained in fruits, nuts and some vegetables, antioxidants are the body's defense against what scientists call free radicals—highly reactive molecules zinging around the body doing all sorts of cellular damage. They are implicated in the initiation of cancer, heart disease and even aging itself—so much so that some scientists feel that the aging process is produced largely by a lifetime of tiny cellular nicks, dents and bumps caused by free radicals as they oxidize various cells.

Antioxidants—as their name suggests—provide the body with a natural defense against these free radicals. That's why nutritionists frequently recommend that you eat foods that are rich in vitamins C and E and beta-carotene.

Sources of vitamin C include citrus fruits, red bell peppers and cabbage. Other good sources are strawberries and tomatoes.

The best sources of beta-carotene are carrots, spinach, broccoli and lettuce.

Vitamin E is found mostly in nut oils such as hazelnut, sunflower and almond—all of which weigh in at more than 100 calories per tablespoon. You could eat the nuts themselves, of course, but you'd have to eat so many to

*(continued on page 15)*

# How Long Will You Live?

The choices you make every day about what you eat, whether you exercise and how stressed you let yourself get combine with any genetic glitches to determine your longevity.

Take the following test to see whether you stand a good chance at longevity. Keep a running tally of your score as you answer the following questions.

## Family History
## (Choose all that apply)

1. −1  One or both parents lived beyond age 75 and did not have cancer or heart disease
2. +2  Cancer in a parent or sibling
3.     Coronary heart disease before age 40 in:
   - +2  One parent
   - +4  Both parents
4.     High blood pressure before age 50 in:
   - +2  One parent
   - +4  Both parents
5.     Diabetes mellitus before age 60 in:
   - +2  One parent
   - +4  Both parents
6.     A stroke before age 60 in:
   - +2  One parent
   - +4  Both parents

## Lifestyle and Health
## (Choose all that apply)

7. +2  Live and/or work in a heavily air-polluted area
8.     Smoking:
   - −1  Never smoked or quit over 5 years ago
   -  0  Quit 1 to 5 years ago
   - +1  Quit within past year
   - +5  Have smoked more than 20 years
9.     You smoke cigarettes:
   - +2  Less than one pack a day
   - +3  One pack a day
   - +5  Over two packs a day

10.      Your alcohol use:
-1   None or seldom
 0   Drink no more than 1½ ounces of hard liquor, 5 ounces of wine or 12 ounces of beer a day
+2   Three or more drinks a day

11.      Your blood pressure:
-2   Below 121/71
 0   121/71 to 140/85
+2   141/86 to 170/100
+4   171/101 to 190/110
+6   Above 190/110

12.      Your blood cholesterol level:
 0   190 or below
+1   191 to 230
+2   231 to 289
+4   290 to 320
+6   Over 320

13.      Your HDL cholesterol level:
-1   over 60
 0   60 to 45
+2   44 to 36
+4   35 to 28
+6   27 to 22

14.      Your weight:
 0   Normal or within 10% of normal
+1   Overweight by 20 to 29 percent
+2   Overweight by 30 to 39 percent

15.      You exercise:
-2   Vigorously, more than 45 minutes, four to five times a week
-1   Vigorously, at least 30 minutes, three times a week
 0   Moderately, at least 30 minutes, three times a week
+2   Moderately, twice weekly
+3   Rarely or never

## Personality and Stress Evaluation
### (Choose all that apply)

16. +2   Intensely competitive

*(continued)*

## How Long Will You Live? —Continued

17. +2  Angry and hostile
18. +2  Don't express anger
19. +2  Work hard without feeling satisfaction
20. +2  Hardly laugh; depressed often
21. +2  Rarely discuss problems or feelings with others
22. +2  Constantly strive to please others rather than yourself
23. −2  None of the above

### Diet
### (Choose all that apply)

24. −2  You eat cabbage, broccoli, cauliflower, carrots or beans three or more times a week
25. −2  You eat high-fiber grains (such as whole-wheat bread, brown rice, bran cereal) almost daily
26. −2  You eat three or more servings of fruits and vegetables a day
27. +1  You go on one or two fad weight-loss diets a year
28. +2  You eat butter, cream and cheese frequently
29. +2  You eat beef, bacon or processed meats frequently
30. +2  You salt food before tasting
31. +2  You eat more than six eggs a week
32. +2  You eat ice cream, cake or rich desserts almost every day

### Other Factors

33. +3  You take birth control pills and smoke
34. +1  You are post-menopausal and do not take estrogen

### Interpreting Your Score

**−16 to 0.** Low risk. You should enjoy a long, healthy life free of cancer, heart disease, stroke or diabetes. Continue your lifestyle.

**1 to 34.** Moderate risk. You are at some risk of developing ill health and can expect to live an average life span. Check the test to see where you can lower your risk.

**35 to 60.** High risk. You are at considerable risk of contracting a life-threatening illness early in life and dying sooner than you should. Use the test to see how you can lower your risk. Seek medical advice.

**Over 60.** Very high risk. Your health is at extreme risk, and you may die prematurely. Use this test to identify your unhealthy habits and consult your physician for further advice.

get much vitamin E that you'd be munching all the time—not to mention getting all that fat, too. As a result, many women prefer to get their vitamin E from a supplement.

# Commit Yourself to Life

"The scientific literature is absolutely unequivocal on one point," says Dr. Evans. "People who have meaningful lives and something that gives them a sense of purpose—a fulfilling career, involvement in community or church work—live longer and live healthier than those who don't."

# Walk in the Moonlight

You may call the effects of sun on your skin tanning, but dermatologists call it photoaging. That's because exposure to the ultraviolet rays in sunlight literally causes the wrinkles, speckles, uneven pigments and age spots that we generally attribute to aging skin. With enough exposure, the skin thickens, sags and develops a harsh, leathery texture. And the fairer your complexion, the more extensive the damage.

You'll also look older than you really are. Dermatologists studied 41 white women, ranging in age from 25 to 51, who'd lived in Tucson, Arizona, for at least a decade. Some were inveterate sun worshippers; others stayed pretty much indoors.

The women's faces were photographed, without makeup, in unflinching close-ups. Then the photos were shown to a panel of female judges who were asked, "How old do these women look?"

There was no difference in perceived age between those who'd exposed themselves to a lifetime of tanning and those who'd shunned the sun in the women who were in their twenties and early thirties. But among the older women (median age 47), the story wasn't so pretty. In fact, the women with sunbaked faces were perceived to be fully five years older than those who'd kept out of the sun.

What's more, since studies have shown that long-term sun exposure increases your risk of cataracts, too much sun can age your eyes as well.

That's why experts say you should stay out of the sun as much as possible and learn to love big shady hats. Wraparound sunglasses and a sunscreen with a sun protection factor, or SPF, of 15 will also help shield your eyes and skin from the sun.

# Avoid Smoke

Smoking cigarettes is a great way to spend a lot of money to age faster, feel worse and get sick sooner.

Although smoking used to be thought of as a man's health problem,

"You've come a long way, baby." And now, if you smoke, you're just as likely to die from lung cancer as a man.

You also get to join the guys in an extra added smoking bonus: For those of you who've actually inhaled, you get "smoker's face," which includes wrinkles at the mouth, nose and eyes that are exclusively due to the facial contortions necessary to drag on a cigarette.

## Work Those Neurons

The best way to keep your mind alert, your intellect sharp and your memory keen is to keep your brain active. That's because brain cells have tiny branches that grow and spread when used—just like the roots of a plant when it's watered—or wither and die when not used.

Researchers have found that the brain cells of rats housed in an intellectually stimulating environment—meaning rat toys and other rats—are more densely packed with these brain cell branches than animals kept in toyless, joyless isolation.

The same may be true in humans. Studies indicate that when one or another area of the brain is used intensively, that area explodes with growth. The area of the brain devoted to understanding words, for example, is much larger in college grads than in high school grads. And the reason is probably due to the fact that college folks spend more time working with words.

In short, keeping your mind working—pursuing an advanced degree, reading on a wide variety of topics, learning a new language or in any way providing the brain with mental stimulation—keeps your neural filaments jangling well into old age.

# Part II
## Stop the Age Robbers

# AGE SPOTS

## *What to Do When the Damage Is Done*

She was a striking woman of a certain age. She was fit and trim, and she had obviously cared for her complexion. You admired her style, her carriage, her makeup. Getting older wouldn't be so bad if you could look that good, you thought. Then suddenly, you noticed her hands. They were covered with brown blotches. Ugh.

These days, you might find yourself glancing worriedly at your own hands. Only a few so far—but there they are. Age spots. Liver spots. Solar lentigos. But it doesn't matter what you call them: They add unnecessary years to your appearance, and they're one reason your hands can give away your age. But nowadays, you can do a whole lot more about age spots than simply count them as they come.

## Sort Your Spots

First, you need to decipher what's an age spot and what's not. There are several types of these unsightly blotches, but one cause is common to all of them, doctors say, and that's sun damage. You may have exposed unprotected skin to ultraviolet rays, whether from a tanning booth, a sunlamp or years of going without sunscreen. In response, your skin has tried to protect itself by producing an overabundance of melanin—the pigmented cells in your skin—in uneven patches.

What's the difference between age spots and freckles? Freckles appear when you're young, they're more numerous in the summer and they tend to fade with age, says Nicholas Lowe, M.D., clinical professor of dermatology at the University of California, Los Angeles, UCLA School of Medicine. Age spots get worse—and they don't go away.

If you've ever gone in the sun while pregnant, you may have developed the "mask of pregnancy"—a light to dark patch on the skin. This is not an age spot. Properly called melasma, these blotches most often occur on the face and might go away on their own.

## Chemical Causes

Certain substances that come in contact with your skin may cause age spots, says Karen Burke, M.D., Ph.D., a dermatologist in private practice in New York City. Chemicals called psoralens are present in foods such as parsley, limes and parsnips. When you handle these foods and then go out in the sun, your skin may be more sensitive and burn more easily where the psoralens touched it. When the little blisters from the burns have healed, age spots may appear in their places.

Antibiotics such as tetracycline (Achromycin), some diuretics (water pills) and antipsychotic medicines such as chlorpromazine (Thorazine) will also cause your skin to produce age spots when it is not protected from the sun, Dr. Burke says.

And if your favorite fragrance or lotion contains musk or bergamot oil, which are common perfume ingredients, it may give you more than a lovely scent. When perfumes or lotions containing these ingredients are applied to sun-exposed areas, they can produce age spots, says Dr. Burke.

## An Ounce of Prevention

The most important thing you can do to stop new age spots from forming is to wear sunscreen—all the time. And an ounce is just about what it takes, dermatologists say.

**Apply it daily.** "Start using an SPF 15 or higher sunscreen on a daily basis," says John E. Wolf, Jr., M.D., professor and chairman of the dermatology department at Baylor College of Medicine in Houston. What's SPF? It stands for sun protection factor. SPF 15, for example, means you can stay out in the sun 15 times longer before burning than you could without the sunscreen.

"Apply it to the backs of your hands and to your face first thing in the morning, before you put on any moisturizer or makeup," says Dr. Wolf. "When you wash your hands, don't forget to reapply your sunscreen. If you see the beginnings of age spots or melasma, switch to a higher SPF sunscreen than the one you are currently using."

And remember that if you're not prepared to use sunscreen every day, year-round, there's really no point in treating your age spots, Dr. Lowe says. Without daily sunscreen, "in a number of months your skin will be back in the same shape," he says.

**Wash up.** Wash your hands thoroughly after handling foods that contain psoralens and reapply sunscreen before going outdoors again, says Dr. Burke.

**Save your scents for the shadows.** Apply your perfume or lotion to areas of your skin that will not be exposed to sun, Dr. Burke suggests.

# Spot Removers

The most important thing you can do about age spots is to first make sure they're not precancerous lesions, says Dr. Wolf. "If a brown spot pops up out of the blue, or an old one suddenly changes shape, becomes raised or bleeds, have a dermatologist look at it to be certain it's not an early melanoma," he says. The number of cases of melanoma, a potentially fatal form of skin cancer, is increasing more rapidly than any other type of cancer. (For more information on melanoma, see Skin Cancer, page 314.)

If you have just a few age spots that are not too dark, you can try an over-the-counter remedy. But for a persistent crop of age spots, your dermatologist has several very effective treatments.

**Bleach them away.** Head for the hair care aisle at your drugstore for nonprescription help. It takes time, but a hair bleaching product that's at least 30 percent hydrogen peroxide may help fade away smaller age spots. The products with the highest percentage of peroxide are those for blonde shades, such as Nice 'n Easy 97 and 98 and Ultress 24, 25 and 26. Dr. Burke suggests dabbing on the peroxide with a cotton swab. You may have to use it daily for several weeks.

**Try a fade cream.** We're not kidding. You heard those ads for "Porcelana, the Fade Cream" when you were a kid. It's still around—and it just may work. Porcelana and other creams, including Esotérica and Palmer's Skin Success fade creams, contain hydroquinone, which interferes with your skin's production of melanin. Dr. Burke says these products work slowly, however. Prescription-strength hydroquinone preparations might work faster.

**Seek a stronger solution.** Melanex and Eldoquin, creams that contain prescription-strength hydroquinone, can go a long way toward wiping out bigger, more stubborn age spots. Tretinoin (Retin-A), which comes in cream or gel, is another potential age spot eraser, although it's normally used against acne and wrinkles. Retin-A gradually returns skin to its normal state, making age spots fade away. It can be used in conjunction with hydroquinone at your doctor's discretion, Dr. Burke says.

**Consider peeling or freezing.** Your dermatologist may try trichloroacetic acid, which is often used for chemical peels and is quite effective on age spots. It would be a good choice for just a few spots that aren't too dark, says Dr. Wolf. Another alternative is freezing the spots with liquid nitrogen. With these treatments, which must be done in a doctor's office, there is some risk that the chemicals will do their job too well, leaving de-pigmented white spots where the age spots have been removed, he says.

**Learn about lasers.** Wielded by a highly skilled physician, a laser is the high-tech solution to age spots, says Dr. Lowe. It's also the priciest. "The great thing about laser treatment for this problem is that in the hands of an expert, you don't run the risk of having white spots where the dark spots had been," he says. Ask your dermatologist whether laser treatment is available. Does it hurt? Only for an instant. And the pain is similar to a rubber band snapped against your skin, Dr. Lowe says.

Remember that with all these treatments, it is essential to keep using sunscreen. Otherwise, new age spots are sure to form.

# ALLERGIES

## *Easing the Sneezing*

**M**other Nature really painted a masterpiece today. Crisp blue skies, fragrant blooming flowers, a gentle spring breeze—perfect for a stroll through your favorite patch of woods.

For all of ten minutes, that is. Then the pollen police take over, stuffing up your nose, making you sneeze uncontrollably and turning your leisurely walk into a mad sprint for a box of tissues. You quickly go from spry spring chicken to grumpy old hen, ready to crawl back indoors, close up the windows and hibernate with a packet of sinus tablets.

Seasonal allergies like this affect an estimated 45 to 50 million Americans, or one in every five, according to the National Institutes of Health. But pollen isn't your only allergy enemy. Dozens and dozens of things can trigger reactions, from dust mites, mold and pet dander to shrimp and peanuts. Even a pair of latex gloves can cause trouble.

And allergies aren't always something to just sneeze at, either. In cases of asthma and severe allergic reactions, they can prove deadly.

"Fortunately, there's a lot you can do to improve things," says Harold S. Nelson, M.D., senior staff physician at the National Jewish Center for Immunology and Respiratory Medicine in Denver and a member of the National Asthma Education Expert Panel of the National Heart, Lung and Blood Institute. "Although they seem terrible when you have them, allergies really don't have to dominate your life."

## A Case of Mistaken Identity

When it comes to fighting disease, your immune system is usually pretty sharp. It can quickly identify harmful foreign substances such as germs and viruses and whip them with lethal efficiency.

But sometimes your body gets a little confused. For reasons nobody quite understands, your immune system can mis-identify harmless substances such as mold, pollen and food by-products and attack them. Mast cells, part of your immune system, attach to these substances, which are known as allergens. The mast cells then release powerful chemicals called allergic mediators, including histamine, to combat the allergens.

The result, Dr. Nelson says, is a classic case of allergy symptoms: a stuffed-up nose, sneezing and watery eyes. In some cases, you can end up with a rash, hives, stomach cramps, nausea or vomiting, too. And 5 to 12 hours later, when other parts of the immune system join the battle, a second wave of similar symptoms can strike.

Heredity plays a big role in many allergies. You can inherit the ability to produce an antibody called immunoglobulin E, or IgE, says allergist David Tinkelman, M.D., clinical professor of pediatrics in the Department of Allergy and Immunology at the Medical College of Georgia in Augusta. If a person doesn't inherit IgE, he says, she is less likely to develop any allergies.

Food allergies are rarer than you may think. Only 0.1 to 5 percent of the population suffers from them, Dr. Nelson says—and most people outgrow them by age three. Still, some adults are highly allergic to nuts, seafood, milk, eggs or other foods. And in some cases, the reactions worsen over time.

Women rarely develop new allergies after age 30, Dr. Nelson says, unless you are exposed to some new allergen such as a pet or a pollen. The good news is that allergies tend to subside at about age 55, says Edward O'Connell, M.D., professor of pediatrics, allergy and immunology at Mayo Medical School in Rochester, Minnesota. That's because your immune system begins to decline, making it less likely to attack an invading mold spore or another allergen.

## More Than a Little Trouble

Allergies are usually just an annoyance. Over-the-counter or prescription medication may ease the symptoms when taken properly, Dr. Nelson says. But some allergies can be much more serious.

In the case of bee stings and other unfortunate insect encounters, about 1 percent of the population can develop a dangerous allergic reaction called anaphylaxis, according to Susan Rudd Wynn, M.D., an allergist with Fort Worth Allergy and Asthma Associates in Texas.

Shortly after a bee sting, you may notice symptoms such as itchy palms, tightness in your chest, hoarseness or even a feeling of impending doom. "If so, get yourself to an emergency room fast," Dr. Wynn says. "Anaphylaxis is not something to mess around with." In fact, she says, as many as 50 people a year die of the reaction—many because their throats swell shut and they suffocate. In rare cases, food allergies can cause anaphylaxis as well, Dr. Wynn says.

There's no test to predict anaphylaxis. But doctors can give adrenaline self-injection kits to people known to have severe allergic reactions. "That can buy you some valuable time, so you can get to the hospital for further treatment," Dr. Wynn says.

There's also some evidence that women with allergies may be at higher risk of developing certain cancers, including breast cancer. A six-year study of more than 34,000 Seventh-Day Adventists in California showed that women with three or more allergies may be 1.25 times more likely to develop breast cancer. The good news is that the study found a slight decrease in ovarian cancer risk for women with allergies.

Researchers don't understand the possible link between allergies and cancer. In fact, Dr. Nelson says other studies have shown that the chances of developing some types of cancer actually seem to decrease in people with allergies. "That whole area is really up for grabs," he says.

## Sniffle Stoppers

The best advice for beating allergies? Avoid whatever makes you sneeze or break out. An allergist can perform simple blood or skin tests to pinpoint your allergies. "Once you know what causes your problems, you can try to stay away from it," Dr. Wynn says. Here are some tips on keeping your allergies at bay.

**Know your medicines.** Two types of over-the-counter medication attack allergy symptoms. Antihistamines relieve sneezing, itching and a runny nose. And decongestants help unclog a stuffed-up nose. Some medicines combine both; read the label to find out what you need.

"The big drawback of antihistamines is that they can make you drowsy," says Edward Philpot, M.D., assistant clinical professor of medicine in the Department of Rheumatology, Allergy and Immunology at the University of California, Davis, School of Medicine. "If all you have is a stuffy nose, just take a decongestant." Or if you need an antihistamine, try one of the newer prescription antihistamines such as terfenadine (Seldane), which don't make you drowsy. If you're unhappy with the effectiveness of one antihistamine, try different brands until you find one that works.

**Strike first.** If you know the pollen count is high, or if you're going to visit Aunt Jane and her hairy cat, take your medication before symptoms arrive. "It's much more effective that way," Dr. Philpot says. "It gives the antihistamine a jump on your allergies." Make sure you take the medicine at least 30 minutes to an hour before you're exposed to allergens.

**Avoid alcohol.** Alcohol can worsen symptoms such as congestion, Dr.

Wynn says, and mixing alcohol with antihistamines can cause serious health problems. Read the label on allergy medication before drinking anything.

**Be doggone careful.** Dander from dogs and cats is a major household allergen. If you're allergic to dander, the simplest way to ease the problem is to send Fido or Fifi packing. But that's hard to do emotionally—and it may be unnecessary. Dr. Nelson says taking these steps might correct the problem and still let Rover stay over:

- Keep pets out of your bedroom.
- Confine them to parts of the house that don't have carpeting.
- Bathe pets weekly to wash the dander away.

**Wipe out dust.** The biggest enemy in your house is also the smallest. The dust mite is a microscopic organism—but under magnification, it looks like the Beast That Ate Coney Island. Breathing these little buggers can cause all sorts of allergy symptoms. To help reduce the problem, the experts suggest these steps:

- Cover your pillow cases and mattress in plastic covers. Wash sheets, mattress pads and blankets every week in water that is at least 130°F.
- Clean house regularly. Vacuum at least once a week, and keep clutter to a minimum—it collects dust.
- Choose hardwood or vinyl floors over carpet whenever possible. A study at the University of Virginia at Charlottesville found that carpeting attracts and keeps allergens at 100 times the rate of bare polished floors. Use washable area rugs instead, especially in the bathroom.

**Starve your food allergy.** The only way you're going to avoid a food allergy is to avoid the food that's causing it. If you're not exactly sure which food causes problems, Dr. Nelson says a doctor can perform tests to check your sensitivity. You can also keep a food diary, noting what you eat each day and keeping track of when you have an allergic reaction. That should help you narrow down the source of the allergy.

**Lay off the latex.** A study of more than 1,000 U.S. Army dentists found that between 9 and 14 percent of people may be allergic to the latex found in gloves. Other studies found similar allergies to rubber products ranging from boots to condoms.

The bottom line? If one brand gives you a rash, try another. Since manufacturers use different additives in their products, Dr. Nelson says it may help to sample brands until you find one that doesn't bother you.

**Sleep in.** Pollen counts usually peak in the early morning, between 5:00 A.M. and 8:00 A.M. If you can stay inside until mid-morning, Dr. Philpot says you'll be better off. And no matter how nice it feels outside, don't sleep with the windows open on high-pollen days. "You'll guarantee yourself a miserable wake-up call," he says.

# Can You Be Allergic to Cold?

You walk down the driveway on a cold winter morning to fetch the newspaper. Two minutes later, you break out in hives. Why?

It's rare but possible to be allergic to sudden drops in temperature, says Martin Valentine, M.D., an allergy expert and professor of medicine at the Johns Hopkins Asthma and Allergy Center in Baltimore. A 30-degree drop—such as when you leave your warm house to fetch the paper—can cause hives and swelling that can last for up to two hours. Drastic changes, such as jumping into a frigid swimming pool, can cause shock in some people.

If you think you're allergic to cold, try placing a sandwich bag full of ice on your arm for 30 seconds to two minutes. An itchy welt will form if you're allergic. Your doctor can prescribe the proper antihistamine medication to help you deal with the problem, Dr. Valentine says.

**Halt the humidity.** Keep your house or apartment dry to cut back on allergens. That means running the air conditioner, which dries the air as it cools it, or using a dehumidifier. A humidifier or vaporizer is a bad idea. "Dust mites just love the extra moisture from a humidifier," Dr. Wynn says. "And so does mold. If you have allergies, just forget the humidifier altogether."

**Uproot your problem.** The American Lung Association says the following plants can cause big-time allergies: oak and walnut trees, juniper, cypress, privet shrubs and all types of Bermuda grass. If you're looking for sneezeless replacements for your yard, try these: mulberry, fir, pear and silk trees; hibiscus, yucca and pyracantha shrubs; and dichondra, Irish moss and bunchgrass lawns.

You can obtain a complete list by writing to the American Lung Association of California, 424 Pendleton Way, Oakland, CA 94621. Enclose a self-addressed, stamped envelope.

**Give it a shot.** If your allergies resist every trick, you may need allergy shots, Dr. Philpot says. Doctors can inject you with small quantities of what you're allergic to, helping your body build immunity to the allergen. This is usually a last resort, since you may need from six months to a year of weekly shots plus another shot each month for up to five years.

"It takes a commitment," Dr. Philpot says. "But it's the only thing that helps some allergy sufferers." Dr. Philpot recommends that you steer clear of corticosteroid injections, which he says can suppress your immune system and linger in your body. "They're like using a bazooka to rid your house of termites," he says. "You'll get rid of the termites, but you'll damage the house pretty badly, too."

# ANGER

## *Find the Calm before You Storm*

Unlike our mothers, we've been encouraged to express our feelings—all of them. Even anger.

"The older generation of women—those ages 55 and older—was raised to believe that nice ladies don't get angry. But young women got a different message—that you don't have to be a 'nice lady' all the time," says anger researcher Sandra Thomas, R.N., Ph.D., author of *Women and Anger* and director of the Center for Nursing Research at the University of Tennessee, Knoxville.

That's good, because suppressing anger is a sure way to make you old before your time. Failing to deal with anger has been linked with numerous physical and mental ills as well as premature death, according to Mara Julius, Sc.D., psychosocial epidemiologist at the University of Michigan School of Public Health in Ann Arbor. For more than 20 years, Dr. Julius has studied how coping with anger affects the health of women and men. In her first study, she found that women who suppressed anger during arguments with their spouses were more likely to die prematurely from cardiovascular disease, cancer and other causes than those who expressed their anger during arguments.

## Equal Opportunity Destroyer

Now that we're expressing our anger as freely as men, we're suffering like them. Men have long had a reputation for venting easily enough—maybe too easily, since their anger is often misdirected. "A man who is angry for one reason or another will come home and kick the dog," says Sidney B. Simon, Ed.D., a counselor and professor emeritus of psychological education at the University of Massachusetts at Amherst and an author who specializes in anger and forgiveness.

And we seem to be following suit, according to a comprehensive new study on women and anger. "We found that women tend to express their angry feelings most frequently to members of their families—especially their husbands—even if their families are not the source of their anger," says Dr. Thomas, who conducted a study of the anger habits of 535 women. "On one hand, this can be viewed in a positive way: More women now feel secure enough in their relationships to express their real feelings without fear that they will end those relationships. But some constraints must be practiced. Yelling and cursing solve nothing and can cause a lot of alienating, especially when they involve children. Little kids don't understand why Mommy is really angry at Dad or the people at work but is yelling at them. When this occurs, and it occurs frequently, it can cause a whole new set of problems—including guilt."

# A Is for Aging

Not that dealing with the A-word has ever been a walk in the park. "When you get angry, there are various physiological changes in the body, because anger triggers the fight-or-flight response," says Christopher Peterson, Ph.D., author of *Health and Optimism* and professor of psychology at the University of Michigan. "The adrenaline gets hyped up, the heart beats faster, the respiration becomes more rapid and shallow and digestion stops."

When they occur often, these changes take a toll on your health. Getting angry frequently has clearly been established as a contributing factor to higher rates of heart disease, high blood pressure and other life-threatening illnesses,

## Eating to Tame Your Temper

The wrong diet can make you feel grumpy as well as look lumpy, according to researchers at the State University of New York at Stony Brook and Oregon Health Sciences University in Portland.

After studying 156 women and 149 men for five years, they noted that people who consumed the typical high-fat American diet were more easily angered than those who changed to healthier diets. Those who switched to low-fat eating showed less anger and were less likely to get depressed.

Researchers believe that reducing the amount of fat in the diet and in the bloodstream plays a role: The less fat there is, the better the overall mood.

especially if you have a Type A personality and get angry easily. "Everything bad that anger does to men it also does to women," says Redford B. Williams, M.D., director of the Behavioral Medicine Research Center and professor of psychiatry at Duke University Medical Center in Durham, North Carolina, and author of *Anger Kills*. Women start out with lower risk of heart disease than men, he says, but hostility increases that risk just as it does for men.

Anger also affects our mental capabilities. "All emotions have some influence on the way we think, but strong emotions can actually slow your ability to rationalize, solve problems and make decisions," says Dr. Julius. "When you're feeling anger, rage or hostility, it overwhelms you. In some people, it slows down the thinking process; in others, it stops the thinking process completely."

Adds Dr. Peterson, "Anger also causes us to lose our sense of humor and to alienate people. It takes its toll on our energy, creativity and all those other things that might keep us feeling young."

## Extinguishing the Ire

So what can we do? After all, we will get angry; everybody does. And surely nobody is advising that we hide the rage, frustration and other feelings that can eat us up inside, because that does even more harm than expressing them.

The answer? Get angry when you're provoked, says Dr. Julius, but don't stay that way. Cool off and identify the source of your anger. Remove the source by identifying the underlying problem.

If anger is handled correctly, says Dr. Julius, all those related health problems—elevated blood pressure, obesity, depression and even future heart problems or cancer—can be avoided. "You become ill during chronic prolongation of anger," says Dr. Julius. "In other words, it's not so much getting angry that hurts. The damage is done when you stay angry. If you get angry and deal with it quickly and effectively, the damage is minimal, if anything."

So here's how to blow your top without blowing it.

**Get busy to chill out.** While men are quicker to fly off the handle, women tend to stew for as much as an hour before their anger is spent, says Dr. Thomas. It's during this time that much of the physical damage is done. "One thing that's really effective is to do something physical during this time," she advises. "Take a walk. Go for a swim. Vacuum or clean out your closets . . . anything physical that you can do will help."

Since anger triggers the fight-or-flight response, your body will want to either fight or move (fly), Dr. Thomas explains. Exercise burns off this adrenaline more positively than does idle stewing, allowing you to think more clearly about how to deal with your anger.

**Take a zen-minute break.** The workplace is one of our most frequent sources of anger, but the office isn't always the best place to unwind by logging some miles or laps. "In situations where you can't exercise, find a quiet spot and

# From Repression to Expression

So you're one of those women who simply can't express their anger? Well, you're not alone. Despite findings that women are having an easier time expressing their anger, "many women, even young women, still feel uncomfortable expressing their feelings," says anger researcher Sandra Thomas, R.N., Ph.D., author of *Women and Anger* and director of the Center for Nursing Research at the University of Tennessee, Knoxville.

If that sounds like you, here are some ways of learning how to express yourself.

**Learn to be assertive.** That's right—it's a learned behavior for many of us. There are various assertiveness training courses that teach women how to deal with anger. Call the local chapter of a mental health agency for a list of courses being offered near you. "Being more assertive initially shakes up the balance in a relationship, even if it will ultimately be helpful," says Emily Rosten, Ph.D., a psychologist in private practice in Salt Lake City.

Be sure to let everyone know about the new you. "Without an announcement of your new attitude, you can bewilder the other person. Even more important, unless you let the person know you want to change, that person will do all kinds of things to make you behave the way you did before," says Dr. Rosten.

**Respond in writing.** Still not comfortable with a face-to-face encounter? Then put it on paper. Nobody says you have to talk to express yourself. "Respond in writing," says Jerry L. Deffenbacher, Ph.D., professor of psychology at Colorado State University in Fort Collins. "That gives you a chance to collect yourself and to get your act together to respond more rationally. And you'll feel in control by halting the immediate confrontation."

**Have a good cry.** "Crying is a very healthy emotional release that helps you get anger out of your system," says Dr. Thomas.

meditate, breathe deeply or practice some other type of relaxation technique," says Dr. Thomas.

**Know your limits.** A lot of our anger is over things we can't do anything about. "Take traffic, for instance," says Dr. Julius. "Everybody gets angry at traffic, so I won't say 'Don't get angry when you're stuck in traffic.' But you don't have to be consumed by that anger if you do what you can but realize that it's all you can do."

In other words, try to avoid traffic by rescheduling your commuting time or taking a bus or train. "But realize that you alone cannot stop traffic, so getting angry about it is a waste of your energy. Instead, channel your feelings into using this wasted time more effectively—by listening to music or audio books in your car, planning out your schedule or some other activity," suggests Dr. Julius.

**And count your blessings.** "It's also important to realize the trade-offs—to count your blessings, so to speak," adds Dr. Julius. "When you're stuck in traffic, think of all the positive things: the fact that you own a car and that along with city traffic come some advantages—museums, good restaurants, parks." It takes some time to do this, but it helps put things in perspective. When you're angry at your kids or husband, thinking about how lucky you are to have them eases your anger.

**Choose your targets.** "It's important that you express your anger, but there are constraints against expression in a lot of situations," says Dr. Thomas. "For instance, it's usually disadvantageous to express your feelings in the workplace to your supervisor or even to your co-workers. Even if you're doing everything right, speaking in a totally rational and low-key manner, the other person is likely to get defensive and later engage in vindictive behavior."

You have to be careful with whom you share your feelings, or they might come back to haunt you. Dr. Thomas's advice: "Pick a close friend, confidante or someone else you can trust—and not necessarily the subject of your anger—to tell how you feel."

**Mind your I's and you's.** It's always better to express your feelings rather than to tell others how they should have behaved, says Roland D. Maiuro, Ph.D., director of the Harborview Anger Management and Domestic Violence Program in Seattle. One way is to concentrate on giving "I" messages. For instance, it's better to say "I was angry that you didn't drop off the car" than "You said you'd drop off the car, and you didn't." "You" messages sound accusatory and put people on the defensive, setting up rather than solving arguments.

**Surround yourself with happy people.** "If you want to not be angry, try to associate with non-angry people," advises Dr. Peterson. "These ways of feeling and acting are contagious. The trick, of course, is to surround yourself not with some annoyingly positive Pollyanna people but with rational people who see solutions to problems."

**Be a joiner.** Some anger stems from loneliness, so adding to your social calendar can help. "Sometimes you have to force yourself to get involved. You may not like everyone, and they might not like you, but being active breaks up depression, and depression can leave many people angry," says Dr. Peterson. "Besides, joining clubs and other groups helps you see the accomplishments in your life, which can defuse feelings of anger, loneliness and depression."

# ARRHYTHMIAS

## *When Your Heart Skips a Beat*

**W**hen was the last time you felt the pitter-patter of rapid or quirky heartbeats inside your chest? Maybe it was just moments before you presented a report at work. Or during a rigorous workout at the gym.

Welcome to the world of arrhythmias, which are disturbances of your heartbeat's normal rhythm.

Your heart may be the ultimate workaholic, beating about 100,000 times a day, year after year, decade after decade. If you had a schedule that rigorous, you'd occasionally blip, bump and jump, too. Fortunately, your heart is smart enough to kick back only briefly. Most of the time, almost faster than you can feel it, the heart sets itself on course, and life goes on as if nothing had happened.

But as we get older, those idiosyncrasies of the heart can sometimes become more than just a harmless nuisance. Certain forms of arrhythmia can sap your energy, leaving you feeling weak and timeworn. On occasion, big disturbances in the heart's rhythm can threaten the heart itself. "In general, when arrhythmias begin later in life, they should be investigated much more carefully and treated more seriously," says Marianne J. Legato, M.D., associate professor of clinical medicine at Columbia University College of Physicians and Surgeons in New York City and author of *The Female Heart*.

## The Plaque Connection

Let's put things in perspective: No matter what your age, the vast majority of ticker tremors aren't a sign of impending doom. "At some time in our lives, everyone has extra beats," says Gerald Pohost, M.D., director of the Division of Cardiovascular Disease at the University of Alabama School of Medicine in Birmingham. "And certainly, the vast majority of these extra beats are harmless."

But if you develop coronary artery disease—in particular, the buildup of plaque, which consists of fatty and other deposits that can play a role in a heart attack—then those arrhythmias might need a little more attention. If plaque deprives your heart of the blood and oxygen it needs, your heart might shake and shudder with arrhythmias that are potentially more serious and may even be life-threatening.

Luckily, premenopausal women have some extra protection against heart problems because our bodies produce the sex hormone estrogen, which guards the heart against disease. As a result, women lag about ten years behind men in the development of hardening of the arteries. But all good things must come to an end. After menopause, women rapidly catch up with men as their estrogen is reduced to a trickle. So as we age, we have a greater chance of heart disease, heart attack and potentially serious rhythm disorders.

If you have had a heart attack, your doctor may have cautioned you that your injured heart muscle is more likely to cause anarchy in the heart's routine electrical impulses, possibly producing dangerous abnormal beats called ventricular arrhythmias. When this happens, the heart can accelerate from a jog to a supersonic sprint, beating at a frantic, chaotic pace of perhaps 150 to 300 times per minute instead of the normal 60 to 100. At its worst, this condition can deteriorate into such serious quivers and quakes that the heart will no longer pump blood adequately—and sudden death may be the result.

## A Woman's Heart Problem

It's not necessarily a worrisome condition, but in some women, it can cause mild chest pain, fainting, dizziness—and irregular heart rhythms. It's called mitral valve prolapse (MVP), a congenital condition that affects about 5 percent of the population—as many as two-thirds of them women.

Just what is MVP? It's a heart valve irregularity in which the leaflets (or flaps) of one of the heart's valves bulge, or prolapse, when the heart contracts. "In women, it's one of the more common causes of palpitations and heart rhythm disturbances," says Richard H. Helfant, M.D., vice chairman of medicine and director of the Cardiology Training Program at the University of California, Irvine, Medical Center and author of *Women, Take Heart.*

If you have MVP and you're concerned about those irregular blips in your chest, talk to your doctor.

This scenario might make you anxious. But don't panic. Remember, most irregular heartbeats are pretty routine—and if you take control of your health, you may reduce your chances of experiencing both the harmless and the more troubling fidgets and flickers in your heartbeat.

# Righting Your Rhythm

Since many of the most worrisome heartbeat irregularities are closely intertwined with coronary disease, probably your best defense against those unwanted shivers and shudders of the heart is to prevent problems such as heart attack in the first place. Even if you've experienced palpitations, you might be able to keep them to a minimum through lifestyle changes. Here are some ways to do that, either by preventing them altogether or by cutting down on their frequency.

**Snuff out smoking.** Too many women—about one-fourth of the female population—smoke. And as a group, we're starting to smoke earlier. These cigarettes are increasing our risk of heart disease and of certain types of irregular heartbeat. But if you nix the nicotine in your life, your heart will have an easier time keeping a steady beat, says Richard H. Helfant, M.D., vice chairman of medicine and director of the Cardiology Training Program at the University of California, Irvine, Medical Center and author of *Women, Take Heart.*

**Learn some stress busters.** Now that more women than ever before are climbing the corporate ladder, there is a greater number experiencing job-related stress. Add to that the tension brought on by women's other roles—wife, mother and homemaker—and it's no wonder that some women feel that they're buckling under the pressure.

Many experts believe that stress plays a role in the development of coronary artery disease as well as contributes to arrhythmias. To take a bite out of stress, try lots of exercise, warm baths, massages and creative hobbies, says Fredric J. Pashkow, M.D., medical director of the Cardiac Health Improvement and Rehabilitation Program at the Cleveland Clinic Foundation in Cleveland and co-author of *The Woman's Heart Book.*

**Avoid the java jitters.** One British study of 7,300 people found that nine or more cups of coffee can make some hearts skip beats. Some smaller studies suggest that lesser amounts of coffee may have similar effects, particularly in those people unaccustomed to drinking lots of caffeine. Play it safe: If you're prone to arrhythmias, go easy on the caffeine.

**Imbibe with caution.** Even if you don't consume alcohol regularly, don't think you're out of harm's way. Binges of heavy drinking—six or more drinks in a day, according to one U.S. study—can increase the risk of very rapid heartbeat associated with an irregularity called supraventricular tachyarrhythmia. Some doctors call this syndrome holiday heart because it often happens in people who consume more alcohol than they're used to during the holidays.

# Professional Beat Keepers

Arrhythmias might be the farthest thing from your mind when you go to the doctor for a physical exam. But with an electrocardiogram—a test that measures the smoothness of your heartbeat—she could confirm a rhythm disorder. She may also diagnose arrhythmias if you show up at her office complaining of palpitations and light-headedness. You have several options when more than lifestyle changes are required to control a seriously irregular heartbeat.

Medications are one. "Medications are able to control many arrhythmias and their symptoms. Some of the newer drugs are quite effective," says Dr. Pohost. These medications can usually relieve you of the fear of sudden death by stabilizing the electrical activity of the heart, but they must be carefully chosen by your doctor, since they may cause side effects of their own, including aggravated arrhythmias, gastrointestinal upsets and low blood pressure. In many cases, people end up taking these drugs for the rest of their lives.

Your doctor might also recommend an implantable cardiac defibrillator. Your doctor will insert this battery-driven device right into your chest or abdomen, where it will monitor your heartbeat. If the beats become dangerously fast or chaotic, it will zap the heart with a shock that might feel like a slap or a thump in the chest. This is meant to startle your heart back to normal activity.

How successful are these devices? One study found that among 650 patients (average age 60 years), the implantable defibrillators kept 60 percent of them alive for at least ten years. The researchers estimated that virtually all of them would have died without this high-tech hardware.

When your heartbeat just won't shape up, doctors have another hi-tech option, called catheter ablation, at their disposal. This treatment is reserved for particular types of rhythm disorder that may be resistant to other therapies. It is particularly useful for conditions in which the abnormal heartbeat originates in the heart's upper chambers. It involves threading a thin tube through one of your veins and into the heart.

Once this catheter is properly positioned, a mild radio-frequency current is activated to kill tiny areas of the heart tissue that are causing the arrhythmias. By destroying cells in a section no bigger than one-fifth inch in diameter, this procedure eliminates the wacky impulses that cause certain types of high-risk arrhythmias.

# ARTHRITIS

## *How You Can Beat the Pain*

**A**n estimated 37 million Americans have arthritis—but often it's not whom you'd expect.

Sure, you might understand if it was your mother or grandmother. After all, about half the people over age 60 have some form of this disease, making it the single most common chronic condition among older Americans.

But arthritis in people your age?

It can happen.

Despite its reputation for being as much a part of growing old as gray hair, arthritis is an equal opportunity deployer—of pain. "Many people aren't surprised to hear that arthritis is the leading cause of disability in people over age 45," says Paul Caldron, D.O., a clinical rheumatologist and researcher at the Arthritis Center in Phoenix. "But they are surprised to learn it's the single leading cause of disability among all ages."

## The Hormone Link

Although there are more than 100 different types of arthritis, the most common are osteoarthritis and rheumatoid arthritis. Women are three times more likely than men to get rheumatoid arthritis, the most debilitating form of the disease.

Unlike osteoarthritis, rheumatoid arthritis typically affects the entire body. It is especially painful and commonly strikes in a woman's twenties and thirties.

"What's really sad is that many people have significant pain and loss of function, and there's nothing you can do to prevent it, since we don't know what causes it," says Arthur Grayzel, M.D., vice president of medical affairs for the Arthritis Foundation. "We know rheumatoid arthritis is an immunological disease, and like other immunological diseases such as asthma, lupus and thyroid problems, women get it at higher rates because they tend to have overactive immune systems. But there are also strong data to support that rheumatoid arthritis is related to hormones."

Researchers speculate that during our childbearing years, some of our hormones are assigned to protect fetuses from immunological attacks, says Dr. Grayzel. In the process, other parts of our bodies are left more vulnerable, and some researchers believe that's why some of us fall victim to rheumatoid arthritis. Even if a woman never bears a child, these hormonal changes still take place, which is why many childless women are among the nearly two million American women with rheumatoid arthritis.

The most common form of arthritis, osteoarthritis, affects 16 million Americans and results when the cartilage in joints deteriorates from stress, overweight or injury, which is often sports-related. "That's not to say that if you play sports, you'll get arthritis. But those who have experienced repeated injury to a joint, no matter how minor, have an increased chance of getting osteoarthritis," says Dr. Caldron. It strikes about 12 million women, who usually get it after age 55. Typical trouble spots include the fingers, feet, back, knees and hips.

## A Burden to Body and Mind

Either form of arthritis can take a toll on an active life. Arthritis can slow down your movements and cause some pain in your muscles, joints or tendons. At worst, it can cause enough agony to require hospitalization or around-the-clock care, says Jeffrey R. Lisse, M.D., director of the Division of Rheumatology and associate professor of medicine at the University of Texas Medical Branch at Galveston. Arthritis can also result in sleeping problems, decreased sexual activity because of pain and a weaker cardiovascular system, since many sufferers stop exercising when they have pain and swollen joints.

But arthritis ages more than just the body. "Depression is almost universal among arthritis patients," says Dr. Lisse. "But a lot of people with arthritis also get what's known as learned helplessness. That occurs when someone starts out healthy and able to do things for herself, but over time, as the pain gets worse, she is less able to take care of herself. Someone else must assume these functions, so the person with arthritis winds up more and more helpless. In fact, some of the youngest patients in nursing homes are people suffering from severe arthritis, who are there because of the inability to care for themselves."

Adds Dr. Grayzel: "I think that society almost expects people to have arthritis when they're old, so when an elderly woman limps or uses a cane, it doesn't really surprise anyone. But when you're young and your body image is very different, the effects can be devastating. The fact is, a lot of people who have arthritis—athletes, movies stars and others in the public eye—won't admit it because it seems to have a negative image. Having arthritis makes you seem old before your time."

# A Smart Strategy

But it doesn't have to be that way. You may not be able to prevent rheumatoid arthritis, but you can lessen its aging effects on you. And you may be able to prevent or lessen the pain of osteoarthritis. Here's how.

**Lose weight.** "Being overweight is a major risk factor, especially for arthritis of the knees and hips," says Dr. Grayzel. "Even when you're in your twenties or thirties, you should try to reduce your weight close to the normal range for your height. If you're 20 percent overweight—about 160 pounds or more for the average woman—you're a prime candidate for osteoarthritis. But any weight loss helps. If you lose just 10 pounds and keep it off for ten years, no matter your current weight, you can cut your risk of osteoarthritis in your knees by 50 percent."

**Watch what you eat.** Various studies show that food plays a crucial role in the severity of arthritis. Norwegian researchers discovered that patients with rheumatoid arthritis saw dramatic improvements in their conditions within one month of beginning vegetarian diets. Other scientists have found that omega-3 fatty acids, abundant in cold-water fish such as salmon, herring and sardines, also ease rheumatoid arthritis pain.

"A diet that's low in saturated fat and animal fat seems to be helpful," says Dr. Caldron. "Eating a lot of fresh fruits and vegetables and non–red meat sources of fat such as fish and chicken may cause the body to produce fewer pro-inflammatory substances. That's not to say a diet will cure arthritis, but it may modify the effects of arthritis.

"Some people react to certain foods, almost like an allergy," adds Dr. Caldron. "It may result from wheat or citrus fruits, lentils or even alcohol. The problem is, there's no way to test for this. But if you notice a significant reaction and more pain consistently within 48 hours after eating a certain food, eliminate it from your diet."

**Get physical.** Regular exercise to build your muscles and flexibility can keep osteoarthritis at bay or lessen its effects. Exercise is also recommended for rheumatoid arthritis, although workouts should be under a doctor's supervision and emphasize range-of-motion exercises.

"Exercise improves strength and flexibility, so less stress is placed on the joints and they can move easier and more efficiently," says John H. Klippel, M.D., clinical director of the National Institute of Arthritis and Musculoskeletal and Skin Diseases in Bethesda, Maryland. "Inactivity, on the other hand, actually encourages pain, stiffness and other symptoms."

Weight lifting is particularly useful because it builds muscle tone, which is especially important for arthritis sufferers. Emphasize building the abdominal muscles to reduce back pain and the thigh muscles for knee pain, advises Dr. Grayzel. Meanwhile, aerobic exercise such as running, bicycling and swimming are also helpful for improving flexibility.

**Slow down when you have to.** When a joint is swollen and inflamed, continuing to use it doesn't help. "Don't exercise through the pain," says Dr. Grayzel. "Otherwise, you'll just hurt more." So even if you're on a regular exercise program, skip a day (or two) when your joints or muscles begin to hurt.

**Get in gear.** "A frequent cause of osteoarthritis is injury, so you should take full advantage of the various protective equipment for athletics," says Dr. Caldron. "By wearing protective gear, you'll lessen the likelihood of injuring or reinjuring joints, tendons and muscles, which reduces the risk of osteoarthritis." That means you should wear padding on your knees, elbows and other likely trouble spots in order to reduce injury. These pads are available at any sporting goods store.

**Turn up the heat.** For immediate relief, many people find that placing warm, moist heat directly on inflamed areas helps reduce pain, says Dr. Lisse. Hot water bottles, heating blankets and hot baths help. But use heat judiciously—no more than 10 to 15 minutes at a time. And be sure to take a break for at least one hour before reapplying. Over-the-counter analgesic balms such as Ben-Gay can also help ease pain when joints are hot, tender and swollen. But don't use them with heat, cautions Dr. Caldron. The two together may cause nasty reactions such as burning and blistering.

**Or chill out to prevent pain.** Ice, meanwhile, is sometimes recommended to prevent pain when joints are overworked or overused. Dr. Lisse suggests that you wrap some ice in a towel and gently apply it to your joints several times a day, 15 minutes on and 15 minutes off.

Also practice the other way to cool off—by finding ways to deal with the stresses in your life. When you're tensed up, you hurt more. But anything you can do to learn to relax—whether it's listening to music, meditating or taking up a hobby—can help, especially when pain is severe.

# BACK PAIN

## *Coping with a Common Ache*

Years ago, you had dance moves that could have tied Patrick Swayze in knots. So when you went to your high school class reunion, you figured you were a cinch to win the limbo contest. But just as you were making your first pass under the bar, you felt a stabbing pain in your back. In an instant, "Twist and Shout" had a whole new meaning, and you felt like a golden oldie.

You recovered in a few days, but that episode was an all-too-painful reminder that your spine isn't made of rubber and that age is tiptoeing into your life through the back door.

"A 30-year-old woman who has an aching back and limited mobility can feel like a 90-year-old," says Joseph Sasso, D.C., president of the Federation of Straight Chiropractors and Organizations.

At least 70 percent of women will suffer from back pain at some point in their lives. Of those, 14 percent will have severe pain that lasts at least two weeks, and up to 7 percent will suffer chronic pain that can last for more than six months, according to Gunnar B. J. Andersson, M.D., Ph.D., professor and associate chairman of the Department of Orthopedic Surgery at Rush-Presbyterian–St. Luke's Medical Center in Chicago. Nearly 400,000 back injuries occur on the job each year, and that results in more lost productivity than any other medical condition. Back pain is the most frequent cause of restricted activity among people under age 45 and the second most common reason (after cold and flu) that we see doctors, according to the American Academy of Orthopaedic Surgeons. It is also the fifth leading cause of hospitalization and the third most common reason for surgery, Dr. Andersson says.

"Sleep, sex, sitting—I can't imagine any activity that isn't affected by the back. It's involved in almost everything we do. You can't get in and out of a car, run, jump or walk. Until you have back pain, you don't realize everything that a back does for you," says Alan Bensman, M.D., a physiatrist at Rehabilitative Health Services in Minneapolis.

# The Age of Opportunity

Many women experience their first bouts of back pain during pregnancy, as the uterus expands to accommodate the growing baby, Dr. Bensman says. Back pain can also occur after menopause, when estrogen production falls and a woman becomes more susceptible to osteoporosis, a loss of bone mass that weakens the back and causes pain. But back pain is particularly common among women between the ages of 30 and 45, says Dan Futch, D.C., chief of the chiropractic staff at Group Health Cooperative HMO in Madison, Wisconsin.

"Those ages are the window of opportunity for back pain," he says. "About the same time you start getting gray hairs, you'll probably start noticing twinges of pain in your back."

The thirties and forties are the years when arthritis and other types of natural degeneration in the small joints of the back begin to catch up with us, says Robert Waldrip, M.D., an orthopedic spine surgeon in private practice in Phoenix. Spinal stenosis, for example, a narrowing of the canal in the vertebrae that surround the spinal cord, puts pressure on nerves in the low back and causes pain. In other cases, the problem is a herniated disk. Disks are small pads made of a tough, elastic outer covering (called the annulus) and a soft center. The disks act like shock absorbers between the vertebrae. Over time, a disk can herniate, meaning that the annulus has torn and the soft center has extended out to press against a nerve root, causing horrible pain. Poor posture also increases strain on the back and can aggravate arthritis and lead to disk problems.

But by far, the most common cause of back pain is muscle and strain. As we get older, many of us get less exercise. As a result, the muscles in the abdomen and back that support the spine weaken and get out of shape, Dr. Bensman says. So things that you used to do with ease, such as hauling a bag of groceries out of your car, lifting a baby out of a crib or raking the leaves, suddenly make you feel like you have a dozen knives sticking in your back.

Lifting something when your back is out of shape is like someone pulling you out of the crowd at the Boston Marathon and forcing you to run the 26-mile course. You're probably going to get hurt, because you're straining your back in ways that it's not prepared for.

Of course, even well-trained athletes can get back pain, but in general, the better conditioned you are, the less likely your spine will cause havoc.

See your doctor if the pain is so intense that you can't move, if it spreads to your legs or buttocks, if your legs or feet feel numb or tingly, if you lose control of your bladder or bowel movements or if you also have a fever or abdominal pain.

# Keeping Your Spine Sublime

Often back pain is easily relieved without surgery or drugs, Dr. Waldrip says. In fact, 60 percent of people with acute back pain return to work within one week, and 90 percent are back on the job within six weeks. Here are some tips for preventing and treating back pain.

**Do an early morning stretch.** "I tell my patients to always start off their days by stretching while they're still in bed," Dr. Bensman says. "Remember that you've been lying prone for eight hours, and if you jump right up, you may be looking at a sore back." So before you get up, slowly stretch your arms over your head, then gently pull your knees up to your chest one at a time. When you're ready to sit up, roll to the side of the bed and use your arm to help prop yourself up. Put your hands on your buttocks and slowly lean back to extend your spine.

**Walk away from it.** Walking and other aerobic exercises such as swimming, biking and running keep your back healthy by conditioning your whole body. They strengthen the postural muscles of the buttocks, legs, back and abdomen. Aerobic exercise may help your body release endorphins, hormones that subdue pain. Try doing an aerobic workout for 20 minutes a day, three times a week, says Dr. Futch.

**You deserve a break.** Sitting puts more strain on your back than standing. If you must sit at your desk for an extended time or you're traveling by plane, train or car, change position often and give your back a break by standing up and walking around every hour or so, says Augustus A. White III, M.D., professor of orthopedic surgery at Harvard Medical School in Boston and author of *Your Aching Back*.

**Leave your luggage lie.** Instead of leaping out of the car or airplane and grabbing your bags, take a couple of minutes to stretch, Dr. Bensman suggests. Slowly bring your knees toward your chest and gently swing your arms around to loosen up stiff muscles. Avoid lifting with overstretched arms and try to keep the bags close to your body. Consider getting a collapsible luggage carrier with wheels.

**Kneel, don't bend.** Avoid bending over at the waist to pick up something. That creates tension in the back and increases your risk of injury, Dr. Futch says. Instead, use long-handled tools and kneel on a cushion or knee pad to garden, vacuum or do other "low-level" activities.

**Let your legs do the work.** If you're lifting something—no matter if it weighs 5 pounds or 50—bend your knees, keep your back straight, and lift with your legs. "The legs are much stronger than the back and can lift a lot more weight without strain," Dr. Futch says.

**Test the load.** "How many of us have strained back muscles when we tried to pick up boxes that we thought were empty but were actually filled with encyclopedias?" asks Dr. Sasso. Always nudge a box with your foot or cautiously lift it an inch or so before really trying to heft it. If it's too heavy for you, ask for help.

**Turn your back on heavy lifting.** If you can't find someone to help you

# Lifting 101: Back to Basics

We all think we know how to do it. After all, you've hoisted, hauled and hefted things for years. But even if lifting seems like a mundane part of life, doing it wrong can send a painful shock wave rippling through the sturdiest of spines. To prevent that, the American Academy of Orthopaedic Surgeons suggests that you follow these guidelines when lifting.

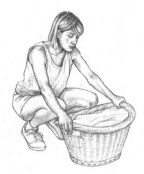

*Stand as close as you can to the object you want to lift. Separate your feet shoulder-width apart to give yourself a solid base of support. Bend at the knees, tighten your stomach muscles and lift with your legs as you stand up. Don't bend at the waist and don't try to lift an object that is too heavy or an awkward shape by yourself.*

*To lift a very light object such as a pencil off the floor, lean over, slightly bend one knee, and extend the other leg behind you. Hold on to a nearby chair or table for support as you reach down for the pencil.*

*When you are holding an object, keep your knees slightly bent to maintain your balance. Point your toes in the direction you want to move. Avoid twisting your torso. Instead, pivot on your feet. Keep the object close to you when moving.*

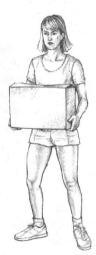

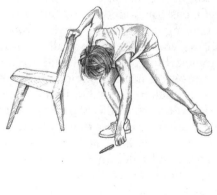

move a heavy object, try this maneuver as a last resort: If the object is sitting at table height, turn your back to it to drag or lift it. You can also use this technique for raising windows. This position reduces the pressure that would be exerted on your spine by forcing you to use your legs for leverage.

**Straighten up.** Maintaining good posture is one of the best ways to prevent back pain, Dr. Futch says. To improve your posture, try this. Stand against a wall or sit in a dining room chair, making sure that your shoulders and buttocks touch the wall or your chair. Slip your arm into the space between your lower back and the wall or chair. If there is a point where your hand isn't touching both your back and the wall or chair, tilt your hips so that the extra space is eliminated. Hold that position for a count of 20 while looking in a mirror to see what your posture looks like. Try to sense what it feels like, so you can maintain that posture for the rest of the day. Do that exercise once a day for three weeks to ensure that good posture will become a habit.

**Don't be a heel.** High heels change your gait, put additional stress on your lower back and adversely affect your posture, Dr. Bensman says. "High heels shouldn't be part of a woman's daily life. They should be worn only for special occasions. In normal daily life, heels should never exceed 1½ inches," he says. If you occasionally wear heels higher than that, wear them for no more than two hours at a time. Always have a pair of tennis shoes or flats available.

**Check your mattress.** Your mattress should provide proper support, be level and not sag. So if you feel like you're sleeping in the middle of a pita bread, it's probably time to get a new mattress, Dr. Sasso says.

**Roll it up.** A lumbar roll, a round foam-rubber pad that can be purchased at most medical supply stores, can help you maintain the natural curve in the small of your spine and prevent lower back pain, says Hamilton Hall, M.D., director of the Canadian Back Institute in Toronto. Whenever you sit, stick the roll between your lower back and the chair.

**Dress for success.** Fitting into a pair of skintight jeans may do wonders for your ego, but it can prevent you from using proper biomechanics such as bending your knees, especially in lifting, Dr. White says. Try wearing looser-fitting clothing for a month and see if that makes a difference.

**Smoking makes backs fume.** Smoking decreases blood flow to the back and can weaken disks, Dr. Bensman says. So if you smoke, quit.

**Drink your milk.** Women in their thirties and forties who exercise regularly and have calcium-rich diets are less likely to suffer from back pain caused by osteoporosis later in life, Dr. Bensman says. The Recommended Dietary Allowance of calcium for women over 25 years old is 800 milligrams a day. That's about the equivalent of one eight-ounce glass of skim milk, 1 cup of nonfat yogurt and ½ cup of cooked broccoli a day. Other good sources of calcium include salmon, sardines, cheese, buttermilk, kale, broccoli, pinto beans and almonds. If you don't eat plenty of calcium-rich foods—and many women don't—talk to your doctor about supplements.

**Do the big chill.** Apply ice to your aching back as soon as possible to reduce pain and swelling, Dr. Bensman says. Wrap an ice pack in a pillowcase or towel (never place the ice directly on your skin) and put it on the sore spot for ten minutes each hour until the ache subsides.

**Then warm it up.** Once ice relieves the swelling—usually within 48 hours—you can begin using heat. Heat increases blood flow to the wound, relaxes tissues and can improve your mobility, Dr. Bensman says. Apply a warm washcloth—it should be about skin temperature—to your back for 5 to 10 minutes every hour, or take a warm 15-minute shower or dip in a whirlpool.

**Reach for over-the-counter relief.** Taking one or two aspirin or ibuprofen tablets every four to six hours can relieve pain and reduce swelling, Dr. Bensman says. Be sure you don't exceed the manufacturer's recommended dosage.

**Put up your feet.** When minor back pain strikes, lie down on the floor and put your legs up on a chair so that your thighs stay at a 90-degree angle to your hips and your calves rest at a 90-degree angle to your thighs. This position relaxes key back muscles and is one of the least stressful for your spine, Dr. White says.

**Keep moving.** Although lengthy bed rest was once recommended for back pain, doctors now believe that the more active you are, the sooner you'll recover. In fact, two weeks of bed rest weakens muscles and the spine, and that can actually slow your recovery and make you more likely to have a relapse, Dr. Hall says. So don't stay in bed for more than two days, and make sure you get up at least once an hour to walk or stretch.

**Get manipulated.** Chiropractors are gaining respectability in the medical community, Dr. Bensman says. An analysis of 25 studies of spinal manipulation—the heart and soul of chiropractic treatment—found that manipulation does provide at least some short-term relief for uncomplicated, acute back pain.

"Sure, chiropractors work," Dr. Bensman says. "They're becoming quite knowledgeable and offering some real benefits." In a typical case, a chiropractor may do a series of thrusts with the heels of her hands along the troubled area of your spine. Ask your doctor for a referral to a chiropractor in your area.

**Belt it out.** If you have back pain during pregnancy, it could be caused by stress in the sacroiliac joint, which joins the pelvis to the spine, Dr. Hall says. To relieve that pain, which tends to be lower in the buttocks and is aggravated by standing or walking, wear a belt around your hips, below your pregnancy, to stabilize the pelvis. "When my wife was pregnant, she had this kind of pain," Dr. Hall says. "I gave her a big, wide cowboy belt from a pair of my jeans. She just cinched that on, and it was quite remarkable in relieving her pain."

**Get a second opinion.** More than 400,000 surgeries, such as spinal fusion and disk removal or destruction, are done each year to relieve back pain, according to the American Academy of Orthopaedic Surgeons. Yet a Blue Cross and Blue Shield study found that almost 13 percent of spine operations are performed for inappropriate reasons. Get at least one other opinion if your doctor has suggested surgery, Dr. White says.

# Eight Exercises to Minimize Back Pain

If you want a large return for a small investment, try these exercises recommended by the American Academy of Orthopaedic Surgeons. By strengthening and stretching your back, stomach, hip and thigh muscles, they will help keep your back feeling strong and flexible.

Check with your doctor before starting any exercise program.

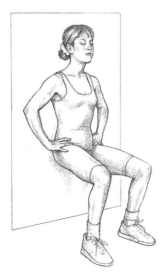

*Stand with your back against a wall and your feet shoulder-width apart. Slide down into a crouch, with your knees bent to about 90 degrees. Hold for a count of five and slide back up the wall. Repeat five times.*

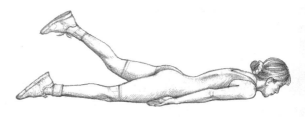

*Lying on your stomach, tighten the muscles in one leg and raise it from the floor. Hold for a count of ten and return your leg to the floor. Repeat with the other leg. Do five repetitions with each leg.*

*Lie on your back with your arms at your sides. Lift one leg off the floor and hold it for a count of ten. Return it to the floor and lift the other leg. Repeat five times with each leg. If this is too difficult, keep one knee bent while raising the other leg.*

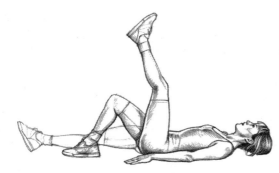

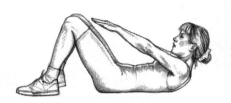

Lie on your back with your knees bent and your feet flat on the floor. Slowly raise your head and shoulders off the floor and reach forward toward your knees with both hands. Hold for a count of ten. Lie back down and repeat five times.

Holding on to the back of a chair, lift one leg backward. Keep your knee straight. Lower the leg slowly and repeat with the other leg. Do five repetitions with each leg.

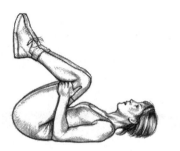

On the floor or on your bed, lie on your back with your knees bent and your feet flat. Raise both your knees toward your chest. Put both hands under your knees and gently pull your knees as close to your chest as possible. Do not raise your head. Lower your legs without straightening them. Start with five repetitions several times a day.

*(continued)*

# Eight Exercises to Minimize Back Pain—
## Continued

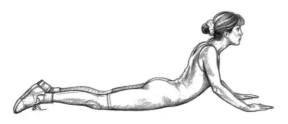

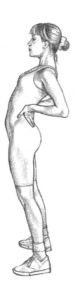

*Lie on your stomach with your hands under your shoulders and your elbows bent. Push up with your arms. Raise the top half of your body as high as possible, allowing your hips and legs to remain flat on the floor or bed. Hold the position for one or two seconds. Repeat ten times several times a day.*

*Stand with your feet slightly apart. Place your hands in the small of your back. Keeping your knees straight, bend backward at the waist as far as possible and hold the position for one or two seconds.*

# BINGE EATING

## *When You Just Can't Stop*

It can start with a single spoonful of chocolate ice cream, a hard-won reward for surviving the weekly spat with the boss. But things get out of hand almost instantly. The spoonful becomes a pint, then a half-gallon, followed by a piece—or two, or three—of coconut cream pie, a half-dozen doughnuts and even a can of tuna.

Two hours later, it finally ends with an uneasy nap, a ton of guilt and the sinking feeling that the whole episode was completely out of your control.

Food binges like these leave an estimated one in two American college women upset about her body and her life—and at greater risk of obesity, with its accompanying risks of heart disease, high blood pressure and diabetes. Robert L. Spitzer, M.D., professor of psychiatry at Columbia University's New York State Psychiatric Institute in New York City, says bingeing can also be a sign of clinical problems such as depression or bulimia, which can require professional treatment.

If you overeat occasionally, it's probably not a big deal, says Dori Winchell, Ph.D., a psychologist in private practice in Encinitas, California. But Dr. Winchell warns that any time you lose control over your eating, when you feel that you simply can't stop eating, there's cause for concern.

## D Is for Danger

Two D words—diet and depression—could be at the root of many binges. If you eat poorly (such as when you're trying a restrictive or fad diet), your body may rebel, says Dr. Winchell.

"I don't think you indulge in binges. I think they're brought on by your body because you don't eat enough of the right things," she says. "When you're lacking nutrients, your body kind of goes haywire and starts a search mission for what it needs."

# When Things Get Serious

If you binge frequently—perhaps two or more times a week—you could be suffering from binge eating disorder.

Robert L. Spitzer, M.D., professor of psychiatry at Columbia University's New York State Psychiatric Institute in New York City, says that as many as five million people in America—most of them women—might have the disorder. He says women with binge eating disorder show many of these signs:

- Eating much faster than normal
- Eating large amounts of food (2,000 calories or more in a sitting) even when not hungry
- Eating alone because of feelings of embarrassment
- Feeling guilty after binges
- Bingeing at least twice a week for at least six months

Dr. Spitzer says binge eating disorder is not considered as serious as bulimia or anorexia nervosa. Still, he warns that the effects of the disorder can be powerful.

"These people tend to be obese, and they are putting themselves at risk for heart disease, diabetes and other problems," he says. "They could also be clinically depressed and in need of treatment."

Doctors typically treat binge eating disorder with a combination of therapy to identify underlying psychological causes for bingeing, counseling about better eating habits and sometimes medication to deal with depression and anxiety.

One more note: If you binge frequently and attempt to purge the food through self-induced vomiting, overuse of laxatives or excessive exercise, you could be suffering from bulimia.

Maria Simonson, Ph.D., Sc.D., professor emeritus and director of the Health, Weight and Stress Clinic at Johns Hopkins Medical Institutions in Baltimore, says the majority of her patients overeat for psychological reasons—to comfort themselves or to forget about other problems.

Dr. Winchell says depression, stress and anxiety can also burn enormous amounts of vitamin C and B-complex vitamins. That, she says, can lead to a nasty cycle: binge eating followed by anxiety or depression about binge eating—followed by another binge.

# Binge Busters

If you're prone to binges, try some of these tips to help regain control.

**Dump that diet.** Dr. Winchell says the best way to eat is to follow a balanced plan that lasts a lifetime. "If you've got the nutrients you need, your body will be happy, and you probably won't binge," she says.

**Drown your urges in water.** Drinking about 64 ounces of water a day, 3 to 4 ounces at a time, is a good way to keep your belly full and your binges in check, according to George Blackburn, M.D., Ph.D., associate professor of surgery at Harvard Medical School and chief of the Nutrition/Metabolism Laboratory at New England Deaconess Hospital, both in Boston.

**Write away.** Dr. Winchell says keeping a private diary can be an enormously helpful way to help overcome binges. Write about your feelings before, during and after a binge. Write about events of the day—what made you nervous, upset or happy. Dr. Winchell says a diary may help you understand yourself better—and help pinpoint the causes of your binges.

"It teaches you more about yourself and how you're feeling," she says. "If you're aware of your feelings, you won't panic when things don't seem perfect." And if you don't panic, Dr. Winchell says, you're probably not going to binge.

**Make your eating habits complex.** Complex carbohydrates—found in pasta, potatoes, rice, corn and many other foods—can make you feel full faster, says James Kenney, R.D., Ph.D., a nutrition research specialist at the Pritikin Longevity Center in Santa Monica, California.

**Question yourself.** Many people convince themselves that they are lazy, lack willpower and fail at everything when just the opposite may be the case. Dr. Winchell says such feelings can cause stress and anxiety and help spark binges.

Asking yourself one simple question—"Is that really true?"—will help dispel many self-generated myths about your shortcomings, Dr. Winchell says. If you blame problems on being lazy, make a list of your recent accomplishments, anything from closing a big deal to cleaning the bathroom. Then ask yourself "Am I really lazy? Is that really true?"

"You'll realize that your life is actually a lot better than you thought it was," Dr. Winchell says.

**Spice it up.** Try as you might, you just can't binge on jalapeño peppers. Dr. Simonson says hot and spicy foods can satisfy hunger faster. There is some evidence that they also speed your metabolism, helping you burn calories quicker.

**Take 20.** If you feel the urge to binge, try hard to hold off for 20 minutes. G. Alan Marlatt, Ph.D., professor of psychology and director of the Addictive Behaviors Research Center at the University of Washington in Seattle, has conducted research that shows food cravings usually disappear within that time. He suggests taking a walk or otherwise distracting yourself until the critical moments have passed.

**Find your triggers.** Identify what causes you to binge—the smell of popcorn, the sizzle of sausage—and try to avoid it, Dr. Simonson says. She suggests keeping high-fat binge foods out of the house, where you won't be tempted by them.

**Get real.** You're not going to become CEO after six weeks on the job. You won't master the piano after three lessons. And you're not going to look like a supermodel after one workout.

"Be realistic," Dr. Winchell says. "You can accomplish amazing things, but only one step at a time."

It's probably best, in fact, to forget the supermodel thing altogether. "Nobody can attain the ideal body image this culture has set," Dr. Winchell says. "If you eat right, exercise a little and have a good outlook on life, you're going to weigh what you're supposed to—and you'll look great."

# BIOLOGICAL CLOCK

## *Ticking toward Wisdom*

Delicate lines extend the curves of your eyes. Support stockings are now more than a way to add shine to your legs.

You're beginning to feel . . . older You heard the first tick of your biological clock at age 30, when a glint of silver appeared in your hair. The ticking grew louder at 35, when crow's-feet made their debut. And it reached a crescendo at 40, when you wondered whether you were fertile enough to get pregnant.

True, your body is beginning to age. But the process may not be as inevitable as you think.

In the past, the physical markers of aging led scientists to believe that the body was one big biological clock that got wound up at birth, never missed a tick through age 29, then spent the next 46 years or so winding down.

Today, scientists suspect that our biological clocks could actually keep on ticking for as long as 120 years. And the only reason they don't is molecular sabotage, says Huber Warner, Ph.D., deputy associate director of the Biology of Aging Program at the National Institute on Aging in Bethesda, Maryland.

Molecules left over from normal body processes such as breathing and eating are the culprits, explains Dr. Warner. They damage all the body's genes, including those responsible for quality control, so that the genes can no longer do their jobs. And with damaged quality control genes less able to check the work of cellular repair squads, mistakes made by the squads start to pile up. Eventually, the body's cells cease to function properly, and the gray hair, crow's-feet, poor vision and saggy breasts that we associate with aging begin.

Of course, no one theory can explain all the complex changes associated with aging, says Dr. Warner. Other factors, such as changes in the levels of key body chemicals that tell various genes when to turn on and off, may also contribute to the aging process.

When human growth hormone, estrogen and testosterone (yes, in women, too) are reduced sometime after age 30, women shrink instead of grow, their egg quality declines and their skin thins and becomes dry. Moreover, immune system fighters that normally target invading microbes apparently lose the ability to tell friend from foe and end up targeting parts of the body that they're supposed to defend—and triggering diseases such as arthritis and lupus in the process.

## Can You Turn Back the Clock?

Scientists are working on various strategies to keep our biological clocks in good repair until our last seconds of life, says Dr. Warner. Some scientists are tinkering with genes to correct genetic mistakes. Some are replacing hormones that affect cell growth. Some are developing compounds that will trap free radicals, the molecules that damage quality control genes. And some are studying lifestyle changes that may help.

Based on animal studies, some scientists suspect that eating radically fewer calories may keep you healthier well into your sixties and seventies.

A second strategy involves taking antioxidants—beta-carotene and vitamins C and E—to reduce the damage done by free radicals.

And one theory, still in the preliminary stages, involves replacing human growth hormone as it peters out.

## Dealing with Reality

Until scientists are able to tell us how to keep our biological clocks running more efficiently for a longer time, at some point all of us must eventually come to terms with the fact that our joints are less flexible, our memory less trustworthy, our vision less acute, our fertility less of a sure thing.

Here's how experts suggest we do it.

**Share.** "Getting together with other women to talk about the changes in ourselves is crucial," says Phyllis R. Koch-Sheras, Ph.D., a clinical psychologist and adjunct professor at the University of Virginia in Charlottesville, particularly since our youth-oriented culture doesn't yet support or appreciate women who are getting older.

Sharing your feelings with other women who are experiencing the same biological changes will help you understand and accept those changes, says Dr. Koch-Sheras. You'll learn to look at yourself differently, without applying incorrect and destructive social attitudes about aging toward yourself.

It's not a case of denial or trying to look through rose-colored glasses, emphasizes Dr. Koch-Sheras. It's a case of putting aging in its proper perspective. You'll learn to appreciate your silver hair as a sign of increasing wisdom and your wrinkles as a sign of having an invigorating outdoor life. And you'll also see the positive reality of growing older—the increased tolerance, energy and assertiveness that allow you more control of your life than you've ever had, not to mention a well-developed sense of humor that allows you to laugh at your own foibles.

**Examine your dreams.** Another way to come to terms with a biological clock that's slowing down is through your dreams, says Dr. Koch-Sheras, who co-authored *Dream On: A Dream Interpretation and Exploration Guide for Women.*

"Dreams are an access to parts of yourself you don't know," she explains. In them, you can identify how you feel about yourself getting older.

Some women might see images in their dreams that indicate they are having difficulty accepting the breakdown of their biological clocks—perhaps the appearance of an old woman who was evil or who was rejected by everyone she met.

The point is to bring these anti-aging feelings out into the light, where you can evaluate them instead of having them subconsciously determine your attitude toward getting older, says Dr. Koch-Sheras. Once in the light, the truth tends to be more obvious.

**Write a letter.** For some women, one of the best ways to come to terms with aging is to write about the biological changes in a letter addressed to a friend or relative, Dr. Koch-Sheras says. You don't have to send the letter to anyone. The idea is to list your feelings on paper, then think about them. It's a process that not only will help you accept the notion that you're getting older, she says, but also will help you get to know yourself better as well.

**Feel you've accomplished something.** "Adjusting to aging is really not that difficult," says I. M. Hulicka, Ph.D., professor emeritus of psychology at Buffalo State College in Buffalo, New York. If you've done things that you're proud of—built a bridge, raised a child, supported friends or family through life's crises, volunteered at a local hospice—then "it's simply a matter of saying 'Well, I like what I've accomplished, I like my life and I'm looking forward to more.'"

Many people who have difficult times accepting their own aging are the ones who believe that they have done little with their lives and are just now realizing that there may not be enough time left in which to do anything they consider significant.

"That's terrible," says Dr. Hulicka. Make sure it doesn't happen to you by taking stock of your life now and establishing goals that, once attained, will give you a sense of accomplishment whenever you look back.

# BLADDER PROBLEMS

## *Taming a Nasty Nuisance*

**Y**our bladder, once as dependable as the Hoover Dam, has lost its reliability. Wherever you go these days, you fear the floodgates will open, embarrassing you beyond belief.

Your social life is wilting. You feel frustrated, angry and humiliated. You're too young for these kinds of problems, you tell yourself. Yet you're too bashful to ask anyone, even your doctor, for help.

"The psychological impact of a bladder problem is tremendous. If a woman between the ages of 30 and 50 begins to urinate more frequently, wets herself or has other bladder problems that she associates with aging, I'm sure that she might think 'This never used to happen to me. My god, I must be getting older. This is the first thing that happened to Aunt Millie when she started her downward slide,' " says Alan J. Wein, M.D., chairman of the Division of Urology at the University of Pennsylvania School of Medicine in Philadelphia.

But in reality, most bladder difficulties are not an inevitable sign of aging. In fact, urinary tract infections and incontinence, the two most common causes of bladder problems, can affect women at any age and can usually be treated effectively or cured, Dr. Wein says.

Here's a closer look at the causes of and remedies for these two nuisances.

## When Bacteria Invade

It may begin with a severe pain every time you urinate. Soon you feel the unmistakable urge to go again, even if you went just a few minutes ago. And when you do go, a surprisingly small amount of urine trickles out. Sometimes your urine has a strong odor and you pass blood. In severe cases, you might also develop back pain, chills, fever, nausea and vomiting.

More than likely, you have a urinary tract infection (UTI), the most common bladder problem among women in their thirties and forties, Dr. Wein says. At least 25 to 35 percent of women between the ages of 20 and 40 have had at least one UTI. Of those, nearly 20 percent will have at least one recurrence, says Penny Wise Budoff, M.D., clinical associate professor of family medicine at the State University of New York at Stony Brook Health Sciences Center School of Medicine. Overall, women are up to 50 times more likely than men to develop UTIs.

That's because a woman's urethra, the tube that carries urine out of the bladder, is less than two inches long. Since it is so short, the urethra is vulnerable to invasion by bacteria that naturally live in the vagina and rectum. Sexual intercourse can drive bacteria up into the urinary tract, where these microorganisms can cause inflammation of the urethra, bladder or kidneys.

Waiting too long to urinate is another common cause of UTIs. If you go for hours without urinating, you can stretch the bladder muscle and weaken it to the point that it can't expel all the urine. This residue of urine increases your risk of infection.

Once an infection strikes, your doctor will prescribe antibiotics, says Jonathan Vapnek, M.D., assistant professor of urology at Mount Sinai School of Medicine in New York City.

While your family physician can treat a UTI, you should see a urologist or gynecologist if you have blood in your urine, recurrent UTIs or a history of kidney infections or stones, Dr. Vapnek says.

In some cases, women with UTIs may develop interstitial cystitis, a chronic disease that causes inflammation of the bladder. Women who have it often feel the urge to void up to 60 times a day. It has no known cause or cure, but its symptoms are often relieved by drugs such as steroids and antihistamines.

Although bladder infections should be brought to your doctor's attention, there are plenty of ways to prevent them in the first place. Here's how.

**Fill 'er up.** Drinking at least six eight-ounce glasses of water and other noncaffeinated beverages every day dilutes urine in the bladder, which makes it more difficult for bacteria to thrive, Dr. Budoff says.

**Urinate often.** Try to empty your bladder at least four to six times a day, Dr. Budoff says. That will help keep your bladder clear of bacteria. Going to the bathroom that often shouldn't be a problem if you drink plenty of fluids.

**Quaff cranberry juice.** This age-old remedy got a shot of scientific validation from researchers at Harvard Medical School, who divided 153 women into cranberry juice drinkers and non–cranberry juice drinkers. Those who drank about ten ounces a day of the tangy beverage experienced bladder infections only 42 percent as often as those who did not. The researchers speculate that cranberry juice may inhibit bacteria's ability to latch on to the bladder wall.

**Let it go after sex.** Urinate soon after intercourse, suggests Deborah Erickson, M.D., a urologist and assistant professor of surgery at the Pennsylvania State University College of Medicine in Hershey. Urinating will flush out any bacteria that were driven into the bladder during sex. If you have recurrent infections, ask your doctor about the possibility of taking an antibiotic after sex.

**Take a close look at your birth control.** Researchers at the University of Washington found a connection between recurrent UTIs and women who use diaphragms in conjunction with spermicide. Women who used this contraceptive method had much greater risk of having *Escherichia coli* bacteria, the most likely culprit to cause UTIs, in their urine. If you use a diaphragm with spermicide and suffer frequent UTIs, consider switching to another form of birth control, says Seth Lerner, M.D., assistant professor of urology at the Baylor College of Medicine in Houston. Consult with your doctor.

**Practice good hygiene.** Washing your hands before and after urinating may reduce your chances of a UTI, Dr. Budoff says. When wiping your bottom, do it from front to back. That will keep potentially harmful bacteria away from your urethra. For extra cleanliness, Dr. Budoff suggests using a large, moistened cotton ball to wipe from front to back.

**Shower, don't bathe.** Soaking in a tub filled with soapy water or bubble bath can irritate the lining of the urinary tract, particularly if you have a history of recurrent bladder infections, says David Rivas, M.D., a urologist at Thomas Jefferson University Hospital in Philadelphia.

**Stick with cotton.** Snug nylon panties can restrict airflow, trap moisture and promote bacterial growth around the urethra, Dr. Rivas says. Instead, wear loose-fitting cotton undergarments that permit better air circulation. If you wear panty hose, be sure that they have a cotton crotch.

# The Horror of Losing Control

When your son throws a baseball through a window or your husband plows the car into a snowbank, you shrug it off because you know accidents do happen. But the accidents that have plagued you lately aren't so easy to dismiss. You may have trouble getting to the bathroom in time or experience an embarrassing leak when you cough, sneeze or even lift weights at the gym.

"Incontinence makes some women feel older because they think it's a sure sign that they're becoming decrepit. It signifies a lack of control and suggests that other valued qualities of life, such as exercising, traveling and even living independently, are at stake," says Katherine Jeter, Ed.D., executive director of Help for Incontinent People in Union, South Carolina.

But incontinence isn't necessarily a sign of aging, Dr. Lerner says. In fact, studies indicate that about one in four women between the ages of 30 and 59 has had at least one instance of incontinence in her adult life. That's about the same rate as for women over 60.

"Incontinence isn't like gray hair. It's not inevitable," Dr. Lerner says. "It usually has an underlying physiological cause that may be treatable."

Older women tend to have incontinence for different reasons than younger women, says Tamara Bavendam, M.D., assistant professor of urology and director of the Female Urology Clinic at the University of Washington Medical

Center in Seattle. Arthritis, for instance, can make it more difficult for an older woman to walk to a bathroom quickly. Older women are also more likely to take medications, and some drugs—such as those used to treat heart disease—can cause excessive urine production that overwhelms the bladder's capacity.

Of the major types of bladder leakage, stress incontinence and urge incontinence are the most common among women in their thirties and forties, Dr. Lerner says. Stress incontinence may result when pelvic floor muscles are weakened or damaged. This can occur because of pregnancy and childbirth, excessive weight or decreased hormonal production. The bladder and urethra sag, and the sphincter muscle can't completely close. So any abdominal pressure, such as a laugh or sneeze or lifting a heavy object, triggers a leak.

Urge incontinence, which can be caused by UTIs or inflammation of the bladder, occurs when irritated or overactive bladder muscles contract uncontrollably. As a result, a woman can feel a compelling need to urinate. If she hesitates, she may lose urine before she gets to a bathroom, Dr. Bavendam says. Sometimes a woman can have a combination of stress and urge incontinence.

In another type of incontinence called overflow incontinence, a woman feels no urge to void, so the bladder fills to the brim and causes so much pressure that the excess urine spills out. Diabetes is one of the primary causes of this type of bladder leakage. But women who habitually hold their urine for more than five or six hours at a time can damage their bladder muscles and develop overflow incontinence, Dr. Bavendam says. Stroke, spinal cord injuries, multiple sclerosis and other neurological disorders can also cause overflow incontinence.

It's important to remember that incontinence is not a disease but a symptom of an underlying ailment, Dr. Erickson says. So if you have a leaky bladder, don't assume that you'll need to wear adult diapers the rest of your life. More than likely, your doctor can help you. Sometimes that may mean taking drugs that will tighten the sphincter muscle or relax the bladder muscle to stop inappropriate bladder contractions. As a last resort, surgery can restore a sagging bladder to its natural position or make the urethra tight. But in most cases, simple remedies such as doing pelvic muscle exercises or making changes in diet or bathroom habits relieve the problem. Here are some ways to keep yourself dry.

**Keep track.** Keep a urinary log for a week or two before you see a doctor, Dr. Vapnek suggests. Note what you eat and drink, when you go to the bathroom and when and where you leak. Were you coughing, or did you feel an urge and not make it to the bathroom on time? The diary will help you and your physician track down the problem.

**Know your drugs.** Some medications, including diuretics, antihistamines, sedatives, anticholinergics such as motion sickness drugs and over-the-counter cold remedies, can weaken bladder control, Dr. Wein says. If you're taking any drug, ask your doctor or pharmacist if it could be contributing to your problem.

**Target your diet.** Some women report that consuming coffee, tea, carbonated soft drinks, artificial sweeteners, chocolate, tomatoes, hot spices and other foods and beverages makes their incontinence worse, Dr. Bavendam says. If you suspect a food may be contributing to your problem, try eliminating it from your diet for a week and see what happens. If your symptoms improve, continue to avoid that food, since it may have been irritating your bladder.

**Puff no more.** Women who smoke are 2.5 times more likely to develop incontinence than women who don't light up, says Richard Bump, M.D., associate professor and chief of the Division of Gynecologic Specialities at Duke University Medical Center in Durham, North Carolina, who studied incontinence among 606 smoking and nonsmoking women. He suspects that excessive coughing, which is common among smokers, weakens pelvic floor muscles and causes stress incontinence. Smoking may also irritate bladder muscles, so they contract more often and cause leaks. So if you smoke, quit.

**Drink up.** "A lot of women will cut back on their fluids in the hope that less in equals less out," Dr. Jeter says. But doing that may make you more, not less, likely to have problems, because highly concentrated urine irritates the bladder and causes it to contract to rid itself of that urine as soon as it can. Restricting fluids can also lead to dehydration, constipation, UTIs and kidney stones. Drink at least six to eight glasses of water, juices or other fluids a day, Dr. Erickson says.

**Loosen up.** Constipation can contribute to incontinence. When your rectum is full of stool, it can put pressure on the bladder and increase the risk of urge incontinence. So be sure to eat a high-fiber diet that includes fruits, vegetables and whole-grain breads and cereals.

Dr. Jeter recommends a recipe of 1 cup of applesauce, 1 cup of oat bran and ¼ cup of prune juice in a bowl. Add spices such as cinnamon or nutmeg for taste, then refrigerate. Introduce the mixture into your diet slowly, building up to two tablespoons each evening as needed, followed by an eight-ounce glass of water. The water is essential, says Dr. Jeter; without it, adding fiber can actually make matters worse.

**Do a double take.** If you feel like your bladder isn't draining completely, try double voiding. To do it, remain on the toilet until your bladder feels empty. Then stand up for 10 to 20 seconds, sit down, lean slightly forward over your knees, relax, and wait until your bladder empties completely, Dr. Jeter says.

**Shed a few pounds.** Excess weight strains the pelvic floor muscles and increases the risk of incontinence, Dr. Vapnek says. "Women who are moderately overweight tell us that the loss of just five to seven pounds means the difference between being wet and staying dry," Dr. Jeter says. Ask your doctor if losing a few pounds might help you.

**Dodge booze.** Alcohol is a diuretic that will make you produce a lot of urine very quickly. So if you have an incontinence problem, drinking alcohol can make it worse, Dr. Rivas says.

**Use those muscles.** Kegel exercises can strengthen the pelvic floor muscles and reduce your chances of a leak, Dr. Erickson says. To do Kegels, squeeze the muscles in your rectum as if you were trying to prevent passing gas. This should also tense the pelvic floor muscles. Feel the sensation of the muscles pulling upward. That's the sensation you want to achieve when doing these exercises. Squeeze the muscles, hold for a slow count of four, then relax for another count of four. Try to do 10 sets of Kegels each day. As these muscles become stronger, gradually increase the time you squeeze until you can hold the position for 25 to 30 sets of ten seconds each. Your bladder control should improve within three to four weeks.

As an alternative, consider using weighted vaginal cones. The cones, which are about the size of a tampon, are available in sets of five increasing weights ranging from ¾ ounce to 3 ounces. When you insert a cone into the vagina, you must squeeze the pelvic floor muscles to hold it in. When the muscles tire, the cone slips out.

"If you can hold the cone in, you know that you're doing your Kegels right," Dr. Erickson says. "You'll probably be able to hold the cone in for just a couple of minutes at first, but as your muscles get stronger, you can hold it in for longer and longer. I tell my patients that when you can hold a cone in for 15 minutes, then it's time to move on to the next higher weight." For more information about the cones, write to Lifestyle 2000, 101 Carnegie Center, Suite 203, Princeton, NJ 08540.

**Balance your needs.** Bladder control is often a matter of equilibrium, Dr. Bavendam says. The average women can go three to four hours without voiding. But if you urinate every hour, for instance, you won't stretch the bladder to its full capacity. On the other hand, if you wait longer than four hours, you may be straining your bladder muscles to the point that they can't hold in the urine anymore.

If you tend to hold your urine too long, don't fight nature, Dr. Erickson says. When you feel the urge to void, do it, even if you have to excuse yourself from an important business meeting. It may prevent an embarrassment later.

If you urinate more often than you'd like, try bladder retraining. To do it, urinate when you first get up in the morning, then set a timer for one hour. When the timer sounds, go to the bathroom, even if you don't feel the urge. Then reset the timer for another hour. Do this every waking hour for a week. Then each subsequent week, add 30 minutes to the time between bathroom trips until week seven, when you should be at four hours. If you feel the urge to void before the time is up, do Kegel exercises or concentrate on a distracting task, such as recalling the phone numbers of ten friends or relatives, until the urge passes.

For more information about incontinence, send a self-addressed, stamped business-size envelope to Help for Incontinent People, P.O. Box 544, Union, SC 29379, or the Simon Foundation for Continence, P.O. Box 835, Wilmette, IL 60091.

# BODY IMAGE

## Looking for, and Liking, the Real You

**A**s you and your husband sit down for a romantic dinner at an elegant restaurant, you catch him checking out the pretty young cock-tail waitress.

"You think I'm fat!" you blurt out.

"What? You're five-foot-three and 115 pounds. You look fine," he says.

" 'Fine' really means you think I'm just okay," you say. "The truth is," you think to yourself, "you probably think that my breasts are sagging, my hips are too big, my legs are flabby, my face is wrinkling and I'm turning into my mother."

No, he probably doesn't think that. But, unfortunately, you do, and no matter how many people tell you how good you look, you just don't believe them. Even now when you look in the mirror, you can see changes looming and wonder how long before your youth vanishes completely.

"Body image has a total impact on how we feel about aging," says Mary Huntington Lehner, clinical director of the Rocky Mountain Treatment Center in Great Falls, Montana. "There's a direct connection between your self-esteem and your body image. The better your self-esteem, the better you'll feel about what is happening to your body as you journey through life."

But even if you have terrific self-esteem, fighting an ongoing battle against gray hair, crow's-feet and extra pounds on the hips and thighs in a society that worships youth and thinness can be demoralizing and make you feel over the hill before your time, says Ann Kearney-Cooke, Ph.D., a Cincinnati psychologist in private practice who specializes in body image problems and eating disorders.

## Model Behavior

From the little old ladies in the TV commercial who are miraculously trans-formed into young sex vixens after drinking beer to magazine covers that proclaim "Perfect Breasts: Yours Can Stack Up," women are bombarded with the message that if you're not tall, thin, young and perfect, you're not worth much, psychologists say.

"In the eyes of society, when you're 20, you're hot; when you're 40, you're not; and when you're 60, you're shot," says Stanley Teitelbaum, Ph.D., a clinical psychologist in private practice in New York City.

That not-so-subtle vision is reflected in the ages and sizes of models. Female models have steadily become younger, thinner and taller in the past 50 years. A generation ago, a model weighed only 8 percent less than the average woman. Today, a model weighs 23 percent less. For perspective, consider that only 5 percent of women can achieve the same weight and proportions of today's models without dieting.

## What Magazines Are Really Telling Us

Women's magazines love perfection. They tell us we can have perfect hair, perfect lips, perfect legs, perfect sex. They show us perfect models wearing perfect clothing and perfect makeup.

So how does all this perfection make us feel? Perfectly rotten, says Debbie Then, Ph.D., a social psychologist in Stanford, California, who studies the effects of media on body image and conducts seminars on the topic.

"Most women who look at those magazines know that they don't look like the models and never will," Dr. Then says. "Yet if you're constantly bombarded with those images, you might begin to consider yourself unattractive when in fact you're actually very good-looking."

In a small study, Dr. Then asked 75 women how they felt after reading their favorite women's magazines. Some said they were motivated to improve their appearance, but nearly 70 percent said the images in the magazines lowered their self-esteem and made them feel worse about their looks.

"I feel like every woman is at least 20 pounds lighter and four inches taller than I am," one woman wrote. "It really depresses me."

"It is impossible to look like the models unless I have a $5 million wardrobe, a personal airbrusher and a makeup artist and I go on (a liquid diet) for ten years," said another.

What to do? Well, a few women found what they considered the perfect solution: They stopped reading the magazines.

"That girl in that stunning dress on the cover of the women's magazine is probably 16 or 17 years old, and most of her flaws have been airbrushed out of the picture," says Debbie Then, Ph.D., a social psychologist in Stanford, California, who studies the effects of media on body image and conducts seminars on the topic. "Then when the middle-aged woman in the grocery store checkout line sees that magazine on the rack, she's going to feel horrible about herself because she doesn't look that way."

Although a few models are bigger these days, Dr. Then says that the message to women remains the same. "The majority of women older than 25 wear a size 12 or larger," she says. "So when the fashion industry starts calling a size 10 a larger-size model, that tells most women that they're overweight, and their self-esteem plummets."

Even the clothing store mannequins project an unreal image to the point that the average American woman would have to lose 30 percent of her body weight to have similar proportions, Dr. Then says.

# Distorted Beliefs

These pressures on women to look thin, youthful and sexy are clearly having an effect. By most measures, a growing number of women believe looking young and attractive is important, but at the same time, more and more of us are displeased with our appearance.

In a 1989 survey of 1,000 women ages 18 to 60, Dr. Kearney-Cooke and Ruth Striegel-Moore, Ph.D., associate professor of psychology at Wesleyan University in Middletown, Connecticut, found that 68 percent of the women believed that being attractive is very important compared with only 32 percent of women in a similar survey conducted in 1973. In addition, 91 percent of the women in the 1989 survey said they wanted to change their bodies.

So what exactly do women dislike about their bodies? Twenty percent are dissatisfied with their faces, 45 percent dislike their muscle tone, 32 percent would like to change their breast or chest sizes, and about 40 percent are dissatisfied with their overall appearance, according to Judith Rodin, Ph.D., author of *Bodytraps* and professor of psychiatry and medicine at Yale University School of Medicine in New Haven, Connecticut.

But the thing most women would change is their weight, because they believe men are attracted to thinner women. In a study of women who were asked to rate their body shapes against the body shape they believed was most attractive to men, women consistently rated themselves as far plumper than a man's ideal. However, their body shapes were actually closer to what men said they found attractive.

The desire to meet the model's ideal is so intense that nearly half of all average-weight women actually consider themselves overweight, according to surveys conducted by Thomas Cash, Ph.D., professor of psychology at Old Dominion University in Norfolk, Virginia. Little wonder, then, that on any given

# What Do You See in the Mirror?

What do you really think of your body, and what does it mean? To find out, take this quiz adapted from *The Body Image Trap* by Marion Crook. Answer these yes or no questions. A key to interpreting your answers follows.

1. Do you think thin women generally are more competent than overweight women?
2. Do you think thin women generally are more able to feel sexual pleasure and excitement than overweight women?
3. Are most of the women you admire slim?
4. Do you want to be thinner?
5. Do you wish parts of your body would disappear?
6. Do you think you would have more choice of sexual partners if you were thinner?
7. Do you think job opportunities would be greater if you were thinner?
8. Do you put off activities or beginning relationships until the time when you will be thinner?
9. Do you think overweight people do not deserve job promotions, sexual partners, admiration or respect?
10. Do you think most women can and should be slim?
11. Do you think most women do not try hard enough to be slim?
12. Do you consider yourself "bad" when you eat certain foods and "good" when you restrict your eating?
13. Do you consider yourself overweight?

## What It Means

If you answered yes more than once to questions 1 through 8, you believe, like millions of women, that your body isn't good enough and that a thinner one would magically create success and opportunity for you.

If you answered yes to any of questions 9 through 12, you have absorbed the message that thin is good and fat is bad. Consider the anxiety that is created by this moral judgment, the criticism, the pressure on self-esteem that comes from believing in the good or bad of a particular size and shape.

If you answered yes to question 13, as most women do, you think you're not good enough as you are. Are you ever going to be good enough? Perhaps instead of changing your weight, you can work on changing your attitude about your body.

day, 25 percent of all women are on diets, and up to one in seven of us has an eating disorder.

## Caught in the Middle

Although almost every woman feels compelled to do something to maintain her looks, women in their thirties and forties may have the most difficulty doing it, says Susan Olson, Ph.D., director of psychological services at the Southwest Bariatric Nutrition Center in Tempe, Arizona.

"Women are in the middle of careers, raising children and possibly caring for their aging parents. So it's hard to find time to focus on themselves," Dr. Olson says. "When they do, they all of sudden realize they're getting older, and that's scary."

So it's probably not surprising that women are keeping plastic surgeons busy. People between the ages of 35 and 50 get about 66 percent of buttock lifts in this country, 58 percent of tummy tucks, 58 percent of collagen injections, 49 percent of liposuctions and 30 percent of face-lifts done each year, according to the American Society of Plastic and Reconstructive Surgeons. Of 394,911 cosmetic surgery procedures that the organization logged in 1992, 343,965—or 87 percent—were done on women.

## Seeking Function over Form

Of course, good looks don't guarantee that you will have a good body image or that you will age more gracefully than others. "The more attractive a person is, the harder aging is on her," Dr. Kearney-Cooke says. "People who are used to getting attention for their looks actually struggle more with aging than a person who is more plain-looking."

While body image can be a problem throughout the lives of many women— Dr. Kearney-Cooke has patients who at age 62 obsess about their appearance— worries about it usually level off for most women as they near their fifties.

"As women get older, they're more concerned about having healthy bodies than looking good," Dr. Kearney-Cooke says. "Instead of worrying if they can still fit into a size eight dress, they're more concerned that their backs will hurt tomorrow if they play golf today."

The ultimate reward for improving your body image at any age is that you'll feel more comfortable with yourself, and as a result, more people will want to be around you. "A good body image can definitely make you feel younger," Dr. Then says. "The more positive you are, the more outgoing you'll be. And that's important, because it's been shown that people who have more friends and acquaintances are healthier."

Here are some tips to help you feel better about your body.

**Take an inside look.** "You aren't your body. You just happen to be in your body," Dr. Olson says. "Try not to look at yourself as just a physical being, because that's going to pass." Find other reasons for liking yourself, such as a solid career or a good sense of humor.

**Find a heroine.** "I used to browse through magazines looking for pictures of women who had features similar to mine," Dr. Olson says. "They weren't perfect, but here they were in these magazines, and that made me feel better about myself." Find a picture of a woman you admire, cut it out, and put it on your mirror for inspiration.

**Give yourself a hug.** Dr. Olson suggests that each time you look in a mirror, say to yourself "I love you; I think you're absolutely beautiful." "That affirmation may seem ridiculous, but it's important, because you're not going to believe those words coming from anyone else until you believe them from yourself," she says.

**Look back.** Find a favorite picture of yourself from each decade of your life. "Looking at those pictures will help you realize that you were a better-looking person than you may have thought you were at the time," says Ann Meissner, Ph.D., a psychologist in private practice in St. Paul, Minnesota. "It will also make you think twice about how accurate your judgments are about yourself now."

**Look ahead.** Conjure up an image of yourself 5, 10 or 20 years from now. How do you look? How does it feel? Keep doing it until you find an image of yourself that feels comfortable, says Rita Freedman, Ph.D., author of *Bodylove*. "Look for role models whom you admire and think are attractive even though they are older and grayer. Put pictures of those people on your refrigerator, and use those images as something to look forward to and grow into."

**Be a comparison shopper.** "When you go to a shopping mall or beach, specifically watch the women there. Chances are most of them aren't going to look like fashion models, and you'll end up feeling better about yourself," Dr. Then says.

**Take note.** "Each day, write a note to a part of your body that you like and a part that you don't like," Dr. Meissner suggests. "For example, you might write 'Hips, I may not love you, but you're a part of me and along for the ride.' If you like your eyes, you might write 'Thanks, eyes. I really value you, because you sparkle and show that I'm alive.' "

**Sweat it out.** Regular exercise such as walking, bicycling, swimming or weight training can help you stay fit—and improve your body image—when you do it for at least 20 minutes a day, three times a week, says Mark Leary, Ph.D., professor of psychology at Wake Forest University in Winston-Salem, North Carolina.

**Please yourself first.** If you do decide to make changes in your body, do it for yourself; you'll enjoy it more. "As we get older, we cling to this idea that your physique has to look like it did when you were 22. In fact, your friends and family probably don't care if you have the body of a 22-year-old. They just want you to have a decent 40-year-old body," Dr. Leary says.

**Try some soul food.** If you're working on changing your appearance, commit yourself to two other goals that aren't related to your body, Dr. Kearney-Cooke says. So if you're trying to lose ten pounds, for example, also take a flower-arranging class or start keeping a journal—or something. "It helps you see yourself as a whole person," she says.

**Dress for success.** "Appearance does count at any age, but you don't have to obsess about it. Just make the most of what you do have," Dr. Then says. "For health reasons, exercise, eat a balanced diet, maintain a weight that is right for your proportions, and practice good grooming. Wear clothes, makeup and accessories that complement your figure, but realize that you don't have to look like a cover girl to have a happy, successful life. Try to be the best possible version of yourself."

# BURNOUT

## *Take Your Brain off Roast*

**Y**ou've been feeling so down and out lately that you're wondering if you've been bitten by a tsetse fly. A friend assures you that African sleeping sickness isn't very common in America, so your next thought is to check your birth certificate to reassure yourself that you are in fact the age you thought you were. Yup. You're still a fairly young woman—at least on paper.

So why are your body and mind behaving as if they had 90,000 miles on them instead of 40,000? Why the sadness? The disenchantment with life? The mysterious aches and pains? The constant fatigue?

It could be burnout.

"Burnout can certainly make you feel old before your time," says C. David Jenkins, Ph.D., professor of preventive medicine and community health at the University of Texas Medical Branch at Galveston. "Burnout tends to drain people of the physiological and mental reserves that are, in youth, typically there to keep them going. Luckily, burnout does not necessarily age people or take years off their lives in a permanent fashion. It can be reversed."

But if you want to stop feeling decades beyond your biological age, you first need to know what's happened to you and why.

## No Variety, No Relief

Believe it or not, burnout was once thought to be a man's problem. Today, we know all too well that it's not. "I'm seeing more and more women coming in with symptoms of burnout," says Herbert J. Freudenberger, Ph.D., author of *Women's Burnout* and *Burnout: The High Cost of High Achievement* and originator of the term *burnout.* "In part, I think this is due to the expanded, multi-role lives they lead as mothers, wives and professionals."

Actually, it is not the number of activities in your life but rather a lack of variety among activities that causes burnout, says Faye Crosby, Ph.D., professor of psychology at Smith College in Northampton, Massachusetts, and author of *Juggling*. "Burnout does not occur by having too many pots boiling on your stove. Many times it occurs because you have only one pot boiling constantly and can never take it over to the sink to fill it up. Eventually, all the water boils away."

Any woman can get burnout, from housewife to corporate president. But those who tackle the responsibilities of both seem most liable. Too often the career woman still ends up acting as the primary nest builder in the home. This means the rejuvenating time she might spend cuddling with her family in front of the fireplace is squeezed out by household duties such as making sure that the kids have clean clothes and that the den doesn't become a permanent resting place for dirty dishes. So while a woman may jump between roles, she still ends up doing goal-oriented activities and has little time for the social, emotional ones, says Dr. Crosby. "In essence, it's still a one-track life."

For many women, the burnout-inducing effects of double duty become most apparent around the holidays. "I have so many women patients who come into my office around the holidays completely frazzled," says Dr. Freudenberger. "One in particular was sobbing because she was up until 4:00 in the morning two days before Thanksgiving—cleaning. This is after a job that she leaves for at 6:00 in the morning and gets home from after 7:00 in the evening. She was actually referred to me by a dermatologist because she had hives, which he'd been treating for years with no success. In fact, the problem was burnout-related."

# Perfectionism Hurts

Another burnout-inducing extreme for women is the concept of all-around perfectionism. "The perfect wife, mother and professional," says Dr. Freudenberger. "I hate the idea because it's exactly the kind of impossible goal that leads to burnout. It's a concept that was widely disseminated in the 1970s and 1980s, and although I'm seeing less and less of it today, there are still many women who buy into this false belief."

The pursuit of perfection is not without its costs. One of the highest burnout ratios to be found is in the air traffic controller profession, where people work under conditions that make anything less than perfect performance a matter of catastrophic possibilities. So great is the pressure they're under not to make mistakes that by the time they reach their mid-forties, many of these people have had to leave their jobs, says Dr. Jenkins, who participated in a definitive study of air traffic controllers and burnout. "And in fact, it seems that the professions most prone to burnout are the ones where constant vigilance is demanded and where the cost of mistakes is horrendous. Nurses who work in the intensive care wards of hospitals come to mind," he says.

But not everyone who suffers from burnout is operating in an environment that demands such perfection. Some people do it to themselves simply by setting impossibly high goals and viewing all harmless mistakes as catastrophes.

# A Thirst for Recognition

Burnout can also occur when there is a lack of positive feedback and re-ward. At work, women are still bumping their heads against the glass ceiling. At home, the task of keeping the household running in an orderly fashion is often a thankless job.

The absence or presence of positive feedback can make all the difference between emotional well-being and burnout. "Some years ago, Massachusetts General Hospital was experiencing a burnout problem among its nurses that manifested itself in a high job turnover rate," recalls Dr. Jenkins. "So they called in some of their psychiatrists and started a support therapy group, which met once or twice a week."

Within this group, people shared experiences with their peers, got a lot of gripes off their chests and received praise and understanding from the psychia-trists. "In terms of employee turnover and increased satisfaction, the results were quite good," says Dr. Jenkins. "And all that was really applied was a little feedback and support."

# Take a Look at Yourself

How do you know if you have burnout? One way to tell is by taking the test on page 74. Another is to listen to whether your friends say you've changed lately. "But you probably won't," says Dr. Freudenberger. "A major coping mechanism that I've noticed in burnout patients is denial—denial that this is happening, de-nial that this is something they need help to overcome." In other words, the person who knows the least about burnout is the one who is suffering from it.

But if you won't listen to your friends, at least listen to your body. "One of the first signs we noticed in the air traffic controllers who were burning out was a sense of fatigue," says Dr. Jenkins. "And I'm talking about a pervasive mental and physical fatigue that a good night's sleep will not get rid of."

Chest pain, gastrointestinal problems, sleep disturbances, headache, back pain and a higher incidence of minor illness such as colds are some of the body's other responses to burnout. So are skin disorders, adds Dr. Freudenberger. "The woman I mentioned who had hives is not an unusual case. I also see a lot of burnout-induced acne and eczema."

On the mental front, a lack of resilience, characterized by a feeling of being whipped, can be a harbinger of burnout. "Our air traffic controllers called it bounce-back," says Dr. Jenkins. "They couldn't bounce back from a taxing pe-riod of heavy controlling and face the next period of activity with any sense of ease, comfort and casualness. They were drained."

Irritability and depression are also possibilities for those who are burning out. "But more interesting is the development of a superperson personality," notes Dr. Freudenberger. "The person feels that she can handle everything, needs no help and may actually become arrogant about it."

# Are You Burning Out?

Feeling like a wrung-out old dishrag lately? It could be burnout.

The following self-test, developed by Herbert J. Freudenberger, Ph.D., and included in his book *Burnout: The High Cost of High Achievement*, may give you the answer. When taking this test, consider changes in your behavior over the past six months. Give yourself about 30 seconds before answering each question and then rate your response from 1 to 5. One means little or no change; 5 means a great deal of change.

1. Do you tire more easily? Feel fatigued rather than energetic?
2. Are people annoying you by telling you "You don't look so good lately?"
3. Are you working harder and harder and accomplishing less and less?
4. Are you increasingly cynical and disenchanted?
5. Are you often invaded by a sadness you can't explain?
6. Are you forgetting deadlines, appointments, personal possessions?
7. Are you increasingly irritable? More short-tempered? More disappointed in the people around you?
8. Are you seeing close friends and family members less frequently?
9. Are you too busy to do even routine things such as making phone calls, reading reports or sending out Christmas cards?
10. Are you suffering from physical complaints—aches, pains, headaches, lingering colds?
11. Do you feel disoriented when the activity of the day comes to a halt?
12. Is joy elusive?
13. Are you unable to laugh at a joke about yourself?
14. Does sex seem like more trouble than it's worth?
15. Do you have very little to say to people?

## Scoring

Add up your answers.

**0 to 25.** You're doing fine.

**26 to 35.** There are things you should be watching.

**36 to 50.** You are a candidate.

**51 to 65.** You're burning out.

**Over 65.** You are in a dangerous place, threatening to your physical and mental well-being.

# Rekindle Your Flame

Whether burnout has made you move, think and feel like a cranky Methuselah on a bad day, or you just want to make sure that you never end up aging 30 years in as many weeks, the following tips will help you "de-burnout" your life.

**Listen to others.** "The first step to curing burnout is to admit the problem exists," says Dr. Freudenberger. "But that's harder than it sounds, because of the denial mechanism people often use to cope with burnout. So listen to your friends and family members. Pay attention when they say you've changed. You may not notice it yourself, but burnout can be very apparent to those close to you as well as to co-workers who can see the transformation."

**Diversify.** "Just as a bank must diversify its holdings so that it doesn't have to depend on one source for its profits, people have to diversify their emotional portfolios," says Dr. Crosby. "This means looking at your activities and making sure that you participate in some that are goal-oriented and some where the aim is to feel good and have fun. I actually encourage people to list them in two columns. If you have 2 items in one column and 40 in the other, things are out of whack, and you need to do some account balancing."

**Stop being perfect.** The trick is to give yourself a little leeway when you can. "Take stock of your situation and see what mistakes you can and can't make," says Dr. Crosby. "Not every miscalculation you make is going to plummet the world into Armageddon. In other words, don't sweat the small stuff." And that goes for all activities, work-related and otherwise.

**Know your needs.** "If you know that you need positive feedback to replenish yourself, then don't just ignore that fact," counsels Dr. Freudenberger. "Actively solicit feedback from family and friends and in the workplace." Tell them that you would occasionally like to hear "Good job!" when you've done something well. Or find a support group that you can share your feelings, achievements and gripes with. It doesn't have to be anything formal. A few people going through the same things as you will do just fine.

A corollary to this rule is: Ask for help. "Especially around the holidays," adds Dr. Freudenberger. "You're busy, things are hectic, and the last thing you need to be doing is scrambling around at all hours doing prep work." Enlist family members to help clean. When you invite people over, have them bring a salad or side dish.

**Volunteer.** "Volunteering is a very important anti-burnout device," says Dr. Crosby. "Whether you're at work or at home, worrying over a set of marketing reports or putting up aluminum siding, you have to drop what you're doing, mentally change gears and go interact with a whole new set of people in a whole new environment."

"It doesn't matter if you work in a soup kitchen twice a week, collect clothes or deliver meals. You receive gratification that you are doing something for someone else," adds Dr. Freudenberger. "You may also receive some very important perspective on your life by seeing those less fortunate than you."

**Take five.** Dr. Crosby prescribes a five-day vacation alone at least once a year. "It's especially important for women not only to get away from the office but also to get away from home," she says. That means leaving the husband, the kids, the dog, the goldfish—everything—behind. They'll get on just fine without you for five days. "As a matter of fact," adds Dr. Crosby, "if you feel that the world will fall apart if you leave for five days, you have a good indicator that you are taking things far too seriously and are probably heading for burnout."

**Take 15.** "You also have to set aside some relaxation time during the course of the day," says Dr. Freudenberger. "And I mean every day, both at work and at home. When people tell me they can't do that, I make them actually take apart their days piece by piece, and they suddenly find all sorts of little opportunities for 15-minute breaks. And that's all it really takes."

**Take off the red cape.** Stop trying to be a superwoman. "No one is going to consistently be the perfect wife, mother and professional," says Dr. Crosby. "The trick is to allow yourself the occasional mistake—to recognize pressure release points where mistakes will not mean the end of the world." In other words, mismatched silver at the dinner party you're throwing isn't going to signal the end of civilization. And handing in that report a day late probably won't push the company into bankruptcy.

# BURSITIS AND TENDINITIS

## *Easing Those Overworked Joints*

You're on the stair climber for an hour. You shovel snow all afternoon. You wallpaper the kitchen over the weekend.

What do these things have in common? They're all terrific ways to get a raging case of bursitis or tendinitis. These painful conditions overlap so often that doctors frequently diagnose them as bursitis/tendinitis, because it can be hard to tell where one leaves off and the other begins.

And they can happen most often to people in their forties, particularly those who haven't worked to maintain their flexibility. Without regular stretching, muscles and tendons get tighter and rub together more, increasing the risk of inflammation.

Once you have bursitis and tendinitis, you move around with the caution of a much older person. And you can forget the joys of your favorite sport, because a sudden motion can feel as though you've just been jabbed with a red-hot poker.

Here's why it hurts.

## The No-Use Syndrome

Your bursae are tiny fluid-filled sacs that cushion the spaces where muscle passes over bone and where two muscles rub together. In your kneecaps and elbows, they form cushions between skin and bone. They can get inflamed when you injure or overuse a joint or when you accelerate your workout beyond what you're used to, says Pekka Mooar, M.D., director of the Delaware Valley Sports Medicine Center in Philadelphia.

If you have tendinitis, it is not really your tendon but a ring of tissue around the tendon where it attaches to a bone or muscle that hurts. The pain is caused by overuse of the tendon, which produces inflammation.

"We all get more aches and pains with age; there's no controversy about that," says Phillip E. Higgs, M.D., a reconstructive surgeon at Washington University School of Medicine in St. Louis. But if you stay limber over the years, a burst of effort is much less likely to bring on bursitis and tendinitis, he says.

It is too little exercise, not aging itself, that increases your risk of these painful ailments. That's what Dr. Higgs and his colleagues concluded after counting cases of bursitis and tendinitis in a study of 157 poultry workers and 118 data processors. Although the workers ranged in age from 20 to 71, the younger workers who got little exercise had nearly the same number of inflammations as older workers who didn't exercise much.

Bursitis and tendinitis vary a great deal from person to person, Dr. Higgs says. For example, one day of all-out sports may cause symptoms in one person, while another may not have trouble until after many years of work on an assembly line.

## Where It Hurts Most

Shoulders, elbows, hips, knees and ankles are especially vulnerable to bursitis and tendinitis. Women tend to get inflammations in the hips more than men do because our hips are set at a wider angle from the pelvis, putting greater stress on the hip joints. For men, shoulders are the usual problem area, because they tend to do more throwing or to have jobs that require a lot of overhead lifting.

Back when we were the only ones scrubbing floors, an inflamed knee bursa was called housemaid's knee. And one form of tendinitis rarely seen in anyone these days used to occur almost exclusively in women's wrists. The cause? Wringing out cloth diapers and cleaning rags. These days, many of us still get other forms of tendinitis from activities such as typing, doctors say. Any job or hobby that requires repetitive motion, from working on an assembly line to sewing, increases the risk.

Bursitis and tendinitis are also caused by overdoing a favorite sport. Tennis can do in elbows and wrists; swimming can irritate the shoulder bursae; running can aggravate ankles and Achilles tendons, particularly if you run on hard surfaces in the wrong shoes. And aerobics, particularly step aerobics, can cause hips and knees to flare up.

Bursitis is often missed as a cause of lower back pain, experts say. And it often accompanies the disorder called fibromyalgia, which causes muscle pain and stiffness throughout the body.

Fortunately, bursitis and tendinitis are very treatable. And you can do a lot to prevent them.

## Safeguarding Your Joints

The most important thing is to get into condition gradually and to ease into vigorous exercise gently, says Stephen Campbell, M.D., a rheumatologist at Oregon Health Sciences University in Portland. Here are some suggestions.

**Stretch before exercise.** "In preparation for vigorous activity, you need to do more stretches of the muscles you'll be using," says Dr. Mooar. "Hold a slow, sustained stretch for ten seconds, and don't bounce. Repeat the stretch three to five times before exercising." And don't do high-speed stretches, or you risk tearing muscle fibers or ligaments, he says. If you're unsure which stretching exercise is best for you, check with a trainer.

**Start new activities slowly.** If you take up a new sport, work at gradually increasing the strength and flexibility of the muscles you'll be using, says Dr. Mooar. If you choose tennis, for example, take it one set at a time at first. "Don't pick up a racket and play lots of sets at once, because your shoulder is going to feel like it's falling off," he says.

**Prepare for work or play.** If your job or hobby calls for repetitive motion, ask a trainer to recommend strengthening and endurance exercises targeted for that motion, Dr. Mooar says. "If you do this," he says, "you can stop bursitis and tendinitis from happening over and over." Many people develop chronic inflammation from reinjuring their joints, he says.

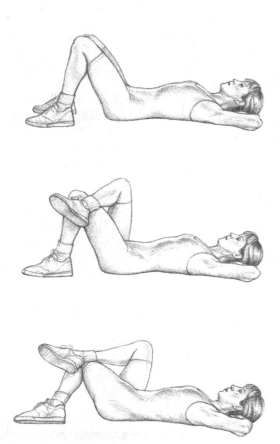

*Lie flat on your back with your knees bent and your feet resting flat on the floor (top). Clasp your hands behind your head. Cross your right leg over your left leg, placing your right foot on the outside of your left leg just below the left knee (center). Do a gentle pelvic tilt (that is, gently press the curve of your back toward the floor). Keeping your shoulders and upper back stationary, use your right foot to steadily pull your left knee toward the floor on your right side (bottom). You should feel a stretch in your left lower back or outer thigh as you try to touch your left knee to the floor. Hold the stretch for six seconds. Return to the starting position. Relax. Repeat the exercise using your left foot on the outside of your right leg (just below the right knee) to pull your right knee toward the floor on your left side. Repeat three to five times, twice daily.*

**Support yourself.** Typing and filing can trigger problems in your wrists and back. Use a keyboard wrist rest for typing, says Dr. Campbell. And check that your chair is well adjusted so that your back is supported and your arms and wrists are level with each other.

**Have mercy on your knees.** There is little but a tiny bursa between your kneecap and the skin over it, says Dr. Mooar. So if you're doing housework or gardening on your knees, kneel on a piece of foam rubber or wear knee pads to

---

# Pain-Free Workouts

There's no need to let bursitis or tendinitis spoil your participation in your favorite sport. Gradual conditioning is the key to prevention— or to staging a careful comeback if bursitis or tendinitis has already hit. Here's some advice for various activities.

*Aerobics.* Learn the routines at your own pace; don't push yourself. Always warm up and stretch before you exercise and cool down after, says Robert L. Swezey, M.D., medical director of the Arthritis and Back Pain Center in Santa Monica, California.

*Tennis.* To avoid serving up wrist pain or tennis elbow, choose a large-handled racquet, decrease the string tension and wear an elastic band around your forearm to support the muscles, says Stephen Campbell, M.D., a rheumatologist at Oregon Health Sciences University in Portland. If your shoulder is the problem, modify your serve to avoid vigorously swinging your arm over your head.

*Running.* Condition yourself very gradually before running longer distances, says Dr. Campbell. Don't run too vigorously if you're just starting, avoid hard surfaces and wear shoes with soft soles and high-quality insoles and arch supports.

*Swimming.* Although swimming is very gentle on most joints, the shoulder can get too much of a workout, Dr. Campbell says. To prevent or heal shoulder bursitis or tendinitis, avoid the freestyle, or crawl, and butterfly strokes, he says. Use the breaststroke or sidestroke or a kick-board instead.

*Returning to training.* After a bout of bursitis or tendinitis, it's crucial to wait until all the pain has gone for restarting vigorous workouts, says Dr. Campbell. When you have your doctor's okay to start again, exercise at a lower frequency and intensity and recondition your injured joint over weeks or months, he says.

cushion them. Many garden centers, sporting goods stores and hardware stores carry foam rubber or knee pads.

# Tips for a Quick Recovery

Ouch. You already have bursitis or tendinitis, and you want relief—quick. The first question to ask yourself is, what have you done differently? "You're overdoing whatever it is," says Dr. Campbell. "First, stop doing it." Then:

**Give yourself an ice massage.** "Apply a paper cup full of ice to the painful area," says Robert L. Swezey, M.D., medical director of the Arthritis and Back Pain Center in Santa Monica, California. Rub the icy bottom of the cup into the sore spot for two to five minutes, three or four times a day, to control the inflammation, he says.

**Alternate it with heat.** After the ice, apply a microwavable heat pack or electric heating pad to soothe the pain, says Dr. Campbell. The microwavable packs are available at most pharmacies, he says.

**Bundle up for bed.** Wear a flannel shirt or a wool sweater at night to keep a painful shoulder extra warm. If you sleep sleeveless in a cool room, your morning stiffness and soreness will be greater.

**Use the right pain reliever.** Choose an aspirin or ibuprofen pain reliever for the pain, says Dr. Campbell. Aspirin and ibuprofen block the production of chemicals called prostaglandins, which contribute to swelling and pain in inflamed tissue. Acetaminophen won't control inflammation because it does not block prostaglandins.

**Swing it.** Sometimes bursitis in the shoulder progresses to a painful condition called adhesive capsulitis, or frozen shoulder. When this happens, the shoulder's range of motion is almost completely restricted, and the joint is nearly immobile. To avoid frozen shoulder, you need to start moving your shoulder as soon as the acute pain has passed, says Dr. Campbell. Lie facedown on a cushioned surface such as a bed, and hang the affected arm over the side. Gently swing your arm like a pendulum, gradually increasing the range until you can swing it in a full circle. Do this for 15 to 30 minutes, three to five times a week, to restore your range of motion, he says.

**Consider chiropractic care.** If your pain won't quit, a technique called friction massage may clear up the problem, says Warren Hammer, D.C., a chiropractor in private practice in Norwalk, Connecticut. When inflammation is chronic, fibrous adhesions don't allow the bursae to glide smoothly. Friction massage can break down those adhesions, says Dr. Hammer, relieving the cause of bursitis pain. "Also, an inflamed tendon becomes thicker and shorter, which creates further inflammation in the bursa it's rubbing over," Dr. Hammer says. "The deep pressure of massage across the bursa and tendon can lengthen the tendon fibers again." Use ice to calm the inflammation before chiropractic treatment, he says.

# Preventing the Freeze

If bursitis or tendinitis lingers too long, you may need to see your doctor for help in battling the pain. Here are some remedies to ask her about.

**Consider prescription relief.** If you have no history of stomach problems, ask your doctor about prescription-strength non-steroidal anti-inflammatory drugs (NSAIDs) for pain, says Dr. Campbell. Like aspirin and ibuprofen, NSAIDs work by blocking the production of prostaglandins. But they can also irritate the stomach like aspirin does, so they are usually not prescribed for long periods.

**Go slow on shots.** Nearly the last resort for pain, steroids are "shortcuts, not cures," says Dr. Mooar. Most doctors recommend injecting a painful joint, tendon or bursa no more than twice a year. Frequent injections can weaken or rupture a tendon.

"Most people are overinjected with cortisone-like drugs," says Dr. Swezey. "Most doctors use 10 to 20 milligrams for bursal injections, but I've found that 2½ milligrams works quite well."

**Make surgery the last resort.** For extremely severe bursitis, your doctor may use a needle to draw fluid off a painful joint or recommend that an orthopedic surgeon remove an inflamed bursa entirely, says Dr. Mooar. But before consenting to surgery, you should seek a second opinion.

# CAFFEINE

## *Beware the Java Jitters*

She shuffles past your office every morning at 9:03, head down, coffee mug in hand, one eye shut, the other half-open.

"Hi, Jenny," you say.

"Hullumph," she mumbles.

By 11:30 A.M., she's sprinting down the hallway and leaping file cabinets.

"Hi, Jenny," you say.

"Oh-geez-hi-how-are-you-nice-dress-have-you-seen-the-boss-I-have-to-get-this-report-done-by-noon," Jenny says.

When it's time to go home, you find her facedown in a spreadsheet, empty cans of cola scattered across her desk.

"Good night, Jenny," you say.

"Grok," Jenny says.

Like Jenny, more than half the people in America use caffeine to jump into the day. A cup of coffee or tea, or even a can of cola, can sometimes clear your head, perk up your body and quickly return you to the land of the living.

But be careful not to overdo it. Too much caffeine can make you like Jenny—fatigued, jittery, irritable or all three at once—and may put you at risk of health and age-related problems, ranging from headaches and insomnia to heart disease.

"Take it easy with caffeine," says Mary Sullivan, R.D., a nutrition support specialist at the University of Chicago Hospitals. "It can really help you sharpen your mind and body when taken in small amounts. But it might also cause some harm if you take an excessive amount in your diet."

## Grounds for Concern

Caffeine stimulates the central nervous system, triggering the release of adrenaline into your bloodstream and raising blood sugar levels. That makes you more alert and focused and reduces fatigue in the short term.

But too much can lead to a condition called caffeinism, more commonly known as coffee nerves. This problem is marked by light-headedness, fidgeting, upset stomach, diarrhea, frequent urination, insomnia and headache. To stop all that, you have to cut back on caffeine.

Studies also warn about possible links between caffeine and elevated cholesterol levels, increased problems with high blood pressure and aggravated symptoms of premenstrual syndrome and fibrocystic breast disease. But test results have been inconsistent and often contradictory. Manfred Kroger, Ph.D., professor of food science at the Pennsylvania State University in University Park, says that's because many studies use coffee to provide caffeine to test subjects, and coffee may contain other ingredients that cause problems of their own.

How much caffeine is too much? It depends. "No two people are the same," says Richard Podell, M.D., clinical professor of family medicine at the University of Medicine and Dentistry of New Jersey Robert Wood Johnson Medical School in Piscataway, New Jersey. "One cup of coffee can cause problems in some women, and other women seem to have a much higher tolerance."

The federal Food and Drug Administration includes caffeine on its "Generally Recognized as Safe" list but warns that people should ingest it in moderation. Americans consume an average of 200 milligrams of caffeine per day, the equivalent of about two five-ounce cups of coffee or four cans of cola. Sullivan says that amount of caffeine probably won't hurt most people.

"Just use your head," she says. "If you're having trouble sleeping or feeling jittery, it's probably a good idea to cut back."

Dr. Kroger warns that no one should be drinking more than two or three cups of coffee a day, no matter how an individual reacts to caffeine. "We just don't know enough about what it can do to you," he says. "Err to the side of moderation."

## How to be Cautious with Caffeine

If you are looking to limit caffeine in your diet but don't want to eliminate it altogether, experts offer this advice.

**Nix the nightcap.** Caffeine stays in your system longer than most other stimulants. Half the caffeine you drink in a cup of coffee may still be coursing through your veins five hours later. So if you're having problems sleeping, Sullivan says you should avoid caffeine starting in the late afternoon.

**Do some decaf.** Can't bear the thought of a coffeeless life? Decaffeinated brands may be one answer, but Dr. Kroger warns that decaf may still contain harmful elements of regular coffee that have yet to be investigated fully. "Switching to decaf is not an invitation to continue drinking ten cups a day," Dr. Kroger says.

You could also try the new half-decaf, half-regular coffees on the market. Or switch to coffee made from arabica beans. These beans can contain about one-third less caffeine than the cheaper robusta beans, which are often used in instant coffees.

**It's not just coffee and tea.** Coffee and tea aren't the only caffeine hide-outs. Soft drinks contain one-third to one-half as much caffeine as coffee. Drinking a caffeine-free brand can cut your caffeine intake by as much as 60 milligrams, Sullivan says.

Be careful with dark chocolate, too. You'd need to eat more than a pound of Hershey's milk chocolate to get the same amount of caffeine found in a cup of percolated coffee—but just three ounces of Ghirardelli dark chocolate is nearly a cup of coffee's worth of caffeine by itself.

Nonprescription drugs may also contain a surprising amount of caffeine.

---

# THE CAFFEINE COUNT

How many milligrams of caffeine are in that beverage or candy bar? Here are the numbers.

| Food/Beverage | Caffeine (mg.) |
| --- | --- |
| **COFFEE (per 5-oz. cup)** | |
| Drip | 115 |
| Percolated | 80 |
| Instant | 68–98 |
| Decaffeinated | 4 |
| **TEA (per 5-oz. cup)** | |
| Tetley | 64 |
| Lipton | 52 |
| Tender Leaf | 33 |
| Constant Comment | 29 |
| **SOFT DRINKS (per 12-oz. can)** | |
| Tab | 57 |
| Mountain Dew | 54 |
| Coca-Cola | 46 |
| Diet Coke | 46 |
| Pepsi | 38 |
| Diet Pepsi | 36 |
| **CHOCOLATE (per 1 oz.)** | |
| Ghirardelli dark chocolate | 24 |
| Hershey's milk chocolate | 4 |

# A HIDDEN KICK

Some over-the-counter drugs contain surprising amounts of caffeine. The following table shows the caffeine content of one tablet of each nonprescription medication.

| Drug | Caffeine (mg.) |
| --- | --- |
| Maximum Strength No Doz | 200 |
| Vivarin | 200 |
| No Doz | 100 |
| Aspirin Free Excedrin | 65 |
| Excedrin Extra Strength | 65 |
| Anacin (regular strength) | 32 |
| Maximum Strength Anacin | 32 |

Some analgesics contain a soft drink's worth or more. And diet pills and pep-up pills such as Maximum Strength No Doz and Vivarin contain as much as 200 milligrams of caffeine.

**Break your routine.** Maybe you're not hooked on caffeine as much as you are hooked on the routine. "If you find yourself picking up a mug of coffee every time you sit down to a task, you probably just have a bad habit," Sullivan explains. "Ask yourself if you really want that cup or whether you can do without it."

You could also try putting something else in your mug (water, perhaps, since most of us don't drink enough anyway).

**Read the label.** Anyone who has ever pulled an all-nighter knows that pep pills such as No Doz and Vivarin are absolutely stuffed with caffeine. That's the whole point. But you may be surprised to find that some analgesics (such as Anacin and Excedrin) contain as much caffeine as a typical can of cola. If you're caffeine sensitive, check the small print on your box of aspirin.

**Back off slowly.** If you decide to reduce your caffeine intake, Sullivan suggests you do it gradually, over the course of a few days. Going cold turkey on caffeine can lead to unpleasant withdrawal symptoms, including headache, anxiety and feelings of depression. Studies show these symptoms occur even in people who are moderate coffee drinkers.

# CANCER

## *How You Can Help Yourself*

When a woman is told she has cancer, a lot of questions zip through her mind: "Am I going to die?" "Will surgery disfigure me?" "Will my husband think I'm less of a woman?" "What am I going to tell my friends and family?" "How are we going to pay the bills?" "Does this mean I won't be able to have more children?"

Cancer is a particularly powerful ager. It's a heartless disease that can cause debilitating pain and suck youth and vigor out of any one of us.

The disease can actually accelerate the aging process by causing chemical changes in the body that lead to painful joints, dulled appetite, weight loss, weakness, fatigue and loss of stamina, says Ernest Rosenbaum, M.D., an oncologist at the University of California, San Francisco/Mount Zion.

"Cancer drains you. If you have cancer, you can feel aged and older very quickly," says Charles B. Simone, M.D., an oncologist in Princeton, New Jersey, and author of *Cancer and Nutrition*.

## The Truth about Cancer

Cancer is life-threatening because its abnormal cells grow uncontrollably, can spread throughout the body and can damage surrounding normal cells, says John Laszlo, M.D., national vice president for research at the American Cancer Society. It is actually not one disease but an array of more than 100 kinds of malignancy that attack different organs of the body in a variety of ways. So lung cancer, for example, may spread to other tissues in a slightly different way than breast cancer.

"There's this perception that cancer is a single entity and that we're going to find some magic pill that will totally prevent the disease or will be the ultimate cure for all forms of cancer. Unfortunately, cancer is more complicated than that," says Ronald Ross, M.D., director of cancer cause and prevention research at the University of Southern California Kenneth Norris, Jr., Comprehensive Cancer Center in Los Angeles.

Researchers suspect that 5 to 10 percent of cancers may be inherited, meaning that the disease is passed on from one generation to another through an abnormal gene. But in the vast majority of cases, cancer develops through a complex series of steps that often includes prolonged exposure to carcinogens, which are cancer-causing substances such as tobacco and asbestos, Dr. Laszlo says. These carcinogens usually affect cells in specific organs. Asbestos, for example, increases a person's risk of lung cancer, while excessive sun exposure is linked to increased risk of skin cancer.

Some researchers believe that carcinogens cause the formation of free radicals, unstable oxygen molecules that can damage the string of DNA molecules that tell cells how to reproduce. Once the DNA is damaged in critical places, a cancer cell may form.

"The free radicals that cause aging are the same things that cause cancer," Dr. Simone explains. "How do we prevent that? We need to decrease our exposure to the things that cause free radicals, including fatty foods, tobacco and alcohol."

Each year, about 576,000 new cases of cancer are diagnosed among American women, according to the American Cancer Society. The most common types of cancer in females are found in the breast, colon and rectum, lungs, uterus, lymph tissue and ovaries. In women who are under age 35, cancers of the breast and skin and lymphomas such as Hodgkin's disease are the three most prevalent.

Cancer kills about 255,000 women annually and is the second leading cause

---

# Seven Signs You Shouldn't Ignore

Here are seven common warning signs of cancer. If you develop any of them, contact your doctor immediately.

1. A lump or thickening in the breast
2. A change in a wart or a mole
3. A sore that doesn't heal
4. A change in bowel or bladder habits
5. A persistent cough or hoarseness
6. Constant indigestion or trouble swallowing
7. Unusual bleeding or discharge

of death for Americans of all ages. By the year 2000, cancer is expected to affect two in every five Americans and will surpass heart disease as the nation's leading killer, Dr. Simone says.

But having cancer isn't an automatic death sentence. In fact, more than half of all Americans diagnosed with cancer survive it, according to the American Cancer Society. If detected early, some types of cancer, such as those of the skin and breast, have five-year survival rates topping 90 percent. If a patient appears free of cancer symptoms for five years, doctors may consider her "cured," although some cancers may relapse after ten or more years.

"We've made slow, steady progress against cancer in the past 50 years. Step by step, we're winning this war," says Harmon Eyre, M.D., the American Cancer Society's deputy executive vice president for research and medical affairs.

Most cancers occur in women older than age 50, and 66 percent of cancer deaths occur after 65. In fact, of the 182,000 cases of breast cancer—the most common cancer among women—diagnosed annually, less than 11,000 are among women under 40.

"For the most part, the young don't have to fear cancer. It's something that lurks in the distant future, sometimes up to 30 or 40 years away," says Carl Mansfield, M.D., professor and chairman of the Department of Radiation Oncology and Nuclear Medicine at Thomas Jefferson University Hospital in Philadelphia.

## What You Can Do

Some cancers, however, can take more than 30 years to develop. So what you do now can have a tremendous impact on your ability to have a long, healthy and cancer-free life, Dr. Lazlo says. In fact, oncologists estimate that perhaps 50 percent of cancers could be prevented if women made just a few simple adjustments in their lifestyles. Here's where to start.

**Become an ex-smoker.** Lung cancer was a rare disease before cigarette smoking became popular. Now it kills about 59,000 women annually and has surpassed breast cancer as the number-one cause of cancer-related deaths in women, says Dennis Ahnen, M.D., associate director for cancer prevention and control at the University of Colorado Cancer Center in Denver. (Breast cancer, however, is still the most common type of cancer women get.) Smokers are ten times more likely to develop lung cancer, and up to 30 percent of all cancer deaths are caused by smoking, says Dr. Rosenbaum, author of *You Can Prevent Cancer*. Studies also suggest that women who smoke are twice as likely to get cervical cancer. So if you don't smoke, don't start, and if you smoke, quit.

**Watch out for passive smoke.** Up to 8,000 lung cancer deaths a year among nonsmokers can be attributed to secondhand smoke, Dr. Simone says. Researchers at the University of California, Berkeley/University of California, San Francisco Preventive Medicine Residency Program found that restaurant workers are exposed to twice as much passive smoke as people who live in households where at least one person smokes. Bartenders are exposed to 4½ times as much passive smoke. Compared with the general population, these food service workers were found to be 50 percent more likely to develop lung cancer, a difference attributable, at least in part, to passive smoking in the workplace. Avoid smoky bars and always ask to be seated in nonsmoking sections of restaurants, Dr. Simone suggests. If people in your household smoke, ask them to quit or establish an area where they can smoke without endangering you.

**Go light on the booze.** Heavy alcohol consumption increases your risk for cancers of the liver, mouth, esophagus and larynx. Studies attempting to link alcohol to breast cancer have had contradictory results, but it's best to be cautious, says Louise Brinton, Ph.D., chief of the Environmental Studies Section at the National Cancer Institute in Rockville, Maryland. Dr. Rosenbaum recommends that you limit yourself daily to no more than one 12-ounce beer, one 4-ounce glass of wine or 1 ounce of liquor in a cocktail or shot.

**Fill up on fiber.** Women who eat lots of fibrous fruits, vegetables and whole grains, such as broccoli, brussels sprouts, cabbage, apples, bananas, mangoes and whole-wheat cereals and breads, may have fewer breast, colon and rectal cancers than those who don't eat these foods, Dr. Simone says. Fiber reduces the amount of estrogen in the blood. Estrogen possibly alters cell structure and promotes breast cancer, Dr. Mansfield says. In addition, fiber helps speed stool through your body and reduce exposure of your digestive tract to carcinogens.

Fiber may also help prevent other cancers. In a study of 399 women with endometrial cancer and 296 disease-free women, Dr. Brinton found that women who ate more than two servings of high-fiber breads and cereals a day had 40 percent less risk of developing endometrial cancer.

The National Cancer Institute recommends that women eat at least 20 to 30 grams of fiber a day. If you start your day with a cereal that has at least 7 grams of fiber per serving, add another 3 grams of fiber by topping your cereal with one medium sliced banana and two tablespoons of raisins. Then you're halfway to the minimum daily recommendation of 20 grams, says Gladys Block, Ph.D., professor of public health nutrition at the University of California, Berkeley. Then all you need to do is make sure you get three more servings of fruits, vegetables and/or grains through the rest of the day. Beans, for example, are particularly high in fiber.

**Go for vegetables.** Eat at least five servings of fruits and vegetables a day, Dr. Rosenbaum says. These foods contain antioxidant vitamins and minerals such as beta-carotene, selenium and vitamins A and E that combat the formation of free radicals.

**Take a supplement.** Supplements containing vitamins C and E and other antioxidant vitamins and minerals can help neutralize certain carcinogens such as the nitrites found in bacon, sausage, hot dogs and cured meats, according to Kedar N. Prasad, Ph.D., director of the Center for Vitamins and Cancer Research at the University of Colorado Health Sciences Center in Denver and author of *Vitamins in Cancer Prevention and Treatment*. Supplements can also strengthen your body's immune system so that it can destroy newly formed cancer cells before they multiply, Dr. Prasad says. He suggests taking 15 milligrams of beta-carotene once a day, 2,500 IU of vitamin A twice a day, 500 milligrams of vitamin C twice a day, 200 milligrams (or 134 IU) of vitamin E twice a day and 50 micrograms of selenium twice a day.

**Trim the fat.** A high-fat diet, like many American women eat, is believed to trigger cancer. Researchers at the University of Hawaii at Manoa compared the fat consumption of 272 postmenopausal women who had breast cancer with that of 296 women who were cancer-free. The researchers found a significant association between breast cancer and eating sausage, processed cold cuts, beef and lamb. Doctors aren't certain why fat promotes tumors, but several factors could play a role, Dr. Mansfield says. Some suspect that fatty foods spark the production of bile acids that interact with bacteria in the colon to form carcinogens. It could also be that fat cells are more susceptible to carcinogens than other cells. Whatever the cause, many experts suggest slashing your dietary fat consumption to no more than 25 percent of calories. To do that, eat more fruits, vegetables and whole-grain foods, trim all visible fat from meats and eat no more than one three-ounce serving of red meat, fish or poultry a day.

**Throw the deep fryer away.** Frying simply adds more fat to food, and fat promotes cancer. Broil, steam, bake or boil your food instead, Dr. Mansfield says. Brown or sauté in nonstick pans, or use vegetable spray or chicken broth.

**Go easy on the barbecue.** The smoke and heat of charbroiling creates several cancer-causing substances, including nitrosamine, one of the most potent carcinogens known, Dr. Mansfield says. If you like to barbecue, do it carefully and sparingly, Dr. Prasad suggests. Place the grill as far above the coals as possible, and wrap aluminum foil around the grill to prevent fat from dripping onto the flame and causing excessive smoke and charring.

**Lose weight.** If you're overweight, you could be producing more estrogen than you need. Excessive amounts of estrogen, a reproductive hormone, are believed to alter cell structure and have been linked to increased risk of breast cancer, Dr. Mansfield says. Keep your weight within the range suggested by your gynecologist or family physician.

In one study, researchers at the Harvard School of Public Health concluded that women who remain physically active throughout their lives are 2½ times less susceptible to cervical and other cancers of the reproductive system. Try doing regular aerobic exercise such as swimming, walking or running for 20 minutes a day, at least three times a week, Dr. Simone says.

**Stay in the shadows.** Skin cancer, one of the most common cancers (it affects more than 700,000 Americans), is caused primarily by sunburn. To prevent skin cancer, avoid prolonged sun exposure, wear hats and long-sleeved blouses, and don't go bare-legged without using a sunblock that has a sun protection factor (SPF) of at least 15. You should apply sunblock to exposed skin when you're outdoors, says Dr. Rosenbaum.

**Don't douche too often.** Researchers at the Uniformed Services University of the Health Sciences in Bethesda, Maryland, found that the cervical cancer risk was four to five times higher in women who douched more than four times a month. Women who douched less had no increased risk. The type of douching liquid made little difference in risk. The researchers speculate that too-frequent cleansing may upset the normal chemical balance, diluting secretions or destroying friendly bacteria that may protect against viral invaders.

**Practice safe sex.** Human papillomavirus (HPV), a sexually transmitted disease, has been linked to precancerous changes in the cervix called dysplasia. Multiple sex partners and unprotected sex are the two major risk factors for HPV. Use condoms and maintain a mutually monogamous relationship, Dr. Rosenbaum suggests.

**Check out your family tree.** Although less than 10 percent of cancers have genetic roots, finding out if cancer runs in your family can help your doctor evaluate your risk and recommend ways to prevent the disease or detect it early, Dr. Rosenbaum says. Include as many relatives on both sides of your family as you can. If someone had cancer, jot down the age at which they were diagnosed and the organ in which it originated.

## Screening Safeguards Your Health

Even if you eat right, don't smoke and don't have a family history of cancer, you can still get the disease. In fact, 75 percent of women who develop breast cancer have no known risk factors, says Charles Taylor, M.D., director of medical oncology in the Breast Cancer Program at the Arizona Cancer Center in Tucson. But the earlier cancer is detected, the more likely you can be cured.

That's why it's important for women to do monthly breast self-exams, to get their first mammograms between the ages of 35 and 40 and to have Pap smears at least every other year.

Here's the lowdown on the mammogram and Pap smear. (For more on the breast self-exam, see Breast Care, page 435.)

## Mammograms: Catching Trouble Early On

A mammogram, an x-ray of the breast, detects lumps that can't be felt by either the patient or the physician, Dr. Taylor says. Here are a couple of tips that can make your mammogram more pleasant.

**Be a pal.** Arrange with a friend to remind each other to schedule and keep your mammogram appointments. Or better yet, go together, suggests Phyllis Kornguth, M.D., Ph.D., chief of breast imaging at Duke University Medical Center in Durham, North Carolina. Afterward, do lunch or go shopping—make it a special time to enjoy each other's company.

**Take charge.** Mammograms can be uncomfortable because in order to find small cancers, the breast must be compressed. But if you have control over the amount of pressure applied, you may find it more comfortable, Dr. Kornguth says. "In fact, studies show that women who compress their own breasts get just as good images with less pain," she adds. At your mammogram, ask "Would you mind if I operated the compression device?" You could also arrange for a verbal signal. Tell the technician "I'll say 'That's enough' when I want you to ease up on the pressure." Most technicians are willing to accommodate you.

## Pap Smears: Checking Your Cell's Health

A Pap smear is a test to detect abnormal cells in and around the cervix, the narrow, doughnut-shaped opening to the uterus. Your doctor collects a sample of cells from the cervix and upper vagina with a wooden scraper, cotton swab or cervical brush and places the sample on a glass slide. The slide is sent to a medical laboratory for evaluation.

About 15 to 40 percent of Pap smears are reported normal when, in fact, cell abnormalities are present. Here are a few ways to improve the accuracy of your results.

**Avoid sex.** Abstain from sexual intercourse for at least 12 hours before a test because semen can interfere with test results.

**Shoot for the midpoint.** Schedule your Pap smear in the middle of your menstrual cycle. The exact timing isn't critical, but you should avoid the days of your menstrual period, since blood can obscure cells on the slide.

**Don't test if you have yeast.** Postpone your Pap smear if you have an active yeast infection. Inflammation from the infection can mask abnormal cells on your cervix.

**Keep them alive.** Don't douche or wear a tampon for at least 72 hours before the test. If you do, you may reduce the number of cells available for examination.

## You Have It—Now What?

Nobody wants to hear her doctor tell her that she has cancer, but if you are diagnosed with it, don't panic, oncologists say.

"For many cancers, cure is clearly possible," says Dr. Eyre. "The majority of individuals in this country who have cancer can expect to live normal life spans."

Treatments include surgery, radiation, chemotherapy and immunotherapy, which consists of injections of proteins and antibodies that assist or stimulate the immune system to fight the cancer. New combinations of treatments are also promising. In many cases, lumpectomy, in which a small part of the breast is removed, combined with radiation is proving to be just as effective a treatment for breast cancer as mastectomy, the removal of the breast, Dr. Taylor says. It's also possible to have a mastectomy and reconstructive surgery of the breast during the same operation.

Which treatments are right for you will depend on the type of cancer, its size, how fast it is growing and if it has spread beyond the original site.

But whatever type of cancer you have, the psychological strain can be enormous.

"It feels unfair," says Karen Syrjala, Ph.D., a psychologist at the Fred Hutchinson Research Cancer Center in Seattle. "They think 'At 30 or 40, how can this be happening to me?' It's not really what you planned to be doing with your life at that point, so it feels like an intrusion. It feels wrong. The whole family can feel that way."

Even the closest of friends and family may start distancing themselves from a woman who has cancer because of their own dread of cancer or fears that she will die, Dr. Mansfield says. As a result, the woman with cancer often ends up socially isolated.

Here are some strategies for coping with cancer.

**Become a know-it-all.** Find out everything you can about your cancer and treatment. Ask your doctors and nurses question after question. "The first thing to do is gather information, so you understand what is happening to you and what your options are," Dr. Syrjala says. "Any time you know that you have options, you're going to feel more in control of the situation."

**Don't blame yourself.** "That's something that women sometimes do," Dr. Syrjala says. "You didn't cause your cancer. Yes, there are things you can do to reduce your chances of getting cancer, but nothing will absolutely prevent it."

**Have a daily laugh.** A sense of humor is extremely important because it can help you cope with the worst aspects of cancer and its treatment, Dr. Syrjala says. Make time to watch funny movies or have a good laugh with a friend.

**Don't be a passive patient.** Treatment shouldn't be something that your doctor does to you; it should be something in which you have an active role. Think about what you can do for yourself that might help you recover, says Dr. Syrjala, and discuss it with your doctor.

**Be honest with your doctor.** Your oncologist won't know if a treatment is bothering you unless you speak up. If you don't have a good relationship with your physician, consider seeing someone else, Dr. Syrjala says.

**Talk about it.** "It's helpful to talk about your fears and sadness, because if you talk about them, you might find out there's something you can do about them," Dr. Syrjala says. "If you don't talk about your fears, you tend to not do anything about them. Sometimes talking takes away the power of your fears." Counseling may help.

**Know you're not alone.** Find a support group for people with your type of cancer. "People in support groups live longer," Dr. Syrjala says. "We don't know why, but clearly, there is something about sharing your experiences with people who are in similar circumstances that can help you live a longer, more fulfilling life." Your doctor or local affiliate of the American Cancer Society should be able to help you find such a group.

**Keep eating.** Up to 40 percent of women who have cancer actually die of malnutrition, Dr. Simone says. That's because cancer cells release a hormone called cachectin that suppresses the appetite. That loss of appetite is compounded by some types of cancer treatment that can cause nausea and vomiting, such as chemotherapy. "The foundation of healing is good nutrition. I tell my patients that even if a meal seems unappetizing, try to eat some of it. Just chew and swallow, because you need that food," Dr. Mansfield says. He suggests eating small meals such as half a sandwich and a glass of orange juice several times a day and nibbling on healthy snacks such as carrots, apples and other fruits and vegetables.

# CELLULITE

## *It's Fat—And Nothing Else*

At the beach, you wrap the biggest beach towel you can find around your hips and thighs.

In the gym, you wear dark, form-fitting Lycra tights under your gym shorts.

And for that formal party, you slip into a slinky gown with a side slit—one that stops at the knee.

What are you trying to hide? Your thighs, of course. And more specifically, the cellulite that first appeared on them sometime around your 30th birthday. Besides looking as though you have cottage cheese burbling under your skin, cellulite makes you feel old, ugly and fat—especially when you're standing next to a 19-year-old in a string bikini at the beach.

But relax. You're not alone.

"Ninety-nine percent of women develop at least some dimply fat after age 30," explains Donald Robertson, M.D., medical director of the Bariatric Nutrition Center in Scottsdale, Arizona.

Part of the problem is genetics. But much of it is simply due to aging. Sometime in a woman's thirties, a natural drop in estrogen levels, along with sun damage accumulated over the years, causes the skin to lose its elasticity, says Ted Lockwood, M.D., assistant clinical professor of plastic surgery at the University of Missouri–Kansas City School of Medicine. The skin sags a little here, bags a little there and generally doesn't have the firm resiliency of youth.

At the same time, the supporting network of fibers that anchors the skin to underlying muscles is also starting to stretch. That, combined with the extra pounds most of us put on as we approach midlife—and which hormones dictate will go directly to a woman's hips, thighs and buttocks—leads to *cellulite*, a fancy word for what is really just dimply fat and skin that has lost its elasticity.

# Is Liposuction for You?

You've been on a sensible low-fat diet and a major aerobics campaign for several years. But no amount of motivation seems to help with your rounded stomach or saddlebag thighs. And they just make you feel older and out of shape. Is there anything a surgeon can do?

The most requested form of cosmetic surgery is liposuction—a vacuuming technique that literally sucks fat cells from beneath the skin. And the change is permanent. As an adult, you can no longer grow new fat cells to replace the ones that have been removed.

"Liposuction can work wonders," says Alan Matarasso, M.D., a plastic surgeon at Manhattan Eye, Ear and Throat Hospital in New York City. "But no surgical procedure can substitute for a healthy diet, exercise and weight loss."

And liposuction is far from an instant weight loss plan. Because removing large amounts of fat can be dangerous, it is best performed on people who are at or near their ideal body weight and who have pockets of stubborn flab that remain despite diet and exercise. And afterward, you should maintain those healthy habits. If you begin to overeat, those excess calories will just be stored in the remaining fat cells on another part of your body, Dr. Matarasso says.

Here's how the surgery goes. While you're under general anesthesia or dozy with a local anesthetic and sedation, a surgeon makes a small incision in your belly or groin. Next, he inserts a blunt-tipped metal tube called a cannula. With vigorous movements, he guides the cannula back and forth under the skin. The cannula is hooked up to a vacuumlike machine that can suck out up to four pounds of fat cells, along with blood.

After the surgery, you're put into a stretchy, girdlelike garment that you wear for one to four weeks to keep swelling to a minimum and your skin smooth. In most patients, bruising fades in about two weeks, and the swelling completely subsides in about six months. The results keep improving with time. You can often return to work after a weekend of rest and to full activity in 7 to 14 days.

Are you a good candidate for liposuction? It's important to be in good health, not significantly overweight (though some surgeons will give you more latitude than others) and under the age of 40 to 50, while your skin is still pliable and stretchy.

It wouldn't be so bad if the men in our lives were sagging and bagging right along with us.

But they're not.

One reason is that men tend to gain weight around their midriffs rather than in their hips, thighs and butts. Another is that men's skin is thicker and more elastic, so it holds the fat beneath it more firmly than ours does. And still another reason is that the fibers that anchor skin to muscle are structured differently in men than in women: While the fibers that support women's skin run in only one direction, men have tight, crisscrossed fibers that form a net to keep their fat firmly in place.

Life is not always fair.

# What to Do about It

While you may not be able to avoid getting cellulite, you don't have to keep it. Because cellulite is fat. And like other forms of fat, you can dump it. Here's how.

**Work it off.** Women who try to get rid of cellulite by doing exercises for only the thighs and buttocks fail miserably. "Spot reducing doesn't work," says Susan Olson, Ph.D., director of psychological services at the Southwest Bariatric Nutrition Center in Tempe, Arizona.

The best way to reduce cellulite—as with fat anywhere else on your body—is with aerobic activity that burns calories throughout the entire body. The best activity is one that gets your heart rate up and keeps it there for 20 continuous minutes at least three times a week.

Running, walking, bicycling, skating, dancing and swimming—all of which stoke up the metabolism for efficient fat burning—are perfect.

Just remember: If you've led a sedentary life, check with your doctor before embarking on any exercise program.

**Pump some iron.** A good aerobic workout will help tone muscles. But building them up through weight training may also help hide dimpled skin. "Bulking your muscles can make a slight improvement," says Dr. Lockwood. "Just don't expect miracles." Check with a trainer at your gym for a program that will help you.

**Ditch the fat in your diet.** Besides exercise, eating a low-fat diet is the best way to keep so-called cellulite to a minimum. "A lot of cellulite comes from eating high-fat foods," says Maria Simonson, Sc.D., Ph.D., professor emeritus and director of the Health, Weight and Stress Clinic at Johns Hopkins Medical Institutions in Baltimore. "So the less fat you have in your diet, the less problem you'll have."

Try limiting your total fat intake to around 25 percent of your calories, adds Dr. Simonson. You can track fat intake by reading product labels and staying away from high-fat fare such as cakes, cheeses, fried foods and processed luncheon meats.

# Cellulite Products: A Big, Fat Lie

Each year, American women spend more than $20 million trying to get rid of cellulite with gels, creams, electrical currents and other too-good-to-be-true products. Unfortunately, the only thinning these products do is to your wallet.

The Food and Drug Administration is now monitoring claims made by the manufacturers of these products, many of which are imported from France, where consumer protection is more lax. But those hawking cellulite products have long been able to promise too much, since *cellulite* is a marketing term—not a medical diagnosis.

A research team from the Health, Weight and Stress Clinic at Johns Hopkins Medical Institutions in Baltimore tested 32 cellulite removal products, says Maria Simonson, Sc.D., Ph.D., professor emeritus and director of the clinic.

Not a single one worked.

**Knuckle under.** "A deep massage using the knuckles may help break up the dimples," says Dr. Robertson. When combined with weight loss and smart eating, a twice-weekly massage helps whittle down the most resistant fat pockets.

**Cream it.** Rubbing any skin cream that contains alpha-hydroxy acids—essentially, acids made from fruits or milk—into your skin will give your body a smoother look. But remember: No cream or lotion will get rid of cellulite.

**Camouflage it.** Use a tanning cream to camouflage cellulite. The darker color will even out your skin tone and make the shadows cast by the lumps of fat beneath the skin less apparent.

**Smear on the sunscreen.** You can't undo the years of sun exposure that paved the way for cellulite by zapping your skin's elasticity. "But by limiting your sun exposure or using a good sunscreen when you're outdoors, you can keep your skin from degenerating further," says Dr. Lockwood. The sun's skin-damaging rays are most harmful between 10:00 A.M. and 2:00 P.M., so it's essential to keep thighs and other vulnerable areas covered during those hours. And whenever you're in the sun, make sure to use a sunscreen with a sun protection factor (SPF) of at least 15.

**Consider a nip and tuck.** If all else fails and you feel that cottage cheese thighs are ruining your life, there is one surgical procedure that may be able to reduce your cellulite, says Dr. Lockwood. By performing nip and tuck surgery—which costs several thousand dollars and is generally not covered by health insurance—a plastic surgeon can stretch the skin of problem areas to hide the fatty deposits underneath. As with any surgery, consider your practitioner's experience and reputation. You may want to get a second opinion before proceeding.

# CHOLESTEROL

## *The Less, the Better*

Sometimes it seems that everybody is talking about cholesterol: How to lower it. How to maintain it. What their latest cholesterol count was.

And it doesn't stop there. Food packages scream their "no cholesterol" proclamations. Items on restaurant menus are often marked with red hearts, reminding you that if you know what's good for you, you'll limit your choices to low-cholesterol dishes.

We have met the enemy, and it is disguised as a white, waxy, fatty substance called cholesterol. Ask the experts, and they'll tell you that high cholesterol is a major contributor to one of America's most dreaded age-related health problems: heart disease. And if you think you can breathe a sigh of relief because heart disease afflicts only men, think again. It's a woman's disease, too.

## Reason for Concern

Yes, your female hormones provide you with some natural safeguards against high cholesterol levels in your premenopausal years. Estrogen can lower the bad (low-density lipoprotein, or LDL) portion of the cholesterol in your blood and raise the good (high-density lipoprotein, or HDL) part. But that kind of protection won't last forever, thanks to the aging process. As your body's production of estrogen wanes in menopause, so does your Teflon-like anticholesterol refuge. Welcome to the real world of women and high cholesterol.

Here are the heartless facts: A good cholesterol level is below 200 milligrams of cholesterol per deciliter of blood. Before age 45, women have an average total blood cholesterol of 190; from ages 45 to 64, those cholesterol figures rise to between 217 and 237. In all, about 55 million adult women have cholesterol levels of 200 or above. And as our cholesterol figures go, so goes the onslaught of heart problems in women.

For example, one major study—the Lipid Research Clinics investigation, conducted in medical centers across the country—showed that women with total cholesterol levels above 235 have a 70 percent higher risk of death than women with lower cholesterol readings.

One in seven women between the ages of 45 and 64 has some type of heart disease or has had a stroke. For those 65 and over, those figures increase to one in three. No wonder the American Heart Association calls heart disease a silent epidemic in women.

But even amid this quicksand of bad news, there is some reason for optimism. We still live longer than men by about seven years, and because of estrogen, we have extra protection against heart disease in our premenopausal years. Still, the lower you can get your cholesterol count, the better. If you take the initiative, you can outsmart cholesterol, no matter what your age, and make those extra years healthier ones.

## The Nature of the Beast

There's some irony to the bad news about cholesterol. After all, some of the cholesterol floating through your bloodstream is actually produced by your own liver. Without cholesterol, your cells could not function properly, and life itself would be threatened.

So while having some cholesterol isn't the problem, having too much of it is. Because cholesterol is consumed in your diet (exclusively from foods of animal origin), it can end up circulating in the blood in excess, joining forces with the cholesterol manufactured by your liver as well as with the saturated fat you eat. And as these substances navigate through your bloodstream, some of them attack and attach to the walls of your arteries, forming plaques that over time narrow your arteries and impede the flow of blood to your heart. This ominous process, called atherosclerosis, can age you before your time, leading to agonizing angina (chest pain) and heart attack.

To outwit cholesterol, the first step is to get your cholesterol checked. Your doctor should measure not only the total cholesterol level in your bloodstream but also your HDL cholesterol level. If these tests show signs of potential trouble, your doctor should check your LDL level, too, since evaluating all these numbers can be important in determining your risk.

Let's look more closely at these cholesterol factions. Cholesterol maneuvers through your bloodstream by catching rides on cooperative molecules called lipoproteins. While the cholesterol transported on the LDL carriers is the instigator of trouble in your arteries, the HDL carriers are the good guys, rounding up cholesterol and booting it right out of the body. In other words, while LDL cholesterol is the bully of your bloodstream, HDL cholesterol is the good Samaritan.

Unfortunately, too many of America's bloodstreams have too many LDLs

# Playing the Cholesterol Numbers Game

Once you've reached the ripe old age of 20, experts say that you're due for your first cholesterol test. After that, you should have one at least every five years.

One of the readings that this test will produce is your total blood cholesterol level. Here's a look at what that number means (all numbers refer to milligrams per deciliter of blood):

Less than 200—desirable
200–239—borderline high
240 and above—high

Even if you are settled comfortably in the "desirable" range, you still need to have your cholesterol measured regularly, along with a check of your HDL (high-density lipoprotein) cholesterol, the good kind. Sometimes a high HDL level will help compensate for a total cholesterol number in the "borderline high" range (although you're still well advised to get your total cholesterol as low as possible). However, if your HDL reading is less than 35, it falls into the "low" category, and you need to work at raising it. Your best options are losing weight, exercising more, quitting smoking and cutting back on how much sugar you eat.

And what about LDL (low-density lipoprotein) cholesterol, the bad kind? If your other tests reveal potential trouble, your doctor should have your LDL level tested, too. Below 130 is generally considered desirable.

Finally, to help interpret what all these numbers mean, your doctor may determine your cholesterol ratio, which is the ratio between your total cholesterol and your HDL number. If this ratio is 3.5 to 1 or lower, you are doing just fine.

and too few HDLs, a combination that gives unhealthy total cholesterol numbers. In the United States, the average total cholesterol is about 206, which is higher than the desirable level of less than 200.

## Turning the Tide

Experts say that by making some moderate lifestyle adjustments, you can dramatically lower your cholesterol. Studies show that for every 1 percent cut in your cholesterol level, you can deflate your chances of a heart attack by 2 percent. With dietary changes alone, you can whittle away an average of 10 percent of your cholesterol reading—and perhaps even more. Margo Denke, M.D., assistant professor of medicine at the University of Texas Southwestern Medical Center at Dallas's Center for Human Nutrition and a member of the nutrition committee of the American Heart Association, says that the higher your cholesterol count, the greater impact a heart-healthy diet can have. For example, a woman with a cholesterol reading of 280 may be able to steamroll 25 percent off the top by eating right. If longevity and anti-aging are your goals, that's a bottom line you can't afford to ignore.

To outmaneuver high cholesterol and the havoc it can wreak, give these cholesterol busters a try.

**Switch fat.** "Decreasing saturated fat is the most effective anticholesterol strategy you can use," says Karen Miller-Kovach, R.D., chief nutritionist at Weight Watchers International in Jericho, New York. That means eating less red meat, butter, cheese, whole milk and ice cream, all which raise LDL and total cholesterol levels. On the other hand, monounsaturated fat, known as the good fat, can actually help decrease cholesterol.

"When you switch from a diet high in saturated fat to one high in monounsaturated fat, and your weight stays about the same, your LDL cholesterol will fall while the HDL cholesterol remains stable," says Robert Rosenson, M.D., director of the Preventive Cardiology Center at Rush-Presbyterian–St. Luke's Medical Center in Chicago. "That's why olive oil is so popular, since it's high in monounsaturates." Better yet, increase your consumption of fatty fish, such as salmon and tuna. The fat in these fish are monounsaturates.

**Eat less cholesterol.** As important as reducing saturated fat can be, don't forget about dietary cholesterol. The cholesterol in your blood that isn't produced by your own body comes from your diet. Here's how to keep it under control.

Try to eliminate organ meats (such as liver) from your diet. Limit the amount of lean meat, poultry and fish to three ounces a day. And when it comes to eggs, limit your consumption of yolks to no more than two a week. Make your own cookies, cakes and pies, and use egg whites and egg substitute when you bake or cook.

Finally, when you're going through the buffet line, reach with gusto for vegetables, fruits and grains, which contain absolutely no dietary cholesterol. But show some willpower in holding out against high-fat salad dressings, sauces and butter.

**Feed on fiber.** Fiber is just what the doctor ordered to help fill the void as saturated fat beats a retreat in your meal planning. Concentrate on soluble fiber, the kind that's jam-packed in dried beans, lentils, citrus fruits, peas and apples. Adding soluble fiber to your diet could help lower your blood cholesterol by 5 to 10 percent.

**Feel your oats.** Oat bran has been on a roll for years. But how much is hype, and how much holds water? Researchers at the University of Minnesota in Minneapolis reviewed all the studies examining the power of oats and reached an artery-cleansing conclusion: Add 1⅓ cups of oat bran cereal (or three packets of instant oatmeal) to your daily diet, and watch your cholesterol level dip by 2 to 3 percent. If your cholesterol level is already high, you'll reap even more benefits, with oat bran skimming 6 to 7 percent off the top.

**Get fit.** This one won't surprise you: Exercise does a body good. In fact, to get your HDL level high, jump into an exercise class and work up a sweat. And don't worry about having to go to extremes. "We've learned that even moderate aerobic exercise (brisk walking, jogging, swimming) raises HDLs, although this often takes six months to a year to occur," says Dr. Rosenson.

**Trim your tummy.** Too many women lead lives of diet desperation, with not much to show for their efforts but a lot of frustration. But a sensible, moderate weight loss program can hit your cholesterol where it hurts. Dr. Denke has found that when young women are carrying around excess body weight, their total and LDL cholesterol levels tend to be higher, and their HDL levels are lower. Losing weight produces the reverse effect.

**Bag the cigarettes.** There are a lot of good reasons to quit smoking, and here's one more: Smoking can lower your HDL reading, something that no health-conscious person can afford to do.

But even if you're a chain-smoker, there's some encouraging news—if you're willing to toss out your cigarettes for good. By stopping smoking, says Dr. Rosenson, you can reverse the decline in your HDL level in about 60 days. It doesn't take years to eliminate smoking's dirty work.

**Make a toast.** Perhaps you've heard reports that a drink or two of any alcoholic beverage each day can raise the HDL component of your cholesterol. Well, you've heard correctly. Even so, approach this cholesterol-fighting strategy cautiously. Alcoholic drinks are brimming with calories, so they can defeat your efforts at losing weight. Even moderate drinking may also increase your chances of developing breast cancer. Finally, if you're pregnant or trying to get pregnant, stay away from alcohol altogether for the health of your baby.

Another option? Drink grape juice—the purple kind. Grape skin contains a cholesterol-lowering ingredient, according to Leroy Creasy, Ph.D., professor of pomology at Cornell University College of Agriculture and Life Sciences in Ithaca, New York.

**Consider estrogen.** Because natural estrogen protects you against cholesterol problems during your premenopausal years, doesn't it make sense that estrogen replacement therapy after menopause might do the same? In fact, that's exactly what research shows: Estrogen replacement therapy can cut your LDL cholesterol and raise your HDL cholesterol by about 15 percent each, according to an American Heart Association report on cardiovascular disease in women.

At the same time, however, estrogen replacement therapy has some red flags of its own, particularly a link to cancers of the endometrium and perhaps of the breast. You and your doctor need to keep these factors in mind when weighing the pros and cons of using estrogen replacement therapy in the war on cholesterol. Fortunately, doctors believe that by combining estrogen with progestin (another female hormone), you may be able to reduce your cancer risk.

# How Magical Is Medicine?

Even the most heroic efforts at lowering high cholesterol may run aground. A possible source of help may be anticholesterol medications, which can cut cholesterol readings by an average of 20 percent. Before you take these medications, however, many doctors advise trying a more conservative approach (diet, exercise, weight loss) for about six months. If that doesn't work, drugs may be the answer, particularly if your LDL cholesterol is still high, you have other risk factors for heart disease (such as family history or high blood pressure) or you already have heart disease.

Nicotinic acid and bile acid binders may be your doctor's first medication choices.

Nicotinic acid (such as Niacor) is one form of niacin, the vitamin that can be purchased without a prescription. But since you need to take nicotinic acid in high doses for it to make a difference in your cholesterol reading, doctors consider it a drug. So should you. High doses can cause serious side effects. Make sure that you take only the prescription form of this drug and relay any problems to your doctor.

"Flushing and stomach upset can occur with niacin," cautions Richard H. Helfant, M.D., vice chairman of medicine and director of the Cardiology Training Program at the University of California, Irvine, Medical Center and author of *Women, Take Heart*. He suggests avoiding niacin completely if you have diabetes, ulcers, liver disease or major heart rhythm problems.

Other medications have potential side effects, too, so your doctor should monitor you closely when you're taking them. Some of these prescription drugs, including the bile acid binders cholestyramine (such as Questran) and colestipol hydrochloride (Colestid), are available in powder form. Most others, including lovastatin (Mevacor) and gemfibrozil (Lopid), come as pills. Some of these drugs—nicotinic acid and bile acid binders—have been around long enough for studies to show that they not only can bring your LDL cholesterol level to its knees but also can decrease your chances of developing heart disease.

Incidentally, even if your doctor prescribes medication, don't think that you're off the hook, Dr. Denke cautions. "Drugs aren't a substitute for healthier eating, losing weight, exercising and other lifestyle strategies that need to be part of getting your cholesterol under control."

# Dental Problems

## *Teeth Can Last Forever*

The camera clicks at your high school reunion, and your lips slam together like cymbals. Why are you greeting the world with a little Mona Lisa smile when you really feel like flashing a great big grin?

Few things can age a woman's appearance more quickly than bad teeth. When you were young, a little dental neglect might have led to an occasional filling. But as you get older, ignoring your teeth can set you up for more serious problems, such as periodontal disease. And if not arrested promptly, long-term neglect can eventually cause you to lose teeth entirely.

But what if you've always been conscientious about dental care? Age still brings changes in the appearance and health of your smile. Years of chewing wears down tooth surfaces and actually shortens your teeth. Gums recede with age and wear. And even careful brushing has its downside if you've used the wrong technique for decades. Hard scrubbing wears down the translucent enamel coating of your teeth so that the yellowish material underneath, called dentin, begins to show through. Many otherwise lovely women as young as age 40 are frustrated by dingy-looking teeth.

As you age, your teeth will also show the telltale signs of years of indulgences. Coffee, red wine, tobacco and food dyes can work their way deep into microscopic cracks in the tooth enamel, resulting in brown or yellowish stains.

## Know the Score

When you were an adolescent, the dreaded cavity count might have been foremost in your mind when you went to the dentist. But these days, your dentist will tell you that the greatest enemy to your mouth is not cavities but gum disease.

There's a little moat around each tooth that forms a tiny crevice between

# Facing the Fear

If you'd rather face a hundred bad hair days than go to the dentist, you are not alone. Plenty of grown women quail at the thought of a session in the dentist's chair.

Wild fears about dentistry abound, says Mark Slovin, D.D.S., director of the Dental Phobia Clinic at the State University of New York at Stony Brook. But most of these fears are unfounded, he adds. Modern dentistry, while not always entirely painless, is no reason for panic. If you do panic, here's how to calm yourself.

**Open up before you open wide.** If you're afraid of the drill, share your feelings. "A good dentist is able to understand the feelings and thoughts of a patient," says Arthur A. Weiner, D.M.D., associate clinical professor at Tufts University School of Dental Medicine in Boston. Don't be shy about shopping around for a dentist you're comfortable with.

**Ask for a demo.** Ask your dentist to explain unfamiliar procedures step-by-step and to demonstrate how he'll use the instruments. Ask what kind of sensations to expect while the work is being done.

**Plan to communicate.** Ask your dentist to alert you to any upcoming pinching or pressure, so you can relax in the meantime, Dr. Weiner says. And agree on hand signals that will tell her when you want to sit up for a minute, pause or rinse.

**Use relaxation techniques.** Try deep breathing, concentrating on a pleasant image such as a day at the beach or listening to your favorite tunes on a headset to soothe your stay in the chair, says Dr. Slovin.

**Ask for more pain relief.** If you need extra anesthesia, go ahead and ask. Sedatives aren't a permanent solution, but they can get you through a procedure you need.

**Seek professional help.** If your fear is overwhelming, call your state dental society for help in finding a dental phobia clinic close to you. Or ask your dentist to recommend a psychological counselor who is familiar with dental phobias.

---

tooth and gum. When bacteria get in and linger, they cause inflammation, which over time deepens the crevices into pockets. As the inflammation simmers, bones, gums and connective tissue may get eaten away, leaving you with less foundation to hold your teeth in place. All that simmering can also cause soreness and bleeding as well as bad breath.

The other enemy is cavities (yes, they still count). Cavities start when a sticky film called plaque builds up on your teeth, trapping bacteria and breeding decay. Even though you may not have gotten many new cavities in your first years of adulthood, hang on to that toothbrush. Many women approaching middle age begin to get cavities along with gum disease. That's because as gums recede with age, the root (which has no protective enamel) is exposed to decay.

# A Daily Plan for a Perfect Mouth

If you want to keep a dazzling, healthy smile as you get older, it will take a new commitment to daily preventive care. That may mean spending more time brushing and flossing than you used to—and being more aware of the foods you eat. The first step is to catch up with the latest cleaning methods and keep an educated eye on what goes in your mouth.

**Brush often, brush right.** Brushing is your number-one defense against dental problems as you get older. "At a very minimum, be sure to brush after breakfast and before you go to bed at night," says Hazel Harper, D.D.S., associate professor of community dentistry at Howard University in Washington, D.C., and vice president of the National Dental Association. Of course, it's best to brush after every meal—with the right technique.

Done correctly, brushing removes the bacteria and plaque responsible for so many dental woes. Correct brushing, says Dr. Harper, means holding the brush with the handle in your palm and your thumb extended to act as a brace. This palm-thumb grasp tilts the brush at an angle, so bristles reach the gums and just underneath the gums as well as the tooth surfaces. Gently vibrate the brush in a small back-and-forth motion, covering only three teeth at a time. Then with a flick of the wrist, roll the brush against the sides of your teeth to sweep debris and bacteria away from the gum line. Finish up by brushing your tongue—your best antidote to bad breath, Dr. Harper says.

**Use the right brush.** Banish that hard-tufted, frayed thing from your toothbrush holder, says Dr. Harper. You need to use a soft-bristle toothbrush, and you should replace it every three months—sooner if the bristles start to fray, she says.

**Pick a proper paste.** Any toothpaste with the American Dental Association's seal of approval will do the job with a minimal amount of abrasion. If you tend to build up tartar, try a tartar control toothpaste. Tartar, or hardened plaque, feels like a rough coating on your teeth, says Richard Price, D.D.S., clinical instructor of dentistry at Boston University's Henry Goldman School of Dentistry. "These pastes reduce the amount of tartar you get, and the tartar that does build up will be softened and easier to remove," he says.

**Don't forget flossing.** Floss daily to be sure of complete cleaning and healthy gums, says Dr. Price. Toothbrush bristles simply can't get into the crannies around teeth. It doesn't matter what type of floss you use—waxed,

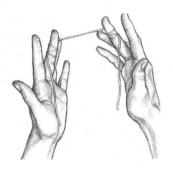 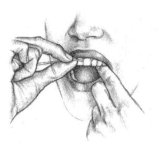 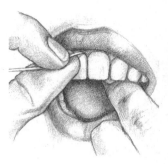

*Break off about 18 inches of floss and wind most of it around one middle finger. Wind the rest around the middle finger of your other hand.*

*Using your thumbs and forefingers, slide about an inch of taut floss between your teeth. Gently curve the floss in a C shape around the tooth at the gum line.*

*Gently slide the floss up and down between the tooth and gum, making sure you go beneath the gum line. Repeat on the rest of your teeth with clean sections of floss.*

unwaxed or flavored; just pick one that feels most comfortable to you, he says.

If you have a touch of arthritis in your fingers, a small mouth or a dexterity problem, try flossing one-handed. Wrap floss around the thumb and index finger of one hand, like you're forming a little slingshot, Dr. Price says. Or ask your dentist about flossing devices.

**Watch out for sticky surprises.** The foods that cling to your teeth are the foods that decay them, experts say. But it's hard to be sure which edibles in the following pairs are stickier: caramels or crackers? Hot-fudge sundaes or bread? Dried figs or puffed-oat cereal? Believe it or not, crackers, bread and cereal are the most likely to cling for long periods. Your best defense is to brush after every single snack, sugary or not. But if you can't get to a toothbrush soon, it's best to avoid the stickier foods.

**Say cheese for dessert.** It's an old custom in some cultures to serve cheese for dessert, and it might help cut cavities when you can't brush your teeth right after a meal. A few studies indicate that certain cheeses, particularly hard, aged ones such as cheddar and Monterey Jack, may reduce cavity-causing bacteria. Just a small slice will do the job—and not add much fat or cholesterol to your diet.

**Swish, swish.** Regardless of what you've just eaten, if you can't brush right away, the next best thing is to find a sink and swish a mouthful of water around your teeth, says Andrew M. Lewis, D.D.S., a dentist in private practice in Beverly Hills. Swishing will remove most debris and also dilute the acids formed by food particles.

# Heavy-Duty Home Care

If your dentist has noticed new cavities or early signs of gum disease, don't give up on your teeth—take charge. There's a lot you can do to turn the tide at any age. Try these home treatments, with your dentist's guidance.

**Use a fluoride rinse.** "If you're prone to cavities, use an over-the-counter fluoride rinse every night," says Dr. Lewis. "You want to rinse and spit it out so that it's the last thing in your mouth just before you go to sleep." Fluoride actually remineralizes teeth, making them stronger and less prone to cavities and root sensitivity.

**Plug in your toothbrush.** Try an electric toothbrush if you have trouble brushing thoroughly by hand or you have gum problems, says Dr. Harper. The gentle vibration of the brush head massages gums as it cleans the teeth, she says. And research at the University of Alabama School of Dentistry in Birmingham has proven that electric toothbrushes can significantly reduce gingivitis. Before you do your shopping, check with your dentist. Many professionals recommend the newer breed of electric toothbrush, with bristles that rotate rather than vibrate. There are several brands for sale, including Interplak and the Braun Oral-B Plaque Remover.

**Try an irrigator.** An oral irrigator such as the Water Pik can help clean debris from between teeth and under gums, but use it cautiously, Dr. Harper says. "Sometimes irrigators aren't adjusted right, and the flow of water is strong enough to damage gum tissue," she says. Slow the flow if your gums feel sore or irritated after using your irrigator.

# Help from the Pros

No amount of zeal at the bathroom sink can substitute for regular dental checkups, Dr. Harper says. To keep your teeth looking younger, see a dental hygienist twice a year for cleaning and your dentist at least once a year for an exam.

Your first stop is at the hygienist's chair for a professional cleaning to remove plaque and tartar, says Dr. Lewis. Once your teeth are squeaky clean, your dentist will examine your mouth. If cavities are cropping up more than they used to, you may be given a fluoride treatment at the office and a fluoride rinse or gel to use at home. But first, your dentist will fill any cavities.

And quicker than you might expect. With new, faster drills, your dentist can usually fill a cavity in about 15 minutes, a procedure that would have taken an hour 20 years ago, Dr. Harper says. What about pain? If reruns of the dental torture scene in *Marathon Man* are running through your head, don't worry—you won't need to outrun anything that awful. Modern dental procedures are light-years ahead of your worst dental memory.

On rare occasions, you may need a root canal to remove the pulp or nerve of a rotted tooth and fill the hole. Despite its painful reputation, a

# Facts about Fillings

Your dentist tells you that you have a few cavities. "Whoaaaa," you say. "Have you inhaled too much of that laughing gas? I'm too old for cavities."

Sorry, sister, but you're never too old for cavities.

Lots of women get them well into their later years, says Richard Price, D.D.S., clinical instructor of dentistry at Boston University's Henry Goldman School of Dentistry. One reason is that old fillings wear out. Although some may last decades, the average life span of silver fillings is about nine years. Beyond that, they tend to chip, crack and wear out.

"They're just replacement parts," says Dr. Price. "Any time you get a tooth drilled and filled, it will need to be drilled and filled for the rest of your life. It's like your warranty wearing out."

Sometimes adult women, even champion brushers and flossers, may acquire new cavities as well. The most common spot for these black holes is at the base of the teeth, where gums receding with age have exposed the sensitive roots to decay, says Dr. Price.

If you do need a filling—either a replacement or a new one—get ready to choose from a number of alternative materials.

Silver is by far the most common of the lot, because it's durable and affordable. The silver is mixed with mercury, which makes it easy to shape. The question has arisen from time to time whether this mercury, a poisonous metal, could leach into the body. Some women have even had perfectly good fillings removed because of the mercury scare.

That's a shame.

Yes, some mercury is released from silver fillings when you chew, but only minuscule amounts. Even less is actually absorbed by your body. "Nothing to worry about," says Joel M. Boriskin, D.D.S., chief of the Division of Dentistry at Alameda County Medical Center in Oakland, California. A number of studies measured the release of mercury from silver fillings and came to the same conclusion: There's no reason to be concerned unless your mouth can hold 1,000 fillings.

But just because silver is safe, that doesn't mean it's always best. Gold, though pricy, is super strong and especially good for jumbo cavities. Fillings made from porcelain, quartz or acrylic, though not as durable as the metals, may be preferable for more visible fillings. They can be colored to match your own teeth.

root canal done right can be no more uncomfortable than any other dental procedure, says Dr. Lewis.

For advancing gum disease, your dentist will refer you to a periodontist, or gum disease specialist. Treatment may involve oral antibiotics, antibacterial ointments squeezed into the gum pockets or, in severe cases, surgical removal of part of the infected gum or diseased bone.

And if stains or crooked teeth are your greatest dental problem, a cosmetic dentist can help. Bleaching whitens stains, and a variety of other techniques can restore the youth and beauty of your smile. (For details, see Cosmetic Dentistry, page 463.)

# DEPRESSION

## *The Sneaky Stealer of Youth*

On most days, Bonnie Brand feels really good. But occasionally, when the pressure of juggling a career and the needs of her family overwhelm her, a dark shadow of depression descends, and she feels age creeping up on her.

"Like most women, I worry about my weight, I worry about my appearance, and yes, I worry about getting older," says the 33-year-old word processing supervisor at a legal firm in Newport Beach, California. "When I feel good, I feel attractive. But when I'm depressed, I definitely feel older. Every ache and pain in my body seems to be magnified when I feel that way."

That wouldn't surprise many doctors who say depression affects the body as well as the mind.

"Certainly, depression can slow you down and make you look and feel older," says Janice Peterson, M.D., a clinical psychiatrist at the University of Colorado Health Sciences Center in Denver. "If you look at some of the major symptoms of depression—lack of energy, lowered sex drive, loss of appetite, difficulty concentrating, changes in sleeping patterns and generalized aches and pains—you'd see some things that you might consider a normal part of aging. So if you saw a person with those problems, you might think 'Oh, she's just getting older' when in fact she has a major depression."

The effects of depression on the body are so powerful that often they can make you appear more than a decade older than your natural age. "Some people who are chronically depressed can look very old and have stooped shoulders, furrowed lines around the eyes and all the other things that make a person looked aged. I've seen some depressed people who look like they're in their sixties when they're actually 35 or 40," says Harry Prosen, M.D., chairman of the Department of Psychiatry and Mental Health Sciences at the Medical College of Wisconsin in Milwaukee.

# What's Getting Us Down

All of us feel sad at one time or another. The death of a loved one, divorce, the loss of a job or another hardship can leave us feeling so down that we doubt we'll ever be up again. While most of us do pull out of it, lots of others don't. During her lifetime, a woman has an 8 to 12 percent chance that she will suffer from a major depression, meaning she has five or more symptoms of depression for at least two weeks, including feelings of worthlessness or thoughts of death and suicide.

Over a lifetime, women are twice as likely as men to be diagnosed as having major depression. That difference mystifies researchers, says Dan Blazer, M.D., Ph.D., professor of psychiatry at Duke University Medical Center in Durham, North Carolina. But heredity, biological differences and a disparity in our society's expectations of how men and women should behave may contribute to the gap.

"There's a theory of depression that revolves around anger," says Kimberly Yonkers, M.D., assistant professor of psychiatry and gynecology at the University of Texas Southwestern Medical Center at Dallas. "According to this theory, women tend to repress their anger, turn it inward and, as a result, get depressed. Men, on the other hand, outwardly express their anger and

## Is It All in the Family?

You're not the only one who gets depressed. Grandma, Mom, Dad and your brother all regularly tumble into a funk that they can't seem to shake. Coincidence, or is there something going on here?

"It's clear that people with family histories of depression are much more likely to suffer from depression than people who don't have family histories of depression," says Alan Mellow, M.D., Ph.D., assistant professor of psychiatry at the University of Michigan Medical School in Ann Arbor. "There is well-documented evidence that like cancer, diabetes and high blood pressure, major depression has a genetic component."

Okay, so you can't choose your parents. But knowing that your family has a history of depression should help you understand why you may feel particularly on the downside more often than other people, Dr. Mellow says. If you are feeling unusually blue, especially if you have a family history of major depression, you should consider seeking counseling and asking about antidepressant drug therapy.

rage by getting aggressive." However, it could also be that women are just more likely than men to talk about their emotions and seek treatment for depression, Dr. Yonkers says.

# The Physical Price

Even mild sadness that lasts only one or two days can make you more susceptible to many of the illnesses and changes in appearance that are considered a part of aging. "Certainly, depression takes its toll on people physically. We don't know all the mechanisms that are involved, but we do know that the general well-being of the body is thrown out of whack when a person is depressed," Dr. Blazer says.

Decreased muscle tone is one of the most immediate physical changes that occurs when you begin to get depressed. "That causes muscles to sag and contributes to the sad facial expressions and poor posture that you see in depressed people," says Elmer Gardner, M.D., a psychiatrist in private practice in Washington, D.C.

But the changes caused by depression can be more than skin-deep. Researchers believe depression can weaken the immune system, accelerate hardening of the arteries and trigger some forms of arthritis.

If you're depressed, your immune cell activity can drop to the levels of a person who is 25 to 30 years older, says Michael Irwin, M.D., associate professor of psychiatry at the University of California, San Diego, School of Medicine. Dr. Irwin has not studied depression in women, but in a study of depressed men in their early forties, he found they had natural killer cell activity that looked remarkably similar to men in their seventies who weren't depressed. Natural killer cells are the part of the immune system that protects you from viruses such as herpes simplex, the cold sore virus, and these killer cells are normally less active as we age.

"Depression triggers a lowered immune response, but we still don't know to what extent that leads to sickness," Dr. Irwin says. "We do know, however, that the viruses that natural killer cells help protect us against are more common in people who are depressed."

Depression can also stimulate atherosclerosis, a buildup of fatty deposits on artery walls that contributes to coronary heart disease, says George Kaplan, Ph.D., an epidemiologist and chief of the Human Population Laboratory of the California Department of Health Services in Berkeley.

Rheumatoid arthritis is yet another disease that can be aggravated or even triggered by depression, says Sanford Roth, M.D., a rheumatologist and medical director of the Arthritis Center in Phoenix. "It's not unusual for a person who suffers a devastating loss of a parent or spouse to develop a disease like rheumatoid arthritis," Dr. Roth says. "Because rheumatoid arthritis may be associated with a genetic root, these people probably had the potential to develop the disease all along. It just took a depressive episode to open it up."

# Are You Really Depressed?

Here's a list of symptoms, according to the American Psychiatric Association, that may help you determine the severity of a depression. If you have five or more of these symptoms in a two-week span, or if you have felt depressed for more than two weeks, you should seek the help of your doctor or a qualified therapist.

- You feel sad most of the day and have lost interest in pleasurable activities, including sex.
- You feel tired or lack energy to do day-to-day chores.
- You feel restless and can't sit still.
- You either have insomnia or sleep more than usual.
- You have difficulty concentrating or making decisions.
- You have fluctuations in your appetite or weight.
- You feel hopeless, worthless and guilty.
- You think about death and suicide.

# Climbing into the Light

So now that you know depression can have a serious impact on how you age, what can you do to prevent or treat it? Plenty, doctors say.

Keep in mind that severe depression—one that persists for more than two weeks—may require a doctor's care and treatment with antidepressant drugs. But if your depression lasts a few days and doesn't appear to be interfering with your activities, here are a few suggestions that may perk you up.

**Keep a goal in sight.** "People who have dreams and visions of accomplishment are less likely to be depressed than those who don't have short- and long-term goals," says Dennis Gerster, M.D., a psychiatrist in private practice in San Diego. Write down a list of goals. Divide the list into sections that include things you want to do this week, this month, within a year and within five years. Put the list in a prominent place, such as on your refrigerator, and check off the goals as you achieve them. Try to update your list at least once a month.

**Get busy.** "If you can keep yourself busy, it will help, because staying active can prevent you from dwelling on whatever is making you feel unhappy," says Linda George, Ph.D., professor of medical sociology at Duke University Medical Center.

**Keep laughing.** Humor is your best ally, Dr. Prosen says. Clip cartoons and funny articles out of newspapers and magazines and put them in a file you can flip through when you feel low.

**Lean on family and friends.** They've helped you survive bad relationships and other disasters; now they can help you through this bleak time. "That doesn't mean you're asking them to solve your problems for you," Dr. George says. "It just means you're asking them to listen, let you get things off your chest and be supportive."

**Put your negative thoughts on paper.** Writing down your feelings when you're depressed can help you recognize faulty thought patterns and help you find ways to replace those thoughts with more uplifting ones, Dr. Peterson says. For every negative thought you write down, such as "I'm the worst person in the world," also write down a positive one, such as "I have imperfections, but I also have a lot going for me." After a while, the positive thoughts may replace the negative ones.

**Stay away from booze.** Although it may be tempting to drown your sorrows in a few glasses of wine, don't do it, Dr. Yonkers warns. Alcohol is a depressant that can drag you further into the dumps. "Excessive drinking will also disrupt your sleep and may drive your friends and family away from you just when you need their support the most," she says.

**Sweat it out.** "Exercise is a fabulous way to relieve depression," Dr. Gersten says. "Aerobic exercise such as walking, running, swimming or bicycling cranks up your brain activity and can reverse the effects of even a major depression." He suggests exercising at least 20 minutes a day, three times a week.

**Keep the credit cards in your purse.** "Some people who get depressed try to break out of it with the credit card prescription," Dr. Yonkers says. "They think that if they go shopping and buy something, it's going to pick them up. But often they end up feeling guilty because they make major purchases they can't afford and that depresses them even more." If you are depressed and do go shopping, set a spending limit before you go, and pay in cash.

**Be a good actress.** A great way to fend off depression is to act happy for an hour, Dr. Yonkers says. Then try it for another hour and so on. By the end of the day, you might be surprised to find you're not faking it anymore.

# DIABETES

## *Disarming a Potential Killer*

Sugar and spice are fine for nursery rhymes.

But when the amount of sugar in your blood is too high, you probably have diabetes, a disease that afflicts nearly eight million American women. It's the nation's fourth leading cause of death, claiming about 160,000 lives each year—about half that number women. Over time, unmanaged diabetes can cause stroke, heart attack and kidney failure even in young people, who normally don't face these problems. Diabetes can also lead to blindness, nerve damage and sexual disinterest.

## No Easy Outs

But even trying to manage this disease can age you before your time. Women with diabetes must adhere to strict diets in both what and when they eat. "Maybe they can have an infrequent piece of cake, on a child's birthday or an anniversary, but that's it," says Audrey Lally, R.D., a certified diabetes educator and nutrition specialist at the Mayo Clinic in Scottsdale, Arizona. "But for the most part, I discourage my patients with diabetes from ever using anything that contains large amounts of pure sugar."

This regimen goes beyond the kitchen. No longer can women with diabetes casually stroll barefoot on a summer's day. Because of nerve damage that could result in a loss of sensation in their legs and feet, they may be unaware of foot injuries. According to the American Diabetes Association, more than 54,000 diabetes sufferers lose their feet or legs to amputation each year because of the disease.

"Any time you change the chemistry of the blood, you're going to change virtually every system affected by the blood," says Steve Manley, Ph.D., a psychologist in private practice in Denton, Texas. "And that would be all of them."

Including your sexual organs. Since diabetes can debilitate both the neurological system and the vascular system, and you need good nerves and blood flow to function sexually, many women lose the pleasure they once found in sex. "Men often become impotent from diabetes, and in a way, it affects women the same way," says Dr. Manley. "The lubrication phase for women is similar to the erection phase for men."

## The Brain Drain

Diabetes can have an effect on your mind in more ways than one. "When your blood sugar is out of control, it has an effect on your cognitive function," says Patricia Stenger, R.N., a diabetes counselor and senior vice president for the American Diabetes Association. "You may have slower response time, and you feel sluggish and fatigued."

Adds Dr. Manley, "In effect, diabetes kicks you into a grief reaction, because you have lost something. Some people feel helpless and hopeless that their bodies somehow revolted against them. Some feel that they are no longer in control of their own destinies. They may lose belief, at least temporarily, that they are going to be okay at some point in the future. The disease begins to interact with their basic personalities."

## A Bitter Sweet

Diabetes occurs when the body doesn't produce enough or properly use insulin, a hormone secreted in the pancreas that's needed to convert food into energy. Much of what we eat for energy is broken down into a sugar called glucose, the fuel that's fed into every single cell to keep us alive. The disease isn't caused by eating sweets, although people with diabetes must limit their sugar intakes because sweets can make blood sugar rise drastically.

In healthy people, glucose is automatically absorbed by cells. The body uses exactly what it needs and stores the rest. But without insulin to unlock a cell's receptors so that glucose can enter, excess amounts of this sugar accumulate in the bloodstream, where it can cause a host of problems. People with diabetes face five times the risk of stroke and two to four times the risk of heart disease compared with people who don't have the disease. One in ten sufferers develops kidney disease, and between 15,000 and 39,000 a year lose their sight because of the disease.

## Subtle Trouble

There are two types of diabetes. With Type I (or juvenile) diabetes, which accounts for only 10 percent of cases, the body completely fails to produce insulin, so daily injections of this hormone are needed. Type I is often diagnosed during puberty, and the symptoms, which can mimic the flu, are sudden and very noticeable: extreme hunger and thirst, sudden weight loss and extreme fatigue and irritability.

In the more common Type II (or adult-onset) diabetes, which usually strikes women after age 45, the pancreas produces insulin, but not enough. There may be some symptoms—slow-healing cuts or bruises, recurring skin, gum or bladder infections or slight tingling or numbness in the hands or feet—but many women don't notice these subtle changes or simply shrug them off. And that's exactly why over half the women with diabetes are unaware of their condition. Diabetes is a subtle disease that just creeps up on people—and with devastating results, says Xavier Pi-Sunyer, M.D., professor of medicine at Columbia University in New York City and past president of the American Diabetes Association.

That's why it's important for you to get a blood screening for elevated glucose levels, especially if you have a family history of the disease, are overweight, are over age 40 or had a baby with a birth weight of over nine pounds. "People may be unaware that they have the disease because they feel fine," says Stenger.

## Beating the Odds

"The best way to avoid diabetes is to watch your weight," says Lally. "That means eating a healthy diet that focuses on fruits and vegetables. Being overweight is the major risk factor for adult-onset diabetes. This is important for everyone but is essential if you have a family history of diabetes or had diabetes during pregnancy."

Even if you're among the 650,000 people diagnosed this year—that's one every 60 seconds—a healthy lifestyle may be all that's needed to get the upper hand on diabetes. Although some people with Type II diabetes require oral drugs or injections to stabilize their blood sugar, most can control the disease simply by adopting healthier lifestyles. By committing yourself to certain lifestyle changes, you may be able to reduce your need for medication—and possibly get off and stay off diabetes drugs for the rest of your life, says James Barnard, Ph.D., professor of physiological science at the University of California, Los Angeles. Here's how.

**Share your feelings.** Learning that you have diabetes can be quite a blow, and many women find comfort in sharing their experiences with others going through the same thing.

Meeting regularly with a support group can help you cope with the disease, mentally and physically; it's also a good way to beat depression. Call your local chapter of the American Diabetes Association for a list of support groups in your area.

**Neutralize stress.** Even if you're not worried about depression, studies by researchers at Duke University in Durham, North Carolina, show that when you're under stress, certain hormones are activated that pump stored glucose into your bloodstream. Conversely, stress management and taking time to relax improve glucose control, a significant factor for those with diabetes. While group therapy is one way to relax, others include meditation and yoga.

**Eat right.** That means low-fat and high-fiber, with at least five servings of fruits and vegetables a day, says Lally. For each extra 40 grams of fat eaten per day—the amount found in one fast-food burger and a large order of fries—your risk of developing diabetes rises threefold, and if you already have diabetes, you face a greater chance of complications, finds a study in the *American Journal of Epidemiology*. The problem: Dietary fat readily converts to body fat, and body fat induces cells to resist insulin, says Frank Q. Nuttall, M.D., Ph.D., chief of the Endocrine, Metabolic and Nutrition Section of the Minneapolis Veterans Administration Medical Center.

Meanwhile, try to consume at least 25 grams of fiber daily from complex-carbohydrate foods, which help put the brakes on glucose entering your blood-stream and also keep cholesterol low—important for people with diabetes, who face higher risk of heart disease. That's between two and three times what most Americans eat. The best sources of complex carbohydrates are potatoes, whole-grain breads, rice, pasta, legumes, oats and barley.

**Time it right.** "If you have diabetes, you need to eat every four or five hours," says Lally. Grazing is best, since large meals make it tougher for your body to meet the increased demand for insulin. The key is to evenly distribute your food throughout the day, so no single meal overwhelms the pancreas.

**Avoid sugar and salt.** It's a given that you should avoid sugar; even in tiny amounts, it can send your blood sugar sky-high. Of course, low sugar and low salt are good dietary rules for everyone to follow, but those with diabetes must be especially careful. Instead, satisfy your sweet tooth with artificial sweeteners such as aspartame (NutraSweet). But also be on the lookout for low-sodium or reduced-sodium products. Salty foods can raise blood pressure, a danger for people with diabetes.

**Get your heart pumping.** Regular aerobic exercise not only helps you control your weight but also makes cells more receptive to insulin. "You need to get your heart going and keep it going for at least 20 minutes," says Stenger. "You don't need to do anything fancy: a brisk walk is fine."

Meanwhile, researchers at Harvard University in Cambridge, Massachusetts, found that exercise is an excellent way to help prevent Type II diabetes. In their Physicians Health Study of 22,000 doctors, researchers noted that those who exercise at least five times a week lowered their risk of developing diabetes by more than 40 percent.

But people with diabetes need to exercise with care. "The main concern for exercise and diabetes is the risk of hypoglycemia, or low blood sugar," says Greg Dwyer, Ph.D., professor of physical education at Ball State University in Muncie, Indiana. To avoid this, he suggests sticking to a routine that requires the same amount of exercise at the same time daily.

**Pump some iron, too.** Weight lifting also plays a role in improving glucose tolerance, the body's ability to metabolize sugar properly, according to a study by researchers at the University of Maryland College Park and Johns Hopkins University in Baltimore. Check with your doctor before starting a weight-lifting program. Resistance training may cause surges in blood pressure.

**Take vitamins E and C.** These two antioxidants tend to be in short supply among people with diabetes—and Italian researchers have found that vitamin E helps improve the action of insulin. Good food sources include wheat germ, corn oil and nuts, but you should take a supplement containing 400 IU each day.

Meanwhile, because those with diabetes are prone to vascular disease, they may need to increase their intakes of vitamin C, suggests Ishwarial Jialal, M.D., assistant professor of internal medicine and clinical nutrition at the University of Texas Southwestern Medical Center at Dallas. The Recommended Dietary Allowance is 60 milligrams a day, but Dr. Jialal suggests a minimum of 120 milligrams of vitamin C daily, the amount you'd find in a guava or a glass of orange juice.

**Pretend you have a headache.** Aspirin can reduce the risk of heart attack and stroke among diabetes sufferers by as much as 20 percent, according to research conducted by the National Institutes of Health on 3,711 people with both types of the disease. "People with diabetes are much more likely to have cardiovascular disease, so the aspirin recommendation is even more relevant for them," says Frederick Ferris, M.D., chief of the Clinical Trials Branch at the National Institutes of Health in Bethesda, Maryland.

Most researchers recommend a daily dosage of one-half of an adult aspirin or one children's aspirin, but check with your doctor first: Aspirin therapy isn't suggested for people taking blood thinners or suffering from ulcers.

# DIETING

## *Deprivation Doesn't Work*

You remember how it's done: Mom was always dieting, especially as she got older. So just like Mom used to do, you head for the kitchen, humming all the way . . .

One big, juicy slab of iceberg lettuce. Top it with a little scoop of cottage cheese. How about half a canned peach? Hmm, let's see. What else? Of course! Melba toast. Take three; they're small. Hey, this isn't so bad—is it? Now add a little artificial sweetener to the coffee, and you're all set. Dig in.

Suddenly, you don't feel like humming anymore.

Diets don't work. Sure, you might lose some weight at first. But eventually, when you're so hungry that you could eat your slippers, you'll go off the diet with a vengeance. And you'll usually regain more weight than you lost, says John Foreyt, Ph.D., director of the Nutrition Research Clinic at Baylor College of Medicine in Houston.

Who hasn't thought that "if I can lose just these last ten pounds, I'll look younger"? But the sad truth is that the net gain of body fat resulting from this cycle of lose and gain puts a tremendous strain on your body. You see it in your skin as wrinkles and sagging, says George Blackburn, M.D., Ph.D., associate professor of surgery at Harvard Medical School and chief of the Nutrition/Metabolism Laboratory at New England Deaconess Hospital, both in Boston.

But what you don't see is the aging on the inside—organs and systems that get old before their time.

## Yo-Yo Illogic

A lifetime of dieting may take a toll on your heart. Research done by Kelly Brownell, Ph.D., a psychologist and obesity researcher at Yale University in New Haven, Connecticut, found that repeated dieting can set you up for heart

124

# The Diet Pill Question

Do diet pills really work, or do they offer only false hope?

"Some antidepressants can help people who have serious weight problems that include binge eating caused by behavioral or psychiatric disorders," says David Schlundt, Ph.D., a clinical psychologist and assistant professor of psychology at Vanderbilt University in Nashville. "But be sure to combine them with some form of psychotherapy."

What about over-the-counter diet pills? Most experts don't recommend them. Their active ingredient, phenylpropanolamine hydrochloride (PPA), is an adrenaline-like stimulant. "For people who aren't that healthy in the first place—who have high blood pressure, heart disease, asthma or diabetes—PPA can cause real problems," says Dr. Schlundt. Even low doses can raise blood pressure and increase heart rate. And large doses can cause anxiety, sleeplessness, even convulsions. PPA also has the potential for abuse, Dr. Schlundt points out. It causes a "high" similar to that of speed or amphetamines that can become addictive.

For seriously overweight people, there may be a promising "fat blocker" pill on the horizon, says John Foreyt, Ph.D., director of the Nutrition Research Clinic at Baylor College of Medicine in Houston. It's called orlistat (Xenical), and it's being tested in the United States and Europe. "Orlistat is not for someone who needs to lose five or ten pounds but for moderate to severe obesity," he says. The drug works by blocking fat absorption.

"But no pill is a magic bullet," Dr. Foreyt says. "Even with orlistat, you still have to follow a low-fat diet and a sensible exercise program."

disease. Dr. Brownell's studies showed that people with big weight fluctuations have a 75 percent greater risk of dying from heart disease than people whose weights stay relatively steady. "A lot of weight fluctuation is required to put you in this category—not five pounds now and then," says Dr. Brownell.

Yo-yo dieting may also cause high blood pressure and redistribute fat to areas of the body where it does more damage, such as from your bottom to your belly. People with lots of abdominal fat, for instance, are more likely to develop heart disease, say experts.

Dieting also makes it impossible for you to reap the full benefits of physical activity. A study at Arizona State University in Tempe found that women who had been on at least four different diets in the previous year used fewer calories during exercise than nondieters. They also weighed more and had more body fat than the nondieting women.

# Listen for the Quacks

The ads trumpet "Lose a Pound a Day!" "I Lost 100 Pounds in Three Months!" "Miracle Weight Loss Pill!" "Mystery Food Melts Pounds Away!" "Low-Carbohydrate Diet!" "High-Protein Diet!"

Sound familiar? Quick weight loss diets simply don't work. You may lose weight rapidly at first, but most of that is water. The moment you stop starving yourself, you'll gain it all right back—plus extra fat.

Here's how to identify a legitimate weight control program as opposed to just another dumb diet plan.

**Fast is false.** Don't fall prey to weight loss schemes that promise speed, says Dr. Blackburn. The greatest virtue for successful weight loss is patience, because the only way to lose weight is slowly. One-half to one pound a week is best, he says.

**Never say never.** Deprivation doesn't work, but lifestyle changes can, says Janet Polivy, Ph.D., professor of psychology at the University of Toronto Faculty of Medicine. A good eating plan—one that is geared toward health, not toward weight loss—doesn't forbid occasional indulgences in high-fat favorites, she says. "If you're told to never eat fried foods, you'll feel terrible when you have some—which is inevitable—and you'll give up good eating because you'll feel like a failure."

**Forget about fad food diets.** "This concept is hogwash," Dr. Blackburn says. "There are no magical foods that cancel other calories consumed, such as grapefruit."

**Don't trust testimonials.** "Testimonials are a major approach of bogus weight loss schemes," says Terrence Kuske, M.D., a nutritionist and professor of medicine at the Medical College of Georgia in Augusta. A typical testimonial might look something like this: "I lost 30 pounds in one month with Diet Dynamite! J. Smith, New York City." Chances are good that J. Smith doesn't exist—or, if she does, that she is related to the owner of the company selling this diet scheme. Weight control programs that work are backed up by scientific studies, not by testimonials.

# DIGESTIVE PROBLEMS

## *Calming the Pain and Rumble*

As if chocolate bars and cheese curls haven't caused us enough problems all these years, now we're getting grief from unassuming eats such as onions, tomatoes and even strawberries. What gives?

Apparently, your digestive tract.

You could understand why men have digestive problems; all you have to do is watch them eat. But lately, you've found yourself reaching for the Di-Gel or Pepto-Bismol a little more often. Why? Because of gas. Or heartburn. Or bloating. Or diarrhea or constipation. Or any number of these problems.

Well, you're in good company.

"Just as it takes longer to recover from a cold or an injury as you grow older, the same happens to your digestive system. Things just kind of slow down, and the repair mechanisms aren't quite the same as they used to be," says William B. Ruderman, M.D., chairman of the Department of Gastroenterology at the Cleveland Clinic Florida in Fort Lauderdale. "You can't tolerate certain foods or the effects of alcohol as well as you used to. It certainly makes you feel your own mortality."

All those belches, rumbles and other internal actions wear on more than just your digestive tract. "You may be hesitant to take a bus or go outdoors in case you have to go to the bathroom. You may not go to certain restaurants because you can't eat certain foods," says Devendra Mehta, M.D., a gastroenterologist and assistant professor of pediatrics at Hahnemann University Hospital in Philadelphia. "This can be very distressing at any age. But when you are young and have these problems, it disrupts your life."

Just because your innards may be out of kilter, however, it doesn't mean they have to stay that way. Whatever the problem, here's how to fix it.

# Constipation: Get Yourself Moving

If you haven't been bothered by constipation, give yourself a few years. "Constipation gets a lot more common as you age," says Jorge Herrera, M.D., associate professor of medicine at the University of South Alabama College of Medicine in Mobile. "For one thing, as they get older, most people tend to eat less and become less active." And many medicines that people tend to take as they age for conditions such as heart disease and diabetes also cause constipation, says Dr. Herrera.

At any age, however, constipation can make you feel older. Whether you have to strain to move your bowels or simply don't feel the urge, constipation occupies your mind with thoughts of what you can't do, and because of that, your body may not feel like doing much of anything. Most women over age 30 can expect at least an occasional bout with constipation—and more as they get older. But here's how to keep problems to a minimum, no matter your age.

**Eat in bulk.** "If you're eating the typical Western diet with a lot of processed foods, that will lead to constipation," says Dr. Mehta. "But a diet with lots of roughage and fiber that centers on plenty of fresh fruits and vegetables is the most important thing you can do to treat or avoid constipation, especially as you get older."

Experts say you need at least five servings a day in order to get the recommended minimum of 25 grams of fiber—about twice what's actually consumed by the typical American. Besides fresh produce, good sources of dietary fiber include whole-grain breads and cereals, pastas, brown rice, beans and bran.

**Work out.** Any type of exercise speeds up gastrointestinal transit time, the length of time it takes food to get from your mouth through the stomach and intestines. But researchers at the University of Maryland College Park found that people who undergo strength training programs can improve their bowel transit times by about 56 percent compared with their pre-pumping days. It seems that the contractions of abdominal muscles done in weight lifting help "squeeze" the waste through the intestines more quickly. Researchers also believe that any type of exercise has an effect on motilin, a gastrointestinal hormone that's related to faster transit time. Exercise also improves blood flow to the intestines, which improves bowel movements.

**Drink water.** "One reason why constipation is more common as you age is that generally, the older people get, the less they drink," says Dr. Mehta. "And the less you drink, the harder and less frequent stools become." Even if you don't have a problem with constipation, you'll help keep yourself regular by drinking at least six glasses of water or other nonalcoholic beverages each day.

Meanwhile, try to limit your intake of coffee, tea and alcohol. While caffeinated beverages actually speed bowel transit time (alcohol has no effect), these beverages are diuretics that can leave you dehydrated, and you need fluids in your system to aid bowel movements. And those with frequent constipation should avoid milk, cheese and other dairy products, which contain casein, an insoluble protein that tends to plug up the intestinal tract.

# Heartburn: Douse the Fire

You probably already know how heartburn makes you feel: lousy. Nothing can take the wind out of your sails—not to mention your appetite—faster than having to rest after each meal until the pain subsides or having to monitor your every bite in order to avoid the pain in the first place.

Heartburn occurs when stomach acids, in a process called reflux, splash up into the esophagus, says Sheila Rodriguez, Ph.D., gastrointestinal laboratory director for the Oklahoma Foundation for Digestive Research in Oklahoma City. Eating too fast or too much is one common cause, but pigging out isn't the only reason for this all-too-common after-dinner ailment. Heartburn can also be the primary symptom of other conditions, such as gastritis, an inflammation in the lining of the stomach.

"It's not that the natural aging process contributes to heartburn per se, but the condition does seem to be more of a problem as you get older," says Dr. Mehta. One reason is that there's a clear association between heartburn and being overweight—and most of us have gained a few pounds over the last few years.

But another, less obvious reason is bacteria. The same bacteria—*Helicobacter pylori*—that cause ulcers have been linked to heartburn symptoms in many women, says Dr. Mehta. Also, after age 40, our esophageal muscles start to weaken, which can contribute to reflux. But no matter the reason, here's how to take the fire out of heartburn.

**Eat smaller.** Many women with heartburn problems find that grazing helps extinguish that internal blaze. When you eat four or five smaller meals instead of three massive squares a day, your stomach churns out less acid, says Frank Hamilton, M.D., director of the Gastrointestinal Diseases Program at the National Institutes of Health in Bethesda, Maryland.

**Down it with water.** Drinking lots of water—especially with meals—helps wash stomach acids from the surface of the esophagus back into your stomach, says Ronald L. Hoffman, M.D., a physician in New York City and author of *Seven Weeks to a Settled Stomach*.

**Know the offenders.** Certain foods are more likely than others to bring on the symptoms of heartburn. According to Dr. Rodriguez, onions, chocolate and mints relax the lower esophageal sphincter, which allows stomach acids to wash up. Citrus fruits such as oranges and grapefruit, as well as tomato products, coffee and fried or fatty foods, can also cause trouble because they can irritate the esophageal lining, adds Dr. Hamilton.

**Sleep on a slope.** If heartburn troubles you often, place wooden or concrete blocks under the headboard of your bed so that you sleep on an incline, advises William Lipshultz, M.D., chief of gastroenterology at Pennsylvania Hospital in Philadelphia. By raising the head of your bed six inches higher, it's harder for stomach acid to flow. That's because it would have to go uphill.

If you must lie flat, lying on your left side might produce less heartburn, says Leo Katz, M.D., a gastroenterologist at Jefferson Medical College of

Thomas Jefferson University in Philadelphia. In tests, he found that people who ate the same heartburn-producing meal usually got more heartburn when they lay on their right sides compared with their left sides. "We think it has something to do with the anatomy of the stomach and gravity," he says.

# Lactose Intolerance: Drink Up—Safely

Dare to eat dairy? Perhaps not. As much as 70 percent of the world's population has some symptoms of lactose intolerance, meaning these people experience ill effects from milk, ice cream and other dairy products. Symptoms include bloating, gas, stomach cramping and diarrhea, which can curtail your activities and hamper your lifestyle. Besides making you feel older, the symptoms often get worse as you grow older.

By about age eight, many of us start losing an enzyme called lactase, which helps us digest lactose, the sugar that makes milk taste sweet. Without the lactase, much of the lactose passes along your digestive system undigested, possibly sending your colon into spasms and churning up gas. "By age 20, lactose-intolerant people pretty much lose the ability to digest milk," says Dr. Herrera.

Lactose intolerance varies from person to person. Some women may feel minor discomfort after a lot of dairy, while others may get major problems from just a sip or two of milk. So checking your individual tolerance, and staying within that range, is the best way to avoid trouble. While there are plenty of lactose-free products—you'll find them in your supermarket's dairy case— here's how you can have your (real) dairy and eat it, too.

**Be a cocoa nut.** Some research suggests that cocoa slows stomach emptying, which reduces the rate at which lactose reaches the colon, says Dennis A. Savaiano, Ph.D., professor of food science/nutrition and associate dean at the University of Minnesota College of Human Ecology in St. Paul. So by drinking chocolate milk or having chocolate ice cream, you may avoid, if not lessen, symptoms. But if you're making your own chocolate milk, use low-fat milk and powdered cocoa, which has no fat; chocolate syrup is loaded with fat.

**Combine dining with dairy.** Some people find they can go symptom-free if they have their dairy products with meals. That's because having food in your stomach slows the release of lactose into your intestines, says Douglas B. McGill, M.D., professor of medicine at Mayo Medical School/Mayo Clinic in Rochester, Minnesota. Still, it's not advisable to load up on several dairy products at one meal.

**Choose the right yogurt.** Yogurt may be one milk product you can eat without worry. But don't assume that all yogurt products are the same. "Some commercial brands add milk products, which can cause you problems," says Dr. Mehta. "The best thing is to make your own yogurt." You can find yogurt-making machines at cooking supply stores.

If you're buying yogurt, make sure you choose a brand whose label says it contains live active cultures. "As soon as the yogurt cultures pass into the intestine, they become active and start to break down the lactose," says Dr. McGill. Sorry, but frozen yogurt won't help, since there are too few bacteria to be helpful.

# Diverticular Disease: Spare Your Colon

It's fine to act refined at the dinner table, but when you eat that way, don't count on your colon to keep its good manners. After decades of living off refined and processed foods and other low-fiber fare and trying to pass the hard, dry stools they create, the colon walls weaken and often develop tiny pouches called diverticula. While this condition, called diverticulosis, won't cause any symptoms for many people, some people may develop gas, cramping, severe indigestion or even constipation or diarrhea.

Since diverticulosis is the result of years of neglecting the needs of your colon, it usually strikes us after age 40—but it can make you feel decades older. Some women change their diets to avoid foods such as popcorn, seeds and nuts, since these can get caught in the pouches and cause pain. Other women, hampered by abdominal pain, reduce their physical activities or make other lifestyle changes.

About 5 percent of cases develop into the worse-case scenario, when diverticula rupture and cause serious infection or when they bleed, which can result in a significant hemorrhage. However, most of us with diverticulosis can control the problem ourselves and stay as young as we should feel. Here's how.

**Bulk up.** Eat more vegetables, more fresh fruits, more whole grains. If you don't eat much fiber now, you should work up to it gradually. "Eating too much fiber too soon can make symptoms worse," says Alex Aslan, M.D., a gastroenterologist in private practice in Fairfield, California. Start by adding a few small servings of fiber-rich foods—fruits, vegetables, pastas, brown rice, beans, bran or whole-grain cereals and breads—to your diet, and gradually include more each day for about six weeks until you consume at least 25 grams of fiber daily. If you can't eat that much fiber, consider taking an over-the-counter fiber concentrate (such as Metamucil).

**Don't smoke.** Besides being the single worst thing for your overall health, smoking is terrible for those with diverticulosis, says Stephen B. Hanauer, M.D., professor of medicine in the Section of Gastroenterology at the University of Chicago Medical Center. Smoking may increase movement in your intestines, but the nicotine decreases blood supply, which causes or increases cramps.

**Work it out.** Any type of exercise helps by increasing activity in your intestines, which improves bowel function, says Dr. Aslan. Shoot for at least 20 minutes of continuous exercise no less than three times a week.

# Irritable Bowel: Take Control

Here's a disease that some experts say might be as widespread as the common cold—and that causes even more misery. Doctors aren't sure what specifically causes irritable bowel syndrome (IBS) or even how to treat it. But IBS—sometimes called a spastic colon—is the diagnosis for people who are regularly annoyed with constipation, diarrhea, bloating, nausea or abdominal cramps, either singly or in some combination and usually with abdominal pain.

The good news (if there is any) is that you will probably outgrow your problem. "IBS is more of a problem in those in their twenties to fifties," says Dr. Mehta. "But at any age, it has some significant aging effects." Many patients find themselves planning their lives around these symptoms, he says. "You don't know whether you'll suddenly need to rush to the bathroom, so you plan your day-to-day activities with this in mind."

But having an irritable bowel doesn't have to put you in that mind-set. While you should see a doctor if you suspect that you have IBS, there are plenty of things you can do to lessen its symptoms.

**Control your sweet tooth.** Limiting the amount of sugar you eat is a key to putting the bite on IBS-triggered diarrhea. That's because sugars—especially fructose and the artificial sweetener sorbitol—aren't easily digested, which can cause the runs, says Dr. Hanauer. These sweeteners are in most sugar-free or low-calorie candy and gums as well as store-bought fruit juices. So if you like juice, make your own with a juicer.

**Chill out.** Being under stress makes IBS symptoms worse, and conversely, not being stressed out can help, adds Dr. Hanauer. He suggests that women under the gun manage their stress with the help of relaxation therapy techniques such as meditation, self-hypnosis, biofeedback and regular exercise. You can also keep a "stress diary" to help you determine the source of your difficulties.

**Warm up.** Abdominal cramps may be relieved with a heating pad placed directly on the painful area, says Arvey I. Rogers, M.D., chief of gastroenterology at the Veterans Administration Medical Center in Miami. Just be sure to place it on the low setting to prevent burning your skin.

Cramps from an irritable gut may not respond to heat. See a doctor if your symptoms are persistent.

**Watch what you drink.** Coffee and other caffeinated drinks can aggravate IBS by speeding up motility, the pace at which stools move through the bowels—bad news if you're prone to diarrhea. Besides that, there's a chemical in coffee that can cause cramping, says Dr. Aslan. Meanwhile, milk may not be much better, because some people with IBS also have lactose intolerance.

**Feast on fiber.** A high-fiber diet tends to quiet that kvetching colon. Fiber increases stool production and reduces intestinal pressure, which can benefit those with either constipation or diarrhea (or both), says Dr. Hanauer. People with IBS are advised to eat up to 35 to 50 grams of fiber a day. Start by adding about three tablespoons of pure bran to your cereal each morning and eating at least four servings of fruits and vegetables each day. Grains and beans are great sources of fiber. Shoot for a cup of beans or other legumes a day. Other fiber-rich foods include whole-grain breads and cereals, pastas and brown rice. But add fiber to your diet gradually to help avoid its gassy side effects.

**Ax fat.** Fatty foods can make your stomach empty more slowly, causing nausea and bloating, says Dr. Aslan. So avoid cheeses, ice cream, rich desserts, fried foods and fatty meats such as hot dogs, sausage and bacon.

# Inflammatory Bowel: Calm the Intestines

*Inflammatory bowel disease* is a catch-all name for two similar conditions: Crohn's disease, a chronic inflammation of the intestinal tract; and ulcerative colitis, in which the large intestine gets inflamed and riddled with ulcers. In each case, the main complaints consist of some combination of abdominal pain, rectal bleeding, cramps, weight loss, diarrhea and sometimes fever along with malabsorption, or the inability to take up and use nutrients from food. This, of course, can leave you feeling weak and fatigued, especially when you consider that a bout with inflammatory bowel disease (IBD) can last two to three weeks or longer.

So what causes IBD? Most research points to either a glitch in the immune system or an inherited genetic defect or weakness in the gut, since IBD tends to run in families. But IBD doesn't have to cost you your youthful vitality. With appropriate measures, you can still stay in the game. Here's how.

**Eat light.** "Avoid great blowout meals," advises Sidney Phillips, M.D., director of the gastroenterology research unit at the Mayo Clinic. The more you eat, the harder your already inflamed intestines have to work.

**Grab some shut-eye.** Never pass up an opportunity to nap. While your symptoms are acting up, it's important to get as much sleep as possible to keep you from getting excessively tired, mentally or physically, says Dr. Phillips.

**Know when to ease off.** If your symptoms are mild, a high-fiber diet is important. Eating plenty of fruits, vegetables and whole-grain breads and pastas can help control constipation and diarrhea by absorbing the extra water in your intestines, says Samuel Meyers, M.D., clinical professor of medicine at Mount Sinai School of Medicine of the City University of New York. But when symptoms get severe, hold off on fiber until things improve. Too much fiber during a bout with IBD can actually make things worse.

**Soothe your symptoms with nonprescription medication.** Many IBD symptoms can be kept in check with over-the-counter antacids and diarrhea medications, says Dr. Phillips. Of course, most women with IBD also need prescription medications to see them through the worst days.

# DOUBLE CHIN

## *Going Neck and Neck with Aging*

**M**other Nature didn't do us any favors when she invented gravity. Since the day we slipped off our prom dresses, it's been tugging, tugging, tugging on us, pulling body parts to places we would never have thought possible in our teens.

And of all our body parts, none is more gravity-sensitive than the neck. Add a few innocent pounds, a few harmless years, and—aarrgh!—here comes a double chin.

"I must say, a double chin really seems to bother some women. It makes them feel like they're aging in a hurry," says Robert Kotler, M.D., a facial cosmetic surgeon and clinical instructor in surgery at the University of California, Los Angeles. "Every time they look in the mirror, they see it. They are conscious of it at parties or at work. And it's telling them that maybe they're not as young as they used to be."

## Jaw Droppers

Three factors contribute to double chins: body fat, anatomy and time. Women store fat on their necks just as easily as on their hips or thighs, Dr. Kotler says. So if we gain a few extra pounds, there's a good chance some of it will settle under our chins.

But overweight women aren't the only ones in danger. Even thin people get double chins, usually because of the shape of the jaw and throat. "The less sharp the angle between the jawline and neckline, the greater the risk of a fleshy neck," says Dr. Kotler. But the lower your Adam's apple is in your neck, the more likely you are to get a sag in your chin.

Age also increases the odds. Women's skin starts to lose its elasticity after 35 to 40 years. Even if you're fit and firm, you may still show a slight double chin simply because of looser skin, Dr. Kotler says.

From a health perspective, none of this really matters. There's nothing dangerous about a double chin unless you're seriously overweight, Dr. Kotler says. Even then, it's a symptom of obesity, not a problem by itself. "Double chins are just an unfortunate part of the aging process," Dr. Kotler says. "In the overall scheme of things, there are more important things to worry about."

# Keeping Your Chin Up

Harmless or not, most women still find double chins unattractive. To help get rid of those extra folds—or at least to hide them a little—experts offer these tips.

**Lose 10.** Or maybe 15—pounds, that is. "The single best way to get rid of a double chin is to lose weight," Dr. Kotler says. "Lots of people come to my office wanting cosmetic surgery. But if they just take off some excess weight, the problem usually diminishes to the point where they don't need any more help."

The standard rules apply. Get regular aerobic exercise. Eat less fat. Avoid crash diets, which usually do more harm than good. And don't rely on miracle "spot-reducing" exercises for your neck. They won't remove the fat—and in some cases have caused dislocated jaws and severely strained neck muscles.

**Get cropped.** Long hair draws eyes to your neck—precisely what you want to avoid. Pageboy cuts that curl under the chin are the worst. "The rule is to keep it short, at or above the jawline," says Kathleen Walas, fashion and beauty director for New York City–based Avon Products and author of *Real Beauty . . . Real Women.*

**Makeup the difference.** To play down a double chin, play up another feature. Walas suggests using blush high on your cheekbones. Or try a brighter, tasteful shade of eye shadow. If you use foundation, apply it one shade darker under your chin and blend it carefully with the foundation on your face. "That will make the rest of your face bright and attractive and your double chin much less noticeable," Walas says.

**Drop that neckline.** Open, broad necklines are more flattering for women with double chins, Walas says. Turtlenecks are a definite no-no. As for jewelry, avoid chokers and try longer necklaces. Dangling earrings—anything below the jawline—can bring attention to your neck, according to Walas.

**Know the skinny on surgery.** Cosmetic surgery is a last resort, Dr. Kotler says. But if you have tried everything else and can't lose that extra chin—and have about $4,500 handy—you can have your neck "sculpted." The surgeon will make a small horizontal cut under your chin, then suck out the fat that has collected beneath the skin. Finally, he will make a vertical incision between the layers of the neck and jaw muscle and sew the edges together, tightening the muscle layer like a corset.

It's a relatively painless procedure that requires two Band-Aids to hide, Dr. Kotler says. Bruising is minimal, and within about ten days you won't see anything except your old single chin. "It's a common procedure," he says. "The technique has become very refined, and the results are quite good." The operation can be performed under either general anesthesia or local anesthesia with sedation.

For an extra $500 or so, the surgeon can also add a chin implant. It's a piece of solid silicone that is slipped between your jawbone and the sheath of tissue that covers the bone. The implant gives you a more prominent jaw and further accentuates the angle between the jawline and neck, Dr. Kotler says. There is no addition to overall recovery time. Surgeons use implants in about one-fourth of all double chin procedures, Dr. Kotler says.

# DRINKING PROBLEMS

## The Keys to Beating the Bottle

She thinks it's her little secret. But everyone knows she has a flask in her briefcase. She tries to hide the alcohol on her breath with loads of mouthwash. Her "lunch" consists of three glasses of red wine. After work, she zips over to her favorite watering hole and hangs out until last call.

That's the classic image of a woman with an alcohol problem. But alcohol abuse has many subtle faces. It could be your business partner, who drinks only on weekends. It could be your neighbor, who continues to drink despite pleas from her children. And yes, it could be you.

"An alcohol problem can strike anyone, at any time, from any walk of life. No one is immune from it," says Donald Damstra, M.D., an addiction medicine specialist and substance abuse consultant in Phoenix.

And no matter what you call it—alcoholism, drinking heavily or "that little problem"—abusing alcohol is a potent and sometimes deadly ager. It can destroy your liver, decimate your heart, dangerously elevate your blood pressure, sap your energy, ravage your stomach, shatter your sex life, decrease your fertility, short-circuit your brain, aggravate diabetes, lower your immunity, increase your cancer risk and trigger depression, stress and social problems, including marital and job difficulties.

"When you see people who have been drinking heavily for a number of years, they tend to look bad. Some women in their forties can look like they're in their sixties. Their skin just looks old, their gait isn't good, they're overweight and often they have lost bone mass—so they look like little old women a lot earlier than they should," says Frederic C. Blow, Ph.D., research director of the Alcohol Research Center at the University of Michigan in Ann Arbor.

# Who Has a Problem?

Almost every woman who drinks has experienced a hangover and the other tortures that occur after one too many. But after we recover from a few of those self-inflicted disasters, many of us learn to moderate our drinking.

"Drinking generally decreases as we age," Dr. Blow says. "It may be related to chronic diseases such as diabetes and high blood pressure or increased use of medications, or it could be that people just don't feel like drinking as much."

## Are You in Alcohol's Grip?

So how do you know if you might have a drinking problem? Melvin L. Selzer, M.D., clinical professor of psychiatry at the University of California, San Diego, and author of the Michigan Alcoholism Screening Test, suggests you ask yourself the following questions. Answer the questions yes or no, then follow the scoring at the end of the test.

1. Do you feel you are a normal drinker?
2. Have you ever awakened in the morning after drinking the night before and found that you could not remember a part of that evening?
3. Does your partner (or parents) ever worry or complain about your drinking?
4. Can you stop drinking after one or two drinks without a struggle?
5. Do you ever feel bad about your drinking?
6. Do friends or relatives think you are a normal drinker?
7. Are you always able to stop drinking when you want to?
8. Have you ever attended a meeting of Alcoholics Anonymous?
9. Have you gotten into fights when drinking?
10. Has drinking ever created problems between you and your partner?
11. Has your partner (or other family member) ever gone to anyone for help about your drinking?
12. Have you ever lost friends or girlfriends/boyfriends because of drinking?
13. Have you even gotten into trouble at work because of drinking?
14. Have you ever lost a job because of drinking?

Women may also drink less as they get older because they find alcohol seems to have a greater kick. That's because as you age, your body is less able to handle alcohol, Dr. Damstra says.

In fact, alcohol consumption in the United States is at its lowest level since 1967, according to the National Institute on Alcohol Abuse and Alcoholism (NIAAA). The average American drinks about 2½ gallons of alcohol each year. That's roughly the equivalent of 1½ 12-ounce cans of beer a day. That's within the range of one to two drinks a day that doctors believe can reduce your risk of heart disease. A standard alcoholic beverage is one 12-ounce beer, a 5-ounce glass of wine or a cocktail made with 1½ ounces (or one shot) of liquor.

Nearly half of all women ages 30 to 44 abstain from alcohol, and most that

15. Have you ever neglected your obligations, your family or your work for two or more days in a row because you were drinking?
16. Do you ever drink before noon?
17. Have you ever been told you have liver trouble? Cirrhosis?
18. Have you ever had delirium tremens (DTs) or severe shaking, heard voices or seen things that weren't there after heavy drinking?
19. Have you ever gone to anyone for help about your drinking?
20. Have you ever been in a hospital because of drinking?
21. Have you ever been a patient in a psychiatric hospital when drinking was part of the problem?
22. Have you ever been seen at a psychiatric or mental health clinic or gone to a doctor, social worker or clergy for help with a problem in which drinking had played a part?
23. Have you ever been arrested, even for a few hours, because of drunken behavior?
24. Have you ever been arrested for drunk driving or driving after drinking?

## Scoring

If you answered no to questions 1, 4, 6 and 7, give yourself 2 points each. If you answered yes to questions 3, 5, 9 and 16, give yourself one point each. Yes answers to questions 8, 19 and 20 are worth five points each. Yes answers to all other questions except 1, 4, 6 and 7 are worth two points each. If you scored five or more points, you may have a drinking problem and should consider seeking counseling.

do drink do it more moderately than men, according to the NIAAA. But in a federally funded study, one in every 20 women reported a significant alcohol-related problem or a symptom of alcohol dependency in the previous 12 months, says Sheila Blume, M.D., medical director of the alcoholism, chemical dependency and compulsive gambling programs at South Oaks Hospital in Amityville, New York.

Problem drinking can cause difficulties such as absenteeism at work and child neglect, to name two. But how much or how often a woman drinks isn't conclusive evidence that she is among the 5 million American women who have serious drinking problems, Dr. Damstra says. That number is probably under-estimated, however, because women are more likely to try to hide drinking problems. So it takes longer for us to seek help, Dr. Damstra says. (By comparison, 12 million men are considered to be serious problem drinkers.)

A key measure, he says, is if drinking is more important than other aspects of a woman's life, including her family, her health and her job.

"There are some heavy drinkers who are not addicted to alcohol. These are the women who quit drinking when their doctors tell them they have ulcers or other compelling reasons to stop. But if you're addicted to alcohol, you'll tell the doctor 'Take the ulcer out, Doc. I have to keep drinking,'" Dr. Damstra says. "When drinking causes serious negative consequences, no matter if they're physical, psychological, social, economic or spiritual, and the woman continues to drink, then her drinking is out of control and is considered alcoholism."

Why some women have problems with alcohol and others don't is still being sorted out. Researchers believe there is genetic predisposition, since women with family histories of alcoholism are more likely to become alcoholic. But predisposition doesn't mean a woman is doomed to be alcoholic, nor are women without family histories immune from drinking problems, says Norman Miller, M.D., associate professor of psychiatry at the University of Illinois College of Medicine in Chicago. Although the process is complex, some researchers speculate that a woman's risk for alcoholism depends on a combination of factors in addition to genetic predisposition, including religious and moral attitudes, self-esteem, depression and peer pressure. But whatever the cause, the result is an addiction that prematurely ages you in tragic and unnecessary ways.

## Dangerous in Big Doses

When you savor a cocktail after a long day at work, you're drinking one of the most unusual substances on earth. Alcohol acts as a source of empty calories and is a drug that affects your judgment and emotions.

Moderate drinking—a drink a day for women, two drinks a day for men—has some benefits, including lowering your heart disease risk. But in larger amounts, alcohol is a poison that affects every cell in the body, says Dr. Blume.

"Alcohol is a very tiny molecule carried in the bloodstream, and unlike other drugs, it's so small that it gets completely inside every cell. So its ability to do harm and mischief is endless," Dr. Blume explains.

In fact, women may be affected by alcohol sooner than men because we usually weigh less and have less of a key enzyme that metabolizes alcohol in our stomachs. So we end up with higher concentrations of alcohol in our blood when we drink.

"All the physical complications progress much more rapidly once alcoholism begins in women," Dr. Blume says. "Women reach a point of serious damage on fewer drinks per day and over fewer years than men."

For example, alcohol can momentarily suppress production of growth hormone, which keeps our cells vigorous and active as we age, says Mary Ann Emanuele, M.D., professor of endocrinology at Loyola University Medical Center in Chicago. "Blood levels of growth hormone in normal adults fall after drinking, and that could be detrimental," Dr. Emanuele says. "Studies show that these changes do reverse after several hours. However, we don't know if continued heavy drinking can cause permanent suppression of the hormone."

Excess alcohol consumption also generates free radicals, chemically unstable oxygen molecules that can damage the heart and liver and accelerate the aging process throughout the body, says Eric Rimm, Sc.D., a nutritional epidemiologist at the Harvard University School of Public Health in Boston.

Drinking heavily, for instance, severely damages a woman's skin. "It causes rhinophyma—that famous big red nose, like W. C. Fields had. It causes blotchiness, puffiness and decreased skin tone, so a woman who drinks heavily will look prematurely aged," Dr. Blume says.

In addition, studies have shown that people who consume three or more drinks a day have a 40 percent greater risk of developing high blood pressure, which has been linked to heart disease and stroke.

Excessive alcohol use can lead to cirrhosis, an incurable disease that stimulates the formation of scar tissue that destroys the liver. But if a woman stops drinking, the progress of the disease is slowed, and her life can be prolonged. Heavy drinking also increases the risk of liver cancer.

"Alcohol is associated with some types of cancer, particularly in those parts of the body that come in direct contact with alcohol, such as the esophagus, throat and liver," Dr. Rimm says. "These types of cancer are usually rare, but among people who drink five or six drinks a day, they become less rare."

Some researchers believe that these cancers are more common in heavy drinkers because alcohol addiction suppresses the immune system and lowers the body's defenses against diseases such as cancer and AIDS.

## The Toll It Takes on Sex

And as if that weren't enough, alcohol use also impairs judgment and lowers inhibitions, so you'll be more likely to engage in risky sexual behaviors and have a greater chance of infection from AIDS and other sexually transmitted diseases. In addition, says Ronald R. Watson, Ph.D., director of the Alcohol Research Center at the University of Arizona in Tucson, evidence from animal studies suggests that if you have AIDS and continue to drink, you increase damage to your immune system, reduce your body's vitamin and mineral levels and speed the progress of the disease.

But if you drink too much, you probably won't have much of a sex life. Heavy drinking can suppress orgasms and lower your sex drive. It can also decrease your fertility and cause birth defects in unborn children, Dr. Blume says.

"A single drink probably isn't going to cause brain damage or birth defects," Dr. Blume says. "The reason women are advised not to drink if they are planning to get pregnant or are pregnant is that the true minimum amount of alcohol that is harmless is not known and may differ from woman to woman. What may not cause damage to one woman's baby may cause serious harm to another. So since alcohol is not a necessary nutrient, the safest course is to not drink at all."

Alcohol can also disrupt menstrual cycles and cause early onset of menopause, adds Judith S. Gavaler, Ph.D., chief of women's research at Baptist Medical Center and a member of the Oklahoma Medical Research Foundation, both in Oklahoma City.

There is little doubt that alcohol abuse can cause blackouts, seizures, hallucinations and brain damage. Up to 70 percent of people entering alcohol treatment programs have difficulties with memory, problem solving and clear thinking. Heavy drinking can cause confusion, slowed reaction time, blurred vision and loss of judgment and muscle coordination, all which lead to injury and fatal accidents.

Men and women who drink more than five drinks in one sitting are twice as likely to die from injuries as those who don't drink that much, according to researchers at the Centers for Disease Control and Prevention in Atlanta. In fact, the National Highway Traffic Safety Administration estimates that between 45 and 50 percent of all traffic fatalities in the United States each year are alcohol-related. And other statistics suggest that an estimated 22 percent of all deaths due to disease, accidents and homicides are alcohol-related.

"Heavy drinkers die younger—there's no question about that," says Michael Criqui, M.D., professor of epidemiology at the University of California, San Diego, School of Medicine.

But even if you've drunk heavily for years, there is hope that you can still lead a long and healthy life if you quit, Dr. Damstra says.

## Seeking Sobriety

Acknowledging that you have a drinking problem is an important first step in the struggle to stay sober. "The sooner that alcoholism is recognized and treated, the less likely the disease will cause permanent damage," Dr. Damstra

# It's Tough to Talk—But It Can Help

It isn't easy telling a friend or a loved one that you are worried about her drinking. But it can be one of the most vital and rewarding conversations you'll ever have.

"If you're going to share your observations and thoughts about their drinking, you need to expect that it's going to be a painful discussion. But painful doesn't mean harmful," says William Clark, M.D., medical director of the Addiction Resource Center at MidCoast Hospital–Bath in Bath, Maine. "It's like surgery. It's painful when it's done, but it saves lives."

Don't label the person by saying "I think you are an alcoholic" or "You have a drinking problem," Dr. Clark suggests. This kind of statement will only increase the person's feelings of irritability, shame and anger.

Instead, use "I" messages that simply express your concerns and observations, says Sheila Blume, M.D., medical director of the alcoholism, chemical dependency and compulsive gambling programs at South Oaks Hospital in Amityville, New York. Say something like "I'm terrified because I know you've been driving under the influence a lot lately. That scares me. I don't want anything to happen to you, so maybe you could sit down with someone who knows more about these things than we do."

"If you enter the conversation respectfully and thoughtfully, they'll listen," Dr. Clark says.

says. "Most alcoholics begin to feel better very quickly after they stop drinking. Many of the physical complications that are caused by excessive consumption begin to heal within two to three weeks."

High blood pressure, for instance, often returns to normal within a week or two, while stomach irritation and some types of liver damage are reversible within a month. But it can take more than a year to recover from some longtime effects of alcohol consumption, such as impaired memory and concentration. Other conditions, such as cirrhosis of the liver and damage to the pancreas, may be irreversible. Here are some tips to help you get a fresh start without alcohol.

**Seek help.** If you believe that alcohol is controlling your life, ask your doctor for help or contact an alcohol treatment program in your area. Or for confidential information, write to Women for Sobriety, Box 618, Quakertown, PA 18951 (include a self-addressed, stamped envelope), or Alcoholics Anonymous, P.O. Box 459, Grand Central Station, New York, NY 10163.

**Tell a friend.** Some studies suggest that if the person with an alcohol problem goes public, it's easier for her to quit, says Dr. Blow. If you tell the people who are important to you—co-workers, family—that you're not going to drink anymore, it does two things. First, it reduces the amount of peer pressure that will be placed on you to drink. Second, it makes it easier for you to stick to the commitment, because you've made it out loud to the world.

**Sobriety begins at home.** In the early phase of recovery, ask friends and family to not drink around you. Ask your partner to participate in your recovery by attending counseling sessions with you, Dr. Damstra says. If he refuses, he may have a problem, too, and you might have to decide if continuing the relationship is worth jeopardizing your recovery.

**Say the three magic words.** If you do go to a party or another gathering and are offered an alcoholic beverage, simply say "I don't drink" or ask for a soft drink, Dr. Blume says. No further explanation should be necessary. If the people around you continue to pressure you to drink, leave.

**Find new pals.** Hanging out with your old drinking companions, even if you swear you won't drink, is a disaster waiting to happen, Dr. Damstra says. First, you need to get involved in a 12-step recovery program. Then find people who are interested in staying sober at your recovery group, church or gym.

**Invest in fun.** Volunteer at a neighborhood school or get involved in a theater group, Dr. Damstra says. The more activities you do, the more you'll realize that being sober is more fun and rewarding than drinking.

**Accept no substitutes.** Stay away from nonalcoholic beers and wines. "It will remind you of the taste of the real thing and, by association, make you crave alcohol," Dr. Blume says.

# DRUG DEPENDENCY

## *Clearing the Mind, Cleansing the Body*

$P$robably nobody you know actually tried to become addicted to drugs. But dependency sneaks up slowly, insidiously, one pill or marijuana cigarette at a time, until a woman is confronted with a problem that she never thought she'd have to handle.

And despite its reputation as an inner-city problem, drug abuse can strike right in your own neighborhood: the old college roommate, dependent on painkillers since an auto accident three years ago; the hard-driving boss, using cocaine to help her endure a 14-hour-a-day work schedule.

Maybe, if we're not careful, even us.

"Not everyone is in danger of becoming drug-dependent," says Joan Mathews Larson, Ph.D., director of the Health Recovery Center in Minneapolis and author of *Seven Weeks to Sobriety*. "But it cuts across all boundaries. You certainly don't have to be a poor urban youth to become hooked on drugs."

Drug use exacts a brutal toll. It can cost our money, our jobs, our friends, our spouses, our dignity. It can ravage and age our bodies. It can make us stop eating or compel us to eat in binges. It can make us forsake exercise or let our hygiene go. We can lose mental capacity. Drug dependency can even be fatal.

"It doesn't have to be that way," Dr. Larson says. "But unless a person takes action, she will likely continue to deteriorate. People dependent on drugs can fall an awfully long way."

## Filling the Void

Studies show how widespread the country's drug problem has become. A large-scale study of residents of five U.S. cities showed that as many as 1 in 20

145

American women either abuse or are dependent on drugs.

And drug dependency is horribly expensive. Figures from the University of California, San Francisco, show that use of illegal drugs in America costs nearly $7 billion a year in treatment, loss of productivity and other costs.

Why do people become drug-dependent, despite the risks? Because drugs make them feel good—at least at first. "Drugs fill a need in a person's life," Dr. Larson says. "Heroin, for instance, can help a person deal with her natural anxiety. Alcohol acts as a depressant in most people. But in others, it actually stimulates them. It makes up for a natural deficiency in some brain chemicals."

The relief, however, is always short-lived. Over time, drug use interferes with production of endorphins, the body's natural "feel-good" chemicals. "That means you have to use more drugs to make up the difference," says Adam Lewenberg, M.D., a New York City physician whose private practice includes addiction treatment. "It becomes a cycle where you crave the drug more and more and eventually become dependent on its use."

And it's not just cocaine, marijuana, heroin and other illegal drugs that are causing the problem. Doctors and researchers have identified scores of over-the-counter and prescription drugs that can cause dependence, including cough syrups, anxiety drugs in the benzodiazepine family such as diazepam (Valium) and maybe even estrogen taken during hormone replacement therapy.

Women, in fact, are at higher risk than men of abusing prescription drugs such as tranquilizers, sedatives and stimulants simply because they are given them more often. They are also less likely to come forward about their abuse, resulting in more advanced drug dependency, Dr. Larson says. "More and more women are coming forward with problems. That's mainly because they're having trouble at work," she says. "But women who don't work tend to be secretive about their problems, and drug dependency can progress to a more out-of-control state."

While anyone can become dependent on drugs, heredity can play a big role. In his book *The Good News about Drugs and Alcohol*, Mark S. Gold, M.D., estimates that one in ten people is genetically predisposed to becoming dependent on drugs. "There's no question that drug dependence, like alcoholism, can run in families," Dr. Larson says. "Unfortunately, we can't test for it. But if you know of alcoholics or drug-dependent people in your family, you have to be extra careful."

Alcohol abuse also increases your chances of becoming dependent on drugs. We've all heard about how alcohol is a "gateway drug," opening the door to further drug abuse. Well, here's the proof: The National Institute of Mental Health interviewed more than 20,000 American men and women over age 18 from five sites across the country. Researchers found that women who abuse alcohol run nearly six times the risk of abusing drugs as well.

The same study found that having a history of mental disorders also raises your risk. People with disorders such as depression could be 4.7 times more likely to abuse or become dependent on drugs. And those with anxiety problems such as panic disorder or obsessive-compulsive behavior are 2.5 times more likely to become dependent on or abuse drugs.

The most important thing to remember about drug dependency, Dr. Larson says, is that it can happen to anyone. "It's not something to be ashamed of. It doesn't mean you have a moral flaw or a character flaw," she says. "No one sets out to become hooked on drugs. But for a variety of reasons, many of them beyond a person's control, it just happens. And then you have to deal with it."

## Stopping before You Start

Clearly, the best way to beat drug dependency is to avoid it in the first place. To help stay out of trouble, consider these tips.

**Know the warning signs.** "When thoughts of a drug fill your mind, you have a problem," Dr. Larson says. If you feel you can't relax, be happy, get to sleep or do anything at all without first using a drug, it's probably time to seek help.

Other signs of trouble include lying to doctors to refill prescriptions, missing work because of drug binges or hangovers, raiding savings to pay for drugs and consistently forsaking food, friendship or family to get and use drugs.

**Shake your family tree.** Look for signs of drug abuse in your family, because it may indicate that you're more prone to dependency. Include alcoholism in your search. And don't overlook things such as Grandpa's painkillers or Aunt Sophie's Valium.

"If you find signs of it in your family, be extra careful," Dr. Larson says. "Don't ever experiment with drugs, because it may take only once for you to get hooked."

**Resolve conflicts.** People use drugs to avoid dealing with problems such as anxiety, boredom, depression, frustration, bad relationships, pressure at work and unemployment. "Meet these problems head-on," Dr. Larson suggests. "Drinking or taking drugs to avoid them isn't going to solve anything. It's just going to add another layer—drug dependency—to the mix."

If you're bored, find a hobby or do some volunteer work. If you're having trouble at work or with your spouse, seek counseling. Whatever you do, don't turn to drugs for temporary comfort, no matter how appealing they sound.

**Stick to the label.** If your doctor gives you prescription drugs, particularly painkillers and tranquilizers, use them exactly the way you're told to. And never try to have them refilled unless the doctor says so. "Prescription drugs don't act differently in your body than illegal drugs," Dr. Lewenberg says. "In some ways, they're more dangerous because they're available and legal. People who wouldn't think of buying cocaine would not see the same problem in misusing a prescription drug. But they should."

When you're done taking a drug, throw away the bottle. If there's some left, don't shove it in the medicine closet, or you or someone else may be tempted to use it later, without a doctor's approval.

**Just say no.** It's a trite phrase, but it still rings true. Avoid illegal drugs. Because for some people, "recreational" drug use can quickly lead to dependency. "You can't become addicted to illegal drugs unless you use them," Dr. Lewenberg says.

# When You Need Help

If you think you may already have developed a drug dependency, experts offer this advice.

**Ask for help.** "I'll say it again: Don't be ashamed," Dr. Larson says. "Tell a trusted friend. Tell your spouse. The sooner it's out in the open, the sooner you'll start dealing with it in constructive ways." You don't need to broadcast your problem to the world. But if there's even one person out there who knows and cares, you'll get the support you need to get back on the right track.

**Find strength in numbers.** Twelve-step groups are great aids to some women. You can find people with similar problems and hopes who can help you make it through the inevitable rough spots of recovery.

Start by looking for a local chapter of Alcoholics Anonymous, Cocaine Anonymous or Narcotics Anonymous. Call or write these groups for more information:

- Narcotics Anonymous, World Services Office, P.O. Box 9999, Van Nuys, CA 91409
- Cocaine Anonymous, 3740 Overland Avenue, Suite G, Los Angeles, CA 90034; 1-800-347-8998
- National Clearinghouse for Alcohol and Drug Information, P.O. Box 2345, Rockville, MD 20847-2345

**Exercise in moderation.** If you've been abusing drugs, you've been abusing your body, too. You may not have gotten any exercise for months, a factor that may only heighten depression or anxiety.

So start working out. Begin with moderate exercise; walking for about 20 minutes a day, at least three times a week, is best. Heavy-duty exercise isn't a good idea at first, according to Dr. Lewenberg. You're probably not in peak shape right now and could easily be injured or discouraged. And it's possible to become addicted to exercise, too, since it stimulates endorphin production. "It's not a bad trade, really—drugs for exercise," Dr. Lewenberg says. "But the idea is to bring your body back to normal slowly."

**Eat right.** Drugs do strange things to your appetite. People dependent on marijuana, for instance, are prone to overeating and obesity. And cocaine abuse can lead to malnutrition and even eating disorders such as anorexia nervosa. "When you're dependent on drugs, eating well is rarely a priority," Dr. Larson says.

Try to eat a balanced diet, whether you feel like eating or not. Replace sweets with fruits and vegetables. "Feeding your body and brain what it needs is a very necessary first step to recovery," Dr. Larson says.

**Consider treatment.** Inpatient and outpatient recovery centers offer people the chance to both detoxify their bodies and address the underlying causes of their drug dependencies. "Where there's addiction, there's depression," says Dr. Lewenberg. "It's not enough to go cold turkey and not deal with the other problems." Dr. Lewenberg's program has included nonaddicting drug therapy to handle depression and even electroacupuncture, which he says helps stimulate endorphin production and make medication more effective.

Many employers and insurance companies will cover the costs of recovery centers.

# EATING DISORDERS

## *When Thin Isn't Thin Enough*

Two thousand years ago, an unknown Greek artist created the world's first supermodel: the Venus de Milo. Though sculpted from stone, her features were hardly chiseled. Her hips were round and ample, her midriff full—proof that the ancients saw nothing wrong with a little bit of marbling.

Today's society worships a much different goddess. The 100 percent fat-free magazine model comes with a neck like a swan's and legs that flow right into next month's issue. And the message she delivers is anything but subtle: the thinner, the better.

For many women, today's standard of beauty is a minor annoyance. But for millions of others, the fight against fat becomes an obsession that ages them prematurely by depriving their bodies of basic nutrients, weakening their hearts and other organs and hurting their physical appearance.

"It's no wonder to me that we see so many women with anorexia nervosa and bulimia," says Vivian Meehan, president and founder of the National Association of Anorexia Nervosa and Associated Disorders. "In our country, people who are fat are shamed. Instead of looking healthy and normal, women are trying to look like something 99 percent of them can't possibly be."

## A Heavy Price to Pay

An estimated seven million American women suffer from eating disorders. Meehan says a high percentage of them are too embarrassed to seek treatment or don't even realize they have problems.

Eating disorders usually start in the teenage years, but many women suffer with them well into adult life. Meehan says she routinely sees women in their thirties and forties—even in their seventies—with anorexia or bulimia. The disorders can also begin in adult women who never showed symptoms in their younger years.

## Do You Have Anorexia?

If you think you might have anorexia nervosa, answer these questions from the American Psychiatric Association:

1. Is your body weight 15 percent or more below normal? (A five-foot-five woman with a light build should weigh at least 127 pounds. Fifteen percent less than that is 108 pounds.)
2. Do you have an intense fear of gaining weight or becoming fat even though you already weigh less than normal?
3. Have you missed at least three consecutive periods?

If this sounds like you, experts say it's time to see a doctor.

Women with anorexia, Meehan says, are often starving, convincing themselves they're fat when they may be 25 percent or more under their ideal weight. Women with bulimia, on the other hand, may eat enormous quantities of food during secret binges, then purge the food through vomiting, laxatives and diuretics or excessive exercise.

"Both disorders have serious consequences," says Janet David, Ph.D., director of community outreach at the Center for the Study of Anorexia and Bulimia in New York City. "Women are simply not giving their bodies what they need to survive."

Dr. David cites a number of potential health and aging problems, including:

• Loss of calcium. If you don't eat enough calcium, or if you purge it before your body can absorb it, you're at risk for early onset of osteoporosis. The brittle bone disease, which usually attacks after menopause, weakens bones and leads to frequent bone fractures.

• Intestinal problems. Depriving your body of food may hurt its ability to digest food. That can cause problems during recovery from anorexia or bulimia, when women who have starved themselves find it difficult to gain weight.

• Heart and kidney trouble. Again, malnutrition weakens your organs, sometimes leading to irregular heartbeat and permanent damage to heart tissue and kidneys.

• Cosmetic problems. These include hair loss, broken nails, dry skin and rashes around the mouth. Women with bulimia sometimes develop ulcers on the backs of their hands caused by stomach bile that touches them when they force themselves to vomit.

• Loss of tooth enamel. Caused by stomach bile that touches teeth while vomiting, this can progress to tooth loss and degeneration of jawbone.

• Amenorrhea. When your body weight drops too far, menstruation stops. Some younger women with anorexia have never had periods.

• Emaciation—and even death. Statistics show that as many as 10 percent of people with anorexia literally starve themselves to death.

• Hypothermia. Without enough fat in your body, you're at risk of losing body heat dangerously fast.

## Breaking the Grip

Anorexia and bulimia are both classified as psychological disorders. Diagnosis can be tricky, Dr. David says, since doctors are not always trained to look for signs of eating disorders.

Even when doctors diagnose anorexia or bulimia, recovery can take months or even years, Meehan says. Some women overcome the disorders without ever seeing doctors or psychologists, though no one knows how many women have beaten anorexia or bulimia by themselves. "It's tough to estimate," Meehan says. "The people who overcome it on their own don't come in for treatment."

Women who seek help can expect to attend a number of therapy sessions with psychologists or psychiatrists in one-on-one, family and group settings. Treatment for anorexia can sometimes require inpatient hospital stays to help women stabilize their bodies and gain weight.

Underlying psychological problems may come to light during therapy, Meehan says. Researchers believe that as many as 50 percent of women with anorexia and 75 percent of women with bulimia suffer from clinical depression. For some women, doctors prescribe antidepressant drugs such as fluoxetine (Prozac), according to Robert L. Spitzer, M.D., professor of psychiatry at Columbia University's New York State Psychiatric Institute in New York City.

Dr. David says many of her patients come from dysfunctional families, with histories of alcoholism and physical or sexual abuse.

## A Tale of Victory

For many women with bulimia and anorexia, stringent eating habits offer feelings of control over otherwise chaotic lives. "When I was 16, I discovered that I could eat all I wanted, purge it and emerge the victor," says Sara, now 40 years old. "Bulimia was an escape for me, a way to forget everything else that was going on."

Sara beat her eating disorder after a decade-long struggle. She now runs a successful health and fitness club in New York City. But it troubles her to see women in the club, many her age or older, battling anorexia nervosa or bulimia, seeking the same control that she once craved.

## Do You Have Bulimia?

These are the key signs of bulimia, according to the American Psychiatric Association:

• Rapid binge eating—consumption of a large amount of food in a discrete period of time
• A feeling of loss of control during binges
• A minimum of two binges per week for at least three months
• Attempts to purge food through self-induced vomiting, use of laxatives or diuretics or strict dieting or fasting, or attempts to prevent weight gain through excessive vigorous exercise

If you meet most or all of these criteria, experts recommend that you see a doctor.

Even after years of therapy, Sara must still fight off cravings and old habits. "The grip is very powerful," she says. "You really have to want to overcome it."

She also admits that the stigma of an eating disorder can be difficult to overcome. She asked that her name not be used in this book, for fear that knowledge of her disorder would harm her reputation and business.

## Taking the First Steps

While recovering from anorexia and bulimia can require outside help, experts say it's often up to women to begin their own healing process. Specialists offer these guidelines.

**Practice good nutrition.** Women shouldn't view food as a foe, says Dori Winchell, Ph.D., a psychologist in private practice in Encinitas, California. "Eating a balanced, proper diet won't make you fat. It will make you healthy," she says. "If you eat right and exercise sensibly, you will become the most attractive person you possibly can be."

**Seek strength in numbers.** For many people with eating disorders, support and self-help groups can offer needed comfort. "You're not the only person out there with an eating disorder," Dr. Winchell says. "Other people have struggled with the same problems, and sometimes it helps to share experiences."

Dr. Winchell and others suggest finding a local chapter of Overeaters Anonymous, a 12-step group patterned after Alcoholics Anonymous. You'll probably meet people with similar problems who may offer support any time you're having trouble coping. Many areas also have support groups specifically for women with anorexia or bulimia.

While these groups may not be for you, Dr. Winchell says you may at least find a friend or two with whom you can talk.

**Be honest.** Dr. David says the majority of women with eating disorders deny that they have problems—sometimes for years. "Anorexic women look at themselves in the mirror and say 'I'm so fat' when they are in fact terribly emaciated," she says. "You have to be true to yourself, to examine your feelings and really look in that mirror, if you're going to help yourself."

If you feel you might have an eating disorder, Dr. David advises you to see a doctor immediately.

"These are serious disorders," she says. "Your long-term health can be at stake."

# ENDOMETRIOSIS

## *Stop It from Taking a Toll*

ndometriosis has always made 35-year-old Allison Mc-
Cormick feel older than she really is.

When she was a teen, the disease caused intense, chronic pain that made
many of the activities she longed to do, such as traveling and long-distance running, off-limits. "It doesn't allow you to do the things people your age would
do," she says.

In her early twenties, McCormick, a clinical research associate from Aliso
Viejo, California, tried to get pregnant, but because of endometriosis, she was
infertile. Then at age 25, she had a hysterectomy to stop the pain and progression of the disease. Not having a child has been the most painful issue to deal
with, she says. Also, the hysterectomy thrust her into premature menopause.
"Talk about aging," she says.

Having endometriosis made her "feel very different. You're having to deal
with your health all the time. Other people my age didn't have to do that," Mc-
Cormick says. "I missed out on a whole lot of years, a whole lot of things."

## The Pain That Wears Women Out

Endometriosis is a chronic, debilitating disease affecting about five million American women of reproductive age. It's caused when tissue similar to
the lining of the uterus, called endometrial tissue, grows outside the uterine
cavity. This can be painful for women, because renegade tissue behaves just
like normal uterine tissue—it can cause cramping, bleeding and discomfort
before and during a woman's period. If it grows on the large or small intestine,
it can cause pressure and pain when a woman goes to the bathroom. And if it's
located in the pelvic area, it can cause discomfort during sex. For some

women, the pain is mild or nonexistent. But for others, it is excruciating—what some describe as knifelike or burning.

The pain of endometriosis often wears women out, says Nancy Petersen, R.N., director of the Endometriosis Treatment Center at the St. Charles Medical Center in Bend, Oregon, leaving them with very little energy or ability to do the activities they want and need to do.

"I think they are very dragged down by the chronic, intense pain that they are dealing with. Most of them suffer substantial fatigue," says Petersen. Many women with endometriosis are "struggling, really, to live their lives. They have to really work at it," she says. And when they can't participate fully, they're often left with a sense of loneliness and isolation.

## The Question of Children

For women who want children, having endometriosis can be a particularly heavy blow, because it can leave them infertile. (In fact, fertility problems can be the first clue that a woman has the disease.) Often the misplaced endometrial tissue attaches itself to the ovaries and fallopian tubes, binding them to each other and to the walls of the pelvis and making fertilization impossible, says Paula Bernstein, M.D., Ph.D., attending physician at Cedars Sinai Medical Center in Los Angeles. "Because everything is stuck to everything else, the tubes don't have the mobility to pick up the egg" and move it down to the uterus properly, she says.

If you have endometriosis, you may not know whether your fertility is affected until you try to get pregnant. And the longer you wait, the more time the disease has to progress. So many women who have endometriosis often find themselves trying to conceive sooner than they'd prefer. "There's a lot of anxiety about it," says Deborah A. Metzger, M.D., Ph.D., director of the Endometriosis and Pelvic Pain Center at the University of Connecticut Health Center in Farmington. "Dealing with the anxiety can be difficult. Women often feel that their options are limited."

## What Your Doctor Can Do

Doctors diagnose endometriosis through a surgical procedure called laparoscopy. It's the only way to know for sure whether you have the disease.

The procedure involves inserting a laparoscope, a lighted metal tube that has some magnification, through the belly button and into the pelvic cavity, where doctors look for the telltale signs of the disease. Doctors can also use the same procedure to remove out-of-place endometrial tissue.

Surgery isn't the only option for treating endometriosis, although it is very effective for many women. Other options include treatment with medications such as danazol (Danocrine) or GnRH agonists, a class of synthetic drugs that are almost identical to the natural brain hormone gonadotropin-releasing hormone, or GnRH. Both danazol and the GnRH agonists prevent ovulation and menstruation. They decrease the pain of endometriosis by stopping menstrual flow.

But they do have their downsides.

Danazol has a host of side effects. "The ones that women generally find most difficult to deal with are weight gain, some mood changes and often muscle cramps, as well as some hot flashes and a little bit of acne or oily skin. Those are the most common complaints," says G. David Adamson, M.D., clinical associate professor at Stanford University School of Medicine in California and director of the Fertility and Reproductive Health Institute of Northern California in Palo Alto.

The thing that's most disturbing to women, says Dr. Adamson, is the weight gain. Women usually gain between 8 and 12 pounds while on danazol, he says. Most of that goes away when a woman stops taking the drug, but she may retain an extra 2 to 3 pounds even after she comes off it.

Danazol can also change a woman's cholesterol profile in ways that may not be beneficial to the heart, says Dr. Adamson. LDL (low-density lipoprotein) cholesterol, the bad kind, tends to go up. "Intuitively, that doesn't seem to be favorable, and potentially, it could be harmful," Dr. Adamson says. But there are no data that say taking danazol will increase the chance of heart disease. "That connection has not been made," he says.

The GnRH agonists also have aging effects. "GnRH agonists create a menopausal state," says Dr. Adamson. The menopause is temporary and reversible, lasting only as long as the woman is taking the agonists, but it can be difficult nevertheless. The major side effect is hot flashes, says Dr. Adamson, and they tend to be more severe with GnRH agonists than with danazol. In one study, 90 percent of women taking the GnRH agonist called nafarelin (Synarel) had hot flashes, compared with 68 percent of women taking danazol. In order to counteract the hot flashes, women are often given another drug, a form of progestin called norethindrone (such as Nor-Q.D.), Dr. Adamson says.

Women taking GnRH agonists are often more irritable and have more headaches than usual. For the headache-prone, that could be a double whammy: You may likely get even more when taking GnRH agonists, says Dr. Adamson.

And as if that weren't enough, GnRH agonists can also cause bone loss, which is why doctors won't prescribe them for women at risk for osteoporosis. Women tend to lose between 6 and 8 percent of their bone mass while on these drugs, which is why GnRH agonists are only a short-term solution for endometriosis. They shouldn't be taken for more than six months, says Dr. Adamson. Once the drugs are stopped, most women regain their bone in 12 to 18 months. If you have normal bone density when you start taking these drugs, they shouldn't put you in any jeopardy for bone problems later on, Dr. Adamson says. But if you've already started to lose bone as a result of osteoporosis, too little calcium or some other bone problem, GnRH agonists may not be an option for you.

# Hysterectomy: The Controversial "Cure"

By far, the most controversial treatment for endometriosis is hysterectomy. It halts the disease because the uterus, where the disease starts and grows, is removed. Sometimes the ovaries are taken as well, putting a woman in a state of premature menopause.

Endometriosis is the second most common reason hysterectomies are performed on women between the ages of 25 and 44. (For women 25 to 34, heavy bleeding and obstetric complications collectively rank first, and for women 35 to 44, fibroids are the number-one reason.) In 1992, about 335,000 hysterectomies were performed on women under 45.

When it comes to aging, nothing can bring it on more abruptly than a hysterectomy in which the ovaries are removed. For younger women, having the uterus and ovaries removed puts an end to their ability to have children. They also experience the common symptoms women go through at menopause—hot flashes, mood swings, weight gain. And although hormone replacement therapy can help alleviate these problems, women still have to deal with the physical and emotional impact of change of life years or even decades too soon.

The aging factor is only part of the reason why hysterectomy is so controversial as a treatment for endometriosis. In some cases, the pain that the surgery is supposed to alleviate may not go away, or it may come back. Approximately 8 percent of women still experience pain after the operation, says Dr. Adamson. For women who opt to keep their ovaries, estrogen can continue to stimulate the disease, causing pain. Endometrial tissue is sometimes found on other organs, such as the bowel, leaving some of the disease in the body when the uterus is removed. Also, the low levels of estrogen still in the body after a total hysterectomy may be enough to stimulate remaining endometrial tissue into painful action—meaning that hysterectomy is no sure cure.

For many women with serious symptoms, Dr. Adamson reports, surgery brings welcome relief. Others regret the decision. So it's not something to be taken lightly. "Every woman needs to explore the issues before surgery," he says.

# What You Can Do

There is no way to prevent endometriosis. But if you do have it, there are steps you can take to keep pain and fatigue from wearing you down.

**Learn to accept.** "Accepting it and talking about it as a chronic disease is really important," says Dr. Metzger. A lot of times, women go from doctor to doctor expecting magical cures, she says. Then when their pain comes back, they are disillusioned.

"I tell them 'Look, this is a chronic disease,'" Dr. Metzger says. "'I will not be able to cure it. I'm going to help you, though, in dealing with it, and we can significantly reduce your pain.'" When women hear that, they often realize that they are hearing the truth about their disease, and they understand that they can and need to take some control over it, she says.

It's important to acknowledge that you have endometriosis and to realize that it's a chronic disease, agrees McCormick. "For a long time, I would not accept the fact that I had a chronic illness. Until you accept it, you can't deal with it," she says. Once you do that, experiment with some coping techniques that give you some sense of control over endometriosis, she advises. "Put some power back in your hands." Things that work for her, she says, are exercise and hot baths.

**Turn up the heat.** Applying a heat pack or hot water bottle, or taking a hot bath, can help relieve the pain of endometriosis, says McCormick. The cramping pain women feel is caused by contractions of the endometrial tissue, and heat can help break the spasm-pain cycle.

**Get some exercise.** Many women find that exercising helps control and relieve their pain. This works, experts say, because exercise releases endorphins, the body's natural painkillers. McCormick says that while running causes her too much pain, lifting weights and riding a bike provide relief. Walking for at least 20 minutes a day can also help, experts say. There's no prescription, doctors say, so find out what works for you.

**Try medication.** Over-the-counter medications that contain ibuprofen may provide relief for women with mild forms of the disease, says Dr. Bernstein. Ibuprofen works against substances in your body, called prostaglandins, that contribute to menstrual cramping. If nonprescription medication isn't sufficient, you can ask your doctor for a prescription drug such as naproxen (Anaprox), ibuprofen (Motrin), piroxicam (Feldene) or mefenamic acid (Ponstel). All these contain nonsteroidal anti-inflammatory agents that provide pain relief by inhibiting the synthesis of prostaglandins.

**Try the Pill.** Many women achieve pain relief by taking low-dose oral contraceptives, says Dr. Bernstein. The Pill relieves some of the discomfort of menstrual cramping by decreasing menstrual flow. Ask your doctor about it.

**Stretch it out and de-stress.** Yoga is an alternative for women whose endometriosis is so severe that aerobic exercise is out of the question, says Petersen. It helps improve muscle tone and flexibility as well as decrease stress, she says. Look for books and classes that can help you get started.

**Watch your diet.** Cutting down on the amount of refined sugar and caffeine in your diet will keep your blood sugar from fluctuating wildly and keep you calmer, so you'll be better able to cope with your pain, says Dr. Metzger.

**Focus on intimacy.** If your disease makes intercourse painful at certain times, remember that there are other ways to be intimate, experts say. Focus on touching, hugging, kissing and oral sex, suggests one woman with the disease. And remember that while one position may hurt for intercourse, another may not, so try to experiment and explore different possibilities with your partner.

**Try acupuncture.** Some women find that acupuncture helps them cope with endometriosis, says Dr. Metzger. The ancient technique involves inserting needles into points in the skin that are associated with pain relief. For information about recommended acupuncturists in your area, contact the American Association of Acupuncture and Oriental Medicine, 4101 Lake Boone Trail, Suite 201, Raleigh, NC 27607.

**Seek support.** Women with endometriosis often find that it helps to talk to other women who have the disease. For more information about the disease and support groups, contact the Endometriosis Association by writing to 8585 North 76th Place, Milwaukee, WI 53223, or calling 1-800-992-3636. If there are no support groups near you, McCormick suggests starting your own.

# FATIGUE

## *How to Restore Your Energy*

You're up at the crack of dawn. You make breakfast. Get the kids off to school. Sprint to work, where you run around like a madwoman for nine or ten hours. Zoom home to rustle up dinner for the starving masses. Do the dishes. Help the kids with their homework. Throw a load of laundry in the washing machine. And somewhere around midnight, when you just can't move anymore, you limp down the hallway and collapse on the bed until the alarm clock rings and the fun starts all over again.

Is it any wonder that your get-up-and-go has gotten up and gone?

Fatigue is one of the top ten complaints doctors get from women. And why not? We cram a lot of living into every 24 hours. And that can leave our batteries drained.

Usually, it's something we can handle, and we have no problem bouncing back. But other times, an overwhelming sense of fatigue can sneak up on us and take us by surprise. We feel weak. Our bodies ache. Our faces droop. Our spirits sag. And before we know it, we've been transformed from active, vibrant lovers of life into washed-up, worn-out zombies who feel 100 years old.

"Fatigue's greatest impact is on human function and activity," says Lt. Col. Kurt Kroenke, M.D., associate professor of medicine at the Uniformed Services University of the Health Sciences in Bethesda, Maryland, and an expert on fatigue. "When you don't have the strength or energy to move, even simple tasks become difficult. You become sedentary, your productivity drops, your motivation suffers. For some, this persistent weariness can be so debilitating that they can't even get out of bed."

Fatigue can take a toll on your mind as well, experts agree. Thinking becomes difficult and confused. Decisions come slowly. Even your outlook on life turns gloomy.

The result is that fatigue can lead to poor work performance, less interaction with friends and family and less participation in the sports and activities you enjoy.

That's bad news if you're used to being an active woman. But the good news is that with a little detective work, you can almost always get to the source of the problem and reclaim your energy and vitality.

# What's Running You Down?

It's easy to shrug off a case of lethargy as just another sign that you're getting older or that you're coming down with something.

But for most of us, it's neither. "Most fatigue is not due to aging or to a serious medical problem," says Dr. Kroenke. "More often it's a signal that the body is getting too much or too little of something, and that's making you feel run down."

Most fatigue is caused by too much work, too much stress, too much weight, too much junk food and not enough exercise, doctors say.

"Most of us live and work in rapid, pressure-filled environments," explains Ralph LaForge, an exercise physiologist and instructor of health promotion and exercise science at the University of California, San Diego. "Much of the fatigue people experience is really due to the inability to pace themselves, to effectively stagger their workloads or to bring a sense of order to the chaos around them."

Just dealing with the pressures of everyday life takes a lot of energy, says Thomas Miller, Ph.D., professor of psychiatry at the University of Kentucky College of Medicine in Lexington. "One of the first things we look at whenever a patient complains of fatigue is stress. Whenever anyone has a hard time coping—with family problems, relationships, job pressure—there's usually a tremendous burnout factor, physically as well as emotionally."

Fatigue also is often a signal that you're not eating right, says Peter Miller, Ph.D., executive director of the Hilton Head Health Institute, a clinic in Hilton Head, South Carolina, that develops personal health programs. "The eating habits we established when we were younger are not suited for our middle years."

"Think of the body as a car and food as the fuel," says Dr. Peter Miller. "When you're young, you can put almost any kind of gasoline in your tank. But as you get older, the body has a harder time running on that low-octane stuff. So you need to fill up with high-test fuel and in the proper amounts."

If you're an overeater, for example, you're going to be storing more fuel than you need in the form of fat. And lugging around that excess body weight can make anyone feel sluggish. At the other extreme, undereating can also cause fatigue by depriving you of sufficient calories to propel your body through the day. That's why many women who go on "crash" or very low calorie diets often find their energy levels crashing: They're like cars running on empty.

Your activity level also has a direct effect on whether you feel fatigued, says LaForge. Lack of exercise can easily create a pattern of inactivity that is difficult to break. "A body at rest tends to remain at rest," says LaForge. "Generally, the more active and fit you are, the more stamina and energy you'll have on a day-to-day basis. Letter carriers, for example, are always on their feet. Yet they complain of fatigue much less than office workers."

On the other hand, too much exercise can have a negative effect. "Overexertion can send your energy level crashing," says LaForge. That's because when we exercise, the body produces lactic acid, a substance that accumulates in our muscles, producing weakness and body aches. This accumulation usually doesn't pose a problem when we avoid working ourselves to exhaustion and we follow our workouts with proper rest, because then our bodies are able to get rid of the lactic acid.

But when we push our bodies during workouts and don't allow our muscles time to recover, lactic acid accumulates faster than we can get rid of it. And this can leave us feeling fatigued all the time.

Other factors that can make us feel tired all the time? Smoking, so-called recreational drugs, alcohol and inconsistent eating and sleeping patterns put enormous strain on the mind and body. Sometimes, experts agree, fatigue is simply your body's cry that your lifestyle is not one that supports a healthy body.

But fatigue is also something that goes with the territory of being a woman. Both pregnancy and the post-delivery period can be the most exhaustive times of any woman's life. The physical and emotional stress of pregnancy and childbirth—plus the associated weight gain, morning sickness and breastfeeding—devour enormous sums of energy. So do the mood swings, headaches, diarrhea and hot flashes that some women experience with the hormonal changes of menstruation, premenstrual syndrome or menopause.

## Get Back Your Vim and Vigor

Fatigue is a symptom of everything from the common cold to cancer. It's a symptom of hepatitis, diabetes, heart disease, tuberculosis, thyroid problems, Hodgkin's disease, multiple sclerosis, anemia, AIDS, anxiety and depression. And it's also a side effect of some of the medications used to treat these conditions.

But fatigue is rarely anything to worry about unless it's accompanied by other symptoms such as pain, swelling or fever or it lasts longer than a week. If your fatigue has lasted that long or you have other symptoms, see your doctor.

Otherwise, here are some tips to re-energize your life.

**Pace yourself.** "Fatigue is the price we pay for pushing ourselves beyond the point where our minds and bodies say no," says Dr. Kroenke. So think about where you might be pushing yourself past your natural limits. Cut back on some of your activities. Don't work or exercise as hard, as fast or as long as you have been. Take frequent breaks. And make sure you get a good night's sleep every night—meaning you sleep well enough and long enough to wake up refreshed.

**Focus your energy.** Agonizing over situations beyond your control only eats up personal energy, says Dr. Thomas Miller. Learn to let go of things you

# Do You Have
# Chronic Fatigue Syndrome?

Chronic fatigue syndrome (CFS) is a rare, debilitating disorder that leaves its sufferers weak, exhausted and barely able to function for months or even decades.

The cause is still a mystery. "Because CFS usually appears after a flu or another illness, it was once thought to be caused by the Epstein-Barr virus," says Nelson Gantz, M.D., a member of the Centers for Disease Control and Prevention (CDC) Task Force on Chronic Fatigue Syndrome who is clinical professor of medicine at Pennsylvania State University College of Medicine in Hershey and chief of medicine and the Division of Infectious Disease at Polyclinic Medical Center in Harrisburg, Pennsylvania. "Today, we're less sure of its origins. It probably doesn't have a single cause but is a combination of viral infections, allergies and psychological factors acting on the immune system."

There is no cure for the syndrome, says Dr. Gantz. Until one is found, people with the disease can find relief through a program of good nutrition, gentle exercise and rest developed with their personal physicians. In severe cases, nonsteroidal anti-inflammatory drugs and antidepressants are used to partially relieve symptoms, according to Dr. Gantz.

How do you know if you have CFS? The CDC task force has developed a preliminary set of criteria. To be diagnosed as having CFS, you must have suffered from persistent fatigue for at least six months. The fa-

---

cannot change and focus your energies on those that you can.

**Clear the clutter.** Does a list of tasks leave you feeling zapped before you even begin? Clear the clutter out of your life bit by bit, says LaForge. Start your day with a list of four or five tasks you can definitely accomplish and work on them alone. The next day, try four or five more. What at first seemed like a mountain you couldn't climb then becomes a series of small hills you step over with ease.

**Play.** All work and no play puts more stress on the mind and body than they can handle, says Dr. Thomas Miller. Mixing your daily schedule with a combination of social experiences and enjoyable activities provides a needed break in the action and relieves those stresses before they can drain your energy systems.

tigue must not have existed previously, must persist despite bed rest and must cut your daily activity level in half for at least six months.

The existence of any other disease, infection, malignancy or condition that may produce similar symptoms, as well as the use of any drugs, medications or chemicals, must be ruled out by a physician.

You must also have had 8 of the following 11 symptoms for at least six months:

1. Mild fever or chills
2. Sore throat
3. Painful lymph nodes (glands on the sides of your neck)
4. Unexplained general muscle weakness
5. Muscle discomfort or pain
6. Fatigue of 24 hours or more after levels of exercise that used to be easily tolerated
7. Unusual headaches
8. Aches and pains (without swelling or redness) that travel from joint to joint
9. Any of these complaints: forgetfulness, excessive irritability, confusion, difficulty thinking, inability to concentrate, depression
10. Difficulty sleeping
11. Extremely swift development of these symptoms, from within a few hours to a few days

**Hit the road.** According to a study by Robert Thayer, Ph.D., professor of psychology at California State University, Long Beach, a brisk ten-minute walk causes a shift in mood that quickly raises energy levels and keeps them high for up to two hours.

And an after-meal stroll can counteract the energy drop you experience after eating a big meal, adds Dr. Peter Miller. Digesting large meals increases blood and oxygen flow to the stomach and intestines, and this draws energy away from muscles and the brain. But a walk will keep blood and oxygen circulating evenly throughout the body.

**Balance your diet.** A junk food diet high in sugar, fat and processed foods gives your body few or none of the basic vitamins, minerals and nutrients it needs to perform at normal levels. And sometimes just the slightest deficiency of any one nutrient is all it takes to send energy levels plummeting.

The answer, says Dr. Peter Miller, is to find a balance in both the amount and the types of food that you eat. "It's important to hit all the major food groups—fruits, vegetables, grains and cereals, dairy, nuts and meats—every day to guarantee that you're giving your body the right combination of fuel and basic nutrients to keep on running at peak levels," says Dr. Miller.

Ideally, every day you should be getting 60 percent (or more) of your calories from carbohydrate-rich foods such as pasta, bread, potatoes and beans, 25 percent (or less) of your calories from the fat found in foods such as canola oil, olive oil and peanut butter and 15 percent of your calories from protein-rich foods such as chicken and fish.

**Focus on the carbs.** Of the three energy-supplying nutrients—carbohydrates, fat and protein—carbohydrates pack the most fatigue-fighting punch. "Carbohydrates provide an efficient, long-lasting energy source," says Dr. Peter Miller. To produce an abundant reservoir of carbohydrate energy, add some of these foods to your plate whenever you sit down for a meal.

**Eat more frequently.** Skipping meals can leave your fuel reserves dangerously low, and digesting big meals can be an enormous energy drain. Unfortunately, the traditional three meals per day may contribute to the problem.

"Your body needs fuel in moderate doses throughout the day to keep performing at optimal levels," says Dr. Peter Miller. He recommends eating four or five small meals each day. "Reducing the amount of food you eat at any one time and spreading your calorie consumption more evenly over the day make more energy available to your body throughout the day," he says.

**Snack wisely.** When your stomach's growling and your energy's waning, the best pick-me-ups are of the natural variety, says Dr. Peter Miller. Fruits, raw vegetables, nuts and unbuttered popcorn—all which are low in energy-draining fat—are some excellent energizers.

**Avoid a quick fix.** Sugar-loaded foods such as candy and soda may zip up your energy level for a while, but they also cause blood sugar levels to increase and then sharply drop. Unfortunately, the result is that your energy level will dip even lower than it was before, says Dr. Peter Miller.

**Drink coffee.** Studies at the Massachusetts Institute of Technology have discovered that the caffeine in a single cup of coffee can boost your energy level for up to six hours, researchers report. But don't overdo it.

**Stay wet.** Feeling run-down is often the first sign of dehydration, says Dr. Peter Miller. Drinking at least six glasses of water every day—more if you're active or trying to lose weight—will prevent this type of fatigue.

**Avoid booze and pills.** Regular use of alcohol, sleeping pills and tranquilizers will make anybody act like a zombie, says Dr. Kroenke. And believe it or not, stimulants and pep pills can take you from way, way up to way, way down after their immediate effects have worn off.

**Check your medicine cabinet.** Antihistamines and alcohol, both which are found in a wide variety of over-the-counter and prescription cold medications, can make you feel groggy, says Dr. Kroenke. Ask your doctor or pharmacist if she can recommend a non-fatiguing alternative.

**Explore alternative approaches.** Many people fight fatigue by going beyond the traditional limits of Western science, says LaForge. Meditation, yoga and massage are just a few of the nontraditional options that practitioners say will energize, refresh and revive both body and mind.

Studies at Harvard Medical School show that taking a deep breath, exhaling, then sitting quietly for 20 minutes as you focus on a word that reflects your personal faith—*God, Allah, Krishna* or *shalom,* for example—will relax and re-energize both mind and body.

Check the Yellow Pages of your local telephone book for organizations that teach these techniques. In many cases, you'll also find them at your local YMCA.

**Ask your doctor about supplements.** In addition to a balanced diet, a multivitamin/mineral supplement should ensure that you're getting all the vitamins and minerals that you need, says Dr. Kroenke. Talk to your doctor about which one is right for you.

# FIBROIDS

## *Taking Action Isn't Always Necessary*

You feel bloated, your back aches, and you have a period that won't quit. You drag yourself into your doctor, who finds that your heart's okay, your lungs are fine, and your blood pressure's terrific.

Then she does a pelvic exam.

"Bingo," you hear from the other end of the stirrups. She presses down on your uterus, up from the vagina, then renders her verdict. "Yep—it's a fibroid. Not too big. It has your uterus pushed out to about the size of a nine-week pregnancy."

She strips off her gloves. "Sit up, and we'll talk about what we're going to do."

It's a common scenario. At some point in their lives, 60 percent of American women will have fibroids, which are benign tumors. Fibroids begin as tiny clumps of muscle cells that grow from inside, outside or within the uterine wall.

The problem is that fibroids can make us old before our time. They can tear up the lining of the uterus and can grow big enough to put pressure on the bowel, the bladder and the tubes that lead from the kidneys to the bladder—all which can lead to infertility, incontinence, kidney damage, constipation, chronic pain and hemorrhoids.

## Watch and Wait

What causes fibroids is still something of a mystery, doctors say.

Fibroids usually occur during a woman's fertile years, after her first period and before menopause, because they thrive on her supply of estrogen. They're most common in pregnant and overweight women and in those who take the types of birth control or hormone replacement pills that expose women to higher levels of estrogen.

But aside from the observation that they seem to run in families, nobody has a clue as to their cause.

"They're always benign," says Alvin F. Goldfarb, M.D., director of education for obstetrics and gynecology at Jefferson Medical College of Thomas Jefferson University in Philadelphia. "They may undergo malignant changes, but the development of a malignant tumor is rare. So in most instances, if the fibroids don't cause symptoms, nothing need be done."

What kinds of symptoms require action? "Backaches, constipation, pressure on the bladder causing frequency and urgency of urination or a uterus larger than a 10- to 12-week pregnancy," replies Dr. Goldfarb. All may indicate the onset of bladder, bowel and kidney problems spurred by the fibroids.

Fibroids also require action if you begin to bleed excessively during your period, if you bleed between periods, if your gynecologist detects a sudden growth spurt in the fibroids between routine exams or if they affect reproduction either by preventing implantation of a fertilized egg or by causing repeated miscarriages, says Dr. Goldfarb.

## Weighing Your Options

Fortunately, only half of women who get fibroids experience any symptoms severe enough to require treatment. Here's what doctors recommend when women do.

**Starve them.** Your doctor can prescribe gonadotropin-releasing hormone (GnRH), which may decrease the size of fibroids by 50 percent. It shuts down production of the ovaries' estrogen, thus depriving the fibroids of what for them is a steady supply of Miracle-Gro.

But women who take GnRH must understand that when the hormone therapy stops, the fibroids will grow back, cautions Mary Lake Polan, M.D., Ph.D., professor and chairman of the Department of Gynecology and Obstetrics at Stanford University School of Medicine in California. And no one should take the hormone alone for more than six months, because it can cause osteoporosis. There are other therapies that combine GnRH initiators with estrogen and/or progestin, a synthetic form of the hormone progesterone. This allows women to use GnRH therapy for years, says Dr. Polan.

One appropriate time to use GnRH is when a woman is close to menopause, says Dr. Polan. It can shrink the fibroids and keep them small until they naturally disappear at menopause.

**Consider removal.** If you want to protect your fertility, you may need to have the tumors removed. The operation is called a myomectomy and is done two ways, Dr. Goldfarb says.

In a laparoscopic procedure, a couple of tiny incisions are made in the abdomen. In one incision, a laparoscope, a tiny instrument used to view the inside of the body, is inserted; in the other, a laser is inserted. The doctor locates the fibroids and zaps them with the laser. Another surgical instrument removes the debris.

This is the procedure that younger doctors are inclined to use, because it's more modern, adds Dr. Goldfarb. It's less invasive than other options, and it does a great job as long as the fibroids aren't large.

Dr. Goldfarb suggests that women considering this procedure make sure their doctors are well versed in it. He says you should ask your doctor how many laparoscopies she performs annually. Aim for a doctor who does at least 50 a year, Dr. Goldfarb says.

The second procedure is an operation in which the entire abdomen is opened up and the fibroids are surgically removed. The surgery is more invasive and requires a longer recovery time.

Dr. Goldfarb advises that whether the fibroids are removed by laser surgery or by an open operation, you should always discuss with your doctor the possible complications of either procedure.

**Discuss the possibility of hysterectomy.** If your tumors are very large, you may have to have a hysterectomy. And often a doctor won't know you need that until a myomectomy is under way, Dr. Goldfarb says.

"I've done many myomectomies where I've taken off as much as four to seven pounds of tumor and saved the uterus, and the women have gone on to have babies," Dr. Goldfarb says. "But you can never guarantee anything until you're in there. If you're my patient, I'll tell you up front: If you have huge tumors and I can't take them off, I want permission to do a hysterectomy."

Before a myomectomy, ask your doctor about the possibility of a hysterectomy and the repercussions of this surgery. Tell her whether or not you would want this procedure.

# FOOT PROBLEMS

## *What's Fitting Is Good for the Sole*

Each day, the typical woman takes as many as 10,000 steps. That's enough walking in your lifetime to circle the world several times over. Unfortunately, much of that globe-trotting is done in footwear designed more for fashion than for function.

The same shoes that give our legs shape, give us height and make us feel young and fashionable can be an Achilles' heel to our feet, causing numerous problems that hound us with pain and age our spirits. According to a 15-year study by Michael J. Coughlin, M.D., an orthopedic surgeon in private practice in Boise, Idaho, 80 percent of foot surgery patients are women, and most of the problems stem from our shoes.

"There's no question that many of the shoe styles that women wear can contribute to debilitating foot problems," says Glenn Gastwirth, D.P.M., deputy executive director of the American Podiatric Medical Association. "And debilitating foot problems make you feel older by robbing you of the vigor and energy you once had. When your feet hurt, you can't perform your normal daily tasks, so you feel worse about yourself."

These problems harm more than just our feet and psyches. "Bad feet can throw your posture out of whack, setting you up for possible knee pain, hip pain, back pain and neck pain," says Marc A. Brenner, D.P.M., a doctor of podiatric medicine in private practice in Glendale, New York.

## Tight Isn't Right

So what's wrong with our shoes? Plenty, say experts. "High heels can be terrible for your feet," says Philip Sanfilippo, D.P.M., a podiatrist in private practice in San Francisco. "They can cause your feet to slide forward, making you prone to bunions and other problems. And many women develop shortening of their Achilles tendons from wearing heels for too long. After time, this may result in tightness of the tendon and the inability to wear flat shoes or to walk barefoot without pain."

Pointy-toed shoes—regardless of heel height—are no better, Dr. Sanfilippo adds. "They cram your toes, which can cause corns, blisters and calluses and aggravate bunions." Pointy-toed shoes can also cause neuromas, pinched nerves surrounded by fibrous tissue that can become very painful.

But the most serious problem—resulting in an estimated $2 billion a year in health care costs, according to Dr. Coughlin's study—is that women's shoes are just too tight. One study found that most women with significant foot pain wear shoes that are a full two sizes too narrow. It's not that we all knowingly squeeze our size B's into size AA shoes. Although according to an American Podiatric Medical Association survey, nearly half the women questioned admitted that they purposely wear uncomfortable shoes for appearance' sake, compared with only 20 percent of men.

"What happens is that as we age, our feet become longer and wider, a process called splaying," says Dr. Sanfilippo. "This occurs as the ligaments in our feet begin to collapse and the arches fall due to gravity and wear and tear. This flattens out our feet. Unfortunately, many people aren't aware of this process—which can occur in your thirties or forties—and they continue to wear the same size shoes they've always worn. And that causes the problem."

Pregnancy can make this splaying occur earlier and be more severe. "When a woman is pregnant, she releases hormones that prepare the connective tissue around the birth canal for delivery," says Dr. Gastwirth. "What this does is weaken some of the connective tissue in other parts of the body. So if you're not wearing supportive shoes or you're doing a lot of barefoot walking during pregnancy, this splaying of the foot may be even more pronounced."

## Getting Your Feet to Toe the Line

But shoes aren't the only reason for foot pain. Besides causing the feet to splay, the natural aging process also wears the fat pads on the balls of our feet, which cushion our steps and absorb shock. "As we age, these fat pads tend to wear out, just like the padding of a carpet. When it's installed, it's nice and cushy. But after 20 years, that padding can get pretty worn," says Dr. Gastwirth. "It's the same with your feet: The moment you begin to walk, you begin the process of wear and tear that could lead to future foot problems."

Another common problem: loss of moisture in the skin of your feet, which frequently occurs after age 30 and can result in itchy feet and make you more susceptible to athlete's foot and other types of fungus. Some women, especially smokers and those with Raynaud's disease, have circulatory problems that take a toll on the feet, causing a loss of sensation, particularly in cold weather. Says Suzanne M. Levine, D.P.M., adjunct clinical instructor at New York College of Podiatric Medicine in New York City and author of *My Feet Are Killing Me,* "Any foot older than 25 is an aging foot."

But it doesn't have to be that way. With a little know-how, you can dance around foot problems and breathe new life into tired tootsies.

# Foot and Heel Pain: Support Yourself

There are several causes of those "unexplained" pains in your foot or heel, and most are the result of long-term use of your feet. They include fallen arches, Achilles tendon stiffness, plantar fasciitis, which is an inflammation in the bottom of the foot, and heel spurs, which are tiny growths of bone that may form from the constant pulling of ligaments through jumping, walking or running. "Usually, these problems result from overuse of your feet," says Richard Braver, D.P.M., sports podiatric physician for teams at Seton Hall University in South Orange, New Jersey, Fairleigh Dickinson University in Rutherford, New Jersey, and Montclair State College in Upper Montclair, New Jersey. No matter what the cause, here are the solutions.

**Get some support.** There's no getting around the deterioration of your feet's fat pads, but you can do something about the pain it causes on the soles of your feet. "Wearing high-quality, supportive, cushioning insoles in your shoes can certainly ease some of your discomfort," says Dr. Sanfilippo. These insoles are available at drugstores and sporting goods shops. If the pain is centered on your heel, a heel cup, also sold in these stores, can help prevent excess heel movement and ease pain. But perhaps more important than insoles and heel cups is wearing supportive shoes.

**Stretch out your calf.** For heel pain, a lot of women find relief by stretching the heel cord, or Achilles tendon, on the back of the foot, says Gilbert Wright, M.D., an orthopedic surgeon in private practice in Sacramento, California. Stand about three feet from a wall and place your hands on the wall. Lean toward the wall, bringing one leg forward and bending at the elbows. Your back leg should remain straight, with the heel on the floor, so you feel a gentle stretch.

**Roll away pain.** For heel spurs and plantar fasciitis, try massaging the bottom of your foot. "Roll your foot from heel to toe over a rolling pin, a golf ball or even a soup can," advises Dr. Braver. "This eases pain by stretching out the ligaments."

**Heat feet in the morning.** "If you feel stiffness in your foot when you wake up, heat it to stimulate blood flow," says Dr. Braver. He recommends placing a warm compress or hot water bottle on the bottom of your foot for about 20 minutes.

**Ice them in the evening.** At nighttime, switch to ice. Suzanne M. Tanner, M.D., assistant professor in the Department of Orthopedics at the University of Colorado Sports Medicine Center in Denver, suggests placing an ice pack on your foot for 20 minutes, removing it for 20 minutes and then reapplying it for 20 minutes. Be sure to wrap the ice in a towel to prevent ice burns or frostbite.

# Neuromas: The Big Squeeze

This is almost exclusively a woman's problem because of our tight and narrow shoe styles. "What happens is that the shoe pushes your foot in tighter and pinches a nerve," says Dr. Braver. "But then tissue grows around this pinched nerve, causing a great deal of pain." Neuromas usually occur between the third and fourth toe or along the sole of your foot. In extreme cases, surgery may be required. But before the pain gets that far, here's what Dr. Braver suggests.

**Pad it.** "Anything that can be done to support the arch will help women with neuromas," says Dr. Braver. "One of the best things you can do is get an arch support pad, available at drugstores, and place it in your shoe. This reduces pressure to the nerve."

**Give it the big chill.** A nightly application of an ice pack reduces swelling and numbs pain, adds Dr. Braver. Remember to wrap a towel around the ice pack and follow the 20 minutes on, 20 minutes off routine (described in the previous section on foot and heel pain).

**Try physical therapy.** "Basic massage won't help, but electrical nerve stimulation and therapies that reduce swelling can," says Dr. Braver. You'll need the help of a physical therapist for this. Steroid injections by a doctor can also ease pain.

# Corns and Calluses: Things That Go Bump

Corns are lumps of built-up dead skin that form on the bony areas of your feet, such as the toes. They're caused by friction, usually the result of wearing shoes that are too tight. Calluses are essentially corns on non-bony places. Both can make you feel as though you're walking on pebbles. Unless you have severe, constant pain, in which case you'll need a doctor's care, you can usually remedy these problems by yourself. And here's how.

**If it doesn't fit, don't wear it.** "If you have good-fitting shoes, you usually won't have corns and calluses," says Jan P. Silfverskiold, M.D., an orthopedic surgeon in private practice in Wheat Ridge, Colorado, who specializes in foot problems.

To make sure your footwear fits, have both your feet measured for length and width each time you shop for shoes, advises Dr. Gastwirth. Be aware that the shape of your foot influences the best style of shoe to purchase. In general, the best styles for the corn-prone include sandals and running and walking shoes, which have roomy toeboxes. "If you must wear heels," Dr. Gastwirth adds, "buy shoes with wide, stable heels that don't exceed two inches and look for comfort-type pumps that provide greater cushion for shock absorption."

**Apply a moisturizer.** Since corns and calluses result from excessive friction, it's best to keep skin soft and well moisturized. Dr. Levine recommends that you apply a skin moisturizer to your feet immediately after your bath or shower. If your skin is already hardened with corns and calluses, scrape it with an emery board or a pumice stone anywhere from once a day to twice a week, adds Dr. Silfverskiold.

**Be careful with the remover.** Over-the-counter corn and callus removers (such as Dr. Scholl's) contain salicylic acid, which will erode lumpy lesions on your feet. But be careful: These medications should be applied only to the affected area, since they can burn healthy skin, Dr. Levine says. But don't use products containing salicylic acid if you have diabetes or poor circulation, cautions Dr. Levine. There are non-medicated cushions available (such as Dr. Scholl's Advanced Pain Relief Corn Cushions) that you can use to protect your corns.

# Blisters and Bunions:
# Bubbles and Bone

Blisters are painful bubblelike rips in the skin that usually fill with fluid because of excessive friction. Bunions are bumps of bone and thickened skin on the side of your foot just below the base of your big or little toe. They can be accompanied by splaying of the foot and drifting of the big toe toward the little toe. Tight shoes, arthritis and heredity can all lead to bunions. As with corns and calluses, wearing properly fitting supportive shoes can prevent blisters and bunions. But if you already have either problem, here's how to fix it.

**Pamper or pop 'em.** Insoles, moleskin or even little balls of cotton stuffed between your toes can alleviate the immediate agony of blisters and prevent them from recurring. When blisters become too large for pads, however, pop them by pushing the fluid to one end of the "bubble" and pricking that area with a needle that's been sterilized with a flame or rubbing alcohol. After draining the liquid, repeat the procedure 12 hours later, and then again 12 hours after that, to ensure that you've removed all the liquid, advises Rodney Basler, M.D., a dermatologist and assistant professor of internal medicine at the University of Nebraska at Omaha. Don't pull off the skin, but if it has been torn off, wash the sore with hydrogen peroxide or soap and water and apply an antibiotic ointment.

**Try a splint.** Bunion pain can be relieved with a toe-straightening splint that's available at most pharmacies without a prescription. The most common version is a rubber plug that "pulls" the big toe away from the second toe, easing pain. While moleskin pads are often used by bunion sufferers, they're not as effective as these splints.

## Athlete's Foot: Fight the Fungus

This fungus, which leaves feet scaly, itchy, cracked and reddened, can be picked up just about anywhere—especially in warm, moist areas such as locker room floors (hence the name). Once you get it, athlete's foot is hard to get rid of because it thrives in your shoes, but over-the-counter medications are the preferred course of action. Lotions are better than creams, since creams can trap moisture. Still, the best way to deal with athlete's foot is to avoid it. And here's how.

**Sock it to 'em.** When you take off your socks, rub one up and down the web of each toe, advises Dr. Basler. This helps keep feet desert-dry. If sock rubbing isn't your style, you can use a hair dryer set on the low setting to dry those trouble areas. And if you have a problem with sweating after your feet have been dried, you can roll some antiperspirant on your feet after showering, he adds.

**Be a shoe swapper.** Try wearing different pairs of shoes as often as possible, says Dr. Basler. That's because shoes are full of moisture after a day of wear and need at least a day's "rest" to dry out. If you don't have many pairs of shoes, spray them with Lysol at the end of the day to help disinfect them and prevent athlete's foot.

**Get cooking with baking soda.** There are plenty of over-the-counter powders to prevent athlete's foot, but baking soda does essentially the same thing for a lot less money, says Dr. Levine. Just sprinkle it on dry daily to absorb excess moisture.

## Ingrown Toenails: Pain That Digs In

All it takes is a teeny bit of nail to cause big-time pain. Once again, tight shoes can contribute to this problem by forcing the nail downward. If your nail is ingrown to the point that you're in constant agony, you may need a doctor to remove it. But here's how to avoid that anguish and keep nails trouble-free.

**Cut nails straight across.** Leave the half-moons for cloudy nights. The best way to cure an ingrown nail and prevent a new one from forming is to cut the nail straight across, not slightly curved or in a half-moon shape as most people do, says William Van Pelt, D.P.M., a Houston podiatrist and former president of the American Academy of Podiatric Sports Medicine. And don't cut it too short; it should be just over the crease of your nail fold. Be sure to soak your feet in warm water beforehand in order to make the cutting easier.

**Take your piggies to market.** There are several over-the-counter products that can soften an ingrown nail and the skin around it, thereby relieving pain. Dr. Levine recommends Dr. Scholl's ingrown toenail reliever and Outgro solution as two common brands. Make sure you follow the instructions carefully. Don't use these products if you have diabetes or circulation problems because they contain strong acids that could be dangerous to women with limited sensation in their feet.

# Nail Fungus: Avoidance is Best

Nail fungus doesn't hurt. It won't harm your health. In fact, people won't even notice those thick, raggedy-looking toenails if you keep your shoes on. But nail fungus is hard to cure. "There is a race among the drug companies for a cure for nail fungus, and so far, nobody's winning," says Dr. Braver, who tests foot products for one leading company. "If I knew the answer for curing nail fungus, I'd be a very rich man."

Some experts believe that nail fungus is often caused by an immune system problem and aggravated by moisture. So keeping your feet clean and dry is essential for keeping nail fungus at bay. While curing it is difficult and needs a doctor's care, especially if your feet tend to be sweaty, here's how to avoid getting it in the first place.

**Loosen up.** "One way to prevent nail fungus is to make sure your shoes are big enough that toes have room to breathe," says Dr. Braver. "Runners, dancers and other athletes often get nail fungus because they get micro-trauma to their toes from their toes hitting the front of the shoes. If you can, wear looser shoes."

**Apply an antiperspirant.** Sweating makes matters worse, so prevent a potential problem by treating your feet like underarms—apply a daily dose of roll-on deodorant, says Dr. Braver. "There is a prescription product called Drysol made especially for this purpose. It's like using a much stronger underarm antiperspirant."

# Foot Odor: The Nose Knows

If you wash your feet and change your socks daily but your feet still smell, you're not alone. Here's how to handle foot odor.

**Have healthy feet.** "Foot odor is usually related to a fungal infection; sweating feet and pimply or peeling skin are the usual warning signs," says Dr. Braver. "So treat foot odor as you would any fungus problem, with an antifungal lotion such as Lotrimin, which is available over the counter."

**Spray away the smell.** Other ways to kill the smell are to apply Lysol to your shoes and an antiperspirant to your feet, adds Dr. Braver.

# Plantar Warts: A Powerful Punch

Like other warts, these ¼-inch nasties that form on the soles of your feet are caused by a virus, which is probably picked up walking barefoot. The problem with plantar warts, however, is that the pressure of walking flattens them until they are covered by calluses. When the calluses harden, you feel the plantar's punch, which is similar to walking on a pebble. "About 13 percent of all plantar warts disappear on their own, with no treatment," says Dr. Braver. "However, several strains of the wart virus have been known to spread rapidly." He advises aggressive treatment to get rid of the warts before this happens. Try these measures.

**Eat your vegetables.** "There is substantial evidence that vitamin A helps protect against warts," says Dr. Braver. While vitamin A in supplement form can be toxic, you can get this added protection by eating more yellow or orange vegetables and fruits such as carrots, squash, sweet potatoes, cantaloupe, apricots and nectarines as well as green leafy vegetables such as spinach.

**Go commercial.** Using an over-the-counter wart or corn remover (such as Occlusal) can rid you of plantar warts, says Dr. Braver. These products are available at drugstores without a prescription.

**Don't go barefoot.** The best way to avoid plantar warts is to wear shoes or sandals, says Dr. Braver. "It's important to keep the soles of your feet covered, especially when you're around pools and other moist areas that are attractive to the virus." If a family member has a plantar wart, prevent it from spreading by keeping floors and showers clean and disinfected.

**See a doctor.** If you have tried the above measures for six weeks and notice little improvement, or if the problems are getting worse, see your podiatrist for care. Professional treatment may include freezing or burning the warts and traditional or laser surgical removal methods.

# GRAY HAIR

## *Rethinking Your True Colors*

**Y**ou roll out of bed, move slowly to the bathroom and turn on the light. You lean toward the mirror for a close, close look.

How many more gray hairs will there be today?

Besides wrinkles and sagging skin, few things say "aging" louder to a woman than gray hair. While some of us love the look and wear it well, a whole lot of us don't. And there's a multi-million-dollar industry out there catering to our needs to keep our changing true colors a secret.

"If you're going gray, I guarantee you're not happy about it," says Philip Kingsley, a hair care specialist based in New York City. "I have seen tens of thousands of people over the years, and none of them wants gray hair. It can really make people feel old before their time."

## The Roots of Your Family Tree

Most of us have about 100,000 hairs on our heads. Before we go gray, every one of those hairs contains the pigment melanin, which gives hair its color. But for reasons doctors don't understand, the pigment cells near the roots of each hair start to shut down as we get older. So when a blonde, brown or red hair falls out, it's often replaced by a gray one.

A white one, actually—though we call it gray because that's what it looks like in contrast to the hair that still has color.

If you're looking for someone to blame, start with Mom, Dad, Aunt Judith or great-grandpa Joe. "There's a very strong hereditary link with gray hair," says Diana Bihova, M.D., clinical assistant professor of dermatology at New York University Medical Center in New York City. "If your family goes gray early, it's very likely you will, too."

# Follicle Fallacies: The Myths of Gray

There are a million tales out there about gray hair—and precious few good, hard facts. While doctors might not know just yet what causes gray, they do know a few things that won't.

**Gray Hair Myth #1: You can go gray instantly because of a shocking event.** It's physically impossible—existing hair does not turn gray. Diana Bihova, M.D., clinical assistant professor of dermatology at New York University Medical Center in New York City, says you get gray only when a regular hair falls out and is replaced by a gray one in the same follicle.

**Gray Hair Myth #2: Your hair can return to its normal color after it has gone gray.** Sorry, but no. When a hair follicle starts producing gray hair, it doesn't change back.

There are a few exceptions, Dr. Bihova says. Your hair could temporarily go gray if you have an endocrine gland disorder, are malnourished, suffer an injury or a disease of the nervous system or have an autoimmune disorder. Even then, hair may not come back in its original color, she says.

**Gray Hair Myth #3: If you pull one gray hair, two more will grow out.** Nope. You go gray follicle by follicle. If you pull out a gray hair, it will be replaced by a gray hair in the same follicle. "You can't stop the process," Dr. Bihova says. "But pulling white hairs isn't going to speed it up, either."

Whatever you do, don't chalk it up to stress. Playing mom, boss, cook, chauffeur, gardener and loving mate all at once won't give you gray hair, Dr. Bihova says—unless the stress is so bad that you deplete your store of some B vitamins. The evidence remains sketchy on this.

Overexposure to the sun might also cause hair to gray early, Dr. Bihova says. The theory is that ultraviolet rays cause pigment cells on your scalp to work overtime, just as they do on your arms or legs when you get a tan. If they work too hard and burn out early, Dr. Bihova says, the result could be gray hair. There's no concrete evidence of this. But Dr. Bihova still suggests wearing a hat or using hair care products that contain sunscreen. "Let's just say it can't hurt," she says.

The average white woman starts developing gray hair at age 34, while the typical black woman gets about a ten-year reprieve. Dr. Bihova says women usually start graying at the sides, then on the crown and finally the back of the neck. The process can go in fits and starts, with more gray hair growing in some years and less in others.

By age 50, however, 50 percent of women will be 50 percent gray, Dr. Bihova says.

Generally, the hair on your head starts to change first, followed some time later by the hair on your legs, under your arms and in your eyebrows and, finally, in your pubic area. But again, everyone's different.

The good news in all this is that there's usually nothing physically wrong with getting gray hair—it doesn't mean you're aging faster than friends who haven't had a single gray strand yet. Studies show that people who go gray at an early age are usually not suffering from anything but a case of unwelcome family genetics.

The bad news is that graying is irreversible.

# For Many of Us, It's to Dye For

The gray is on the way, like it or not. That leaves you with two choices. You can accept it as an inescapable, even desirable, part of maturing. Or you can put it on hold for a while, using some form of hair dye.

"Some people grow to be quite comfortable with gray hair," Kingsley says. "The most important point to remember about gray hair, or hair in general, is that you have to be comfortable with it. If it makes you feel wise or dignified, that's fine."

Here's some advice from the experts on how to handle that gray.

**Crop it.** If you do decide to stay gray, Kingsley suggests keeping your hair cut short. "It's really simple," Kingsley says. "If you don't want gray hair or you're not sure about it, then short styles leave less gray to show."

**Condition it.** As time passes, your hair and scalp may get dryer. To keep your gray looking healthy, Kingsley suggests using a conditioner each time you shampoo. And he suggests letting your hair air-dry once in a while, instead of using a blow dryer.

So try the gray look for a little while. If you don't like it, you can go for some color. Here are some options that you can try at a salon or at home.

**Bring on the highlights.** Highlighting, in which scattered strands of hair are dyed, can subtly blend away some of the gray. Choose a color that's a couple of shades lighter than your natural hair.

Lighter dyes also help you avoid unsightly gray roots. When your hair grows out, the gray won't show as much.

**Go all the way.** The experts call this process color, and it means that all your hair will be dyed one shade. If you opt for this, stay away from the darkest shades, which tend to make your hair look flat and unnatural. "Black colors don't really work well," Kingsley says. "All the hair is colored exactly the same, and you can instantly see that it's dyed."

There's also some question about whether dark hair dyes can cause cancer. Some studies have linked use of such dyes to increased risk of bone cancer and lymphoma.

The bottom line? "There isn't one yet," says Sheila Hoar Zahm, Ph.D., an epidemiologist at the National Cancer Institute in Rockville, Maryland. "The risk of getting cancer from hair dye isn't as high as getting lung cancer from smoking. But we definitely need to study the relationship further."

Kingsley says you should be wary of progressive dyes that promise to slowly hide your gray hair. He says these products can give your hair an unnatural, yellowish green tint. They can also dry out your hair, making it unmanageable and brittle.

And once you start using them, it's hard to switch over to a regular dye. "That can turn your hair all sorts of colors that you would never want hair to be," Kingsley says.

Semipermanent dyes that wash out over several weeks offer somewhat better color but are not as good as permanent dyes. If you want to try a slow route to darker hair, Kingsley suggests doing it with increasingly darker permanent dyes.

# HAIR LOSS

## *Winning over Thinning*

**Y**our hairstylist has been able to hide it so far. Those short, frizzy 'dos keep your locks looking full, and no one can tell the difference.

Still, it's getting hard to deny that just like 20 million other American women, you're starting to lose your hair. Now you're worried sick, checking the mirror constantly—and feeling older by the minute.

"Hair is very much part of a woman's body image," says Dominic A. Brandy, M.D., medical director of Dominic A. Brandy, M.D., and Associates, a permanent hair restoration practice in Pittsburgh. "Losing it can cause a great deal of stress and, in some cases, can make women lose a certain amount of respect for themselves."

It doesn't help that hair loss typically begins between ages 25 and 40, before you even reach middle age. "That doesn't seem quite fair," Dr. Brandy says. "You're supposed to be at your peak, and something's already happening that makes you feel old. It can make some women worry that their youth is slipping away fast."

## Not for Men Only

Heredity plays a role in as much as 85 percent of hair loss in women. If your mother, grandmother or aunt had thinning hair, you might, too, says Marty Sawaya, M.D., Ph.D., assistant professor of dermatology at the University of Florida Health Sciences Center in Gainesville.

Unlike men, who first lose their hair on the crown and at the hairline, women are more likely to lose hair evenly over the entire scalp. Where a woman once had five hairs, she may now have only two. She may also develop a widow's peak, with a slightly receding hairline and more noticeable hair loss around her temples.

No one is quite sure what causes hair to stop growing. Research shows that women with high levels of male sex hormones—and those with scalps that are sensitive to even normal hormone levels—are more likely to lose their hair. Whatever the cause, individual hair strands thin gradually, and follicles eventually stop producing them altogether.

The sad truth is that short of prescription drugs or hair transplants, there's really not much you can do to stop your hair from thinning. Ken Hashimoto, M.D., professor of dermatology at Wayne State University School of Medicine in Detroit, stresses that miracle hair treatments—massages, topical creams, megavitamins and the rest—do absolutely no good.

But don't give up just yet. You have some options.

# It's Not All in Your Head

You can tackle a number of nonhereditary factors that can cause women to lose their hair, Dr. Sawaya says. She lists:

• Fad and crash diets. Diets deficient in protein (such as grapefruit-only schemes or plans that leave out beans, lean meats and other protein sources) can rob the body of a vital building block for hair.
• Anemia.
• Childbirth.
• Drugs, including birth control pills, anabolic steroids, beta-blocker blood pressure drugs and drugs derived from vitamin A.
• Conditions such as arthritis, lupus (a skin disease characterized by lesions) and polycystic ovarian syndrome, which causes ovaries to fill with small cysts.
• Major stress events, such as a divorce or the death of a loved one. Poor diet can also stress your body.

Dr. Sawaya says some of these nonhereditary causes may result in temporary hair loss. A thorough medical exam, better diet, stress management and medical treatment might spur regrowth in some cases, she says.

# Short Cuts to Thicker Hair

There's no reason why you have to put up with hair that's too thin or too limp, no matter what the cause. You can put body back into your thinning hair. Here's how.

**Do the wave.** The fastest way to hide thinning hair is with a curly perm, according to David Cannell, Ph.D., corporate vice president of technology with the Redken Product Laboratory in Canoga Park, California.

"With a wavy pattern, individual hairs push against each other," Dr. Cannell says. "The overall effect is that they push up and out, making your hair look fuller."

Dr. Cannell also advises women to avoid hairstyles that require small curlers

---

## Are You Really Losing It?

Don't panic if you're finding a couple of hairs in the sink or on your brush every day. Women typically lose 50 to 100 hairs each day, according to Marty Sawaya, M.D., Ph.D., assistant professor of dermatology at the University of Florida Health Sciences Center in Gainesville. That's not many—adults have more than 100,000 hairs on their heads.

If you're afraid you're losing hair, try this simple test. Grab a bunch of hair in one hand and give a firm but gentle pull. If more than a half-dozen hairs pull out, you may be starting the early stages of hair loss.

Don't worry about some hair falling out when you wash your scalp. That happens to everyone.

---

or tightly pulled hair. The more pressure you put on your hair, the more likely it is to pull out.

**Get in condition.** Avoid oily hair dressings and other products that advertise "creamy-rich" results. Dr. Cannell says these tend to weigh down and flatten hair, which can make your hair look thin.

He suggests trying a lighter, leave-in conditioner that may add a microscopic amount of thickness to individual hairs.

**Give yourself a pat on the head.** After showering, dry your hair carefully. Pat it lightly with a towel instead of rubbing.

**Comb with care.** Dr. Cannell says to be gentle with brushes and combs. Never brush your hair when it's wet (pulling on a tangle is always a no-no). Try using a comb with widely spaced teeth instead.

And forget the 100-stroke gospel your great-aunt used to preach. Dr. Cannell says you should brush your hair only as long as it takes to get it styled the way you want it.

**Lighten up.** Choose a new, lighter hair color. Shades that closely match your skin tone are best, Dr. Cannell says, since they blend with your scalp.

"The worst thing you can do is dye your hair jet-black," Dr. Cannell says. "That really shows your scalp, which is the last thing you want to do."

**Keep your hands off.** Drop nervous habits such as tugging on your hair or curling it with your fingers. You may be pulling on it more than you realize, since you're conscious of how it looks.

"Even when a hair is ready to fall out, it will stick around for quite a while—if you leave it be," Dr. Cannell says. "The more you manipulate it, the faster it will go."

# Growing It Back—Sometimes

If you've just noticed that your hair has started to thin, remember this: Minoxidil—the hair loss cure that comes in a topical prescription formula—isn't just for men.

"Women can achieve significant results with the use of minoxidil," says Dominic A. Brandy, M.D., medical director of Dominic A. Brandy, M.D., and Associates, a permanent hair restoration practice in Pittsburgh. "In fact, in some of my patients, the results seem to be better than with men."

Minoxidil is the active chemical ingredient in the topical medication sold under the brand name Rogaine. Clinical tests have shown that Rogaine can help women return some fullness to their hair. But there are limits to Rogaine's effectiveness in women, just as there are in men.

No one is quite sure how Rogaine works. Researchers speculate it may increase blood flow to the scalp, stimulating hair growth.

Dr. Brandy says Rogaine won't grow hair at the frontal hairline or in areas that are completely bald. At best, he says, it will slightly thicken existing hair and return a fuller look to your locks.

"But in most cases, it simply retards the progression of baldness," Dr. Brandy says. "That's what I tell most people to expect. Anything more is a bonus."

One more thing to think about: Rogaine is expensive. Treatments typically cost $500 to $700 per year, and you have to use Rogaine forever. If you stop, you'll lose everything you had gained within six months.

The Upjohn Company, which manufactures Rogaine, continues to refine it. At the same time, other researchers are looking at new treat-

**Know you're not alone.** More than anything else, Dr. Brandy says, you should try to remember that other women are facing the same problems as you.

"Millions of women have thinning hair," he says. "You shouldn't feel singled out, and you shouldn't feel like you don't have options for dealing with it."

# The Surgical Route

If your problem is hereditary and there's no chance your hair will bounce back to its youthful look by itself, you might want to consider hair replacement surgery. Years ago, hair transplants were easy to spot and often not worth the ex-

ments for thinning hair. But the biggest problem facing hair loss researchers is the fact that no one is sure why women start losing hair in the first place.

"We're not taking shots in the dark with these treatments. They're based on theory," says Ken Hashimoto, M.D., professor of dermatology at Wayne State University School of Medicine in Detroit. "But we really don't know the exact mechanism that causes baldness."

Researchers are evaluating these alternative treatments. Some may not be available yet.

*Aromatase.* People with thinning hair appear to be deficient in this enzyme—which, when present in normal levels, causes follicles to grow hair. Marty Sawaya, M.D., Ph.D., assistant professor of dermatology at the University of Florida Health Sciences Center in Gainesville, and other researchers are working to refine a method of restoring natural aromatase levels.

Dr. Sawaya predicts effective hormone treatments could be available to the public by the year 2000.

*Tricomin solution.* Karen Hedine, vice president of business development for the drug's maker, ProCyte of Kirkland, Washington, says this drug appears to work by stimulating the growth of new follicles in the scalp and by preventing existing follicles from becoming dormant.

*Diazoxide.* Like Rogaine, this drug appears to work by dilating blood vessels in the scalp.

*Electrical stimulation.* Tests involving low-current doses of electricity to men's scalps have shown promise in Canadian tests. Researchers predict treatments could be available in the United States in a few years.

pense. But technology and technique have improved dramatically, Dr. Brandy says. And yes, women are having them done, even though the majority of patients are still men.

"When done properly now, you don't see the artificial cornrow or 'doll's hair' look anymore," Dr. Brandy says. "The process may be expensive for some, but the results look quite good."

Doctors are performing three main types of cosmetic surgery on women, Dr. Brandy says.

*Hair transplants.* They've been around for about 35 years. The old practice involved moving large plugs of hair follicles (8 to 20 at a time) from the back of a patient's head, then embedding them in a balding area. This often resulted in uneven, unnatural hairlines.

Dr. Brandy says new micrografting surgical techniques allow doctors to transplant as few as one hair at a time. Dr. Brandy says this procedure is especially good for women, who usually don't have large bald spots to cover.

Total costs can range from $3,500 to $10,000.

*Hair-lifts.* These aren't often used for women, since they are designed to cover large bald spots. The procedure involves cutting away bald scalp, then stretching hair-covered scalp from the sides and back of the head over the woman's crown. The procedure can cost between $3,500 and $5,000, Dr. Brandy says.

*Scalp reduction.* This is a scaled-down version of the hair-lift. It involves removing smaller bald spots by stretching hair-covered scalp over the bald areas. Cost is about $2,500 to $3,000.

*Hair weaves.* These are cosmetic treatments, not surgical procedures, in which technicians splice natural or synthetic extensions to existing hair to make it look fuller. While they may be cheaper than surgery in the short run, Dr. Brandy says they must be adjusted every four to six weeks as hair grows.

# HEARING LOSS

## Fending Off
## the Sounds of Silence

Kathy Peck loved head-banging music. A bass player and lead singer in an all-female punk rock band, she always figured the louder the music, the better.

For nearly five years, her group, the Contractions, rehearsed four times a week in a tiny room filled with gigantic speakers and performed onstage in the San Francisco area at least three nights a week without wearing earplugs.

"At punk clubs in those days, somebody would probably have beat you up if you dared to wear earplugs," she says.

But after the band got its big break as the opening act for Duran Duran at the Oakland Coliseum, Peck noticed her hearing was fading fast. "After that show, I had ringing in my ears, and when I tried to talk with friends, I could see their lips move, but I couldn't hear any sound. I was basically deaf for days."

Soon afterward, testing revealed that she had a suffered a 40 percent hearing loss. Depressed, Peck worried about her career and wondered if Father Time was catching up with her, even though she was only in her early thirties.

"I lost confidence, and I didn't feel I was good at what I was doing anymore. I felt like I was aging. Like a lot of other people, I thought hearing loss was something that happened to older people," says Peck, co-founder and executive director of Hearing Education and Awareness for Rockers (HEAR), a San Francisco–based nonprofit organization that encourages high-decibel musicians and fans to turn down the volume and wear earplugs.

But as Peck and many other women are discovering, hearing loss in the thirties and forties is all too common. "Hearing loss is occurring at younger and younger ages and is more prevalent than is generally thought," says J. Gail Neely, M.D., professor and director of otology, neurotology and base of skull

# The Five-Minute Hearing Test

Suddenly, everyone around you mumbles, mutters or whispers. Could it be that you have a hearing problem? To find out, take this quiz prepared by the American Academy of Otolaryngology–Head and Neck Surgery. Your choices are almost always (A), half the time (H), occasionally (O) and never (N).

1. I have a problem hearing over the phone.
2. I have trouble following conversation when two or more people are talking at the same time.
3. People complain that I turn the TV volume too high.
4. I have to strain to understand conversations.
5. I miss hearing some common sounds, such as the phone or doorbell ringing.
6. I have trouble hearing conversations in a noisy background, such as at a party.
7. I get confused about where sounds come from.
8. I misunderstand some words in a sentence and need to ask people to repeat themselves.
9. I especially have trouble understanding the speech of women and children.

surgery at Washington University School of Medicine in St. Louis.

Overall, about 10 million American women have significant hearing impairment, and over 2.5 million of those women are under age 45, according to the American Speech-Language-Hearing Association. In a survey of 2,731 people with hearing impairment, nearly 57 percent said they first noticed the problem before age 40, says Laurel E. Glass, M.D., Ph.D., professor emeritus and former director of the Center on Deafness at the University of California, San Francisco, School of Medicine.

The toll of that hearing loss is enormous, doctors say. It can lead to social isolation, limit your job prospects, complicate your sex life, rob you of your self-esteem and make you feel as if life's parade is passing you by.

## Hear Ye, Hear Ye

Before looking at why Kathy Peck and other women have hearing problems, it's important to understand how your ears work. When your best friend

10. I have worked in noisy environments (on assembly lines, with jackhammers, near jet engines and so on).
11. I hear fine—if people just speak clearly.
12. People get annoyed because I misunderstand what they say.
13. I misunderstand what others are saying and make inappropriate responses.
14. I avoid social activities because I cannot hear well and fear I'll reply improperly.
To be answered by a family member or friend:
15. Do you think this person has a hearing loss?

## Scoring

Give yourself three points for each time you answered "almost always," two points for every "half the time," one point for every "occasionally" and no points for every "never."

**0 to 5.** Your hearing is fine.

**6 to 9.** The academy suggests that you see an ear, nose and throat specialist.

**10 and above.** The academy strongly recommends that you see an ear, nose and throat specialist.

tells you the punch line to her latest joke, the sound of her voice enters your ear canal and strikes the eardrum, a cone-shaped elastic membrane stretched across the end of the canal. As the eardrum vibrates, it causes tiny bones in the middle ear to move back and forth. These movements trigger small waves of fluid in the inner ear that ripple through a snail-shaped organ called the cochlea. Inside the cochlea, 30,000 hairlike cells transmit impulses to the auditory nerve, which carries the sounds to the brain. There they are interpreted as the funniest joke you've ever heard, and you laugh.

Some hearing loss is a natural part of aging, says Debra Busacco, Ph.D., audiologist and coordinator of the Lifelong Learning Institute at Gallaudet University in Washington, D.C., the world's only liberal arts university for the deaf. The eardrum stiffens with age, thereby reducing its ability to vibrate. Age-related changes to the bones in the middle ear, such as the degeneration of joints and calcium deposits in those joints, cause the middle ear system to become stiffer, resulting in less effective transmission of sound. Over time, irreplaceable hair cells in the inner ear are damaged by a combination of aging, noise exposure, medication, decreased blood supply to the ear and infection. And once they're damaged, the auditory nerve becomes less efficient. But most of those changes don't occur until a woman is at least 60 years of age.

If symptoms of hearing loss appear at an earlier age, the cause could be something as simple as excessive earwax or the very rare side effect of a medication. It could also be caused by a shattered eardrum, a head injury, high blood pressure, an ear infection, meningitis or a tumor. Some types of hearing loss run in families, such as otosclerosis, a disease that causes excessive bone deposits in the middle ear and prevents the middle ear from conducting sounds to the inner ear, says John House, M.D., associate clinical professor of otolaryngology at the University of Southern California in Los Angeles.

But the most common cause of hearing loss in adults under age 50 is excessive noise exposure, says Susan Rezen, Ph.D., professor of audiology at Worcester State College in Massachusetts and author of *Coping with Hearing Loss*. This still is usually a man's problem because of greater exposure to noise on the job and at play. But as women's lives change, the prevalence of noise-induced hearing loss is expected to increase. "The effects of noise exposure are long term," says Dr. Rezen. "They don't show up right away. But when people are continually exposed, their ears wear out faster, and the effects of aging show up earlier."

"There are no continuous loud sounds such as rock concerts or jackhammers in nature. Our ears were designed to be sensitive, so our ancestors could hear a twig snap, which might mean food or danger was nearby. So when you go into a noisy environment, you're putting yourself into an environment that your ears simply weren't designed to handle," says Flash Gordon, M.D., a primary care physician in San Rafael, California, and co-founder of HEAR.

Sudden loud noises close to the ear, such as firecrackers or gunshots, can cause immediate hearing loss. But usually, noise-induced hearing loss happens gradually, over years. In general, the longer you expose yourself to sounds louder than 85 decibels, whether it's a rock concert or a leaf blower, the more likely you are to destroy cilia in the inner ear and damage your hearing, Dr. Rezen says.

## How Loud Is Loud?

Decibels are how hearing experts measure sound intensity (sound pressure), beginning with the softest sound a person can hear in a laboratory setting, which is 0 decibels. Using this system, 20 decibels is 10 times more intense than 0, 40 decibels is 100 times more intense, 60 decibels is 1,000 times more intense, and so on.

So how loud is 85 decibels? It's about the same amount of noise as a vacuum cleaner, a blender or a power lawn mower. In contrast, a normal conversation is about 65 decibels. Noise levels at some rock concerts come close to exceeding 140 decibels, a level that can cause rapid and irreparable hearing damage in some sensitive ears. Even symphony orchestras can generate sounds louder than 110 decibels, which can cause ear discomfort and pain in some people.

In fact, just one two-hour rock concert can potentially age a woman's hearing by nearly 2½ years if she doesn't wear ear protection, according to calculations by Daniel Johnson, Ph.D., an engineer who tests hearing protectors for the military at Kirtland Air Force Base in Albuquerque, New Mexico. Based on that, he estimates that after 50 concerts, the same woman could have a decline in hearing similar to a woman 16 years older who hasn't been exposed to high noise levels. In addition, if a 30-year-old woman who doesn't wear earplugs began working eight hours a day near machinery that produced noise averaging 95 decibels, by age 40 she could have the high-frequency hearing loss of a 70-year-old.

## Louder Isn't Better

But of course, most of us have gone to loud concerts, stood by passing trains or worked near noisy equipment such as chain saws. So what exactly are those noises doing to your hearing?

Try this the next time you go to a rock concert or another loud event, Dr. Gordon suggests. Before you leave your car, tune the radio to a talk radio station and turn down the volume to a point where you can just barely understand all the words. Then after the concert but before starting your engine, turn on the radio. Chances are the voices that were understandable before the concert won't be then.

That's what doctors call a temporary hearing threshold shift. Basically, it means that the noise has overstimulated the hair cells in your inner ear. As a result, the hair cells aren't functioning as efficiently as they usually do, so sounds have to be louder for you to hear them, Dr. Neely says. Researchers at the University of Manitoba in Manitoba, Winnipeg, for example, tested the hearing of ten women before and after a 2½-hour rock concert. For most of the women, the threshold of their ability to hear was ten or more decibels higher after the concert than before.

That may not sound like much, but for several hours you'd probably have difficulty hearing rustling leaves or whispered conversation. Fortunately, your hearing would return to normal within 24 hours.

But a temporary threshold shift is a warning sign that your hearing is at risk if you continue to expose yourself to loud sounds. Some people never experience temporary threshold shifts and mistakenly assume that they are immune to the dangers of loud noise, Dr. Neely says. In truth, repeated exposure to loud noises can gradually kill off hair cells and permanently damage your ability to hear, particularly high-frequency sounds such as the consonants *sh, ch, t, f, h* and *s*, which are frequently used in conversation.

"If you miss hearing those high-frequency sounds, the remaining part of a word won't make sense to you," Dr. Neely says. "You literally won't know if people around you are talking about fish or tin cans. That can be very confusing and frustrating."

# When the Ringing Won't Quit

At 31, Elizabeth Meyer was finding her way in life. She was taking marimba lessons and theater classes and looking forward to a career as a musician. Then the morning after an African music concert in Portland, Oregon, she noticed a ringing in her ears; over the next few weeks, she also developed an intense sensitivity to sound.

Soon she could speak on the telephone only if she held a pillow between her ear and the receiver. Before she gave up going to the movies, she was wearing two pairs of earplugs and industrial-strength earmuffs like airport baggage handlers wear. She couldn't travel for more than 15 minutes in a bus because the noise and the ringing in her ears overwhelmed her.

"Overnight, I felt like I'd aged 30 years," says Meyer, now 36. "I literally felt like I was 60. It has gotten a bit better, but the first year I spent just trying to stop myself from jumping up and banging my head against the wall every 30 seconds. At first I went through a suicidal period. Finally, I realized that although my condition might not improve, my ability to cope with it certainly would."

Meyer is one of the 3.5 million American women who endure chronic tinnitus, an annoying ringing, humming or buzzing in the ears that can be a symptom of everything from excessive earwax to high blood pressure to heart disease. One in three women who has tinnitus, like Meyer, also develops hyperacusis, which is an extreme sensitivity to sounds. Both tinnitus and hyperacusis can also be signs of noise-induced hearing loss caused by damage to the cilia, hair cells in the inner ear that help conduct sound to the auditory nerve in the brain, says Christopher Linstrom, M.D., director of otology and neurotology at the New York Eye and Ear Infirmary in New York City.

# Defending Your Ears

Although most of us will suffer some hearing loss due to aging, you can keep your hearing sharp well into your golden years if you protect your ears from noise now. "Imagine that your hearing is a big barrel of sand," Dr. Gordon says. "Either you can empty it out gradually with a teaspoon, so it will last a long time, or you can use a shovel and run out of it a lot sooner." Here are some ways to prevent hearing loss.

**Turn it down.** You probably can't do much about traffic noise, jackham-

Hyperacusis, for instance, causes individual hair cells, each of which is normally stimulated only by certain frequencies, to react to the same range of sounds. As a result, more and more hair cells vibrate in unison, and that can make the quietest noises seem loud and jarring. When this damage occurs, sounds that are quite tolerable to many people can be painful to you, says Lt. Col. Richard Danielson, Ph.D., supervisor of audiology in the Army Audiology and Speech Center at Walter Reed Army Medical Center in Washington, D.C.

In some cases, tinnitus can be treated with drugs or surgery, particularly if it's caused by excessive fluid in the middle ear, high blood pressure, a partially blocked artery in the neck or allergies. But in most instances, there is no cure for either tinnitus or hyperacusis, Dr. Linstrom says.

Once tinnitus or hyperacusis is diagnosed, you should avoid loud noises and wear earplugs to prevent more hearing damage that can make these conditions worse. Masking devices that produce pleasant sounds such as raindrops or ocean waves can help people with tinnitus drown out the ringing, Dr. Linstrom says. Caffeine and nicotine aggravate both conditions, so quit smoking and avoid coffee, tea and chocolate, he says. Some medications such as aspirin, antibiotics and anticancer drugs can also cause tinnitus and hearing sensitivity. A hearing aid might help, because the better you hear, the less noticeable the ringing may be, says John House, M.D., associate clinical professor of otolaryngology at the University of Southern California in Los Angeles.

If you have questions about these hearing problems, see your physician or write to the American Tinnitus Association, P.O. Box 5, Portland, OR 97207.

mers and many other sources of excessive sound. But you can turn down the volume on your stereo, says Stephen Painton, Ph.D., an audiologist at the University of Oklahoma Health Sciences Center in Oklahoma City. Some sound systems can produce noise equal to the loudest rock concerts. Here's a way to tell if your stereo is too loud. Turn it on, then walk outside your home and close the door. If you can hear the music, it's too loud. The same rule applies to your car radio. And if you use headphones or a personal stereo, the person standing next to you shouldn't be able to hear the sound.

**If you have to shout, get out.** If you have to raise your voice to be heard by someone standing a foot or two away from you, that's a clear warning that the noise level may be dangerous, and you should get away from it as soon as possible or wear ear protection, Dr. House says.

**Keep plugs handy.** Stuffing cotton or pieces of shredded paper napkin into your ears does virtually nothing to minimize damage to your hearing. Instead, get in the habit of carrying earplugs with you, Dr. Busacco says. Most earplugs are small and can easily be carried in your purse or pocket. That way, she says, you'll be prepared for unexpected noise, such as an unusually loud movie. The foam rubber types are good because they are inexpensive and available over the counter at most drugstores and they can be quickly rolled up and placed in your ears. Look for the noise reduction rating on the side of the box, Dr. Painton says. This will tell you how many decibels of sound the earplugs will muffle. Buy plugs that have a rating of at least 15. Those plugs will reduce noise by 15 decibels and slash the chances that your hearing will be damaged. If you want better protection, an audiologist can design a pair of custom-made plugs for about $80 that reduce noise by about 35 decibels, Dr. Busacco says.

**Take time-outs.** The longer you expose yourself to loud sounds without a break, the more likely you are to cause permanent damage to your hearing, even if you're wearing earplugs. So give your ears a 5- or 10-minute break from noise every 30 minutes, Dr. Gordon says. "It's like putting your head underwater for 20 minutes. You can do it if you hold your breath for a minute at a time, then take a 10-second break. But if you'd try to do it in two 10-minute segments, you'd be dead. If you give your ears an occasional break, they can rest and recover from the excessive work that loud noise makes them do."

**Spread out the noise.** Placing several loud appliances or power tools near each other will compound your noise problem. So if your TV set is in the same room as your dishwasher, for example, you might be tempted to turn up the TV volume excessively when you do a load of dishes. Instead, move the television into a quieter room, says Lt. Col. Richard Danielson, Ph.D., supervisor of audiology in the Army Audiology and Speech Center at Walter Reed Army Medical Center in Washington, D.C.

**Swab the deck, not your ears.** Attempting to clean wax out of your ears with a cotton swab, matchstick or anything else smaller than the Love Boat does more harm than good, Dr. House says. Earwax is actually good for you. It repels water and helps keep dust away from your sensitive eardrum. Sticking small objects in your ear pushes the wax farther into your ear and can cause infection. "The best thing to do about earwax inside the ear canal is leave it alone," Dr. House says. If it becomes bothersome, see your physician or get an over-the-counter earwax removal kit that contains drops that will soften the wax and allow it to flow naturally out of your ear.

**Muzzle your medication.** Taking six to eight aspirin a day can cause ringing in your ears and temporary hearing loss, Dr. Gordon says. Antibiotics such as gentamicin (G-Mycin), streptomycin and tobramycin (Nebcin) can also damage your hearing, says Barry E. Hirsch, M.D., a neurotologist at the University of Pittsburgh School of Medicine. If you are taking any drug and develop hearing problems, ask your doctor if the medication could be causing it.

**Puffing hurts your ears.** Smoking reduces blood flow to the ears and may interfere with the natural healing of small blood vessels that occurs after exposure to loud noise, Dr. House says. In a study of 2,348 workers exposed to noise at an aerospace factory, researchers at the University of Southern California School of Medicine found that smokers had greater hearing loss than nonsmokers. So if you smoke, quit.

**Slash the java.** Like nicotine, caffeine cuts blood flow to the ears, increasing your chances of hearing loss, Dr. House says. Drink no more than two eight-ounce cups of coffee or tea a day. If possible, drink decaffeinated brews.

**Balance your diet.** The same fatty and cholesterol-laden foods that are bad for your heart also endanger your ears, according to Dr. House. High blood pressure and atherosclerosis, a buildup of plaque on artery walls, not only cause heart disease but also can reduce blood flow to the ears and gradually strangle your hearing, Dr. House says. So cut the fat with a balanced daily diet that includes at least five servings of fruits and vegetables, six servings of breads and grains and no more than one three-ounce serving of lean red meat, poultry or fish.

**Exercise.** Walk, run, swim, or do any other aerobic exercise for 20 minutes a day, three times a week, Dr. House suggests. It will stimulate blood circulation, lower your blood pressure and help keep your ears in peak condition.

## Making the Best of It

The average person waits five to seven years after first noticing a hearing problem to seek help for it. Those can be years of unnecessary social isolation and frustration, Dr. Busacco says, because the earlier you seek help, the sooner your hearing problem can be diagnosed and treated.

"People are a lot more self-conscious about their hearing than they are about their vision," Dr. Hirsch says. "It's often an issue of vanity. Wearing a hearing aid somehow implies aging, while wearing glasses doesn't."

If you suspect that you have a hearing problem, particularly if you have ringing in your ears or develop a sudden sensitivity to loud noises that didn't bother you in the past, see your doctor or a physician who specializes in diseases of the ear, nose and throat. Some hearing problems such as Ménière's disease, a disorder that causes ringing in the ears and dizziness, can be treated with prescription medication or surgery. Other conditions, such as perforated eardrums and otosclerosis, may be corrected with surgery.

Even if the loss can't be fully corrected, powerful but inconspicuous hearing aids—some small enough to fit inside the ear canal—are available to help you get back in touch with the world. Prices range from about $550 for a basic hearing aid to more than $2,500 for top-of-the-line computerized models.

An audiologist, a professional trained to fit hearing aids, can help you choose one that fits your needs.

Here's how to recognize if you have a hearing loss and how to cope with it.

**Tune in to your turn signal.** Sure, it's annoying when you drive down the road and realize that your turn signal has been on for miles, but it could also be a clue that you have a hearing problem. If you snap on your turn signal and can't hear the accompanying clicking sound in your car, it's time to get your hearing checked by an audiologist or doctor, Dr. Painton says.

**Don't be shy about it.** If you have difficulty hearing or understanding people, tell them, says Philip Zazove, M.D., assistant professor of family medicine at the University of Michigan Medical School in Ann Arbor who has had profound hearing loss since birth. Simply saying "I don't hear as well as I used to," "Could you repeat that?" and "Talk a little slower" can prevent a lot of misunderstandings, frustration and anger, he says. If necessary, ask the person to repeat herself, or if you have trouble with a key word, have her write it on a piece of paper.

**Light up your sex life.** Hearing loss can cause havoc in the bedroom. Those whispered sweet nothings you used to enjoy so much when you were making love are often the first casualty. Leave in your hearing aid if there is any possibility of sex, or ask your partner to leave on the light so that you can see well enough to lip-read, Dr. Rezen suggests. Talk about what you want sexually before you go into the bedroom. If necessary, develop your own secret code, such as "Two taps on the back means kiss me." "If you don't plan, you may lose the opportunity altogether," she says.

**Find a quiet spot.** If you really want to talk to an interesting man at a party, pull him away from the middle of the room and into a secluded corner. Not only is that more intimate, you can concentrate on what he's saying and don't have to compete with laughter, music and other background noise that just makes it that much harder to hear, Dr. Zazove says. At home, consider turning off the television, radio or other noisy appliances before you try to listen to someone.

**Laugh it off.** A good sense of humor is vital if you have a hearing problem, Dr. Painton says. So what if you misunderstand a word or two and say something inappropriate? Enjoy the moment and join the laughter.

**Do your homework.** If you're attending an important business meeting or conference, get there early and try to nab a front row seat facing the person who you think will do most of the talking, Dr. Zazove says. If possible, tell the speaker about your hearing loss and ask her to avoid turning away from you. Maintain eye contact with the speaker. Try to get a written summary of the topic or agenda, so you'll be prepared for words or phrases that might come up. That way, if you do miss a few words, you'll have a better chance of filling them in accurately.

# HEART ATTACK

## *Don't Ignore the Possibility*

Every so often you hear about a woman cut down in her prime by a heart attack. So you wonder "Can it happen to me?"

Don't panic. Until menopause, most women have natural protection against heart attacks. In fact, experts say that just over one-half of 1 percent of heart attacks occur in women ages 44 and under.

But while heart attacks are uncommon among premenopausal women, that doesn't mean you shouldn't do everything you can now to make sure you don't have one.

Few things in life can age you as rapidly as a heart attack.

It can strike like lightning, though the stage may have been set with years of fatty deposits forming in your coronary arteries.

## When Luck Runs Out

By definition, a heart attack is a reduction or blockage of blood flow in a coronary artery that causes potentially life-threatening damage to the heart. And although our society tends to think of heart attack as a man's problem, more than 500,000 women have heart attacks each year, often visited by the crushing chest pain, heavy sweating and shortness of breath that are signs of a sudden clot in a coronary artery and its effect on the heart. One-third of these heart attacks are fatal. Four in five heart attack deaths occur in those ages 65 and older.

When it comes to our hearts, women are much luckier than men. In our premenopausal years, the female sex hormone estrogen provides natural protection against the sinister forces of heart attack that begin striking men in large numbers in their middle years. But once we go through menopause, those natural defenses just about vanish. As we grow older, our hearts and the blood vessels that nourish them begin to show and feel their age, even without the dramatic intrusion of a heart attack. The heart gradually starts to pump a little less efficiently, and the walls of the arteries become a little stiffer and less flexible.

And then there's the heart attack itself. In just minutes or hours, it can take a devastating toll upon your body, as though you were adding 20 or 30 years to your age overnight. As the supply of blood to your heart is impaired, the heart cells can become severely injured. The longer this blood flow is interfered with, the greater the chance of irreversible damage, producing cell death and the demise of part of the heart muscle.

But there's good news, too. Most heart attacks are preventable, no matter what your age, if you adopt lifestyle habits that can slow the buildup of fatty deposits in your coronary arteries. Yes, there are exceptions to this rule. On rare occasions, stress might set off a heart attack, even in a young woman without heavily clogged blood vessels. "Coronary arteries can go into spasm in stressful situations, which can reduce the blood flow to the heart," says James Martin, M.D., a family physician with the Institute for Urban Family Health at Beth Israel Medical Center in New York City. "If the spasm lasts long enough—for about seven to ten minutes—you can have a heart attack."

But that type of scenario is extremely rare. Chances are you have a lot of control over the health and longevity of your heart.

# Fight the Good Fight

So where do you begin? Here are some crucial strategies to keep in mind.

**Know yourself.** "It's important to know where you stand," advises Richard H. Helfant, M.D., vice chairman of medicine and director of the cardiology training program at the University of California, Irvine, Medical Center and author of *Women, Take Heart*. That means being aware of the risk factors that may increase your chances of having heart problems. As a woman, you have estrogen as one of your greatest allies in fighting off heart attack—but your body's production of estrogen dwindles after menopause. Also, if close relatives have had heart attacks at early ages—less than 55—you need to be extra cautious. And if you have conditions that increase your risk that you can change—high blood pressure, an elevated blood cholesterol level, diabetes or a cigarette habit—you need to attack and control them before they attack your heart. Talk to your doctor about how to do that.

**Toe the line.** No one is asking you to be a fanatic. You don't have to swear off red meat or work out at the gym until you can't see straight. But if you live a reasonably careful, energetic lifestyle, you can keep your heart beating with the vigor of a much younger woman, with less worry about the Big One.

**Get active.** If you're one of those women who feels more comfortable with a TV remote control in her hand than with a tennis racket, it's time for a change of heart. Regular exercise, such as brisk walking for just 30 to 45 minutes three times a week or some laps in the pool, can turn that pump in your chest into a mean machine.

"Exercise is beneficial for your heart in a number of ways," says Stephen Havas, M.D., associate professor of epidemiology and preventive medicine at the University of Maryland School of Medicine in Baltimore. "It can boost your HDL (high-density lipoprotein) cholesterol, which is the protective component of your blood cholesterol level. It also can modestly decrease your blood pressure and help you control your weight." It can help keep your heart fit and conditioned, too, just as it gets the other muscles in your body into shape.

**Eat right.** It's not a magic bullet, but proper diet can be the heart and soul of any personalized cardiac care program. According to Fredric J. Pashkow, M.D., medical director of the Cardiac Health Improvement and Rehabilitation Program at the Cleveland Clinic Foundation in Cleveland and author of *The Woman's Heart Book*, research shows that the best way to keep your heart out of danger is to slash the fat and cholesterol in your diet. That means when it comes to menu planning, choose fish more often than steak, skim milk more frequently than whole milk, egg whites rather than whole eggs and low-fat frozen yogurt instead of ice cream. Keep your daily dietary fat intake to 25 percent or less of total calories.

**Consider hormones.** Estrogen replacement therapy can cut your risk of heart attack by as much as one-half to one-third, according to Dr. Helfant.

But you must talk over your options with your doctor. "There's a potential downside to hormonal therapy," says Dr. Helfant, "such as an increased risk of endometrial cancer and perhaps breast cancer, too." If you have a family history of endometrial or breast cancer or other risk factors, you and your doctor may decide that hormonal therapy isn't for you.

## After You've Been Struck

Prevention may sound good, but what if you've already endured the terrifying experience of a heart attack? Well, count your blessings that you survived it—and then make a commitment to some health habits that might keep you from going through it a second time and that might put you on the fast track to a zestful, healthful life. If you've bought into the belief that a heart attack will permanently impair your mobility, activity level, job function or sex life, it's time to dispel those myths. Despite your heart attack, your best years can still be ahead of you.

With lifestyle changes, you should be able to reduce your risk of having another heart attack, says Dr. Helfant. "These changes will also allow you to take control of your health and live a purposeful, meaningful life while protecting yourself to the maximum degree possible."

So what kind of action should you take? The recommendations may sound familiar, but here's the specific impact they can have when a heart attack is part of your medical history.

**Eat healthfully.** After something as major as a heart attack, you might think the damage that has been done to your heart makes simple measures such as healthier eating about as helpful as applying a Band-Aid to your chest. But when researchers at the National Heart, Lung and Blood Institute conducted an analysis of studies of heart attack survivors, they found that people could significantly decrease their chances of having another heart attack by reducing their high blood cholesterol readings. Various studies have shown that declines in blood cholesterol levels of 10 percent cut the risk of having a second heart attack by between 12 and 19 percent. A key to lowering blood cholesterol is cutting back on saturated fat (the kind found in animal products and tropical oils) and dietary cholesterol (found in most animal products).

**Move it.** In many programs for heart attack recovery, physical activity is the center of attention, often beginning at very modest levels even while women are still hospitalized. Most cardiac rehabilitation programs recommend exercising for 15 to 30 minutes at least three times a week.

"People who have done no exercise in the past would certainly be better off doing even a little bit now," says Peter Wood, Ph.D., professor of medicine emeritus and associate director of the Stanford University Center for Research in Disease Prevention in Palo Alto, California. By gradually increasing the amount of physical activity you do—with your doctor's guidance—your heart will reap even more benefits, Dr. Wood says.

**Take aspirin.** In this age of high-powered, high-priced medications, can a simple aspirin make you the picture of health? An American Heart Association team of researchers analyzed six studies in which patients were given aspirin after heart attacks. This inexpensive white pill reduced the death rate from heart disease between 5 and 42 percent and cut the rate of subsequent nonfatal heart attacks between 12 and 57 percent.

One other piece of good news: You needn't go overboard on aspirin dosages. "A baby aspirin a day is all that's necessary," says Dr. Helfant. Nevertheless, some people should probably stay away from aspirin completely, despite its potential benefits. "If you have a bleeding disorder or an ulcer, for example, taking aspirin is not a good idea," says Julie Buring, Sc.D., principal investigator of the Women's Health Study and associate professor of ambulatory care and prevention at Harvard Medical School in Boston. She suggests talking with your doctor before taking aspirin.

# HEART DISEASE

## The Sooner You Act, the Better

There's a myth that says heart disease is a man's problem. A lot of women believe it—and so do many of their doctors. But it couldn't be more wrong.

True, heart attacks usually strike women later in life—an average of seven to ten years later than men. But when they hit, they hit with a vengeance. Heart disease kills more women than any other illness—nearly six times as many as breast cancer and nine times as many as lung cancer.

## The Menopause Connection

When it comes to women and heart disease, age is a key factor. The chances of developing heart disease increase steadily after menopause.

The presumed reason: estrogen. Throughout most of a woman's life, this female hormone stands guard over her heart and coronary arteries, defending them against the fatty deposits that can embed themselves in the arterial walls, clogging the bloodstream and making her more vulnerable to heart attack.

"We are now beginning to think that estrogen's protective effect is related to its influence on the HDL (high-density lipoprotein) cholesterol level," says Richard H. Helfant, M.D., vice chairman of medicine and director of the Cardiology Training Program at the University of California, Irvine, Medical Center and author of *Women, Take Heart.* "There's growing evidence that estrogen increases the amount of this good cholesterol, which we know protects the arteries from infiltration of fatty deposits." At the same time, estrogen may propel your LDL (low-density lipoprotein) cholesterol into a downward spiral, which is just where you want it to head.

After menopause, of course, that protection does a quick retreat. As the natural estrogen produced in your body crops, you're left to fend off the attack of

# If the Worst Happens

Sometimes even the most conscientious efforts at prevention just aren't enough. If you start to feel the warning signs of a heart attack— such as pressure or squeezing sensations in the chest, pain shooting into the shoulders, arms or neck or shortness of breath and nausea— you need to respond rapidly.

Because women tend to think that heart attacks are something that only their husbands, fathers and brothers get, we may not be as quick to react to our own symptoms. But as the American Heart Association warns, "Delay can be deadly!"

Clot-dissolving drugs called thrombolytics are administered in the emergency room and can restore blood flow, thus minimizing damage to the heart muscle.

But time is crucial. "The later you come in to the emergency room, the less likely a thrombolytic is going to be effective," says Gerald Po-host, M.D., director of the Division of Cardiovascular Disease at the University of Alabama School of Medicine in Birmingham. "The first two hours are the best time, but as time passes, the success of these drugs diminishes."

heart disease with one less weapon in your arsenal. At about age 45, your LDL cholesterol level will generally start to climb, along with your total cholesterol count. As it does, so will your risk of heart disease.

It may sound grim. But there's no need to resign yourself to a life of anxiety. True, you can't change your age or keep your natural estrogen flowing, although research indicates that hormone replacement therapy (a combination of estrogen and progestin) given to women at menopause can have a protective effect. Nor can you alter any inherited tendency toward heart disease. But that doesn't mean there are no other risk factors you can alter.

## Committing to Change

Heart disease doesn't happen overnight. Most heart disease results from a narrowing of the coronary arteries, known as atherosclerosis, over decades. What makes arteries narrow? Largely, it's the way we Americans live our lives. In some other countries, where lifestyles are simpler, arteries are healthy and wide open, even in the very elderly.

The encouraging news is pretty straightforward: Progression of heart disease can be slowed, and in some cases even reversed, without drugs or surgery. But don't think you have to go to extremes or have a will of steel to do so. "Moderate changes go a long way," advises Dr. Helfant. "You don't have to be a fanatic or be perfect to make a difference in your health."

Let's look at some strategies that can keep your heart pumping as though it inherited an extra decade or two of life.

**Give up the cigarettes—now.** Okay, maybe you've smoked for years and even tried to quit with no luck. But a lot of ex-smokers successfully stopped only after their second, third or even sixth attempts. So don't give up.

Why not? When you smoke, your blood vessels constrict. That places extra strain on your heart. But that isn't all. Cigarette smoke forces your heart to beat more rapidly and raises your blood pressure

The result is as brutal as it comes: According to the American Heart Association, cigarettes directly cause nearly one-fifth of all deaths from heart disease.

If you smoke and take oral contraceptives, you're asking for trouble. Together, they make you up to 39 times more likely to have a heart attack than a woman who uses neither.

**Cut your cholesterol.** Everyone needs at least some of this substance in her body for some essential body functions to take place. But the fact is that your own liver produces all the cholesterol your body requires.

If your diet leans too heavily on high-fat, high-cholesterol foods, your total blood cholesterol readings may get up to 240 milligrams per deciliter of blood (mg/dl) or above, a perilous level that will double your chances of heart disease. By making some leaner food choices, however, you can take back control and get yourself on a heart-healthy track—perhaps even reversing atherosclerosis. A total cholesterol of below 200 mg/dl is what you need to shoot for.

When Dean Ornish, M.D., president and director of the Preventive Medicine Research Institute in Sausalito, California, put people on a comprehensive lifestyle program that included a very low fat diet, moderate exercise, smoking cessation and stress management training, 82 percent of them experienced a significant regression of the fatty deposits that had clogged their coronary arteries after one year.

But don't think that to prevent heart disease you need to adopt a deprivation diet that's just a step above a hunger strike. "No one ever got a heart attack from a steak or a piece of pie," says Dr. Helfant. "We're talking about an overall change in lifestyle and not worrying about an occasional slip." The trick is to adhere to recommendations to limit fat intake to no more than 25 percent of calories over the long term.

**Tip the triglyceride scale.** As if cholesterol weren't enough to worry about, you and your doctor should keep tabs on your triglycerides, too. They are a type of fat in the bloodstream, and though they appear to play a role in heart disease, their exact role in that process is still not as clear as the link between cholesterol and heart problems.

Many experts say that a triglyceride level above 200 mg/dl should serve as a warning flag. What's one of the best ways to temper your triglycerides? Regular exercise, says Peter Wood, Ph.D., professor of medicine emeritus and associate director of the Stanford University Center for Research in Disease Prevention in Palo Alto, California.

**Maintain your best weight.** In a country that seems obsessed with slogans like "Thin is in," a lot of us could never be mistaken for being undernourished. About 19 million American women are a bit more than pleasantly plump (approximately 20 percent or more over their desirable weights). It's a little like playing Russian roulette with their hearts. In the Nurses' Health Study at Harvard Medical School, 40 percent of heart disease cases were attributed to the buildup of excess pounds.

So whether or not you consider flab to be unattractive, it's clearly hazardous to your heart. "If you're obese, the heart has to work harder to move nutrients to the additional cells in your body," says James Martin, M.D., family physician with the Institute for Urban Family Health at Beth Israel Medical Center in New York City. That extra strain on the heart can be particularly worrisome if you already have other risk factors that can contribute to heart disease, such as high cholesterol or high blood pressure. Set some goals for shedding extra pounds by relying more on low-fat foods and getting more exercise.

---

# Are You an Apple or a Pear?

In the fruit basket, pears tend to age somewhat faster than apples. But when it comes to your heart—and "pear" and "apple" are describing different body shapes—the pear definitely ages slower.

Fortunately, most obese women tend to be shaped like pears (with their extra weight around their hips) rather than apples (with their fat tucked into the midsection). But that isn't always the case, particularly in women after menopause. Studies clearly show that an apple shape creates a higher risk of heart attack (as well as of diabetes, stroke and high blood pressure).

Why is a jelly belly so malicious? One theory is that abdominal fat is more easily converted to cholesterol.

No matter what the cause turns out to be, make an effort to trim the size of your own "apple" by losing a few of those extra pounds. Here's a guideline for you to keep in mind: To cut your risk, your waist measurement should not be more than 80 percent of your hip measurement.

**Sweat a little.** Sure, it's tempting to toss out the exercise shoes, cancel your health club membership and spend every weekend entrenched like Gibraltar in front of the television or camped out on the beach with a best-selling novel. If that's your idea of Shangri-la, you're not alone—but you are paying a price. In fact, almost 60 percent of American women don't get any exercise, a lifestyle choice that greatly increases their risk of heart attack.

Exercise can do more than just get you some fresh air and make you feel more invigorated. "It strengthens the heart muscle," says Dr. Wood. "With regular exercise, the heart becomes a more efficient pump. As a result, the heart rate becomes slower for a given amount of effort." Each beat is more efficient, he says, and so the heart doesn't need to work as hard as it would if you were out of shape.

Exercise is particularly important if you're trying to lose weight. "When women lose weight, their HDL cholesterol levels tend to decrease," cautions Robert Rosenson, M.D., director of the Preventive Cardiology Center at Rush-Presbyterian–St. Luke's Medical Center in Chicago. "To maintain your HDLs at the same level or even produce a slight increase, you need to exercise while you're losing weight through diet."

**Deflate your blood pressure.** High blood pressure is called the silent killer, quietly doing sinister work that puts so much extra strain on the heart and arteries that it can ultimately provoke a heart attack (not to mention a stroke or kidney failure).

But by pulling the plug on your high blood pressure—which you can do by reducing sodium in your diet, losing weight, exercising and (if necessary) taking one of many available medications—you can give your heart a breather. Here are some comforting statistics: For each one-point decline you can achieve in your diastolic blood pressure (the bottom number), you can cut your risk of a heart attack by 2 to 3 percent. And with proper therapy, it's not uncommon for people with high blood pressure to lower their diastolic readings by 20 points or more.

**Consider aspirin.** It may not be the Fountain of Youth, but the drug that can keep your heart vital may be as close as the medicine cabinet in your bathroom. Aspirin, the tiny white pill that has been relied on a zillion times to zap headaches and other mild pain problems, appears to be a heart-saver as well.

Again, the Nurses' Health Study has given us the crucial information. Over a six-year period, women who took from one to six aspirin tablets per week had about a 32 percent decreased chance of having a first heart attack compared with women who took no aspirin. Women over age 50 seemed to get the most protection. But particularly if you're prone to bleeding problems, consult your doctor before self-prescribing aspirin, since it's a medication that discourages blood clotting in your body.

**Get your vitamins.** For decades, mainstream doctors have considered vitamin supplements just a small step away from quackery. But not anymore. A study published in the *New England Journal of Medicine* involving more than

87,000 women concluded that women who took vitamin E supplements for more than two years had about a 40 percent lower risk of major heart disease than those who did not take supplements.

What's the secret of vitamin E? The vitamin is an antioxidant, meaning that it protects cells from malicious molecules called free radicals that trigger a process called oxidation, which can contribute to the clogging of arteries.

"I'm giving vitamin E to my patients in standard doses that do not pose risks," says Marianne J. Legato, M.D., author of *The Female Heart* and associate professor of clinical medicine at Columbia University College of Physicians and Surgeons in New York City. Dr. Legato advises supplements of 400 IU of vitamin E, along with 1,500 milligrams of vitamin C and 6 milligrams of beta-carotene, both of which are also antioxidants. She also advises 1,500 milligrams of supplemental calcium, which studies have shown may help prevent heart disease.

**Seek hormonal help.** Your doctor has the option of prescribing supplemental estrogen in your postmenopausal years, which can empower you to take a bite out of heart disease before it bites you. A study at Harvard University in Cambridge, Massachusetts, of more than 48,000 women found that estrogen replacement therapy could slash the risk of major coronary disease and fatal cardiovascular disease by more than half.

But there's an important caveat to keep in mind: There has been concern that estrogen could increase your risk of cancer of the endometrium (the lining of the uterus) and perhaps of breast cancer. But by prescribing lower doses of estrogen and combining estrogen with progestin (the synthetic form of another hormone called progesterone), your doctor may be able to counteract these threats. You and your doctor need to weigh the pros and cons before deciding whether estrogen alone or in combination with progestin is right for you.

# A Multitude of Treatments

The good thing about heart disease—surely the only good thing—is that it most often gives you warning signs before striking hard. The most common warning sign is angina, chest pain caused by inadequate blood flow to the heart. Should you experience angina, your doctor might prescribe nitroglycerin to relax the blood vessels and allow the heart to get more blood. Or for chronic angina, she might suggest other medications, such as beta-blockers, calcium channel blockers or ACE (angiotensin-converting enzyme) inhibitors.

"The choice of drugs will depend on your own particular situation," says Dr. Martin. "If you have high blood pressure as well as heart disease, there may be a single drug that can help both of these conditions. If you have heart failure in addition to heart disease—that is, if your heart isn't pumping as efficiently as possible—an ACE inhibitor is a good choice. Some patients do need to be placed on more than one medication. So it's an individualized decision."

If the blockage of your coronary arteries has become severe, then your doctor might recommend an open heart operation (coronary bypass surgery) or angioplasty. Approximately 30 percent of these heart operations are performed on women. Angioplasties and bypass surgery are about equally common.

In angioplasty, a tiny balloon-tipped catheter is guided into the coronary arteries, where the balloon is inflated to flatten the fatty deposits that are causing the obstruction.

Although angioplasty successfully opens the arteries in up to 90 percent of patients, these arteries can become clogged again, sometimes within months of the procedure. At that time, angioplasty needs to be repeated, or the doctor may suggest bypass surgery instead.

In a bypass operation, healthy blood vessels (often transplanted from the leg or the chest) are grafted onto the heart to bypass the obstructed portions of the coronary arteries. Although it is a more major procedure, its benefits tend to last longer. Dr. Legato says that surgery is usually chosen for so-called three-vessel disease, in which three or more of the major coronary arteries are obstructed, severely interfering with blood flow to the heart.

If you wind up opting for either medication or surgery, it is still important— perhaps doubly so—to maintain a healthy, active, low-fat lifestyle.

# HEMOCHROMATOSIS

## Ironing Out the Problem

Lately, you've felt as lifeless as a bowl of soggy cornflakes. Anemia, you thought. But after you started taking iron supplements, you felt even more drained. Now your joints are stiff, and your belly aches. You feel like your body is rusting from the inside out.

This is exactly what's happening to the 1 in 200 American women who has hemochromatosis, a genetic disease that causes the body to horde excessive amounts of iron, which then attacks organs such as the liver, heart and pancreas. It may be one of life's most insidious and catastrophic agers. Unless it's detected and treated early, the disease can also lead to arthritis, diabetes, cancer, even premature death.

"Hemochromatosis can certainly slow you down prematurely. If it causes fatigue, you can feel like you're 80 when you're only 40," says Jerome L. Sullivan, M.D., Ph.D., a pathologist and director of clinical laboratories at the Veterans Affairs Medical Center in Charleston, South Carolina.

## The Family Connection

Hemochromatosis occurs when a woman inherits a pair of abnormal genes from her mother and father. Once considered a rare ailment, it is now believed to be one of the most common inherited diseases, afflicting more people than cystic fibrosis, Huntington's disease and muscular dystrophy combined, according to Randall Lauffer, Ph.D., assistant professor at Harvard Medical School in Boston and author of *Iron and Your Heart*. About 500,000 women in the United States may have the disease.

What happens when you have it? Normally, you store small amounts of iron in your body and stop absorbing it when you have enough in reserve. If you

210

have hemochromatosis, however, your body doesn't know when it has enough iron. So you keep absorbing the mineral—often to the point where you can actually set off metal detectors. Symptoms of hemochromatosis can appear at any age. It has been detected in children as young as age 2 and in men as old as 101.

Once iron is in your body, it's there to stay—unless you bleed (iron is a major component of red blood cells). That may be why many women don't develop symptoms of hemochromatosis until after they go through menopause and stop having their periods, which help rid their bodies of at least some excess iron, says William H. Crosby, M.D., director of hematology at Chapman Cancer Center in Joplin, Missouri. If you don't lose iron through bleeding, your body will cram the mineral into every major organ to the point that some women with hemochromatosis have up to 100 times more iron concentrated in their livers, 15 times more iron in their hearts and 5 times more iron in their kidneys than an average person.

In excess amounts, iron generates free radicals, chemically unstable oxygen molecules that can damage the heart and liver and accelerate the aging process throughout the body, Dr. Lauffer says.

"That excess iron is a true poison and can increase your risk of cancer," says Sylvia Bottomley, M.D., a hematologist at the University of Oklahoma Health Sciences Center in Oklahoma City.

Women with hemochromatosis, for example, are 200 times more likely to develop liver cancer than an average person. In addition, excess iron can lead to cirrhosis, an incurable ailment that causes scar tissue and eventually destroys the liver, Dr. Sullivan says.

Excess iron also interferes with the pumping ability of the heart and leads to a form of heart disease called congestive cardiomyopathy, which causes enlargement of the heart muscle. This condition is 300 times more fatal among women with hemochromatosis than among the population at large.

Hemochromatosis can also turn the skin bronze and damage the pituitary gland, causing lowered sex drive, infertility and a disruption in the menstrual cycle.

Fortunately, some complications of hemochromatosis, including heart disease, are reversible if the disease is diagnosed and treated early. But hemochromatosis often does much of its damage before symptoms appear.

"It's an insidious disease. It comes on gradually. It's like being a lobster in the pot. You're cooked before you realize you're in the pot and water is boiling," Dr. Sullivan says.

Even when symptoms are present, hemochromatosis often eludes detection because it has no standard pattern of onset.

"It hits a lot of different organs, so the first symptom may be different in different people," Dr. Sullivan says. "There really isn't a reliable initial symptom of it. The classic findings are heart disease, diabetes, cirrhosis, fatigue and bronzing of the skin. But I've met a woman whose first symptom was just hip pain. It's unpredictable and very confusing."

Doctors are often confounded by the disease. Some may treat the complications, such as diabetes or arthritis, without realizing that hemochromatosis is the underlying cause, Dr. Crosby says. In some cases, women with hemochromatosis end up seeing several physicians before getting proper diagnoses.

# Getting the Iron Out

Once it has been diagnosed, hemochromatosis is treated by removing blood. Bleeding works because a pint of blood contains about 200 milligrams of iron and because it forces the bone marrow to draw on the body's iron stores in order to replenish removed red blood cells with new ones.

Depending on the amount of excess iron, a woman may need to have bleedings, called phlebotomies, once or twice a week for up to three years to get her iron stores down to normal levels. After that, she will need to have phlebotomies every three or four months for the rest of her life in order to prevent new iron buildup, Dr. Bottomley says.

Women who have phlebotomies early, before damage to their vital organs is widespread, can have normal life expectancies, Dr. Crosby says. Skin color usually returns to normal, and fatigue and heart disease are often relieved. In addition, bleeding can sometimes alleviate the symptoms of diabetes and correct liver function.

"If you need 150 phlebotomies to get rid of iron in your body, you can see it's going to be an arduous road, but it's very doable," Dr. Bottomley says. "When you start having phlebotomies, you're not going to feel better tomorrow, but you should within a few months."

For more information, contact the Iron Overload Disease Association, 433 Westwind Drive, North Palm Beach, FL 33408, or the Hemochromatosis Foundation, P.O. Box 8569, Albany, NY 12208. In addition, here are a few things that can make this disease easier to live with.

**Get tested.** By the time symptoms show up, there may be permanent damage to your vital organs. So detecting hemochromatosis early is critical, particularly if you have a parent or sibling who has the disease, says Margit Krikker, M.D., founder and president of the Hemochromatosis Foundation. Ask your doctor to do a blood test called transferrin saturation index, which shows how much iron is in your blood.

**Stay away from supplements.** Never take iron supplements without your doctor's permission, Dr. Sullivan advises. Some women assume that when they feel worn down, they have iron-poor blood. But hemochromatosis can also cause fatigue, and taking supplements could make your symptoms worse.

**Eat a healthy diet.** While avoiding iron-rich foods may seem to be sensible, it isn't that practical or wise, says Dr. Krikker. That's because many iron-laden vegetables and meats such as potatoes, broccoli and tuna also have other indispensable nutrients. Other important foods are fortified with iron, such as cereals and grains.

Keep in mind that iron is actually a small part of your diet and that you store it very slowly, says Dr. Krikker. It's the total accumulation of it over the years that causes problems. Once you begin having phlebotomies, many of those problems should be behind you.

So eating a balanced diet that includes poultry, fish, grains, fruits, vegetables and dairy products such as cheese and milk is still your best bet.

# HIGH BLOOD PRESSURE

## The Silent Thief of Youth

**W**rinkles we can see. Sore muscles we can feel.

But there's a hidden aging problem out there, one that's far more dangerous than varicose veins, farsightedness or gray hair. High blood pressure, also called hypertension, is directly linked to the deaths of more than 18,000 American women each year—and it contributes to the deaths of untold thousands more. It can make us 12 times more likely to suffer strokes, 6 times more likely to suffer heart attacks and 5 times more likely to die of congestive heart failure. It's also a major risk factor for kidney failure.

And it's more common among younger women than many of us think. One in ten American women between the ages of 35 and 44 has high blood pressure. One in four of us develops high blood pressure before her 55th birthday. And after that, our risk is actually higher than that of men. Experts think hormonal changes play a role in the later development of high blood pressure in women.

Yet nearly half the people in this country with high blood pressure don't even know they have it. "There really aren't any noticeable outward signs. But if you have high blood pressure, it is doing damage," says Patrick Mulrow, M.D., chairman of the Department of Medicine at the Medical College of Ohio at Toledo and chairman of the American Heart Association's Council for High Blood Pressure Research.

"We could save lives if people discovered they have high blood pressure and then took measures to control it," Dr. Mulrow says. In many instances, it's just a matter of going to the doctor and having your blood pressure checked once or twice a year, cutting back on salt and fat and breaking a sweat a few times a week. That's really a small price to pay, Dr. Mulrow says, considering that it could add years to your life.

# Try to Remember

If we have to keep reminding you to control your blood pressure, then maybe it's already too high. That's because high blood pressure may weaken your memory.

A study of 100 adults found that people with higher blood pressure scored lower in a process called short-term memory retrieval. That means it took longer for them to remember whether a number shown to them had been part of an original set of numbers that they had seen earlier.

No one's sure why high blood pressure fogs your memory. It may be related to the way blood circulates in the brain or to a reduction in the amount of oxygen that reaches the brain. "Whatever the mechanism, this is just another reason to keep your blood pressure under healthy control," says David J. Madden, Ph.D., professor in the Department of Psychiatry at Duke University Medical Center in Durham, North Carolina.

# Pressure Builders

Doctors take two measures when they check your blood pressure. The first is called the systolic reading. It indicates how hard your heart pumps to push blood through your arteries. The second measure, called the diastolic reading, shows how much resistance your arteries put up to the blood flow. Blood pressure is measured in millimeters of mercury, or mm Hg, and a reading of about 120 mm Hg systolic and 80 mm Hg diastolic is considered healthy. We read that simply as 120/80.

Everyone's blood pressure varies widely throughout the day. Generally, it will rise when we're exercising and drop when we're asleep. But when your baseline, or resting, reading creeps up to 140/90, you have borderline high blood pressure. That means your heart is working too hard to pump blood, either because your arteries have narrowed or stiffened with plaque or because you have too much blood in your system due to water retention or other problems. The result of the extra stress can be heart disease or dangerous blood clots that can cause stroke or heart attack.

Blood pressure tends to rise with age. A combination of factors causes this, including reduced physical activity, extra body weight and hormonal changes, according to Robert DiBianco, M.D., director of cardiology research at the

Washington Adventist Hospital in Takoma Park, Maryland.

In 90 to 95 percent of cases, Dr. Mulrow says, the exact cause of high blood pressure is unknown. But researchers have identified a number of risk factors that may increase your risk of developing high blood pressure. Family history is one. If several members of your immediate family have high blood pressure, you're more likely to develop it. Black women and members of other minority groups are at higher risk than white women. Obesity is another major factor. Studies show that 60 percent of people with high blood pressure are overweight.

# The Sodium-Stress Link

The amount of sodium in the foods we eat is one of the biggest contributors to high blood pressure, experts say. Sodium makes us retain water, Dr. Mulrow says, which increases the volume of blood in our bodies and makes our hearts work harder to pump it. There's also evidence that sodium in some way damages the linings of blood vessels, making scarring and clogged arteries more likely.

The vast majority of our sodium intake is from the salt in our foods (table salt is about 40 percent sodium). After analyzing dozens of studies on sodium and high blood pressure, one British research team found that cutting salt by 3,000 milligrams per day—that's a little less than a teaspoon's worth—could prevent 26 percent of all strokes and 15 percent of heart attacks caused by blood clots.

Some people are more sensitive than others to the effects of salt or, more specifically, of sodium, Dr. DiBianco says. "Maybe you can eat a lot of salt, process and get rid of it quickly and not have to worry about it," he says. But maybe not. There's no reliable test for salt sensitivity. If you are overweight, don't get a lot of exercise or have a family history of high blood pressure or diabetes, Dr. DiBianco says you're probably more at risk and need to limit your salt intake.

Psychological factors can also play a role in high blood pressure. A study of 129 college students at the University of British Columbia in Vancouver showed that women who felt they got little social support from friends, family members or co-workers had slightly higher systolic readings. Researchers are not sure why this is. Job stress may lead to high blood pressure, too. Another study of 129 working adults found that women with high-status, high-pressure jobs showed significantly bigger increases in blood pressure during the workday than those with less demanding jobs.

Scientists have found that the combination of too much sodium and high stress can create a powerful pressure problem. A study of 32 students at the Johns Hopkins University School of Medicine in Baltimore showed that people who ate high-sodium diets and faced high-stress conditions for a two-week period saw their systolic blood pressure readings jump more than 6 points. The

# How Low Can You Go?

When it comes to blood pressure, the lower, the better.

"It doesn't really matter how low your reading is, even if it's something very, very low, like 85 systolic. As long as you're not feeling any ill effects from it, that's just fine. In fact, you should feel good knowing you're in a low-risk group," says Robert DiBianco, M.D., director of cardiology research at the Washington Adventist Hospital in Takoma Park, Maryland.

The landmark Framingham Heart Study, which took a decades-long look at the health of more than 5,200 residents of Framingham, Massachusetts, found that people with systolic blood pressure readings below 120 mm Hg (millimeters of mercury) had the least chance of suffering heart attacks. The risk rose steadily with increased pressure. People with the highest readings, 170 mm Hg or above, were more than three times more likely to die of heart attacks than those at or below 120 mm Hg.

Still, there are a couple of problems to watch for with low blood pressure. As people age, they're more likely to suffer from a form of temporary low blood pressure called orthostatic hypotension—the sensation you get when you hop out of bed and suddenly feel weak, like the room is spinning or the lights are dimmed. "If you have ever fainted from that, or if it happens more than very, very rarely, you should see a doctor," Dr. DiBianco says. The problem could be caused by mild dehydration, a reaction to medication, fever, illness or heat exhaustion, he says.

For some people, especially the elderly and people with diabetes or heart disease and possibly those being treated for high blood pressure, readings that fall too low may be a particular risk. If you fit in one of these groups, consult your doctor, Dr. DiBianco says.

---

high-sodium, low-stress people, by comparison, saw increases of just 0.6 point, and the low-sodium, high-stress people showed increases of just 0.1 point.

There's also a link between birth control pills and high blood pressure in some women, Dr. Mulrow says. The newer low-dose oral contraceptives have greatly decreased the problem of elevated blood pressure, although smoking and taking the Pill will increase your chances of high blood pressure, according to Dr. Mulrow.

Then there's alcohol. Scientists have long known that excess drinking can contribute to high blood pressure. But a study from the Research Institute on Alcoholism in Buffalo, New York, shows that how often you drink may be as important as how much you drink. Researchers looked at 1,635 residents of Erie County, New York, and found that people who drank every day had systolic readings 6.6 points higher and diastolic readings 4.7 points higher than people who drank only once a week. But the study found no significant relationship between blood pressure and the total amount of alcohol consumed.

## Easing the Pressure

Lots of prescription drugs help reduce high blood pressure. Diuretics flush excess fluids from the body. Beta-blockers reduce the heart rate and the heart's total output of blood. Vasodilators widen arteries and allow easier blood flow. Sympathetic nerve inhibitors also prevent blood vessels from constricting.

But drugs should be a last resort. They can cause fatigue and inhibit your sex life, among other problems. The trick is to avoid high blood pressure in the first place—and the tips below will get you started. Even if you already have mild high blood pressure, the advice could reduce your dependence on drugs and maybe even let you control things naturally.

**Have it tested.** There's only one way to know for sure if you have high blood pressure: Have your doctor check your blood pressure. Once a year should be sufficient, unless your doctor orders more tests. It's a quick, painless procedure. The doctor puts an inflatable cuff around your arm and checks your pulse with a stethoscope. If you show a borderline high reading, the doctor may order several retests over a couple of weeks or months.

You can even find do-it-yourself blood pressure monitors in pharmacies, grocery stores and shopping malls. These can give you a rough estimate of your blood pressure, but Dr. Mulrow warns that the machines aren't a substitute for an annual doctor's visit. Some machines are not well calibrated and provide grossly inaccurate results. Too many external factors—have you been walking, or are you wearing a thick sleeve?—can interfere.

**Lighten up.** If you're overweight, even moderate weight loss may help lower your blood pressure, says Marvin Moser, M.D., clinical professor of medicine at Yale University School of Medicine in New Haven, Connecticut, and senior adviser to the National High Blood Pressure Education Program. In some cases, he says, weight loss of 10 to 15 pounds may be enough to lower slightly elevated blood pressure to normal and help you avoid medication.

A nationwide study of 162 overweight women, ages 30 to 54, showed how well weight loss can work. Over a 12-month period, the women on a weight loss program lost an average of six pounds. Their systolic readings fell an average of 3.7 points, while diastolic readings fell 4.1 points.

**Move it.** Exercise, combined with a low-fat diet, is the best way to lose weight and keep your arteries clog-free. Research shows that people who don't exercise are 35 to 50 percent more likely to develop high blood pressure. And the American College of Sports Medicine says that regular aerobic training can reduce systolic and diastolic blood pressure by as much as ten points.

You don't have to be a marathon runner to reap the benefits, either. In fact, some studies have found that lower-intensity workouts such as walking are as good or better at lowering blood pressure than running or other heavy-duty aerobic activities. Many experts recommend working out at least three times a week for 20 minutes a pop.

**Shake it off.** Remember that not everyone is sensitive to the effects of sodium. But until doctors can reliably tell who is or isn't, it's a good idea to limit your intake. "It certainly isn't going to hurt anyone to cut down on salt and probably will be of real value if you're successful," Dr. DiBianco says.

Cut salt from your diet wherever you can. Most of us are eating about 2½ times more than we should. Swearing off the table shaker will have some effect. But research shows that three-fourths of all the salt we eat comes from processed foods such as cheese, soup, bread, baked goods and snacks.

"You have to read labels," Dr. Mulrow says. Check for sodium content, and shoot for a daily total of about 2,400 milligrams. When shopping, look for labels that say "low sodium." That means they contain no more than 140 milligrams of sodium per serving. And spend some extra time in the produce aisle. Almost every fruit and vegetable is naturally low in sodium.

Be careful when you eat out, too. You'll be surprised how fast sodium can add up. A hamburger from your favorite fast-food restaurant, for instance, may give you almost half a day's total.

**Pile on the potassium.** Studies have shown that eating 3,500 milligrams of potassium can help counteract sodium and keep blood volume—and blood pressure—down. And it's easy to get enough. A baked potato packs 838 milligrams of potassium all by itself, and one cup of spinach has 800 milligrams. Other potassium-packed foods include bananas, orange juice, corn, cabbage and broccoli. Check with your doctor before taking potassium supplements. Too much may aggravate kidney problems.

**Meet your magnesium needs.** Researchers seem to have found a link between low magnesium intake and high blood pressure. But just how much magnesium you need to combat high blood pressure remains unclear. For now, Dr. DiBianco says, your best bet is to get the Recommended Dietary Allowance (RDA) of about 280 milligrams.

Unfortunately, America's intake of magnesium has been dropping for a century, since we started processing foods and robbing them of their trace elements. Good sources of magnesium include nuts, spinach, lima beans, peas and seafood. But don't overdo it by taking supplements; Dr. Mulrow says too much magnesium can give you a nasty case of diarrhea.

**Keep up your calcium.** The link between calcium intake and blood pressure is controversial. Some studies show that extra calcium can lower blood pressure, while others show that it has no effect.

But experts aren't yet convinced that large doses of calcium are going to help. Dr. Mulrow says getting the RDA of 800 milligrams per day—three eight-ounce glasses of skim milk provide more than enough—and keeping your other risk factors under control is the best advice for now. Other calcium sources include low-fat cheeses, canned salmon and other canned fish with bones. If you want to take calcium supplements, see your doctor, since too much calcium can cause other problems, such as kidney stones.

**Fill up with fiber.** A Swedish study of 32 people with mild high blood pressure found that taking a seven-gram tablet of fiber each day helps lower diastolic blood pressure by five points. No one is sure why; perhaps it's because of weight loss due to people being fuller and eating less or because they eat less sodium. Whatever the reason, seven extra grams of fiber is easy to find. There's almost that much in a bowl of high-fiber cereal.

**Drink in moderation.** "A little alcohol isn't going to hurt," Dr. Mulrow says. "But drinking every day, and drinking to excess, could mean trouble." For women fighting high blood pressure, three ounces of alcohol a week seems to be about the limit. A 12-year study of 1,643 women, with a mean age of 47, showed that both systolic and diastolic pressure readings begin to rise steadily after that. That means six 12-ounce beers, six 4-ounce glasses of wine or six cocktails containing 1 ounce of hard liquor a week.

**Stop smoking.** Smoking markedly increases your risk of developing a stroke or blood vessel damage from high blood pressure, says Dr. Mulrow. When you smoke, it encourages your body to deposit cholesterol within your coronary arteries. This decreases the size of your vessels and forces your heart to work harder. "Anyone with high blood pressure should stop smoking immediately," advises Dr. Mulrow.

# HYSTERECTOMY

## *Know the Facts*

**M**ost of us wouldn't knowingly choose an operation that triggers early menopause. We wouldn't knowingly choose an operation that accelerates the aging process and makes us vulnerable—a full decade earlier—to heart disease, osteoporosis and urinary incontinence. Yet that's exactly what more than a half-million American women do every year when they schedule hysterectomies.

The tragedy is that the surgery may not be necessary.

"I'd say 80 percent of hysterectomies not done for cancer can be avoided," says Herbert A. Goldfarb, M.D., clinical instructor of obstetrics and gynecology at New York University School of Medicine in New York City and author of *The No Hysterectomy Option.* They're done to solve problems for which other solutions exist.

Thirty percent of the 567,000 procedures performed annually are done to eliminate fibroids, harmless estrogen-dependent growths that pop up in half of all women of reproductive age and that regress on their own at menopause, according to research from the National Center for Health Statistics.

Just over 19 percent are done to eliminate endometriosis, a condition in which clumps of the uterine lining drift outside the uterus and take up residence in the abdominal cavity.

Nineteen percent are done for reasons that include bleeding between periods, pelvic pain and obstetric complications.

About 16 percent are done to correct a prolapsed or droopy uterus, a common consequence of several pregnancies.

Only 15 percent of all hysterectomies are done to treat cancer or precancerous conditions. Yet except for cancer, says Dr. Goldfarb, "there are effective treatments for most of these problems without cutting out the female organs."

# Instant Menopause

Why are so many hysterectomies done in non-life-threatening situations?

"Many doctors have been taught in medical school that the uterus has no purpose beyond being a receptacle for a fetus," says Dr. Goldfarb. So when gynecological problems arise in a woman in her thirties or forties when childbearing is complete, removing the uterus seems to be a "neat and tidy solution—the panacea for all pelvic problems," says Dr. Goldfarb.

The problem is that it's not—not when it thrusts women into old age before their time.

There are four types of hysterectomy. A partial hysterectomy removes most of the uterus, leaving the cervix intact. A total hysterectomy removes the entire uterus, including the cervix. A total hysterectomy with a bilateral salpingo-oophorectomy also excises the fallopian tubes and ovaries. And a radical hysterectomy removes all the above plus the upper part of the vagina and some lymph nodes.

Which operation a woman has depends on which problem a doctor is trying to solve and how he has been trained.

All forms of hysterectomy are major surgery, says Dr. Goldfarb. But the one in which the ovaries are removed—representing about half of all hysterectomies—is probably the toughest because it instantly deprives the body of its major source of the hormones estrogen and androgen.

Androgen is what gives us our sex drive. So without the ovaries, women experience a significant loss of libido, says Dr. Goldfarb. And estrogen is that magic elixir that keeps our skin soft, the vagina lubricated, our arteries flexible, our bladder openings taut and our bones strong. It can even contribute to a peaceful night's sleep.

Normally, the ovaries begin to slow their production of estrogen around age 35. Month by month, year by year, the amount of estrogen slows to a trickle, usually cutting off completely three to five years after menopause.

But when the ovaries are removed and the entire body is suddenly deprived of estrogen, the body overreacts. "Hot flashes are hotter, longer and more frequent" than they would be during the gradual withdrawal of estrogen that naturally occurs, says Dr. Goldfarb.

What's more, the sudden absence of estrogen instantly accelerates various problems that a woman wouldn't expect for another decade. The bone-thinning process that leads to osteoporosis occurs twice as fast, and a study at Harvard Medical School involving 121,700 women indicates that those who had their ovaries removed doubled their risk of heart disease—unless they took estrogen supplements.

# Talk, Don't Cut, First

Women should never agree to a hysterectomy until they are fully informed about the alternatives to and consequences of the surgery, adds Nora W. Coffey, president of Hysterectomy Educational Resources and Services (HERS), a Bala Cynwyd, Pennsylvania–based nonprofit consumer group that offers information on hysterectomy alternatives to women around the world.

A study at Cornell University Medical College in New York City indicates that more than half of all second opinions on hysterectomy find that the procedure is inappropriate. And it is not an innocuous procedure. About one in seven women who have the operation needs repeat surgery for complications due to the operation.

So before you schedule an operation that could age your body and increase your risk of disease, consider these options.

**Seek support.** Even though there are millions of women who have had hysterectomies, many faced it alone—unnecessarily. But if you're considering this procedure, you can get help from HERS. "We offer free counseling about the alternatives to hysterectomy that many women may not know about as well as counseling to women who have undergone hysterectomies," says Coffey.

**Check with another specialist.** Maybe the problem really isn't your uterus. In a study of 200 women with normal-size uteruses referred to a San Diego clinic, researchers found that 80 percent of the women who were told they should have hysterectomies to alleviate their chronic pelvic pain actually had gastrointestinal or other non-gynecological problems. "You can have your uterus removed and still have pain," says Francis Hutchins, M.D., clinical associate professor of obstetrics and gynecology at Thomas Jefferson University Hospital and vice chair of gynecology at Graduate Hospital, both in Philadelphia. So if you have pelvic pain, have a thorough evaluation for various causes before you assume the cause is gynecological, says Dr. Hutchins.

**Exercise your pelvic muscles.** Rather than having a prolapsed uterus removed, try exercising it, says Dr. Hutchins. Ligaments supporting the uterus frequently get weak after childbearing. But Kegel exercises, particularly when combined with an estrogen cream vaginally applied, can help increase the tone of the supporting ligaments.

To build both the uterus and the ligaments, simply tighten your muscles for several seconds as though you were holding urine and then release. Do the exercise up to 20 times a day, says Dr. Hutchins.

**Ask about a scrape.** If your problem is abnormally heavy bleeding—which can result from fibroids, hormonal problems or other causes—ask your doctor about scraping away a portion of your uterine lining to control it. This procedure, which stops heavy bleeding by "cleaning out" the part of the uterus that has a rich blood supply, is done in two ways:

• Dilation and curettage (D & C) is a procedure in which the cervix is dilated and the uterine lining is scraped and removed with a long spoon-shaped instrument.

• Endometrial ablation is a newer procedure that uses a hot coiled instrument called a resectoscope to destroy the lining of the uterus. There's less pain and faster recovery than with a hysterectomy, but it can lead to infertility, and studies show that it's completely successful only about half the time.

# Planning for the Aftermath

Experts say you shouldn't rush into a hysterectomy without complete information on side effects, recovery time and the physical and emotional changes you can expect.

If a hysterectomy is necessary for you, here's how to make the most of it.

**Ask about a vaginal hysterectomy.** In many hysterectomies, the uterus can be removed through the vagina rather than through an incision that's four to six inches long across the abdomen. When a laparoscope is used to help this procedure, it is called a laparoscopic assisted vaginal hysterectomy (LAVH). LAVH leaves no visible scar and can sometimes be handled on an outpatient basis, says Joseph Gambone, D.O., associate professor of obstetrics and gynecology at the University of California, Los Angeles, UCLA School of Medicine.

LAVH requires a well-trained surgeon, so when getting referrals from your primary physician, ask for surgeons who are board-certified in gynecology and obstetrics and who have experience in this procedure, advises Dr. Hutchins. And don't be shy about interviewing more than one surgeon. Keep talking until you find one with whom you're comfortable.

**Fight for your body.** Some doctors who perform hysterectomies advocate removing ovaries as a preventive measure against ovarian cancer. But unless you have cancer or a family history of the disease, don't be talked into it: A woman's lifetime chances of dying from ovarian cancer are only about 2 in 100, says Dr. Gambone. Meanwhile, removing your ovaries without adequate hormone replacement therapy can double your risk of developing osteoporosis and heart disease—the number-one killer of women.

**Ask about low-dose estrogen.** If you must have your ovaries removed, estrogen replacement therapy (ERT) is the best way to protect against heart disease and symptoms of osteoporosis, says Dr. Hutchins. But ask your doctor about the lowest possible effective dose, since ERT may increase your risk of breast cancer and other conditions, says Dr. Goldfarb. Fortunately, doctors believe that by combining estrogen with progestin (another female hormone), you may be able to reduce your cancer risk.

**Start a regular walking program.** If a family history of cancer makes you a bad candidate for ERT, it's essential that you get regular exercise and plenty of calcium in order to slow the bone loss that can lead to osteoporosis. Australian researchers found that a brisk 30-minute walk at least three times weekly helped slow the rate of bone loss in postmenopausal women when coupled with 1,000 milligrams of supplemental calcium each day.

That's because weight-bearing exercises such as walking help build bone mass. Exercise is also a great way to keep your heart healthy, since estrogen deprivation can change the way your body processes cholesterol and can cause hardening of the arteries.

**Include your partner.** If you're considering a hysterectomy, talk with your partner and consider including your partner in discussions with your gynecologist about its effects. With the uterus gone, women will notice changes in their orgasms. The earth-shaking contractions that affect the uterus at climax will be missing, although other tissues will still be just as volatile. Including your partner in a discussion of how your physical sensations may change may prevent future problems in the bedroom, says Dr. Hutchins.

# INFERTILITY

## *When Nature Needs a Boost*

**W**hen she got married in her early twenties, Carla Harkness thought she had plenty of time to have children.

"We wanted kids, but we wanted to get a home and our careers going before we started a family," says Harkness, a 43-year-old freelance writer in Berkeley, California, and author of *The Infertility Book*.

But as she approached 30 and she and her husband, Bob, decided the time was right, nature didn't cooperate. "We tried for about a year, and nothing happened," Carla recalls. "Meanwhile, everyone in our age group seemed to be getting pregnant. Our friends and family started asking us what the problem was—why were we waiting so long? There was this feeling that we didn't have much time left to try. I really felt like my biological clock was my enemy and I was aging fast."

Carla and Bob's story is typical of the 10 to 15 percent of American couples who struggle with infertility. Like many other couples, they watched months turn into years and hope melt into disappointment. Sex became a chore, and each month that Carla didn't conceive made her feel a little more over the hill.

"Infertility is devastating. One of the major aspects of a woman's sense of youthfulness is her ability to reproduce," says Reed C. Moskowitz, M.D., founder and medical director of the Stress Disorders Medical Services at New York University Medical Center in New York City and author of *Your Healing Mind*. "There's nothing more devastating to a woman than struggling with the realization that she can't conceive a child. Psychologically, it can damage her self-esteem and make her feel like she is really getting old and decrepit."

## What Is Infertility?

Most likely, you learned the ABCs of making babies in a high school sex education class. You probably remember your teacher droning on about how nor-

## How to Talk to Your Mate

Your dream of cuddling your baby in your arms and his hope of coaching your kid in Little League is fading. Your sex life has all the excitement and spontaneity of frozen waffles. Then one day your frustration mounts and explodes into a raging argument.

No matter how caring you are, the strain that infertility places on your relationship can be enormous. Fortunately, you can alleviate the tension if you maintain good communication and use this problem to strengthen your bond rather than tear it apart, says Reed C. Moskowitz, M.D., founder and medical director of the Stress Disorders Medical Services at New York University Medical Center in New York City and author of *Your Healing Mind*.

"Accept that it is not you or he that has the problem. As a couple, you have a problem together. It affects both of you," Dr. Moskowitz says. "It's irrelevant who has the physical difficulty. Remember that both of you have the psychological pain because both of you want that little darling."

Try to focus on the positive aspects of your relationship and realize the quality of your life together can continue to improve even if you don't overcome the infertility, says Vicki Rachlin, Ph.D., psychologist and co-director of the Womankind Counseling Center in Concord, New Hampshire. You should also encourage your mate to share his feelings with you.

"Men aren't given much of an opportunity in this culture to express feelings other than anger or frustration," Dr. Rachlin says. "So a woman might say to the man in her life 'It's okay to be sad about our infertility problems. It's okay to feel vulnerable about this.' That may help him get in touch with the range of his emotions."

---

mally during intercourse a man ejaculates millions of sperm into the woman's vagina and these sperm travel up into the fallopian tubes. There, if the couple happens to have sex during the one or two days a month when a woman's egg is released from the ovary and is traveling down one of the tubes, the sperm and the egg meet. If one of the sperm penetrates the egg, fertilization occurs, and pregnancy begins. If conditions are ideal and the couple doesn't use contraception, there is a one in five chance of pregnancy each month.

But your teacher probably didn't tell you what could go wrong. Infertility is

## Searching for the Cause

It's been a year, and you're still not pregnant. It's definitely time to see your physician.

First, your doctor will review your medical history and order a complete physical. If this doesn't identify the problem, you and your partner will undergo diagnostic tests. Here's a look at what a woman might expect.

*Blood test to check for progesterone levels.* These rise after ovulation and stimulate the development of the uterine lining in preparation for receiving a fertilized egg. This test is scheduled for the 20th or 21st day in a 28-day cycle. A low progesterone level may mean that the endometrial lining has not developed sufficiently for a fertilized egg to implant.

*Postcoital or Sims-Huhner test.* Examines the quality of cervical mucus and the ability of sperm to penetrate it and checks for any signs of sexually transmitted disease or bacteria. Within a few hours of intercourse, a small amount of cervical mucus is removed with a syringe. A normal test shows large numbers of healthy, active sperm.

*Endometrial biopsy.* Tests a sample of uterine lining for any abnormalities and to determine if ovulation has occurred. After the 21st day in a

usually diagnosed after a couple has had intercourse without contraception for 12 months or more and has failed to conceive. Infertility can occur even if you've had children in the past. About 40 to 50 percent of the time, doctors determine that the woman has problems in her reproductive tract, says Frederick Licciardi, M.D., assistant professor of obstetrics and gynecology at the New York University School of Medicine in New York City. In another 40 percent, they can pinpoint that the man is the cause of the problem. Sometimes both the man and the woman have difficulties that are interfering with pregnancy, and about 10 percent of the time, doctors can't determine the cause.

For a woman, the basic problem usually is that she isn't ovulating (producing an egg) or that her fallopian tubes are blocked or damaged so that the egg and sperm can't meet. There are many causes for these two conditions, including hormone deficiencies, pelvic infections, fibroid tumors, cysts, sexually transmitted diseases such as gonorrhea and chlamydia and endometriosis, the disease that caused Carla Harkness's infertility. Endometriosis occurs when cells from the uterus begin growing on the ovaries and in the fallopian tubes, causing inflammation and scarring.

28-day cycle, a sample of uterine tissue is surgically removed during an exam similar to a pelvic exam. The tissue should be spongy. Although new instruments make this test almost painless, some women still find it uncomfortable. Ask about local anesthesia.

*Hysterosalpingogram.* Checks if both fallopian tubes are open and inspects internal contours of the uterus. About a week after menstruation, dye is injected into the uterus during a pelvic exam. An x-ray shows the outline of the uterus and tubes. Most women feel cramping during this procedure, so ask for an anti-inflammatory before the test. A slower injection paced to the woman's tolerance is less painful.

*Laparoscopy.* Checks for any abnormalites, endometriosis and scarring and blockage of the uterus, fallopian tubes and ovaries. In this surgical procedure, a telescope called a laparoscope is inserted into the abdomen through an incision in the navel, so organs can be inspected closely for abnormalities. Minor adhesions can be removed during surgery, which is performed under general anesthesia but does not require hospitalization. You may feel some pain afterward due to the incision.

"At least 50 percent of women who come to an infertility clinic have endometriosis," says Donald I. Galen, M.D., director of the In Vitro Fertilization and Reproduction Medical Division at San Ramon Regional Medical Center in San Ramon, California. "No one really knows why it happens, but it definitely interferes with fertility."

Endometriosis and pelvic infections can also cause ectopic (tubal) pregnancies. About 1 in every 100 pregnancies is ectopic, meaning that instead of traveling on to the uterus, the fertilized egg implants itself and starts to grow on the fallopian tube or ovary or even in the abdomen. An ectopic pregnancy must be ended because, untreated, the growing fetus can endanger the life of the mother or severely damage the fallopian tubes and prevent future pregnancies, according to Niels Lauersen, M.D., Ph.D., a founding member of the New York Society of Reproductive Medicine in New York City and author of *Getting Pregnant.*

Impaired cervical mucus, a discharge that usually helps carry sperm into the uterus, is another cause of infertility. If cervical mucus is thickened or is reduced in quantity, sperm may be prevented from reaching the fallopian tubes, says Eli Reshef, M.D., a reproductive endocrinologist at the University of Oklahoma Health Sciences Center in Oklahoma City. Fertility experts suspect some women can also develop antibodies that mistakenly identify sperm as harmful invading organisms and that reduce sperm's capacity to reach or penetrate the egg.

Smoking, alcohol abuse, drugs, stress and exposure to pollution, chemicals and radiation can also reduce a woman's fertility, Dr. Galen says.

## When Time Marches On

But for many women, the real problem is time, because as a woman ages, her fertility—that all too real biological clock—gradually winds down.

"Age 40 is a critical time for women, because that's when we start to see dramatic declines in their fertility rates," Dr. Galen says.

"Infertility occurs in less than 1 percent of couples in their teens," says Sherman Silber, M.D., a fertility specialist at St. Luke's Hospital in St. Louis and author of *How to Get Pregnant with the New Technology.* "In the twenties, it rises to 13 to 15 percent and climbs steadily until 35, when it takes a dramatic turn upward. Twenty-five percent of couples between the ages of 35 and 40 are infertile, and after 40, nearly 50 percent will not be able to conceive."

So although infertility is usually considered a possibility after one year, couples older than 35 who have tried unsuccessfully to conceive for six months should seek medical help, Dr. Licciardi says.

"After six months, come in and at least get some testing started," Dr. Licciardi suggests. "It doesn't mean you have to do anything at that point, but at least you'll get rolling with the diagnostic process."

## Beating the Clock

Overcoming female infertility often requires the help of a gynecologist or reproductive endocrinologist, who, after testing, may suggest fertility drugs or high-tech wizardry (more on that later). But there are some natural ways you can try to boost your chances of having a child. Here's how.

**It takes good timing.** Make sure you're ovulating when you try to get pregnant. Remember that you produce only one egg a month and that it can be fertilized only during the one or two days after you ovulate. "Yes, most woman know approximately when they ovulate, but sometimes they're not exactly sure," Dr. Licciardi says. To find out if the time is right, you can keep track of your basal body temperature. Each day, take your temperature when you awaken, before you do anything else. Your temperature should drop just before ovulation and rise after an egg is released. If that seems like too much hassle, then consider getting an ovulation predictor kit, an over-the-counter urine test that changes colors if you're about to ovulate. It's available at most pharmacies.

**Soothe your stress.** "Stress can disrupt ovulation and cause spasms of the fallopian tubes, which interfere with the passage of the egg down the tube," Dr.

Moskowitz says. Practicing stress reduction techniques such as biofeedback or progressive muscle relaxation can help.

**Make sure you're turned on.** Women who are really aroused produce higher hormone levels, and that may increase their chances of getting pregnant, Dr. Lauersen says. Allow at least 20 minutes for foreplay, he suggests.

**Close the escape hatch.** Immediately after intercourse, lightly press the lips of your vagina together with your fingers for several minutes, Dr. Lauersen suggests. Doing this will help keep sperm inside you and give them a chance to begin swimming toward the fallopian tubes.

**Don't move.** After sex, lie on your back with a pillow under your pelvis for 20 to 30 minutes. This will encourage sperm to move toward your fallopian tubes, Dr. Lauersen says.

**Try cough medicine.** Cough medicines containing the active ingredient guaifenesin (such as Robitussin) thin out cervical mucus and help sperm swim through it easier, Dr. Lauersen says. Take one or two teaspoons a day, beginning three or four days before you ovulate.

**Put a cap on lubricants.** Jellies and other lubricants may make sex easier, but they can impair the sperm's motility even if they don't contain spermicides, says Wolfram Nolten, M.D., associate professor of endocrinology at the University of Wisconsin–Madison Center for Health Studies.

**Ease up on extreme exercise.** Intense exercise such as running 40 or more miles a week may cause irregular periods and disrupt ovulation, says Mary Jane De Souza, Ph.D., an exercise physiologist at the University of Connecticut Health Center in Farmington. The reasons are still unclear, but torrid exercise may suppress production of reproductive hormones.

However, moderate aerobic exercise such as walking, swimming or biking, three times a week, 20 to 30 minutes a session, shouldn't affect your ability to get pregnant, Dr. Reshef says.

**Whack the weed habit.** If you smoke, your chances of becoming a mom may literally be going up in smoke, Dr. Galen says. Women who smoke produce fewer eggs. Even if she does get pregnant, a woman who smokes is more likely to have a miscarriage than a woman who doesn't.

**Steer clear of carbon monoxide.** Studies suggest that carbon monoxide may drive down fertility rates. That's another reason to quit smoking and to stay away from secondary smoke, since both produce large amounts of carbon monoxide. Wood-burning stoves and fireplaces also create carbon monoxide, so make sure that your flues are clear and that your rooms are well ventilated, says Jarnail Singh, Ph.D., professor of biology and environmental toxicology at Stillman College in Tuscaloosa, Alabama. The federal Environmental Protection Agency also recommends that you have your home heating system checked annually to make sure that the exhaust system is working properly.

**Get your protein.** Of course it's hard to avoid all the places where there are high concentrations of carbon monoxide, but a protein-rich diet can be a good way to fight back, Dr. Singh says. In laboratory studies, Dr. Singh found that mice exposed to carbon monoxide and fed a diet that was only 8 percent protein were five times less fertile than mice in the same environment that were fed 16 percent protein. "The best suggestions I could make for women who are trying to get pregnant are to increase the amount of protein in their diets and to avoid any kind of environment where carbon monoxide is present," he says.

If you want to boost the protein in your diet, a typical day's menu might include a cup of oatmeal and a cup of yogurt for breakfast, a tuna salad sandwich and a cup of navy bean soup for lunch, a cup of yogurt for an afternoon snack and a cup or two of lasagna for dinner. Avoid traditional sources of protein such as fatty beef and other red meats because they're loaded with saturated fat and cholesterol, which contribute to heart disease.

**Keep your weight in line.** Reproductive hormones, including estrogen, are thrown out of balance if you're too skinny or overweight, and that will make getting pregnant much harder, Dr. Lauersen says. For maximum fertility, try to maintain a weight within the range suggested by your gynecologist.

**Curb your caffeine.** Coffee, tea, colas and other beverages containing caffeine may increase your risk of some types of infertility, says Francine Grodstein, Ph.D., an epidemiologist at Harvard University School of Public Health in Boston. In a study comparing the caffeine consumption (prior to conception) of 3,833 women who had recently given birth and 1,050 women who had infertility problems, Dr. Grodstein found that women who drank more than two cups of caffeinated coffee or four cans of cola per day had greater risk of having tubal damage or endometriosis. She speculates that caffeine either constricts blood flow and damages the fallopian tubes or stimulates estrogen production, which can lead to endometriosis.

**Dissect your drugs.** Although most medications do not affect your chances of conceiving, some prescription drugs such as antidepressants and illegal ones such as marijuana and cocaine increase your risk of infertility and other sexual problems, according to Dr. Lauersen. Discuss any over-the-counter, prescription or illegal drugs you are taking with your gynecologist.

**Limit your liquor.** Excessive amounts of alcohol can cause irregular ovulation. "Drink in moderation," Dr. Galen says. "I'd say no more than one or two alcoholic drinks a day."

# High-Tech Conception

Okay, so like Carla Harkness, you and your partner have tried everything natural, and you're still not parents. Don't give up hope yet. In most cases, experts can pinpoint and treat infertility problems with dramatic advances in drugs and surgery. More than half the couples seeking such treatment will get pregnant. RESOLVE, a support group for infertile couples, can refer you to a specialist in your area. Write to 1310 Broadway, Somerville, MA 02144-1731.

So what will a doctor do? After thorough testing, he may prescribe fertility drugs such as clomiphene (Clomid) or menotropins (Pergonal) to stimulate ovulation. If you have endometriosis or blocked fallopian tubes or have had an ectopic pregnancy, your doctor may recommend corrective surgery. In Carla's case, she had two surgeries over five years to remove her endometriosis and tried several medications. Within three years, she had a daughter, then a son seven years later.

If there has been scarring of the fallopian tubes or a patient doesn't respond to fertility drugs, doctors will suggest one of the many high-tech fertilization methods.

These aren't cheap—they can cost more than $15,000—and often aren't covered by insurance. Here's a sample of some of the most successful high-tech options.

*Artificial insemination.* Semen is deposited directly into the vagina or uterus. If the man's sperm is of poor quality, the couple could try donor sperm.

*In vitro fertilization (IVF).* Eggs are surgically removed from a woman's ovaries, transferred to a petri dish and mixed with her partner's sperm for fertilization. After a two-day incubation, usually a few fertilized eggs (or embryos) are placed into the uterus.

*Gamete intrafallopian transfer (GIFT).* Eggs and sperm (gametes) are inserted into the fallopian tube, where, it is hoped, fertilization takes place.

*Zygote intrafallopian transfer (ZIFT).* As in IVF, eggs and sperm are combined in a petri dish and incubated for two days. But rather than being placed into the uterus, the embryo, or zygote, is placed into the fallopian tube. From there it will travel a natural course down the tube and into the womb for implantation. The advantage of this procedure over GIFT is that you know fertilization has taken place.

*Zona drilling.* In this laboratory test-tube technique, a surgeon uses chemicals, a laser beam or a needle to open part of the outer layer of the egg, or the zona pellucida, so that sperm have a better chance of penetration.

*Microinjection.* In this procedure, which is in the experimental stage, a thin needle is used to insert a single sperm into an egg.

# INJURIES AND ACCIDENTS

## *They're Easy to Avoid*

T he ice pack is doing its job. The pain has receded, the swelling is down, and your knee—except for an interesting configuration of cuts and colors—looks the way it's supposed to.

But it's going to be a few days before you're up and around. And right now, confined to a chair, feeling stiff and sore, you know that the next time you take a shortcut from one trail to another, you won't scramble across an outcropping of rock as though you were related to a mountain goat.

Nothing is more likely to make you feel like your body is 110 years old than an injury that lands you on your back or confines you to a chair. But whether the injury is caused by a car accident, a fall or a tricky move in a game of volleyball, just about everyone is at risk for an injury at one time or another.

According to the National Safety Council, injuries kill approximately 83,000 Americans every year, primarily through traffic accidents or falls. Despite what you might think, the risk isn't reserved for the elderly. In fact, more than half of all accidental deaths occur among men and women who are between the ages of 25 and 44.

But most of us won't die from injuries or accidents; we'll be temporarily sidelined. And for people between the ages of 25 and 44, the usual cause is a strained or torn muscle from a sports injury.

## The Sports Connection

Sports injuries result in 6,000 deaths a year. Nonfatal injuries in recreational activities such as baseball and softball, basketball, football and bicycling put more than two million people in the emergency room every year. Add to that the mammoth numbers of strains and sprains that are treated in locker rooms, plus injuries suffered in dozens of other sports, and you can understand why the National Safety Council estimates that the total number of sports injuries exceeds three million each year.

People between the ages of 25 and 64 account for more than 74 percent of all emergency room visits for scuba-diving injuries, 68 percent for squash, racquetball and paddleball injuries, 51 percent for horseback-riding injuries, 45 percent for fishing injuries, 44 percent for tennis injuries, 42 percent for volleyball injuries and 40 percent for weight-lifting injuries.

Why are so many people in this age group getting hurt? "By age 25, people have become 'weekend athletes,' " explains Stephen J. Nicholas, M.D., associate team physician for the New York Jets and associate director of the Nicholas Institute of Sports Medicine and Athletic Injuries at Lenox Hill Hospital in New York City. "They're getting more involved with work, and social demands begin to take precedence over physical well-being.

"It's like putting your body in a cast and taking it out only on weekends," says Dr. Nicholas. "The muscles get short, weak and stiff. And they're no longer able to function at their optimal levels."

Studies show that women are most likely to experience ankle injuries, says Christine Wells, Ph.D., a member of the National Collegiate Athletic Association's Committee on Competitive Safeguards and Medical Aspects of Sport and professor of exercise science and physical education at Arizona State University in Tempe. The shoulder and knee also are frequently injured by women—the shoulder primarily from volleyball spikes and pitching, and the knee from a variety of stretches and twists.

Since men and women are equally likely to taper off their sports activities after age 25, both are liable to have bodies that are not quite up to extreme athletics on weekends.

Unfortunately, they still might think they're in peak condition, says Dr. Nicholas. So when they play sports such as tennis on the weekend, they push their bodies the way they used to when they were playing several times a week.

The result? The muscles fatigue, cramp, strain, then pull to the point where they can actually tear, says Dr. Nicholas.

## How to Reduce Your Risk

It's difficult to rein yourself in when you're going for that extra mile or point, Dr. Nicholas adds. But here's how you can help your body keep up—and reduce your risk of injury.

**Take a high school exam.** If you're over age 25 and participating in weekend sports, schedule a physical exam with a family physician who does the local high school's team physicals, suggests Rosemary Agostini, M.D., a staff physician at the Virginia Mason Sports Clinic and clinical associate professor at the University of Washington, both in Seattle.

Ask her to give you the same type of physical that she gives the local football or basketball team, including a review of any previous sports injuries. Combined with a "weekend warrior" approach to sports, old injuries have a way of coming back to haunt you—sometimes on a chronic basis, says Dr. Agostini. A physician can evaluate the likelihood of that happening and make specific suggestions to avoid reinjury.

**Balance your diet.** "Some women athletes get so into exercise that they don't eat appropriately," says Dr. Agostini. "They don't end up with eating disorders, but they do have disordered eating patterns," in which they'll eat only pasta and vegetables one week or only fruits another.

But you can't build muscle or improve performance without eating a balanced diet, explains Dr. Agostini. A lack of calcium to build strong bones, a lack of iron to build red blood cells or a lack of protein to build and maintain muscle can not only sabotage your performance but set you up for injury as well.

Ask the doctor who does your physical to recommend a local sports nutritionist. Then work with her to develop an eating program that suits your particular needs.

**Watch your periods.** Some women will cease to menstruate when they reach certain exercise levels, says Dr. Agostini. The level is different for everyone, but it signals a hormonal imbalance that should be evaluated and corrected. If it's not, says Dr. Agostini, you're at increased risk for stress fractures or premature osteoporosis. So see your doctor if your periods stop for more than three cycles.

**Turn in your shoes every 500 miles.** Shoes need to provide good support and shock absorption to prevent injuries, says Dr. Agostini. Replace them every six months or 500 miles, whichever comes first. And remember that your foot size will probably be larger after pregnancy. So treat yourself to a new pair of shoes once the baby is born.

**Keep moving.** "You'll be able to minimize injuries if you go on a regular exercise program—one that involves 30 or 40 minutes every day or at least three or four times a week," says Dr. Nicholas. The point is that your body not be allowed five or six days in a row in which to stiffen up.

**Stretch.** Begin your exercise program with at least 25 minutes of stretching every time you work out, Dr. Nicholas says. The muscles in the back and front of your thighs—the hamstrings and quadriceps—plus those in the lower back are the most important to loosen up.

"They usually don't get any stretching during the day unless you specifically set out to do it," says Dr. Nicholas. "Yet one of the most common causes of lower back pain is a hamstring tightness that causes a pelvic tilt.

"If you can maintain your hamstrings in a loosened fashion," he adds, "you might minimize not only the number of hamstring pulls or lower extremity injuries you get but also the amount of lower back pain you develop in the future."

**Make your body work.** After you stretch, do any aerobic exercise—walking, running, jumping—that accelerates your heart rate and keeps you breathing hard—hard, not panting—for 20 minutes, says Dr. Nicholas.

The only exception is during the last trimester of pregnancy, he adds, when "the body releases a hormone called relaxin, which relaxes the body's soft tissue structures to prepare for childbirth." Unfortunately, it also loosens up all the ligaments holding your joints together.

Carrying on your regular aerobic exercise is fine as long as you have been cleared to exercise by your physician, says Dr. Nicholas. But you don't want to try for some new personal best during this period, because the increased stress on your relaxin-loosened joints makes you vulnerable to injury.

**Lift.** Strengthen your muscles by lifting at least a minimal amount of weight, says Dr. Nicholas. Get an athletic trainer to review your doctor's exam and recommendations and then to prescribe the specific weights and number of repetitions you should do. And don't forget to stretch before your workout.

Women in the last trimester of pregnancy should avoid weights altogether. Relaxin plus the joint stress from weights could predispose them to injury.

**Activate your relationships.** "I was talking to a friend of mine the other day, and we admitted that as we get older, there's always something that gets in the way of exercise," says Dr. Nicholas. "You have to meet someone for a drink, or you're trying to deal with a mortgage, a patient or the kids."

But if you arrange to meet friends for a game of tennis instead of a drink or you take your kids to the ice rink instead of a movie, he says, you're much more likely to get the extra exercise you need to stay loose and injury-free.

# When You Make a Mistake

No matter how carefully you keep your body in shape, every once in a while you're going to pull or strain something when you twist the wrong way, intensify your exercise program or simply fall over your own two feet.

So here's what Dr. Nicholas advises you to do about a pulled or strained ligament, tendon or muscle.

**Apply RICE.** RICE may be the sports world's most important acronym. It means *r*est, *i*ce, *c*ompression and *e*levation. And that's exactly what you should do for any new injury, says Dr. Nicholas. The idea is to minimize the amount of inflammation that occurs. It's inflammation that produces the swelling that causes the pain, which can then limit your movement.

"Put ice on the injury for three or four days," Dr. Nicholas says. "Apply it for 20 minutes of every hour you're awake." Wrap an elastic bandage around the injured area afterward, then elevate the injured muscle.

**Take ibuprofen.** "I also tell people to take Advil if they don't have any stomach problems," says Dr. Nicholas. That also reduces inflammation. Just follow package directions.

**Use wet heat.** Once you have RICE'd yourself for three or four days, it's time to work on getting your normal function back and preventing the injured area from becoming a chronic problem, says Dr. Nicholas.

The difficulty is that after three or four days, dried blood from torn or traumatized muscle fibers is sitting at the injured site.

"We need to get it out of the area," says Dr. Nicholas. "So we start what we call the wet heat program. We wrap a warm, wet towel around the injured area, put plastic—the kind of plastic bag you get at the dry cleaner's—around the towel to provide insulation, then put a heating pad on top.

"We leave it that way for about an hour and a half, three times a day, being careful not to burn the skin," he adds. "It will liquefy the dried blood in the injured area, bring the blood to the surface and help the body absorb it.

"It also helps with the healing process by loosening up the muscles."

**Restretch the injured muscle.** Once a muscle has been injured, both it and the surrounding muscles have contracted into shorter lengths, says Dr. Nicholas. So before you can resume your normal workouts, you have to restretch the muscles until they achieve their normal resting lengths. Ask an athletic trainer which stretches she suggests for your particular injury.

"If you don't achieve that resting length, you're more subject to chronic pulls that can occur again and again," says Dr. Nicholas.

# Falling Down on the Job

Sports injuries may be costly in terms of time, pain and aggravation, but falls are more likely to kill. And not just older people. Nearly 1,100 men and women between the ages of 25 and 44 fell to their deaths in one year.

While falls that occur in the home are most likely to involve older folks with failing eyesight or wearing floppy footwear, falls by men and women between the ages of 25 and 44 are more likely to occur on the job, says researcher John Britt, R.N., state injury prevention program coordinator at Harborview Hospital in Seattle.

People fall when they're moving from one height to another on everything from stairs and stages to ladders and girders, according to safety experts at the Occupational Safety and Health Administration (OSHA) in Washington, D.C. Railings may stop unexpectedly before the last step, movable sets may not be clamped into place on stages, safety ropes may be torn or frayed on ladders, tools may inadvertently be left on girders.

Want to make sure you're not the next one to go bottoms up at work? Here's how Britt says you can reduce your risk.

**Find the fall guy.** Every company has someone whose job it is to make detailed reports of accidents to insurance companies, safety committees and workers' compensation, says Britt. Find that person. Then ask when and where every injury took place during the past 12 months. Then make sure you don't fall into the same traps that others did.

**Make the invisible visible.** People tend to pay attention to the little things and ignore huge ones, says OSHA. They see the tiny X-Acto blade that might slice their fingers in the art room but not the pool of ink on the floor that can cause them to slip.

Walk into any room at your workplace, stand in a corner, and look for anything that can trip you up or hurt you in any other way. Then either report the hazard to management or take care of it yourself.

**Leave the high heels at home.** If your company suggests you wear flats, nonskid soles, boots or other special footwear designed to keep you from falling down on the job, do it.

# Be a Road Scholar

Many of the men and women who survive the ten million or so traffic accidents in the United States each year can no longer expect friends and co-workers to automatically extend their sympathies.

Instead, says Britt, their accident recitals are just as likely to be met with the question "Were you wearing your seat belt?" or "Did you stop by the bar before you drove home?"

"There's been a subtle shift in public opinion about motor vehicle accidents in the past couple of years," Britt explains. People used to feel sorry for accident victims. But today—partly due to national safety programs and citizen groups such as Mothers Against Drunk Driving—there's more of a sense that accidents are preventable.

What can you do? Here are three safety strategies that Britt feels will help you prevent—or survive—motor vehicle accidents.

**Banish booze.** Safety studies indicate that between 40 and 50 percent of all fatal accidents involve drunk drivers, says Britt. Alcohol is most likely to be involved in fatal crashes with adult male drivers between the ages of 20 and 55. And the more violent the crash, the more likely a drunk was at the wheel. So don't drink before you drive.

**Stay alert on Fridays and Saturdays.** One-third of all fatal crashes occur between 6:00 P.M. and 6:00 A.M. on Fridays and Saturdays, researchers report. So stay particularly alert during those times.

**Use lap/shoulder belts.** Many people simply won't wear safety belts in the mistaken belief that they have less chance of injury if they're "free" to get out of the car quickly. Unfortunately, these are the people who are least likely to get out of their vehicles at all. A study by the National Highway Traffic Safety Administration indicates that when they're worn carefully, lap/shoulder belts reduce the odds of occupant death in a crash by 45 percent.

# MEMORY

## *Forget This Myth of Aging*

**B**oy, is this going to be a day. At 10:00 A.M., you have to see Barb about the Bonner project. At 11:00 A.M., it's Bob and the Bagelman account. This afternoon, the boss has booked a briefing with Bonny in Boston about the Bledsoe bookkeeping blowup.

And so you call Barb at 10:00 A.M. to talk about Bonner. But Barry butts in with a bulletin about the Browning building. By then you have to rush to call Bob about the Bledsoe books—or was that Bonny with the Bagelman account? Belinda with Borghoff? Oh, brother. How bad can it get?

A few years ago, you probably could have kept it all straight. But you're having more trouble remembering things now, like birthdays, clients' names, phone numbers. Wait. Isn't forgetfulness a sign that age is creeping up on you?

"There's no doubt: When you forget things, it makes you feel like your mind is slipping away on you," says Douglas Herrmann, Ph.D., a memory researcher at the National Center for Health Statistics in Washington, D.C., and author of *Super Memory*.

But Dr. Herrmann says there's plenty of room for optimism. You may need to pay a little more attention to your memory, but it's probably still fully functional. "In all likelihood, you're not losing your memory," he says. "With a little focus and a little work, your memory will be just as good as it was in your teens and twenties—maybe even better."

## Still a Gray Area

Experts still don't really know how we store and recall information. One theory holds that people may keep memories in holographic, three-dimensional

## Be Predictable

Always losing your keys? Designate a spot for them in your house or office. If you put your keys—or glasses or other things—in the same place every day, you'll always know where they are, says Douglas Herrmann, Ph.D., a memory researcher at the National Center for Health Statistics in Washington, D.C., and author of *Super Memory*.

form, using networks of neurons and electrochemical reactions to gain access to the system. Researchers do know that you can reach the same memory through a number of different paths. Smells can trigger a memory, as can a familiar sight, word or phrase.

Most scientists break down memory into three parts. First is the working memory, also called the scratch-pad memory. Dr. Herrmann says people use this to recall phone numbers or other information they need for a very short period of time—usually about a minute. Then it's usually just forgotten.

The mid-range, or intermediate, memory keeps all the information you've consciously and unconsciously absorbed within the past few hours or days. Eventually, you either forget that stuff because it's not important (what did you have for breakfast three days ago?) or transfer it to long-term memory. There you store permanent recollections, such as important addresses and names, Mom's apple pie recipe and memories of childhood Christmas mornings.

For years, studies kept showing that scratch-pad and mid-range memories start declining relatively early in life—even in your forties. But the research was flawed, Dr. Herrmann says. New evidence shows that you probably won't suffer serious memory loss until well into your sixties or seventies, he says.

So why are you forgetting things more than you used to? Stress could be the culprit. "Your ability to concentrate and make decisions, along with short-term memory, may be one of the first areas of mental functioning hit by stress," says Paul J. Rosch, M.D., president of the American Institute of Stress in Yonkers, New York. And try not to worry about forgetting things; Dr. Herrmann says anxiety about memory makes it even harder to remember.

Then there's just plain old sensory overload. When life pulls you five ways at once, Dr. Herrmann says, you're less likely to concentrate on details. "And the less you pay attention, the less you're going to remember," he says.

For most women, memory loss never becomes a serious problem. But some diseases, most notably Alzheimer's, lead to direct memory trouble. If you forget significant appointments at work, can't recall the names of family

# Byte Off What You Can Chew

Computers remember information in small pieces, or bytes. That's the best way for you to do it, too, according to Francis Pirozzolo, M.D., a neuropsychologist at the Baylor College of Medicine in Houston.

The process is called chunking. Since your mind remembers items in groups of five to nine, break down lists into segments of that size. It's much easier to remember five groups of 5 items than it is to remember a list of 25 items, Dr. Pirozzolo says. And if you can group similar things together—fruits on one list, paper products on another—you'll do even better.

members or good friends or become severely disoriented or confused, see a doctor, warns Francis Pirozzolo, M.D., a neuropsychologist at Baylor College of Medicine in Houston.

# Hold That Thought

Your brain is not a computer. You can't just run to the store and buy more memory; you have to learn to use what you have.

Fortunately, you already have plenty of storage space. Here's how to take better advantage of it.

**Jog your mind.** Regular exercise may give you a memory boost. In one study, people who took a nine-week water aerobics class scored better on general memory tests than a similar non-exercising group. "The aerobic exercise may have increased oxygen efficiency to the brain," says the study's co-author, Richard Gordin, Ph.D., professor in the Department of Health, Physical Education and Recreation at Utah State University in Logan.

Dr. Gordin stresses that the results are preliminary. But other studies are coming up with similar findings. And then there are the added benefits of lower risk for heart disease and stroke and all the other helpful side effects of exercise.

**Pay attention.** This is the most basic—and most forgotten—memory aid. Don't expect to memorize a client's product line while you're talking to another client long distance. Don't expect to remember a person's name if you're thinking about what you're going to have for lunch when you make your introductions.

"It's simple," Dr. Herrmann says. "Focus, focus, focus. If it doesn't register in your brain initially, you have no chance of remembering it." So when there's key information to recall, drop what you're doing and spend a couple of minutes concentrating. Then move to the next task at hand.

**Sleep on it.** A good night's rest will do wonders for your memory. Research shows that people who are awakened during dream sleep fail to process memories from the day before and thus forget more. Dr. Herrmann also says that regular sleep allows your entire body to recharge, making you more alert and more attentive to detail. "And avoid sleeping pills," he says. "You don't get the same quality sleep, and you're less likely to remember things during the following day."

One more hint: if you're studying or working into the night, go to sleep as soon as you're done. Going out afterward for a drink or a cup of coffee, or staying up to watch the news, makes it harder to remember the information the next day.

**Be selective.** We have invented telephone books, address books, computer files, pencils, pens and those little yellow sticky pads—all to help us remember things. So use them. "Why spend time trying to memorize giant shopping lists when you can just write them down?" Dr. Pirozzolo asks. "If you are a busy person with lots to remember, making lists frees up your memory to recall more important items."

**Break the stereotype.** Studies show that many women believe members of their gender are good at remembering "female things" such as grocery lists—and bad at remembering "male things" such as directions. Untrue. Dr. Herrmann's research shows that women and men have similar memory ability but sometimes apply it differently because of lingering social stereotypes. If you want to improve on any area of your memory—with shopping lists, directions or

## Be a Slow Learner

You'll remember information longer if you absorb it gradually rather than all at once, according to Harry P. Bahrick, Ph.D., professor of psychology at Ohio Wesleyan University in Delaware, Ohio. In an eight-year study, he found that people who practiced their Spanish vocabulary once a month remembered four times more words than people who practiced daily. Dr. Bahrick says the principle works for physical skills, too. "If I was learning how to golf, I'd practice an hour a week for seven weeks rather than an hour a day for seven days," he says.

# GLAD You Can Remember

You have to buy *g*as, pick up the *l*aundry, get some *a*pples and make a bank *d*eposit. To remember the list, try forming a word using the first letter of each item—in this case, GLAD. It's called mnemonics, according to Francis Pirozzolo, M.D., a neuropsychologist at the Baylor College of Medicine in Houston. If you convert information into a familiar form, such as a simple word, you're more likely to remember it, he says.

anything else—Dr. Herrmann suggests practice. "That's the only way to get better at it," he says.

**Mind your minerals.** There's nothing better for your memory than a balanced, healthy diet with lots of fruits and vegetables, Dr. Herrmann says. There's also some evidence that keeping up your intake of zinc and boron can revive your memory, according to James G. Penland, Ph.D., research psychologist with the U.S. Department of Agriculture's Grand Forks Human Nutrition Research Center in North Dakota. One study showed that women on low-zinc diets scored lower on short-term memory than they did when they got their Recommended Dietary Allowance of 12 milligrams. A half-dozen steamed oysters gives you a whopping 76.4 milligrams of zinc. Other good sources include wheat germ, lean meats and pumpkin and squash seeds.

The same held true for boron, which your body needs in trace amounts. Women who ate high-boron diets of about three milligrams per day scored higher on tests of attention and memory. That's the same amount you'll find in three apples. Other good boron sources include prunes, dates, raisins and peanuts.

Dr. Penland points out that these studies show that you're better off with recommended levels of boron and zinc than you are at low levels. But that doesn't mean taking high doses of the two will improve memory further; proving that will take more study.

**Can the coffee.** Caffeine is a proven memory killer, Dr. Herrmann says. More than one cup during the workday is probably going to overstimulate you and make it harder to concentrate. "It's an out-and-out myth that coffee helps you remember. It may keep you awake, but by wrecking your sleep you'll remember even less," Dr. Herrmann says.

Smoking causes the same problem with overstimulation, Dr. Herrmann says. And alcohol, even one drink, reduces the ability of individual brain cells to process and store information. Long-term drinking also kills brain cells, Dr. Herrmann says.

**Ignore miracle cures.** Lots of pills and powders advertise themselves as "miracle memory boosters." They don't work, according to Thomas H. Crook, Ph.D., a clinical psychologist and president of Memory Assessment Clinics, based in Bethesda, Maryland. There has been promising research into memory enhancement drugs, but Dr. Crook says nothing on the market today will help. "They're really just nutritional supplements masquerading as cures," he says.

## Tune Out

Are you sometimes forced to remember information amid the chaos at home or work? Practice will help. Turn on the television loudly and then try to concentrate on something else for a few minutes, such as reading a book or memorizing a phone number. This will help you overcome the background noise and pay attention, says Douglas Herrmann, Ph.D., a memory researcher at the National Center for Health Statistics in Washington, D.C., and author of *Super Memory*. You could also try watching two televisions at the same time. That forces you to pay attention only to important information and helps you hone your concentration.

# MENOPAUSAL CHANGES

## *They're Bound to Happen Sometime*

**Y**our girlfriend called the other day, and you still can't get the conversation out of your mind.

"I've noticed some changes in my body lately," she said. "And I can't help wondering if I'm starting."

"Starting what?" you asked, half distracted by thoughts about your upcoming vacation.

"Menopause."

Menopause! That sure caught your attention. Here was your best friend—the one that's only a few years older than you—talking about a health issue that you didn't think you had to worry about yet. You knew it would happen to both of you eventually. But not now. Not so soon. Neither of you is even 50 years old yet. Menopause was meant for your mother and your great-aunt. It's something for . . . older women.

For most women, menopause is a landmark of aging, says Ellen Klutznick, Psy.D., a psychologist in private practice in San Francisco who specializes in women's health issues. How women respond to it varies greatly.

While women who've already gone through menopause often see it as a new beginning, younger women who aren't there yet tend to feel more anxious about the transition, says Dr. Klutznick. "They are worried about how they are going to feel when they are 50 and about feeling old. They see it as aging," she says.

First, menopause marks the end of a woman's reproductive years. "The biological clock is ticking away for a lot of these younger women, and it's frightening," says Dr. Klutznick. For them, menopause is about the loss of their fertility, and in a society that places great emphasis on youth, beauty and reproduction, this can be difficult, she says. The loss of the potential to have children can be hard even for women who are finished having children or for those who never planned to, agrees Brian Walsh, M.D., director of the Menopause Clinic at Brigham and Women's Hospital in Boston. "They have lost the ability to choose. A door has been closed," he says.

Women are also concerned about how menopause is going to affect their physical appearance. They're worried that their bodies and skin won't be the same—that their breasts will sag, their faces will wrinkle and their waists will thicken, says Dr. Klutznick. And all that is tied to their sexuality, she says. They worry that when they walk into bars or restaurants, men won't be looking at them—they'll be eyeing the younger women in the room or the football game on television, she says. Aging in a youth-worshiping society makes some women feel invisible and devalued, says Dr. Klutznick. It is not that the women feel old physically but that society sees them as old. Women in this age group ask Dr. Klutznick "What do I have to look forward to but getting old? Who's going to want me?"

# Understanding Menopause

Literally speaking, menopause refers to a woman's last period. Technically, a woman must not have menstruated for an entire year to be menopausal. The average age for menopause in the United States is 51, although women can go through it earlier. About 1 percent of women experience menopause before they reach age 40.

Women who have their ovaries removed during a hysterectomy become menopausal virtually overnight, says Joan Borton, a licensed mental health counselor in Rockport, Massachusetts, and author of *Drawing from the Women's Well: Reflections on the Life Passage of Menopause*. They often feel as if they were propelled into menopause without any preparation. Women who have undergone chemotherapy can also go into early menopause.

In natural menopause, a woman's final period is surrounded by a number of years in which other physical changes occur. This is what is known as the climacteric or perimenopause. It generally begins several years before menstruation ends, says Dr. Walsh. During this time, women can experience a whole range of physical changes, including hot flashes, night sweats, sleep difficulties, vaginal dryness, skin changes, hair loss, mood swings, depression and weight gain. Hot flashes, which are often the symptom of most concern to women who are approaching menopause, affect approximately 75 to 85 percent of postmenopausal women.

All these changes, and the loss of the periods themselves, are triggered by decreasing levels of estrogen, one of several hormones produced by the ovaries.

As a woman ages, her ovaries do, too; they shrink in size, stop releasing eggs and produce less estrogen.

# Your Risks down the Road

Estrogen also boosts bone quality and strength, so its decline at menopause can place women at increased risk for osteoporosis, a disease in which bones become brittle and fragile. Osteoporosis results in an estimated 1.5 million fractures per year. One-third of all women over age 65 experience spinal fractures, and one in three women in their nineties fracture their hips (compared with one in six men). Overall, between 25 and 44 percent of women experience fractures after menopause due to the disease.

The decrease in estrogen that accompanies menopause increases the risk of heart disease, the number-one killer of American women. That's because estrogen is a natural protector against heart disease. Without it, women and men are equal in their efforts to avoid heart disease. This means a woman's risk for heart attack and stroke goes up after menopause. Before age 65, one in nine women will experience a heart attack, according to the American Heart Association. After 65, that rate skyrockets to one in three.

# Planning Ahead

You can't avoid menopause. But there are some things you can do now, before you get there, that can make the whole experience a little easier for you. Menopause doesn't have to be a trying time, and it doesn't have to make you look and feel older. Here's what you can do.

**Get a move on it.** Exercise is one of the best things women can do ahead of time in order to fare better during their menopausal years, says Dr. Walsh. Exercise places stress on bone, increasing its density and strength. Women's bones lose density after menopause—at the rate of about 4 to 6 percent in the first four to five years. So the stronger they are to start off with, the better. Weight-bearing activities such as walking and running are best, experts say. Exercise also helps keep your cholesterol levels down, offering protection against heart disease.

**Eat right.** Get on a nutritious diet low in saturated fat, says Dr. Walsh. This will help reduce cholesterol and the risk of heart disease, he says, both of which go up after menopause. Experts recommend that you keep your fat intake to 25 percent or less of the total calories you consume.

**Keep an eye on PMS.** If you have premenstrual syndrome, or PMS, keep a log of your symptoms and pay attention to any changes. Sometimes PMS symptoms become far more intense as women enter menopause, says Dr. Klutznick, and they can serve as a signal for you that you are becoming menopausal. Some possible changes you might notice are PMS symptoms that last longer than usual and a feeling that your mind is fuzzy, she says. If you notice changes, tell your doctor. She can perform a simple blood test called the FSH test, which measures the amount of FSH, or follicle-stimulating hormone. Before menopause, your body produces enough FSH to help follicles develop and trigger ovulation. At menopause, however, you have fewer follicles, and it takes more FSH to get one to mature and ovulate. So your body pumps out more of the hormone than it used to. If your test shows a high FSH level—say, above 40—that means you are officially in menopause.

**Quit smoking.** If you stop smoking at a younger age, that can help you experience a gentler menopause, says Dr. Walsh. Smokers are more likely than nonsmokers to have menopausal symptoms, he says. Smokers also have a tendency toward lower bone mass, putting them at greater risk for osteoporosis. Smoking can cause you to experience menopause earlier, experts say. They think it's because nicotine may somehow contribute to the drop in estrogen. So stopping smoking now could delay menopause a bit.

**Get your calcium now.** While the decrease in bone mass accelerates at menopause, it begins around age 35. After 35, women lose 1 percent of their bone mass per year. So be sure to consume enough calcium. The current Recommended Dietary Allowance for adults is 800 milligrams of calcium, but some experts suggest 1,000 milligrams a day for premenopausal women and 1,500 milligrams for postmenopausal women.

Unfortunately, most women consume only about 500 milligrams a day through diet. You can come closer to the protective amounts by adding low-fat dairy products and canned fish with bones (such as salmon) to your daily diet. For example, one serving of low-fat milk gives you 300 milligrams of calcium, and one serving of low-fat yogurt contains 415 milligrams.

You can up your calcium intake through nondairy foods, too: Three ounces of canned sockeye salmon contains 203 milligrams of calcium, and ½ cup of raw tofu contains 258 milligrams.

Another way to increase your calcium intake is through supplements. The amount that you should take and the type of tablet you use—calcium carbonate, calcium lactate or calcium citrate—will depend on your individual health needs, so consult your doctor.

**Know your cholesterol levels.** Get your cholesterol levels checked, says Dr. Walsh. Menopause can cause levels of HDL (high-density lipoprotein) cholesterol, the "good" kind, to decrease and levels of LDL (low-density lipoprotein) cholesterol, the "bad" kind, to rise. So the better your cholesterol profile before menopause, the greater your chances of keeping it low once you hit menopause. Experts say that the best measurement to use is the ratio of total cholesterol to HDL cholesterol. A ratio of less than 3.5 is considered low, between 3.5 and 6.9, moderate, and over 7, high.

**Talk to your mom.** Women often follow the same patterns as their mothers, says Dr. Walsh, particularly if they have similar health experiences. So ask your mom about when she started menopause and what it was like for her.

# When the Time Comes

If you think you may be entering menopause, or if you're there already, here are some things you can do.

**Get support.** "The most valuable thing is gathering together with other women," says Borton. By talking with other women, either one-on-one or in support groups, you can learn about various symptoms and gather information about doctors and health care professionals whom other women go to, like and recommend, she says. "Talking with other women and sharing experiences helps women feel supported and not so isolated," agrees Dr. Klutznick. One option is to join a support group. Call your local hospital to find out about groups in your area. Or talk to other women.

**Find the right doctor.** Menopause will bring lots of physical changes and lots of questions, particularly about hormone replacement therapy (HRT). HRT is recommended to help replace missing estrogen and keep bones strong. But it is also controversial, mainly because it may increase your risk of certain cancers. "The key is to get a doctor who will work with you—one who will honor your decision," says Borton. Ask your friends about their doctors. And don't be afraid to shop around until you find a doctor you like.

**Choose a mentor.** Find a woman 10 to 15 years older than you who has been through menopause and whom you admire and respect, says Borton. "Spend time with older women, exploring with them what it is that holds meaning in their lives," she says. "Numbers of us feel that doing this has helped us cross the threshold into seeing ourselves as older women and embrace it in a way that feels really wonderful." In addition to identifying or finding women who can serve as mentors in your day-to-day life, look for older women in the public eye whom you can follow and learn from, she says.

**Stay lubricated.** The decrease in estrogen that women experience with menopause can cause vaginal dryness. The elasticity and size of the vagina changes, and the walls become thinner and lose their ability to become moist. This can make sex painful or even undesirable, says Dr. Klutznick. Surveys indicate that this happens in 8 to 25 percent of postmenopausal women. While premenopausal women can generally lubricate in 6 to 20 seconds when aroused, it can take one to three minutes for a postmenopausal woman.

Women can stay lubricated by using water-based vaginal lubricants such as K-Y jelly, Replens and Astroglide, which are available over the counter, says Dr. Klutznick. Steer clear of oil-based lubricants such as petroleum jelly; studies indicate that they don't dissolve as easily in the vagina and can therefore trigger vaginal infections. HRT can also help alleviate the problem, says Dr. Klutznick.

**Stay sexually active.** Studies indicate that women who stay sexually active experience fewer vaginal changes than those who don't. Sexual activity promotes circulation in the vaginal area, which helps it stay moist. For women without partners, masturbation helps promote circulation and moistness in the vagina, she says.

**Keep it cool.** The hot flashes women experience during menopause can range from a warm sensation to a burning-hot one in which a woman flushes and sweats. It can help to dress in layers and to keep the environment cool, experts say. Some women suck on ice cubes and drink cold liquids or visualize themselves walking in the snow or swimming in a clear lake. Hot liquids and spicy foods can trigger hot flashes, so keep those to a minimum. Experts don't completely understand what causes hot flashes, but they think that the decline in estrogen somehow upsets the body's internal thermometer.

# METABOLISM CHANGES

## A Different Kind
## of Energy Crisis

**R**emember when you could diet for a few days and drop an easy ten pounds? Well, nowadays it's not so easy. Oh, sure, you're eating less than you did back in your twenties and making a habit of passing on dessert and that mid-afternoon candy bar. But for some reason, you're a few dress sizes larger. And the pounds are piling on.

Here's what's happening: Your metabolism—how your body converts food into energy and then burns that energy as calories—is slowing down. This is a natural process that begins at about age 30. From then on, your body burns energy about 2 to 4 percent slower every ten years. So fewer calories are burned, and more are stored as fat. You can see that if you do nothing to counter this trend, you'll become heavier and less energetic. And you'll put yourself at greater risk for serious health problems such as high blood pressure and heart disease. Hardly a recipe for a youthful life.

Some of what's happening is beyond your control. You naturally burn calories slower than a man does. And your body also has a higher fat content than a man's, with your percentage of body fat inevitably increasing with time. "Metabolism changes are a direct response to changes in body composition," says Robert Kushner, M.D., director of the Nutrition and Weight Control Clinic at the University of Chicago. "As we age, we tend to lose muscle and gain fat. Since muscle burns a lot of energy, our energy needs diminish as we lose muscle, and our metabolism slows."

But most of this metabolic slowdown is our own doing. Yes, we lose some muscle as we age, but "the major cause of this muscle loss is inactivity," says Eric T. Poehlman, Ph.D., associate professor of medicine at the University of Maryland at Baltimore Department of Medicine. "The more inactive we be-

# It's Tougher for Us

Did you ever wonder why the men you know eat twice as much as you do and hardly gain a pound? Call it biological sexism: The average man burns calories more efficiently than the average woman—and over the same amount of time and with the same amount of physical activity, he'll lose more weight than you will.

Men burn calories faster for two reasons. One, they are usually heavier and are burning more calories all the time. Two, they have a greater proportion of fat-burning muscle. As a result, the average basal metabolic rate in women is 5 to 10 percent lower than in men.

Men are also more likely to put on fat around the belly, which happens to be the easiest location to lose fat. But thanks to estrogen, women tend to carry fat in the thighs, hips and buttocks—those hard-to-slim-down spots. This further slows down our metabolism.

Estrogen, which sends fat to areas where we don't want it, plays another role in our metabolism, because it also influences our appetites. Researchers have observed that food intake drops at the time of ovulation, when estrogen levels are at their peak, then increases in the second half of the menstrual cycle.

come with age, the less lean muscle we have. The less lean muscle we have, the more inactive we become. Over the years, the two feed on each other, and our metabolism plummets."

How do you break out of this trap? Unless you have thyroid disease, which can play havoc with how your body burns energy, you can get your metabolism cranked up again by making some lifestyle changes. But first, here's what's going on inside.

## Overfueled and Underactive

Add up all the energy needed to power the activities in a resting body—everything from breathing and digestion to the activity of nerve cells during thinking—and you have your basal metabolic rate, the minimum energy requirement you need to stay alive. For most women, this is about 1,000 to 1,200 calories per day.

Then add the calories you need to power your additional activities—everything from playing jacks with your kid to jumping jacks in aerobics—and you

# What's Your Calorie RDA?

If you knew exactly how many calories your body burns in the course of a day, you'd know how many calories you need to eat to maintain or lose weight. Here's a handy formula for balancing your energy equation.

First, multiply your weight by ten. This is your basal metabolic rate, the minimum number of calories that you need to keep your system running.

Next, determine your activity level from the table below and multiply your basal metabolic rate by the appropriate percentage. This gives you the additional calories you require for the day.

Sedentary activity refers to the time you spend sitting around the house watching television, reading your favorite magazine or talking on the phone. Light activity includes things such as housework, cooking and a stroll around the block after dinner. Moderate activity includes swimming or walking at a brisk pace while able to talk without gasping for breath. Strenuous activity includes heart-pounding exercise such as running or aerobics.

have the total number of calories you require every day.

This means, of course, that two women may have the same basal metabolic rate but burn very different amounts of calories every day. For example, a very active 125-pound woman can easily burn 2,200 calories a day, while a sedentary 125-pound type can barely burn 1,750.

Which takes us to the punch line of this brief lesson in calories—the metabolic formula for not gaining weight. Calories in must equal calories out. The calories that aren't "out" are stored in your body as fat. But if you burn more calories than you take in, stored fat is burned, and you lose weight.

So the way to not gain weight as you get older is simple: Cut back on calories. Pretend you like rice cakes. You know the routine. But there's a small problem. Your body doesn't know you're on a diet; it thinks you're starving to death. So instead of burning fat, your metabolism goes into famine mode, trying to preserve your fat stores.

"Very low calorie dieting can decrease your basal metabolic rate by 15 to 30 percent, making weight loss even more difficult," says Dr. Kushner. A very low calorie diet is one that consists of fewer than 600 calories a day. Because your body is trying to save you by keeping your fat level intact, it chooses another source of fuel: muscle. You've heard the phrase "Diets don't work." Now you know why.

| Activity Level | Percent |
|---|---|
| Sedentary | 30–50 |
| Light | 55–65 |
| Moderate | 65–70 |
| Strenuous | 75–100 |

Add these two numbers together, and you have your total calorie needs for the day. If you're a 120-pound woman whose daily activity level is on the low end of the strenuous scale, you would need 2,100 calories.

$$120 \times 10 = 1,200$$
$$1,200 \times 0.75 = 900$$
$$1,200 + 900 = 2,100$$

This figure is only an estimate, however. Your metabolism can be measured much more accurately by an exercise physiologist or a physician specializing in weight loss and metabolism.

Your metabolic rate doesn't return to normal after you stop dieting, because your body thinks another famine might be around the corner. Dieting actually prevents long-term, permanent weight loss.

And dieters typically add one more insult to metabolic injury: They cut calories without paying much attention to what kind of calories they're cutting. One gram of fat contains twice the calories of one gram of carbohydrates—and carbohydrates have the added benefit of burning faster than fats. So instead of cutting back on calories across the board, you'd be better off not cutting calories and maintaining a low-fat, high-carbohydrate diet that emphasizes fruits, vegetables, pasta and grains. "The fat you eat is much more likely to become the fat you carry," says Dr. Kushner.

## Exercise: Your Metabolism's Best Friend

Okay, dieting isn't the answer. So what can you do when your age causes your body's metabolism to shift into a lower, slower gear?

Exercise.

Aerobic exercise—walking, riding a stationary bike, aerobic dancing, any activity that boosts your heart rate for 20 minutes or more—is the best way to burn calories. And the benefits of exercise just keep going and going. Exercise sets your metabolism at a higher rate, so calories are incinerated for hours after you've stopped.

But the best way to boost your metabolism is to participate in an aerobic activity and a regular period of a strength training, such as weight lifting. "The major reason one person burns 1 calorie per minute and another burns 1.5 is that the second person has more muscle mass, and muscle is an extremely energy-hungry tissue," says Dr. Poehlman. "Strength-building exercises such as weight lifting will add muscle mass at any age. And the more you do such exercises, the better for your metabolism."

To prove that point, Dr. Poehlman and his associates measured the basal metabolic rates of 96 people: 36 did aerobic activity, 18 did weight lifting, and 42 did nothing. The aerobic group had a 13 percent higher metabolic rate than the sedentary group; the strength group's metabolic rate was 18 percent higher than the sedentary group's.

This study, says Dr. Poehlman, shows that either aerobic exercise or strength training may provide a metabolic boost.

## Maximize Your Metabolism

Convinced that exercise is the best way to beat the middle-age bulge? Here's what you can do to rev your engine.

**Step up the pace.** An easy way to burn more calories in the same amount of time is to put a little more speed into your current aerobic workout. Suppose you're a walker who covers a mile in about 15 minutes (about 4 miles per hour), burning roughly 365 calories per hour (or about 90 calories per mile). If you bump up your speed to a 12-minute mile (5 miles per hour), your calorie burn increases to about 585 for the same hour. That's a bonus of 27 calories a mile. That extra calorie burn each day can translate to a weight loss of about 15 pounds in less than a year.

**Go longer.** If you're already working out at your top speed, don't go any faster, but try to go longer. "Just like a car, your body will burn more fuel—in this case, fat—the longer it is engaged in an activity," says Dr. Kushner.

**Work your arms and legs.** Exercises that vigorously use both arms and legs are better fat burners than those that involve only your legs. "Cross-country skiing rates highest in lab tests for burning the most calories per minute because you're using your legs, upper body and even your torso," says Wayne Westcott, Ph.D., strength-training consultant for the International Association of Fitness Professionals. Stationary rowers and bikes with moving hand levers also rate high.

**Start your day with breakfast.** Experts say your body burns calories at a slower rate as you sleep. Breakfast acts as your metabolism's wake-up call, kicking it into the calorie-burning mode. If you don't eat something in the morning, you may ultimately burn fewer calories during the day. And it's more likely that when you do eat, you'll grab the first high-fat snack you see.

**Spread out your meals.** Eating small meals throughout the day instead of your standard three squares may be better for fat burning. After you eat, your body releases the hormone insulin, which causes your body to store fat. The larger the meal, the more insulin your body releases. But smaller, more frequent meals keep insulin levels lower and more stable. The less insulin you have in your blood, the more fat you burn, and the less you store.

**Don't skip meals.** Skipping meals and then eating one big meal at night can be a triple whammy, says Dr. Kushner. First, it puts you into a slow burn mode during the day. Second, the big meal provides an energy overload: The body can metabolize only so much food at one time, so the excess is likely to become fat. Third, most of the metabolizing will take place while you sleep—when your metabolic rate is at its lowest.

**Exercise after you eat.** A moderate workout right after a meal gives you a fat-burning bonus. A brisk three-mile walk on an empty stomach burns about 300 calories. But walking on a full stomach will burn about 345 calories. That's because eating gives your metabolism a boost; add exercise, and your metabolism gets a double boost and burns even more calories.

**Spice up your life.** Keeping an eye on your metabolism doesn't mean you have to give up tasty foods. In fact, hot, spicy foods such as mustard and chili may even shift your metabolism into high gear for a short period. In a study by British researchers, spicy food was shown to increase basal metabolic rate by an average of 25 percent.

**Stay away from stimulants.** Caffeine, alcohol and other stimulants may raise your metabolic rate, but once they're out of your system, your metabolism crashes back to normal or below. The wise move, says Dr. Poehlman, is to avoid any artificial means of raising your metabolism unless it's prescribed by a doctor.

**Have your thyroid checked.** An underactive thyroid causes the body to burn energy at a slower rate than normal, and an overactive thyroid has the opposite effect. More women than men have thyroid disease. So if you suspect yours is out of whack, have it checked by your doctor. If a thyroid hormone deficiency exists, it can often be regulated with prescription drugs.

# MIDLIFE CRISIS

## *It Doesn't Happen to Everybody*

For years you've balanced career and family with the grace of a ballerina. You danced around doubts and pirouetted past problems. But now this choreography seems out of touch with your life.

You suddenly feel old, uncertain and vulnerable: "Who am I?" "Why am I here?" "Where am I going with my life?"

You're questioning career choices, re-evaluating commitments to friends and family, worrying about fading looks and mourning the passage of youth.

Welcome to a midlife crisis—that uncomfortable time when you no longer feel secure about your life as it is, but you can't look backward without regret or look forward without foreboding.

"There are three wake-up calls in midlife. First, you realize that you're not going to live forever. Second, you realize you're never going to be president of the company, or if you are president of the company, you're not enjoying it as much as you thought you would. Finally, you realize your family life doesn't look like 'Ozzie and Harriet,' " says Ross Goldstein, Ph.D., a San Francisco psychologist and author of *Fortysomething: Claiming the Power and Passion of Your Midlife Years*. "That's the drumbeat of midlife, and the question is, what do you do about it?"

How you cope with those realizations can literally make you feel older or younger than your years, says Leonard Felder, Ph.D., a psychologist in Los Angeles and author of *A Fresh Start: How to Let Go of Emotional Baggage and Enjoy Your Life Again*.

"Some women become more discouraged because they realize that they've set some goals they're having trouble following through on or made choices they're not comfortable living with," Dr. Felder explains. "But many who go through a midlife crisis get motivated to do what they've always wanted to, and that gives them more energy and a greater sense of being alive."

## Beyond the Myths

Although most of us will experience some degree of anxiety and upheaval between the ages of 30 and 60, the average woman doesn't suddenly dash to a fat farm, have plastic surgery, take up belly dancing, buy a fur coat or have an affair with her tennis instructor. Instead of a complete overhaul, midlife for most people is like a minor tune-up, says Gilbert Brim, Ph.D., a social psychologist and director of the John D. and Catherine T. MacArthur Foundation Research Network on Successful Midlife Development, headquartered in Vero Beach, Florida.

So instead of leaving the husband and kids to "find herself," a typical woman in her forties may make a subtle change, such as taking up volunteer work, beginning a fitness program to tone up her aging body or getting her finances in order for the first time, Dr. Goldstein says.

"Most people look at midlife challenges as an opportunity," Dr. Brim says. "They tell us things like 'Yeah, I got fired, but that wasn't a crisis. It was a chance to get a better job' or 'Yes, my mother died, and I miss her, but it was a release of a burden.' "

In fact, only about 10 percent of women go through what we view as a midlife crisis, Dr. Brim says in his book *Ambition: How We Manage Success and Failure throughout Our Lives.* But researchers suspect as few as half of them suffer severe psychological symptoms such as confusion, anxiety, suidical thoughts, substance abuse and doubts about family choices and career. And of those women, most have had difficulty handling stress and trauma throughout their lives.

"If you had chronic troubles in your relationships or on the job earlier in your life, you're more likely to have trouble dealing with midlife events," Dr. Brim says.

Some psychologists even see similarities between adolescence and midlife. "At both times, everything gets tossed in the air, and you find yourself rebelling against the phase of your life that just occurred. So if you're 16, you don't want to be treated like a 12-year-old. If you are 40 and want to take a leading role in the business, you don't want to be treated like a junior partner. In both instances, you want a new relationship with the people around you," says Edward Monte, Ph.D., director of the Couple and Family Therapy Program at the Crozer Chester Medical Center in Upland, Pennsylvania.

## Recognize the Triggers

Unlike adolescence and menopause, midlife crisis isn't believed to be linked to hormonal changes. In fact, at least 40 common stressful midlife

# The Telltale Signs

Are you heading for a midlife crisis? To find out, we asked Ross Goldstein, Ph.D., a San Francisco psychologist and author of *Fortysomething: Claiming the Power and Passion of Your Midlife Years*, to develop this test. Answer the following statements yes or no. Scoring follows.

1. My future looks as positive now as it always has.
2. My life is as rewarding to me as I expected it to be.
3. Security is becoming more important to me.
4. Sometimes I feel excitement is missing in my life.
5. I am more flexible in my values today than I was ten years ago.
6. I get angry about the struggle to find "satisfaction" in life.
7. It feels like time is running out on me.
8. I wish there was an effective way of making all the tension and stress go away.
9. I am more sure of who I am today than ever before.
10. Balancing my work and family is becoming more difficult.
11. Sometimes I feel exhausted from the struggle of "making it."
12. I have a hard time accepting that I am as old as I am.

events, including death of a parent, divorce and job change, can combine to unleash a crisis, Dr. Brim says. Even fear of menopause and anxiety about approaching old age can transform a mild midlife transition into a crisis, Dr. Monte says. The budding sexuality of your children doesn't help, either.

"If you're a woman in your forties who is noticing the aging process, you might unfortunately buy into the myth that this means a decline in sexual desirability. If in addition you have an adolescent daughter in the throes of discovering her own sexuality, you may experience a dramatic increase in self-doubt and anxiety. It is essential that you separate your own issues from your daughter's. This will enable you to give solid support to your daughter while taking care of yourself," Dr. Monte says.

In addition, because we are taught to question ourselves and to be introspective throughout our lives, women often have midlife traumas earlier than men, he says.

"Women often start having signs of a midlife transition around age 35 or 40, while men may not have any signs of it until they're 45 or 50," Dr. Monte says. "It hits women sooner because from birth they've been taught to acknowledge

13. I miss the excitement and adventure of my earlier years.
14. My work is as satisfying as it has always been.
15. I am more aware of my health as I grow older.

Give yourself two points for each "yes" to questions 3, 4, 6, 7, 8, 10, 11, 12, 13 and 15 and two points for each "no" answer to questions 1, 2, 5, 9 and 14. Total your score.

**0 to 8.** Your life is running smoothly. Your philosophy: If it isn't broke, why fix it?

**10 to 16.** Occasionally, you yearn for a day at the beach, but in general, you feel secure and comfortable with your life. Your outlook: You're ready to make a few minor midlife course adjustments, but you don't yearn to sail off to Tahiti with a co-worker.

**18 or more.** Who is that worn-out woman in the mirror, and why is she still working at a job that seems as grueling as watching an IRS agent audit a tax return? Your dilemma: how to make significant changes in your life without sacrificing the best of what you have. Career counseling may help.

their feelings, while men are taught to ignore those feelings. So women know when they're unhappy with their lives a lot sooner than men do."

The ever-present ticking of the biological clock is another reason we confront midlife issues before men do. "Women in their late thirties and early forties realize that they're approaching the end of their childbearing years," Dr. Monte says. "They may not be at that point yet, but they sense the opportunity to bear children is escaping them. So often the crisis isn't about youth, career or even sexuality; it's about children."

# Damage Control

A midlife transition doesn't occur overnight, and navigating through it can take you years, Dr. Monte says. But if you prepare yourself, you can sail through just fine.

"You can come through midlife feeling better about yourself, more alive and younger in some ways," Dr. Goldstein says. "Midlife is an opportunity to have a new beginning. It's a chance to pursue some of the dreams, passions and hopes you didn't have time to explore at earlier points in your life."

Here are a few ways to avoid a crisis and help you make a smooth midlife transition.

**Rediscover the wonder years.** What did you like to do as a child? If you had a favorite book when you were young, reread it. If you liked to play field hockey, go to a high school game. "It may sound silly, but it has a real psychological purpose," says Susan Olson, Ph.D., director of psychological services at the Southwest Bariatric Nutrition Center in Tempe, Arizona. "Doing these childlike things will help you realize that you really don't have to mourn your youth because it's still within you to a certain extent. Once you realize that, your energy levels will literally surge."

**Get a little help from your friends.** Contact your best friend from high school or college, Dr. Olson suggests. "It will rekindle old feelings and bring perspective to your current life," she says. "It may help you realize that you're mourning a time that wasn't as ideal as you once believed."

**Do lunch.** Take at least one person who you know has been through a midlife crisis to lunch. Ask her which of the urges she resisted and which ones she followed through on and why, Dr. Felder recommends. It may give you some insight into your own situation.

**Keep a half-full glass.** Think positive, because being older can be neat, says Stanley Teitelbaum, Ph.D., a clinical psychologist in private practice in New York City. Instead of concentrating on lost energy or sex appeal, consider what you have now that you didn't have at 20, such as a satisfying career, a loving marriage, a supportive family or independence. "Life really does begin at 40 for many people. Yes, you're older, but the things you have now may outweigh or counteract the things you had in the past," he says.

**Switch gears.** One good way to be a leader, help others and build your self-esteem is to become a role model to others—whether it's a young colleague at work or your own children. A woman who is an editor at a daily newspaper could help a young female reporter polish her writing skills and groom herself for a future management position. "Instead of being the star of the show, why not get satisfaction from helping others shine in the spotlight?" Dr. Teitelbaum says.

**Share your feelings.** While many women are more comfortable about expressing their feelings than men, it is particularly important to keep the lines of communication open with loved ones during this crucial time, Dr. Monte says. In fact, if you can't articulate what you want from your relationship, you're likely to destroy it.

Arrange a time each week to discuss your feelings in a non-threatening way. If, for example, you fantasize about other men, you might say "I love you, and I'm attracted to my co-worker. It doesn't mean I love you less, but maybe it means something is missing in our relationship. Can we talk about it?" Dr. Monte explains: "The key is to discuss the topic in a way that doesn't cause either of you to panic and think your relationship is doomed."

**Say happy birthday to you.** So your fortieth birthday is approaching, and you dread it. Don't, Dr. Goldstein says. Instead, embrace the moment. Rituals such as birthdays, anniversaries and class reunions help us unleash feelings, reflect on who we are and where we are going in life. Use these natural pauses to rest, observe the vista, chart or correct your course and move on, he suggests. It's also an excellent time to share feelings and seek the support of family and friends.

**Don't panic.** "Making impulsive decisions during the midlife almost always ends up creating a bigger mess and, in some cases, disaster," Dr. Felder says. "If you think you need to resolve these midlife issues in the next two weeks, you're not going to get happy solutions. You need a plan that will allow you six months or a year to experiment with new options and that has room in it for you to stumble and fall at least a couple of times."

To get started, take a sheet of paper and divide it into three columns, Dr. Olson suggests. In the first column, list the goals you had as a child, such as "I want to be on the Supreme Court." In the second column, write down which of those goals you should abandon, such as "I'll never be judge." In the last column, list new goals that you'd like to accomplish in the next five years, such as "I'd like to resign from my firm and start my own private practice."

# MIGRAINES

## *Avoid Getting a Trigger-Happy Headache*

It's Friday night at last—time to pamper yourself after a stressful week of work. You sit on the balcony and soak up the sunset, sipping red wine and nibbling on some nice French cheese. You order take-out Chinese food, then crawl into bed to watch the late, late movie. And when the hero finally rides off into the sunset, you yawn and decide to sleep until noon.

But the relaxing evening you cooked up turns out to be a recipe for a very painful migraine. As the first light of day creeps across the windowsill, you wake up dizzy, clammy and nauseated, with throbbing pain covering half your head. Your pleasant weekend has come to an abrupt end.

Eighteen million Americans suffer regularly from migraine headaches, and most of them are women between the ages of 30 and 45. Stress, certain foods and beverages and an upset in sleep patterns cause migraines, but 60 percent of all migraines suffered by women are related to the menstrual cycle. These headaches are caused by hormone shifts before and during menstruation, says Seymour Diamond, M.D., director of the Diamond Headache Clinic in Chicago and executive director of the National Headache Foundation. More than half of all female migraine sufferers will stop having the headaches after menopause, he adds.

But no matter what the cause, millions of us are spending the most productive years of our lives living in fear of a migraine onslaught. When the dreaded pain strikes, we find ourselves curled up in a dark room for hours or even days, wishing for a return to those youthful days when we could eat and drink whatever we wanted, stay up to watch the sun rise and never have to pay the piper.

"A migraine is painful, unwelcome and often debilitating," says Dr. Diamond. "People aren't able to do much at all until it goes away."

# The Pain: An Open and Shut Case

Migraines start when blood vessels in your head constrict for a period of 15 minutes to an hour, then rapidly expand, Dr. Diamond says. The culprit in this process is believed to be serotonin, a hormonelike substance produced by blood platelets.

When you trigger a release of serotonin—by eating certain foods, drinking certain beverages, stressing out or sometimes just oversleeping—the blood vessels in your head narrow. As your kidneys process the serotonin and the level of this hormonelike substance drops, the vessels dilate rapidly, pressing on surrounding nerves and causing pain and inflammation. Dr. Diamond says the ache can last for hours or days because the swelling lingers after the blood vessels return to normal.

About one in five migraine sufferers will experience an "aura" minutes before the onset of a headache. Women report seeing flashes of light and zigzag patterns and sometimes experiencing speech impairment, confusion and numbness in their faces and limbs, according to Dr. Diamond.

# Heading Off the Ache

Migraine treatments have come a long way over the past 8,500 years or so. (Yes, migraines have really been with us forever.) In ancient Egypt, people with migraines used to nibble on parts of trees—wormwood and juniper were the favorites—to try to relieve the pain. As medical science progressed, doctors began to prescribe treatments such as placing hot irons on painful spots, cutting a patient's temple and rubbing garlic on the wound and even wrapping an electric eel around a sufferer's head.

Fortunately, such "solutions" are no longer in vogue. If you're looking for ways to stop migraines before they start, experts offer these tips.

**Watch what you eat.** Many foods can cause the body to boost serotonin levels. Dr. Diamond says these include red wine, aged cheese, processed meats such as hot dogs and sausages, citrus fruits, lentils, snow peas and foods prepared with the flavor enhancer monosodium glutamate, or MSG. For MSG, watch the labels on the foods you buy. Chinese food often has MSG, so ask the restaurant to leave it out of your order if you're sensitive to it.

Foods affect people in different ways, so it's a good idea to keep a log that lists what you ate in the hours leading up to a migraine. Dr. Diamond says you might be able to see patterns emerge and to identify your own trigger foods.

**Take an aspirin.** A study of 22,000 American male doctors found that taking one 325-milligram aspirin tablet every other day may help ward off headaches. The doctors in the study who took aspirin reported 20 percent fewer migraines than those who took placebos.

Researchers are trying to find out if women will get the same results. For

# The Relaxation Prescription

That pounding between your ears may be telling you something: Relax.

The National Headache Foundation reports that about 50 percent of migraines occur immediately after a period of unusual stress. To combat stress, doctors can prescribe hypnosis, biofeedback (where you're wired to a monitor and taught to relax parts of your body) and other relaxation techniques, according to the foundation's executive director, Seymour Diamond, M.D., who is also director of the Diamond Headache Clinic in Chicago.

If you're looking for a way to beat stress, Dr. Diamond suggests this at-home relaxation exercise, which should take four to five minutes to complete.

Settle comfortably into a chair. Let all your muscles go loose and heavy.

**1. Frown and furrow.** Wrinkle up your forehead, then smooth it out. Picture your entire forehead and scalp becoming smoother as the relaxation increases.

now, experts say you should see your doctor before taking aspirin regularly because aspirin can cause upset stomach, internal bleeding and other complications that may put you at risk for other health problems.

**Reconsider the Pill.** Birth control pills may cause migraines in some women, Dr. Diamond says. Check with your physician about whether you should discontinue use of the Pill or switch to a different dosage.

**Try some heavy metal.** A study from Henry Ford Hospital in Detroit found that magnesium is in short supply in the brains of most migraine sufferers. So eating foods rich in magnesium, including dark green vegetables, fruits and nuts, might bring some relief.

Kenneth Welch, M.D., chairman of the Department of Neurology at Henry Ford Hospital, stresses that the data are very preliminary. More work is needed before researchers make a positive link between migraines and magnesium. Still, eating a few more servings of fruits and vegetables won't hurt.

**Sleep on a schedule.** Irregular sleep patterns also contribute to migraines, although Dr. Diamond says the exact reason isn't clear. "We see lots of weekend migraines, when people decide to sleep late," he says. "You

Now frown, crease your brows, and study the tension. Let go of the tension again. Smooth out your forehead once more.

**2. Close and clench.** Now close your eyes tighter and tighter. Feel the tension, then relax your eyes. Keep your eyes closed gently, comfortably, and notice the relaxation.

Now clench your teeth. Study the tension throughout the jaw, then relax.

**3. Rock and roll.** Press your head back as far as it can go, and feel the tension in your neck. Roll your head to the right and feel the tension shift; now roll your head to the left.

Straighten your head, bring it forward, and press your chin against your chest. Let your head return to a comfortable position and study the relaxation.

Shrug your shoulders and hold the tension. Drop your shoulders and feel the relaxation. Bring your shoulders up, forward and back. Feel the tension in your shoulders and in your upper back. Drop your shoulders once more and relax.

should try getting the same amount of sleep every night, even on weekends."

**Control your caffeine.** Too much caffeine—anything more than three cups of coffee within an hour or so—can constrict your blood vessels and trigger a headache, according to Dr. Diamond. But he says drinking a cup of coffee or tea just at the start of a headache might keep your vessels from expanding too much and could ward off a migraine.

**Chill out—then see your doctor.** Once a headache flares up, Dr. Diamond says, nothing short of prescription drugs can stop it. He suggests riding out the pain by reclining in a quiet, dark room. Never try to exercise during a migraine episode, since an increased pulse only makes the pain worse.

You might also want to put your headache on ice, says Lawrence Robbins, M.D., assistant professor of neurology at the University of Illinois at Chicago and at Rush Medical College of Rush University, also in Chicago. You have at least a 50-50 chance of getting some pain relief within two to three minutes of applying a soft cold pack and moderate pressure to your head. Soft cold packs are sold at pharmacies and medical supply stores.

Sometimes, Dr. Robbins says, a migraine may be so painful that putting something on your head will make it feel even worse. In that case, forget the cold pack.

If you can't control migraines by yourself, see your doctor. A combination of biofeedback, relaxation exercises and medication may solve your problem.

## A Drug to Dispel the Agony

A new drug, sumatriptan (Imitrex), shows great promise in fighting migraines. One study showed that 70 percent of patients who took sumatriptan during a migraine episode reported mild or no pain an hour later. The prescription drug is also free of most side effects common to migraine medication, such as sedation, nausea and vomiting.

"It's one of the great discoveries in migraine research," Dr. Diamond says. "It really offers great hope to people who suffer from frequent migraines." Unfortunately, it's not for those who have high blood pressure or heart problems. Ask your doctor if you would make a good candidate.

# OSTEOPOROSIS

## *Don't Give Your Bones a Break*

Your bones seem like steel girders—strong, permanent, a structure you can depend on.

But for one in every four women, this skeletal structure is eroding, the girders weakening and wearing away.

The cause is osteoporosis.

Osteoporosis is a disease of thinning bones, fractured hips and hunched spines, a disease of aging that you can prevent—if you start today.

Now you can't stop your bones from thinning. Every woman loses some bone over time, usually at the rate of 1 percent a year. But in women with osteoporosis, the loss is a lot faster than normal, and bones can become so brittle and fragile that they break when you step off a curb or bump your hip on the edge of a table. In fact, the bones in your spine—your vertebrae—can even break under their own weight.

Besides making you look older, osteoporosis can make you feel that way. "Suddenly, women are afraid to go outside, take walks, wash the windows, clean out the tub. They're afraid that if they trip or fall, they'll break a bone," says Clifford Rosen, M.D., director of the Maine Center for Osteoporosis Research and Education in Bangor.

Dr. Rosen says "women" because osteoporosis strikes four women to every man. Women have less bone to start with, and during menopause, there's a drop-off in the production of the female hormone estrogen, which holds calcium in your bones like a dam.

But your bones may start to thin too fast even before menopause arrives, a slow and symptomless draining of your body's interior strength that begins in your thirties or forties. If you don't do anything to stop it—things such as taking in calcium, doing exercise, trying hormone replacement therapy or taking other preventive actions discussed later—it becomes osteoporosis. And that's serious.

Some women with osteoporosis become hunched and shorter as the bones in their spines break. These fractures might be painless or misinterpreted as back problems (at least at first). "A woman may have back pain that hurts for a while and then goes away. She may attribute it to a muscle spasm when she really has a compression fracture," says Dr. Rosen.

Some women break their wrists, another vulnerable spot.

And some women break their hips. Of these women, 10 to 20 percent will die in the next year.

## Are You a Candidate?

If your mother has osteoporosis, you may also be prone to these frightening fractures, says Dr. Rosen. "Up to 70 percent of your peak bone mass, which you reach in your twenties, is determined by heredity," he says. Very small or thin women are also more susceptible to osteoporosis, he adds, since they have less bone mass than other women.

One of the biggest causes of osteoporosis is too little calcium in your diet. Although estimates of how many women are short on this basic bone-building nutrient vary from 10 to 25 percent, experts agree that calcium deficiency is extremely common. Another nutrient vital to bone health is vitamin D, because it aids in the absorption of calcium. If you're not getting enough vitamin D, your body won't be able to take advantage of even generous amounts of calcium.

And if your exercise isn't the kind that stimulates bone growth, your bones will become more porous—and more easily broken.

Other factors that also contribute to osteoporosis are smoking and heavy drinking, experts say. Certain prescription medicines may also erode bone strength, particularly if taken for many years or in extremely high doses.

But you don't have to sit back and surrender to osteoporosis. You can minimize your risks and take definite steps to build stronger bones. What matters most is that you start now.

## Banking Bone

Picture your bones as a kind of bank account. Throughout your life, your body is constantly depositing bone in and withdrawing bone from your skeleton. When you're young, you deposit more bone than you withdraw, says Dr. Rosen. But by the time you reach your mid-thirties, the trend is reversed—you withdraw more than you deposit. To prevent bone bankruptcy, you need to deposit as much bone as possible before menopause.

But what if you're only a few years away from menopause or you're already there and you don't really know how much bone is in your account? Although all doctors don't agree that every woman should be tested for osteoporosis, Dr. Rosen recommends that you play it safe and get a bone density measurement of your hip and spine when you are between the ages of 45 and 55, when thinning

## What's Your Risk?

It's not difficult to evaluate your risk of developing osteoporosis, says Susan Allen, M.D., Ph.D., assistant professor of internal medicine at the University of Missouri–Columbia School of Medicine. Start with the following questions:

1. Do you have a small, thin frame, or are you Caucasian or Asian?
2. Do you have relatives with osteoporosis?
3. Have you reached menopause?
4. Have you had an early or surgically induced menopause?
5. Do you take high doses of thyroid medication or cortisone-like drugs for asthma, arthritis or cancer?
6. Do you avoid eating many dairy products and other sources of calcium?
7. Are you not getting regular weight-bearing exercise such as brisk walking?
8. Do you smoke cigarettes or drink alcohol heavily?

If you answered yes to two or more of these questions, your risk for developing osteoporosis is high, Dr. Allen says. It's time to talk to your doctor about developing a lifelong prevention plan.

bone is first detectable. The best test is called dual energy x-ray absorptiometry, or DEXA, and costs about $100 to $250. Most community hospitals and all large city hospitals should have DEXA scanners, Dr. Rosen says. But if a DEXA machine is not available in your community, your doctor can assess your bone health with a computerized axial tomography (or CAT) scan instead.

Doctors agree that women at greatest risk for the disease—women with family histories of osteoporosis or personal histories of smoking or heavy drinking—should be tested before age 45.

If your test shows a higher than normal level of bone loss, don't despair—it's probably not too late to start building bone.

## Healthy Habits for Life and Limb

Here are the best ways to strengthen your skeleton.

**Pump up your calcium.** Calcium is to your bones what air is to your lungs—the element they need to be healthy. Ninety-nine percent of the calcium in your diet goes straight to your bones. If you don't get enough calcium, you can't make enough bone—it's as simple as that.

Although the Recommended Dietary Allowance (RDA) for women is 800 milligrams a day, you need more calcium in adolescence and after menopause, Dr. Rosen says. Women should get at least 1,000 milligrams before menopause and 1,500 milligrams after menopause. Although food is the best way to get calcium, what matters most is that you take in the recommended amount, says Dr. Rosen. If that's through food, fine; if it's through a combination of food and calcium supplements, fine. Just make sure the numbers add up.

Ounce for ounce, milk and milk products are the best sources of dietary calcium. One eight-ounce serving of nonfat yogurt provides about 450 milligrams of calcium. One cup of skim milk offers more than 300 milligrams. Many other foods contain calcium, but the nutrient isn't as easily absorbed from these foods as it is from dairy products.

**Don't forget the D.** Bones don't absorb calcium unless they have plenty of vitamin D, says Michael F. Holick, M.D., Ph.D., director of the Vitamin D, Skin and Bone Research Laboratory at Boston University Medical Center. Without vitamin D, your body absorbs about 10 percent of the calcium it takes in; with vitamin D, it can absorb 80 to 90 percent. "Vitamin D tells the small intestine 'Here comes the calcium. Open up and let it in,' " explains Dr. Holick. The RDA for vitamin D is five micrograms or 200 IU—easily found in fortified foods such as milk, breads and cereals.

Besides getting some of your daily vitamin D through food, your body can make it from sunshine, which triggers a vitamin D manufacturing process in your skin. Five to 15 minutes of bright sunshine every day, before you apply sunscreen, will supply your needs, says Dr. Rosen. If you live north of New York City, however, you can't depend on the sun. In that case, you'll need to be sure you're getting enough vitamin D from dietary sources. (If you're getting plenty in your diet, you won't need time in the sun at all.)

**Review your medication.** Certain medications—thyroid medications, anti-inflammatory steroids such as hydrocortisone (Locoid), cortisone (Cortone Acetate) and prednisone (Key-Pred 50), anticonvulsants such as phenytoin (Dilantin), depressants such as phenobarbital (Barbita) and the diuretic furosemide (Lasix)—can cause osteoporosis, particularly when they're taken regularly in high doses over a number of years. Thyroid medications in normal doses should pose no problem, however, says Dr. Rosen, and the risk from diuretics can be offset by taking additional calcium. The most serious osteoporosis risk is from steroids, Dr. Rosen says. If you require long-term steroid medication, your doctor may recommend additional anti-osteoporosis medication such as calcitonin (Cibacalcin) or hormone replacement therapy in addition to calcium and vitamin D supplements, he says.

**Keep 'em dry and healthy.** "Alcohol actually poisons the cells that build bone," says Susan Allen, M.D., Ph.D., assistant professor of internal medicine at the University of Missouri–Columbia School of Medicine. A beer or glass of wine now and then probably won't cause you much harm. But avoid drinking to excess, she says—more than two to three drinks a day.

**Don't puff.** Smoking lowers your levels of estrogen, says Barbara S. Levine, Ph.D., associate clinical professor of nutrition in medicine and director of the Calcium Information Center at Cornell University Medical College in New York City. And lower estrogen, she says, means less protection against bone loss.

**Consider hormone replacement therapy.** For some women past menopause, hormone replacement therapy can thicken bones. Ask your doctor whether you're a candidate for it.

# Interior Bodybuilding

An exercise program builds muscle and bone, says Gail Dalsky, Ph.D., director of the Exercise Research Laboratory at the University of Connecticut Health Center in Farmington. "The bone density of women who are good exercisers is 5 to 10 percent higher than that of other women," she says.

And exercise not only increases bone density but also improves your dexterity and reflexes, so you're less likely to fall and break a bone, says Dr. Allen.

**Enjoy weight-bearing exercise.** To strengthen bones, you need activities in which you're bearing weight on your bones, Dr. Allen says. Weight-bearing exercises include brisk walking, jogging and dancing, which actually stimulate bone cells to build more bone, particularly in your back and hips, where you most need it, Dr. Allen says.

You're doing a weight-bearing exercise if your feet are hitting the ground with at least the impact that brisk walking produces, says Dr. Rosen. "Basically, you can count on any exercise that makes heavy use of gravity," he says. "Swimming doesn't, for example, but most aerobics classes and tennis do."

Pumping iron is also an ideal way to build bone strength, because it increases the weight of gravity on your bones. It's good sense to make weight lifting part of your weight-bearing exercise. Any lifting done in a standing position is particularly helpful for the spine and hips. If you've never used weights before, be sure to get your doctor's clearance and a trainer's advice on the safest routine.

**Do it regularly.** Once you've found the weight-bearing exercises you like, keep at them for 30 minutes to one hour three to four times a week, Dr. Allen says.

**Concentrate on the back and hips.** If you're exercising for weight loss and muscle tone, you're probably doing something for your upper body, and that's good. But remember, says Dr. Allen, the bones that are most vulnerable to osteoporosis are the hips and the spinal vertebrae in the mid- to lower back. Walking, jogging and aerobic dancing are particularly helpful for your back and hips, she says.

# Spine-Strengthening Exercises

Doing exercises that stretch your spine as straight as possible will strengthen the vertebrae most vulnerable to osteoporosis. Try these back extension exercises suggested by Susan Allen, M.D., Ph.D., assistant professor of internal medicine at the University of Missouri–Columbia School of Medicine.

"Do as many of these exercises as you can, once in the morning and once at night," says Dr. Allen.

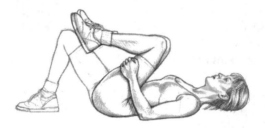

*Lie on your back with your knees bent. Bring both knees as close as possible to your chest and hold (with your hands supporting your knees) for five seconds, then lower your feet slowly to the floor. Then bring one knee up to your chest as far as you can, hold for five seconds and lower it slowly to the floor. Alternate right and left legs for ten repetitions each.*

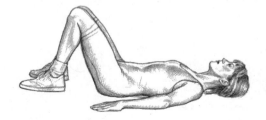

*Lie on your back with your knees bent. Press the small of your back against the floor and hold for five seconds. Repeat ten times.*

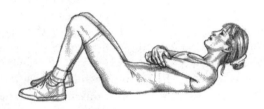

*Lie on your back with your knees bent. Place your arms across your middle, cupping the opposite elbow with each hand. Raise your head and shoulders as far as you can without sitting up. Hold for three seconds. Repeat ten times.*

*Lie on your back with your legs straight and your arms at your sides. Raise your head and shoulders as far as you can without sitting up. Hold for three seconds. Repeat ten times.*

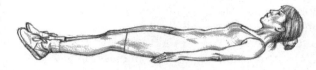

# OVERWEIGHT

## *Getting Yourself Down to Size*

**S**ee that slender woman leading the aerobics class? There used to be 200 pounds on her five-foot-five frame. Can you believe it?

Those were heavy days for Karen Faye, a nurse in her forties who got in shape and is now the owner of Body Basics Aerobics Workout in Tyngsboro, Massachusetts.

"I was mentally and physically exhausted all the time, which just added to the burden of being overweight," she recalls. Like many women, she struggled with her weight from adolescence on. "I remember that when I was sixteen and went to the beach with my mother, the boys whistled at my mother, not at me. I didn't feel like the young person I was supposed to be."

That feeling of being older than her years stayed with her well into adulthood, for as long as she was overweight, Faye says. "Mentally, I was a young person—I had three little children and a thin husband who could still fit into his Marine uniform. But physically, I felt like my own grandmother, and I couldn't believe what was happening to me. I felt the real me was trapped in an older person's body."

For years, Faye thought that her thyroid problem was the cause of her weight. But when she hit 200 pounds, she says, "I saw the handwriting on the artery wall. And it was my artery." She went on a low-fat eating and exercise regimen. Within eight months, she lost 80 pounds, became fit for the first time in her life and has maintained her weight for 11 years.

After she got her weight under control, she became a fitness consultant and opened Body Basics Aerobics Workout. In August 1993, she won the physical fitness award at the Mrs. United States pageant, competing with some women who were in their twenties.

As Faye knows, overweight is a burden on body and soul. You feel you've lost your youth and vitality. And you've opened yourself up to ailments of aging

276

such as heart disease, high blood pressure, diabetes, arthritis and high choles-terol—not to mention the backaches and other pains caused by carrying around more than you should.

There is a cancer connection as well. "When you're overweight, you also have increased risk for several cancers, including cancer of the endometrium, uterus, cervix, ovaries and gallbladder," says John Foreyt, Ph.D., director of the Nutrition Research Clinic at Baylor College of Medicine in Houston.

## Bigger Isn't Better

Most studies of the connection between overweight and heart disease have been limited to men. But that's beginning to change. In one study of 116,000 women, researchers at Harvard University in Cambridge, Massachusetts, found that the relationship of overweight to heart disease is just as strong for women as it is for men. Being overweight was the cause of heart disease in 70 percent of obese women in the study and 40 percent of other women who were above their ideal weights.

High blood pressure has a strong link to overweight. When a heart has to work overtime to carry extra pounds, blood pressure shoots skyward.

Type II diabetes is also tied to being overweight. Carrying those extra pounds directly affects the body's ability to utilize blood sugar. Many over-weight people with diabetes who need regular medication find that once they drop 20 or more pounds, they may also drop their prescriptions.

The connection between overweight and arthritis is fairly obvious: The more pounds you carry, the more pressure you put on your joints. The Fram-ingham Knee Osteoarthritis Study, using data gathered from the more than 5,200 residents of Framingham, Massachusetts, in a landmark heart study, showed that overweight women who lost just 11 pounds reduced their risk of developing arthritic knees by almost 50 percent.

And when it comes to cancer, particularly breast cancer, losing those extra pounds may give you extra protection. Research from the federal Centers for Disease Control and Prevention in Atlanta shows a particular danger for women who are 25 percent or more over their optimal weights at the time their breast cancer is diagnosed. These women face a 42 percent greater risk that the cancer will return.

Being overweight may also increase a woman's risk of developing breast cancer, says Dr. Foreyt. "A high-fat diet leads to obesity, and fat in the diet is associated with an increased risk of breast cancer," he says.

## Aging Ups the Ante

Most of us have already realized that it's getting harder to lose weight. That's because our metabolism, the process by which our bodies burn calories, slows down over time. Reubin Andres, M.D., clinical director of the National

# What's a Healthy Weight, Anyway?

You don't need to be a slave to the scale. "Your healthy weight is what's produced by healthy eating and healthy exercise," says John Foreyt, Ph.D., director of the Nutrition Research Clinic at Baylor College of Medicine in Houston. "That's your goal, period."

But maybe you'd feel better with a weight range to aim for. If so, the chart below, from the federal government, will give you a general idea of where you should stand. These guidelines were prepared for both men and women; women will generally fall toward the lower end of each range.

| Height | Weight (lb.) | |
| --- | --- | --- |
| | Age 19–34 | Age 35 and up |
| 5'0" | 97–128 | 108–138 |
| 5'1" | 101–132 | 111–143 |
| 5'2" | 104–137 | 115–148 |
| 5'3" | 107–141 | 119–152 |
| 5'4" | 111–146 | 122–157 |
| 5'5" | 114–150 | 126–162 |
| 5'6" | 118–155 | 130–167 |
| 5'7" | 121–160 | 134–172 |
| 5'8" | 125–164 | 138–178 |
| 5'9" | 129–169 | 142–183 |
| 5'10" | 132–174 | 146–188 |
| 5'11" | 136–179 | 151–194 |
| 6'0" | 140–184 | 155–199 |
| 6'1" | 144–189 | 159–205 |
| 6'2" | 148–195 | 164–210 |
| 6'3" | 152–200 | 168–216 |
| 6'4" | 156–205 | 173–222 |
| 6'5" | 160–211 | 177–228 |
| 6'6" | 164–216 | 182–234 |

Institute on Aging in Bethesda, Maryland, believes it is harmless to gain about five pounds each decade after age 20—but only if you are in good health to start with and remain free of ailments such as diabetes and heart disease. But many experts say any weight gain should be avoided throughout the years.

But it's best to keep the weight off. After following a group of Harvard University alumni for 27 years, researchers found the lowest mortality rate among men who were 20 percent below the average weight for men of similar age and height. This finding held firm even after the researchers accounted for underweight from smoking or illness, which they believe may have distorted the results of previous studies.

The study also showed that men who were only slightly overweight—2 to 6 percent over their desirable weights—still had a significantly greater chance of dying from heart disease and that men who weighed 20 percent more than their desirable weights actually doubled their risk.

But regardless of where you fit on the charts, if you feel you're struggling with more than a few extra pounds and you don't have thyroid or other health problems, you may be eating too much—particularly fatty foods—and exercising too little.

What to do about it? Well, you could put yourself on a crash diet. But that probably won't get you anything but frustration. "Diets just don't work," says Janet Polivy, Ph.D., professor of psychology at the University of Toronto Faculty of Medicine. "Diets become popular because they work for a week or two and everyone says 'You gotta try it.' Well, speak to those people in a year or two, and you'll find they've failed." When you fall for one of those speedy five-pounds-a-week programs, you lose it, all right—but you lose pounds of fluid, not fat. And as soon as you abandon the diet, the weight comes right back on.

In the long run, what works best to achieve a healthy weight is to modify your eating habits and to get more exercise.

It worked for Karen Faye. "Now I'm 45 and really a grandmother," Faye says. "But since I've lost the weight, when people see me with my 25-year-old son, they think he's my boyfriend! If I can do it, you can do it."

# Setting the Stage

The first step toward successful weight loss is accepting yourself as you are right now, says Thomas A. Wadden, Ph.D., associate professor of psychology and director of the Weight and Eating Disorders Program at the University of Pennsylvania in Philadelphia. Then you have to draw up a strategy for taking control of your weight. Here's how.

**Make a long-term commitment.** The key to healthy and successful weight loss at any age, experts say, is to make the changes gradually. Losing no more than ½ pound a week is ideal, says George Blackburn, M.D., Ph.D., associate professor of surgery at Harvard Medical School and chief of the Nutrition/Metabolism Laboratory at New England Deaconess Hospital, both in Boston. So aim to attain a healthy weight a year from now, not next week, he says.

**Don't try to be a model.** Never mind that professional models are often as skinny as straws. Many of them are teenagers in heavy makeup. "You have to recognize that you can't look like those skinny little models in the magazines, and middle age is a good time to do this," says Dr. Wadden. Once you let go of unrealistic fantasies and accept the notion that it's unfair to model yourself after an adolescent, then you can get on with a healthy and attainable weight loss plan, he says.

**Surround yourself with support.** A good support system is a key to successful weight loss, says Dr. Foreyt. Ask your family and friends to cheer you on. Maybe they could join you in eating low-fat, healthful meals.

"Form a neighborhood group that walks together, or look to the YMCA, the Jewish Community Center or your local church or college for weight loss support groups," Dr. Foreyt says. "And groups such as Weight Watchers, which teach self-maintenance, can be very, very useful." If you tend to lose control and overeat compulsively or go on big food binges followed by a sense of shame, an Overeaters Anonymous group or professional counseling can be a tremendous help, he says.

**Pay attention to your emotional needs.** Sometimes you can confuse hunger with other feelings, especially if you're feeling depressed or stressed or just responding to a luscious photo spread in a gourmet food magazine. If it's not your stomach talking, you need to figure out what kinds of emotions or discomforts are triggering your urge for food, Dr. Foreyt says. Then develop a problem-solving approach. "How can you answer that need without eating? Walk around the block, call a friend, meditate, take a bath, brush your teeth, or gargle with mouthwash," he says. "This breaks the chain and develops an alternate behavior pattern."

**Boycott the fat box.** If you watch more than three hours of television a day, you double your risk of being saddled with extra pounds, says Larry A. Tucker, Ph.D., professor and director of health promotion at Brigham Young University in Provo, Utah. Slouched on the couch, you're not burning many calories, and you're likely to be taking in more by eating fattening snacks. So turn off the tube (plus the junk food habit that usually comes with it) to boost your weight loss campaign.

# How to Eat and Lose Weight

The latest nutrition research shows that there really is a whole new way to lose weight—without dieting and without hunger. It's based on understanding which kinds of food revitalize you and give you real energy and which foods go right to your thighs. You may be surprised to find that the most crucial changes don't require that you eat less—just differently. Here's how.

**Forgo excess fat.** Dietary fat makes us gain weight because it's stored in the body far more easily than either carbohydrates or protein, says Peter D. Vash, M.D., assistant clinical professor of medicine at the University of California, Los Angeles. The body burns those for fuel almost immediately, while the more calorie-dense fat burns slower and is more likely to be left over—on you.

# Trimming the Tummy That Won't Quit

Even when you've been watching your weight diligently, you still may have a stubbornly protruding stomach. It's often a natural consequence of aging for both women and men, research shows. For women, it's often due to repeated dieting—regained weight tends to be deposited on the belly, researchers say. Or it may be a lingering reminder of pregnancy. You can flatten your stomach without complicated exercise gizmos and gadgets, however. Here's how.

**Don't belly up to the bar.** There really is such a thing as a beer belly, and cutting your alcohol intake may be the key to flattening it. In a large study, women and men who drank more than two alcoholic drinks a day had the largest waist-to-hip ratios, which is how doctors quantify potbellies.

**Stamp out the cigs.** In the same study, researchers at Stanford University School of Medicine in Stanford, California, and the University of California, San Diego, detected a similar effect for smoking. There were twice as many fat abdomens among those who lit up as among nonsmokers. See your doctor for help in quitting.

**Start huffing.** Maybe belly dancing is just what that belly needs. To burn off a belly, exercise must do two things, says Bryant Stamford, Ph.D., director of the Health Promotion Center at the University of Louisville in Kentucky. First, it must start out vigorously to trigger a substantial adrenaline release, which frees fat to be used for fuel. You can get this effect from brisk walking, he says. Then the vigorous activity must be followed by prolonged aerobic exercise that will burn up the liberated fat. Walking at a comfortable pace fits the bill. So could a spate of hard housework followed by some steady raking. "Just step up the pace now and then to boost adrenaline output," he says.

**Firm it up.** Once the fat is whittled away by low-fat eating and aerobic exercise, daily abdominal exercises can really help to improve your shape, Dr. Stamford says. Start with isometric squeezes: Tense your abdominal muscles to the maximum and hold for six to ten seconds. Relax, then repeat several times. Later, he says, you can move to crunches: Lie on your back with your legs apart and knees bent. Cross your arms on your chest. Lift your head up toward the ceiling. Keep going until you can lift your shoulder blades slightly off the ground. Hold for two seconds, then lie back down. Build up gradually to ten repetitions a set.

Start by cutting fat in the obvious places: Eat fewer fatty meats, fried foods, high-fat dairy products and desserts. Also, beware of salads slathered in oil or other fatty dressings. It's recommended that you keep your total calories from fat to 25 percent or less of your daily diet.

"A high-fat diet has been linked to obesity, which in turn is associated with an increased risk of various cancers. Prudence says that a high-fat diet is a factor in so many illnesses that it only makes sense to eat low-fat foods instead," says Dr. Foreyt.

**Drown it.** "Drinking generous amounts of water is overwhelmingly the number-one way to reduce appetite," says Dr. Blackburn. Not only does water keep your stomach feeling fuller, but also many people think they're having food cravings when in fact they're thirsty, he says. So aim for 8 cups of fluids daily, sipping ½ cup at a time through the day.

When you're sipping away through the day, keep in mind that caffeine—in cola, coffee or tea—has its drawbacks. Caffeine is a diuretic, which removes water from the body. For that reason, most doctors recommend that people on weight loss programs drink no more than three caffeinated beverages a day.

**Count on carbs.** Don't go hungry. When you replace the excess fat calories you've been eating with foods such as carbohydrates, you can actually eat more and still lose pounds. In one study at the University of Illinois at Chicago, people on moderately high-fat diets were told to maintain their weights for 20 weeks while switching to low-fat, high-carbohydrate diets. They ate all they wanted and still lost more than 11 percent of their body fat and 2 percent of their weight. So enjoy plenty of carbohydrate-rich pasta (without fatty sauces), low-fat cereals, breads, beans, crunchy fresh vegetables and fruits to fill you up while you're losing weight.

**Allow a few splurges.** If you feel that all you're saying to yourself about food is no-no-no, you may eventually let slips turn into a downhill slide, says Susan Kayman, R.D., Dr.P.H., a dietitian and consultant with the Kaiser Permanente Medical Group in Oakland, California. That's why she advocates following the 80/20 rule. If you eat low fat 80 percent of the time, then when you're dining with friends, out on the town or over at the in-laws, enjoy an occasional higher-fat treat without beating yourself up about it, she says.

**Break up the deadly duo.** That's fats and sweets. When the body gets a jolt of sugar, it releases lots of insulin in response. Because insulin is a storage-prone hormone, it opens up fat cells, preparing them for fat storage. So when you eat sugar, keep your fat intake low. Also, fats and sugar taken together can turn up your appetite to unmanageable levels. Eating sweets leads to an increase in the amount of sugar in the blood, which, because of a chain of reactions in the body, pumps up your appetite, says Dr. Wadden. So soothe your sweet tooth with a juicy fresh fruit or bowl of low-fat sugared cereal instead of doughnuts and candy bars.

**Stay with it.** Here's a fat-fighting tip to hang on to: If you stick with it, you'll actually lose your taste for high-fat foods after a while. A four-year study of more than 2,000 women at the Fred Hutchinson Cancer Research Center at the University of Washington in Seattle showed that women who limit their fat intakes lose their taste for fat in six months or less, eventually finding fatty foods unpleasant to eat.

**Eat often.** Some researchers support the idea of grazing—eating numerous small meals throughout the day instead of three larger meals—to control appetite and prevent bingeing. "But you cannot graze on M&M's, potato chips and Häagen-Dazs," says James Kenney, R.D., Ph.D., a nutrition research specialist at the Pritikin Longevity Center in Santa Monica, California. "But if you graze on low-fat, high-fiber foods that aren't packed with calories, such as carrots, apples, peaches, oranges and red peppers, you'll keep your appetite down."

**Turn up the heat.** Be lavish with hot spices such as cayenne pepper and horseradish to boost your metabolic rate, which may help your body burn more calories, says Dr. Kenney. "When people eat hot foods, they often sweat, a sure sign of increased metabolic rate. And the faster the metabolic rate, the more heat produced by the body. Remember, whatever warms you up in turn slims you down," he says. But be sure to avoid high-fat dishes, even if they're loaded with spices.

**Start with soup.** A soup appetizer tends to reduce the amount you eat at a meal, several studies suggest. In one study from Johns Hopkins University in Baltimore, people who had soup before a meal ate 25 percent fewer calories of the entrée than those who started the meal with cheese and crackers. It may be the volume of space that soup takes up in the stomach or the fact that most of soup's calories come from carbohydrates rather than fat, researchers say. Or there may be a psychological factor at work, Dr. Kenney says. "Hot soup is very relaxing if you have a nervous, gnawing appetite."

**Ride out a craving.** When the urge strikes for a chocolate eclair, don't confuse the craving with a command, says Linda Crawford, an eating behavior specialist at Green Mountain at Fox Run, a residential weight and health management center in Ludlow, Vermont. Though many people think cravings keep getting stronger until they're irresistible, research shows that food cravings actually start and escalate, then peak and subside. Distract yourself with a walk or something else incompatible with eating, Crawford says, and ride out the craving. "Just like with surfing," she says, "the more you practice riding a craving wave, the easier it becomes." But if you still have the craving after 20 minutes, go ahead and satisfy it with a small portion—and enjoy it, she advises.

# A Woman's Weight Loss Workout

Adopting a healthier diet will help you lose weight, but you'll acquire a firmer figure faster—and keep it—if you combine your healthy new eating habits with exercise.

Exercise also strengthens your heart and arteries, and it boosts your self-confidence—in short, it will counteract many of the harmful effects of over-

# The Batwing Problem

A beautiful sundress catches your eye. Uh-oh . . . wait a minute. It's sleeveless. You give your flabby upper arms a squeeze, just to make sure they're still with you.

Charmingly dubbed batwings by doctors, these slabs of skin and fat have three main causes, says Alan Matarasso, M.D., a plastic surgeon at Manhattan Eye, Ear and Throat Hospital in New York City. First, you may have inherited a tendency to deposit fat on the underside of your upper arms. Second, if you've gained and lost weight repeatedly over the years, your skin has stretched and contracted so many times that it has lost some of its elasticity. Third, that's loose, thin skin under there. It's as sensitive as the delicate skin on your inner thigh, Dr. Matarasso says. "It's thinner and looser than skin on the outer arm or abdomen," he says.

How to trim your wings? Any exercise that strengthens your triceps muscle—the one running along the back of your arm from underarm to elbow—will help, Dr. Matarasso says. Any trainer will be able to show you several, he says, but here's one to try.

*In a standing position, hold a dumbbell weighing between three and five pounds vertically in front of you with both hands, with your elbows slightly bent (right). Slowly raise the dumbbell straight up over your head (far right). This is your starting position. Bending your elbows, lower the dumbbell to the back of your neck, then raise it back up to the starting position above your head. Continue to raise and lower the weight slowly, working up to sets of ten repetitions.*

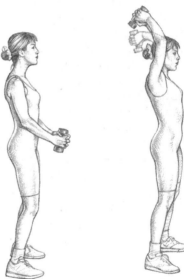

weight. Exercise can even help to curb your appetite.

If you're unaccustomed to exercising, see your doctor before you get started. After you have her okay, you'll be ready. Here are some tips to get you going.

**Keep it up.** "The best predictor of long-term weight management is regular aerobic activity, which boosts your heart rate," says Dr. Foreyt. "Brisk walking is a great choice because it's very easy for most people to do on a regular basis. But the effectiveness of any aerobic activity for weight control has been proven repeatedly." Any kind of daily exercise helps. Thirty minutes of aerobic exercise burns flab and tones muscles—as long as you do it regularly.

**Burn by building.** Aerobic exercise should always be part of your weight loss plan, but when you add resistance training such as weight lifting, you'll keep your weight down with the help of "hungry muscles. Muscle tissue needs more calories," says Janet Walberg-Rankin, Ph.D., associate professor in the Exercise Science Program in the Division of Health and Physical Education at Virginia Polytechnic Institute and State University in Blacksburg. "So if you increase muscle mass while you lose fat, you boost your ability to burn fuel." It's later in the day, when you're in a meeting or waiting in line at the bank, that your new, ravenous muscle is grinding away calories, she says.

"Resistance training isn't just about lifting barbells," adds Dr. Foreyt, though that's great for firming the arms. To really work the different groups of muscles, your best bet is to go to a gym and ask a trainer there to show you how to circuit-train, he says. You use a series of different weight machines to press weights against muscles in the neck, arms, chest and legs. You can accomplish the same thing by working with free weights at home, he says. "Putting your muscles against something that doesn't yield—that's resistance."

# THE PILL

*It's Changed, and So Have You*

Remember when you and your girlfriends first sat around drinking coffee and talking about the Pill? Telling them you were on it made you feel adult and mature. It meant that you were sexually active, that you had a boyfriend, that you were having passionate, romping sex whenever you wanted to.

Now, years later, you once again find yourself talking to your girlfriends over coffee about the Pill. Only now the conversations make you feel like you're growing old. You talk less about the sex and more about what impact the Pill might have on your long-term health. While you once blessed the Pill for its ability to prevent pregnancy (by ceasing ovulation), now you're concerned about what it doesn't protect you from—namely, the threat of sexually transmitted diseases. You're also worried about the possible risks that have been associated with the Pill's long-term use, such as heart disease, cancer and fertility problems.

If nothing else, the conversation alone is showing your age. You find yourself talking about cervical cancer, high cholesterol and AIDS instead of multiple orgasms and foreplay. Yes, you're older now, but you're smarter, too—about your body. Your questions and concerns about the Pill no longer have to do with its ability to prevent pregnancy. It's now a question of health.

Sometime around their mid-thirties, women begin to question their doctors about the wisdom of being on the Pill, says Edward Linn, M.D., chairman of obstetrics and gynecology at Lutheran General Hospital in Park Ridge, Illinois.

And the good news is that there doesn't appear to be as much bad news about the Pill as there used to be. In fact, there may be more benefits than risks. Many experts believe that for women in their thirties and forties, the pros outweigh the cons—if they are healthy and don't smoke.

# Matters of the Heart

When it comes to aging and the Pill, smokers face the greatest risks. Smokers in general are at greater risk for heart attacks, and taking the Pill boosts that risk dramatically. Statistics show that women over age 30 who smoke between 1 and 24 cigarettes a day are three times more likely to have heart attacks if they take the Pill than if they don't. And women over 30 who smoke 25 or more cigarettes a day increase their risk of heart attack ten times by taking the Pill.

The Pill and cigarettes are also a bad combination when it comes to your risk for a stroke. The figures are similar to those for heart attack: Women over age 30 who take the Pill and smoke between 1 and 24 cigarettes a day increase their risk for stroke three times, and women who smoke 25 or more cigarettes a day increase their risk for stroke by almost ten times.

But if you don't smoke and you're otherwise healthy, you can consider the Pill relatively safe. Studies show that the Pill of the 1990s poses little threat to your overall health.

This message is dramatically different from the one women received in the early days of the Pill, which made its debut in the 1960s. That's because synthetic estrogen, the ingredient that gives the Pill its protective action, is lower in content than ever. Researchers have discovered that it takes only a small percentage of the hormone levels used in earlier days to make the Pill effective. And this small dosage has been found to have positive effects.

At these lower levels, estrogen appears to decrease the levels of LDL (low-density lipoprotein) cholesterol, the bad cholesterol that contributes to clogging up the arteries. Estrogen also appears to increase levels of HDL (high-density lipoprotein) cholesterol, the good cholesterol that helps prevent clogged arteries by transporting bad cholesterol away from vessel walls. And even when bad cholesterol is present, studies show that estrogen may act on the vessel wall in a beneficial way that can help prevent plaque buildup.

# The Era of STDs

It's a relief to know that the Pill is no longer the health threat that it used to be. And it's also comforting to know that when it's used correctly, the Pill offers virtually certain protection against what it was originally intended for: pregnancy. But back in the 1960s, AIDS and sexually transmitted diseases (STDs) weren't the major concern to women that they are today.

When used alone, with no condom or other barrier method, the Pill offers no protection against the human immunodeficiency virus, which causes AIDS, or against sexually transmitted diseases such as chlamydia, gonorrhea and human papillomavirus (HPV), or vaginal warts. For women between the ages of 25 and 44, AIDS is the fourth leading cause of death in the United States overall, and in certain areas of the country, it is the number-one cause. The disease is spreading four times faster among women than among men.

Each year, sexually transmitted diseases are thought to be the cause of an estimated 150,000 cases of infertility in women and 45,000 life-threatening ectopic pregnancies, in which the egg is fertilized in the fallopian tubes instead of the womb. Certain strains of HPV, or vaginal warts, have been associated with cervical cancer, which kills more than 4,500 women a year. So by using the Pill with no other protection, a woman can jeopardize her life and her health.

The Pill does offer some protection against one sexually transmitted disease, however. Research indicates that the Pill may actually reduce the risk of pelvic inflammatory disease, or PID, a disease in which sexually transmitted organisms infect a woman's fallopian tubes and uterus and can cause infertility. By some means that researchers don't completely understand yet, the Pill may help prevent lower genital tract infections such as chlamydia and gonorrhea from ascending to the upper genital tract and causing PID.

# Questions about Cancer

You may be asking more questions than you used to about the Pill and cancer. You've heard that breast cancer is the cancer most prevalent in women, and you want to know what role, if any, the Pill can play in its development.

Unfortunately, some questions about breast cancer and the Pill are still unanswered. Several studies, including the cancer and steroid hormone, or CASH, study conducted by the Centers for Disease Control and Prevention in Atlanta, do provide some clues.

The CASH study looked at the effect of Pill use on cancer in 10,000 American women. The results indicated that women 35 years of age or younger were 1.4 times more likely to develop breast cancer if they took the Pill than women of the same age who never used oral contraceptives. Women 35 to 44 who took the Pill were 1.1 times more likely to develop breast cancer than women who didn't take it. And women over 45 were actually at slightly lower risk—they were 0.9 times as likely to develop breast cancer as women their age who never used the Pill. In other words, taking the Pill may increase the risk of breast cancer slightly.

While the jury is still out on the breast cancer/Pill connection, the verdict is in on the Pill's culpability in other female cancers—namely, ovarian and uterine. The verdict: not guilty.

In fact, the Pill is believed to actually help protect against these cancers. Studies show that after a woman has been on the Pill for one year, her risk for both forms of cancer decreases by about 50 percent, says Herbert Peterson, M.D., chief of the Women's Health and Fertility Branch of the Centers for Disease Control and Prevention. And the protective effect extends well after a woman stops taking the Pill, he says.

# Is Fertility Affected?

Another concern for women in their thirties and forties is whether taking the Pill will affect their fertility. "Fertility declines naturally as a woman ages, regardless of whether she's on the Pill," says Dr. Linn. But oral contraceptives have not been shown to increase infertility, he says.

Several studies indicate that oral contraceptive use may slightly delay a woman's ability to conceive, but the delay is generally a matter of a couple of months.

In a study in Oxford, England, women who used oral contraceptives experienced conception delays of about two months. The older women were when they discontinued the Pill or any other method—say, age 35 compared with 30—the longer it took them to get pregnant, though often it took only a month or two, says Carolyn Westhoff, M.D., associate professor at Columbia University in New York City and one of the researchers on the British study. But, she said, the delay may be more a matter of age than taking the Pill.

Another study conducted at Yale University in New Haven, Connecticut, also reported delays in conception in women who took the Pill. Again, the delay was only a matter of a couple of months. Women who used other methods of contraception took nearly four months to conceive, while those who used the Pill generally took closer to six months.

# Your Best Protection

If you are on the Pill or plan to start, here's what you need to know.

**See your doctor annually.** Your decision to start, stay with or get off the Pill should be based on your own health history. So you should see your doctor on an annual basis. Don't hesitate to ask questions and get her opinion. Don't be afraid to seek a second opinion. Remember that a lot of doctors feel that the benefits generally outweigh the risks for healthy, nonsmoking women.

**Know your family history.** If anyone in your family has had heart disease, breast cancer, high blood pressure, ovarian cancer or uterine cancer, discuss it with your doctor. These factors should be taken into consideration, but they won't immediately prohibit you from taking the Pill, says Dr. Linn.

**Protect yourself.** The Pill may protect you from pregnancy, but it won't protect you from sexually transmitted diseases or AIDS. One answer is condoms. Latex condoms containing the spermicide nonoxynol-9 are most effective against sexually transmitted diseases, experts say.

**Practice prevention.** Performing a monthly breast self-examination is always important, but if you're on the Pill, make certain you do it routinely. Doctors also recommend that you have your first mammogram between the ages of 35 and 40, then one every two years during your forties and one every year thereafter.

# PREMENSTRUAL SYNDROME

## Getting Along in Spite of It

I have PMS."

You've probably said it to your friends at one time or another. They've probably said it to you. None of you has to say much more. The three-word statement, kind of a universal among American women, says it all.

It says you're feeling out of sorts, anxious and moody.

It says that you feel ugly and fat and that it's probably a bad hair day.

And it also says you're feeling less than your usual youthful self. You feel old, tired, achy, irritable, bloated, depressed and withdrawn. You're having trouble concentrating. Your back hurts. You don't feel too much like doing anything or seeing anybody.

Your zip for life has been zapped.

## Defining PMS

The term *PMS* (premenstrual syndrome) has become part of the American vernacular; women use it to refer to how they feel before their periods. And many do experience premenstrual symptoms that are uncomfortable, disturbing and difficult. But not all women who say or think they have PMS necessarily do.

There's lots of disagreement among experts about how PMS should be defined, but most agree that for a woman to officially have PMS, her symptoms must recur in two of every three menstrual cycles. And the period of premenstrual symptoms must be followed by a symptom-free period. The symptoms— and there are more than 150 that women may experience—also interfere with her ability to function.

An estimated 20 to 95 percent of all women in their childbearing years experience some premenstrual symptoms. The condition varies from woman to woman and even from one month to the next. But only 3 to 5 percent are said to suffer severely enough to have it interfere with daily living.

"Women with PMS describe themselves as feeling different—not themselves," says Kathleen Hubbs Ulman, Ph.D., an instructor at Harvard Medical School in Boston. "For some, these changes come on slowly, over a day or a few hours. Others say they wake up one morning and feel like a different person." Some women say they want to jump out of their skin. Others are exceptionally sad, slowed down, tired and depressed. They also "feel very irritable," says Dr. Ulman. "It's hard for them to bite their tongues. They're apt to start fights with their husbands or criticize their children more quickly. But those are feelings. Women who feel that way don't have to act on these impulses." With correct diagnosis and counseling, women can work to find ways to experience the feelings without acting on them impulsively and destructively, she says.

# The Controversial Condition

Controversy surrounds PMS. While experts agree on the bare essentials of the condition, the complete definition is a matter of opinion. Some prefer to view PMS as consisting of several different subtypes organized around which symptoms women get. PMS-H women are those whose predominant symptoms are weight gain, swelling of the hands, feet and ankles, breast tenderness and abdominal bloating. PMS-A women are those who tend to suffer most with nervous tension, irritability and mood swings. Others designate levels of PMS based on severity and pattern of symptoms. Women with milder symptoms that don't change throughout the cycle fall into a low symptom (LS) category. Those with consistently severe symptoms, such as chronic low mood or irritability, that get even worse premenstrually have a pattern known as premenstrual magnification (PMM). Women with classic PMS have symptoms that are mild or unnoticeable after their periods but that get increasingly worse as their next periods approach.

Another matter of contention is whether PMS should be classified officially as a psychiatric illness. Mild PMS is not included in the American Psychiatric Association's manual of mental disorders. However, PMDD (premenstrual dysphoric disorder), marked by depression severe enough to interfere with daily living, is included in the manual's appendix. According to the American Psychiatric Association, this does not officially designate PMDD as a mental disorder. Opinions over this are divided; some feel that while this classification may help women with severe premenstrual symptoms get the medical help they need, others feel it may stigmatize women by linking mental disorders to the biological process of menstruation.

There's also disagreement over what causes PMS. Theories range from hormone levels to nutritional factors such as lack of Vitamin $B_6$ or magnesium to the impact of fluctuating levels of hormones on brain neurotransmitters such as serotonin and dopamine to psychological factors such as stress.

## Why Women in Their Thirties?

PMS tends to appear less often during a woman's teens and early twenties. "I see more women in their thirties, definitely. A lot are even in their early forties," says Marcia Szewczyk, M.D., director of the PMS Clinic at the Bowman Gray School of Medicine of Wake Forest University in Winston-Salem, North Carolina.

And researchers have ideas about why that's so.

One is that PMS is the result of hormonal imbalance—specifically, a drop in the ratio of progesterone to estrogen. Progesterone is believed to have a tranquilizing effect. So the belief is that if the ratio of progesterone to estrogen is too low, increased tension, anxiety and irritability may result.

In addition to this, one of the primary reasons women in their thirties get PMS is that they have a number of opportunities to have hormonal swings, such as pregnancy, miscarriage or going on or off the Pill, says Stephanie DeGraff Bender, clinical director of a PMS clinic in Boulder, Colorado, and author of *PMS: A Positive Program to Gain Control* and *PMS: Questions and Answers.*

Other researchers, including Nancy Fugate Woods, Ph.D., of the Center for Women's Health Research at the University of Washington School of Nursing in Seattle, say that stress plays a large role in the development of PMS and that the reason we may see more PMS in women in their thirties and forties is that women's lives tend to get more complex as they get older, says Dr. Fugate Woods. For women between the ages of 30 and 45 today, there are incredible expectations, she says. They may have kids, be supporting their parents, be working two or three jobs or be single parents, she says. "Focusing only on women's biology is to do them a disservice. We need to begin by grounding research in women's lives," she says.

## Preventing PMS

Whatever causes it, if you think you have PMS and you're worried about the toll it's taking on your youthfulness—in both mind and body—there are some things you can do to try to keep symptoms to a minimum. Here are some suggestions.

**Get up and go.** "Women who exercise on a regular basis find that it really does help their PMS," says Dr. Szewczyk. The type of exercise women choose depends on their preferences and fitness levels, she says. Walking, jogging and playing tennis are just a few possibilities. Exercise helps boost endorphins, the body's natural painkillers, so it may help fend off cramps and improve moods. It can also give women a sense of control, says Dr. Szewczyk. There are lots of opportunities to exercise that we often overlook, adds Bender. Simple activities such as taking a walk, riding a bike or turning on a tape player and dancing fast to two or three songs can do the trick, she says.

**Cut back on the sweet stuff.** Avoid sugar in your diet, says Dr. Szewczyk. This means things such as cookies, candies and chocolate, she says. Keeping your sugar intake low will keep your blood sugar levels from fluctuating wildly. Your energy levels will be more stable, and you'll be better able to cope with whatever discomfort you do have.

**Control the caffeine.** "I tell people to avoid caffeine," says Dr. Szewczyk. Caffeine stimulates the nervous system, leading to anxiety and mood swings. Women should cut back slowly, basically weaning themselves off caffeinated coffee, she says. One trick that often works is to mix proportions of decaffeinated and caffeinated coffee until you're drinking all decaf, she says.

**Shake the shaker habit.** Reducing your salt intake can help reduce symptoms of bloating and water retention. Read the food labels carefully. Anything that begins or ends with *sodium* is a salt, so if there are more than three ingredients with that term, chances are the food is high in salt, says Bender. And watch out for hidden sources of sodium, such as salad dressing, she says. If you have to eat out, opt for vinegar and oil over other dressings whose contents you can't find out.

**Reach for calcium.** Boosting your calcium intake above the Recommended Dietary Allowance of 800 milligrams (for women over age 24) may help decrease your premenstrual symptoms, researchers say. In a small study of women with PMS, increasing calcium helped decrease mood problems and poor concentration, says James G. Penland, Ph.D., a research psychologist at the U.S. Department of Agriculture's Grand Forks Human Nutrition Research Center in Grand Forks, North Dakota, where the study was conducted. Other studies of women with PMS found similar effects from increasing calcium, he says.

Calcium is thought to play a role in the regulation of some types of muscle, and it also affects neurotransmitters, brain chemicals that may influence mood. Most women consume about 600 milligrams of calcium a day, says Dr. Penland. All they have to do is add one eight-ounce glass of 1 or 2 percent milk and a cup of yogurt, and they'll boost their calcium intakes to about 1,200 milligrams, he says. "The data suggest that if someone experiences unpleasant menstrual symptoms, there may be an immediate benefit from increased calcium intake," he says.

**Notice your symptoms.** A lot of women say that keeping a symptom diary helps, says Ellen Freeman, Ph.D., director of the PMS Program at the University of Pennsylvania Medical Center in Philadelphia. This helps women see the pattern of their monthly symptoms, she says, which can help them learn to anticipate when they'll feel bad. Women "can be the best experts on their bodies—they can be the best diagnosticians," agrees Dr. Fugate Woods.

**Take time to relax.** Women with PMS can take advantage of multiple relaxation methods, says Dr. Freeman. These range from "listening to music to doing yoga and meditating to retiring and reading a book," she says. "Whatever works for you is okay." Look for books to get you started, or take a class in relaxation techniques.

**Try reflexology.** Applying manual pressure to specific points on the ears, hands and feet may relieve some of the symptoms women experience with PMS, says Terry Oleson, Ph.D., chair of the Department of Behavioral Medicine at the California Graduate Institute in Los Angeles who completed the first controlled study of the use of reflexology. Women can perform reflexology on themselves, he says. Press different spots on your ear between two fingers until you find ones that are sensitive, he says. Once you locate them, apply firm but gentle pressure for 30 seconds to one minute, then release. Repeat up to three times if you like.

**Address PMS ahead of time.** Talk to your partner about having PMS, how it makes you feel, how you might behave, what you're doing about it and what he can do to help, says Bender. Do this at a time of the month when you are symptom-free, she says. Communicating about PMS "needs to be taken care of in non-PMS time," Bender says.

**Communicate with your kids.** It's important to tell your children that you have a health problem and that you are dealing with it, says Bender. She suggests saying to your child "I have this imbalance in my body, and I'm working on getting it fixed. But when it's there, I may not play with you as much, and I may not talk with you as much. And even though I look the same, I may not be acting the same."

Provide signals to your child about what days your PMS is a problem. For younger children, place smile-face magnets on the refrigerator; on days when you have PMS, turn the smile faces upside down. This lets your child know you're not feeling well. For older children, mark off on a calendar the days you expect to be feeling under par. Bender also recommends telling your children that they can help. Offer to let them help find low-sugar foods, for instance.

**Get a diagnosis.** While you may think you have PMS, it's necessary to see a doctor to have it officially diagnosed. You will undergo a medical history, physical exam and psychological evaluation and be asked to fill out a symptom diary for three months. Many women who think they have PMS turn out not to when they track their own symptoms, says Dr. Fugate Woods. Women often find that the symptoms correspond to factors other than their menstrual cycles, such as events or relationships in their lives, she says.

# REACTION TIME

## *Turning Around the Big Slowdown*

There was a time not too long ago when in almost every situation, your response was as quick as a cat's. If you were playing tennis and your opponent hit a smash down the line—*whoosh*! You'd return it, no problem. If you knocked a piece of china off the counter—*zoom*! You'd catch it before it hit the ground. If someone asked you a question—*bang*! You had the answer in an instant.

But lately, there has been a lot less woosh, zoom and bang in your life. Tennis balls are flying past. Family heirlooms are hitting the floor. And TV quiz show contestants are hitting their buzzers while you're still trying to figure out what the heck the question was.

What's happening here?

Well, you're getting older—and probably a little slower. While you're not ready for the nursing home yet, it's an undeniable fact that your reflexes aren't what they used to be.

But don't worry. It happens to all of us. And there's a lot we can do about it.

## The Secret to Speedy Reflexes

Even the fittest of the fit will eventually join the ain't-what-I-used-to-be group. "Everyone, including great athletes, reaches her peak fitness levels in the mid- to late twenties and then gradually declines," says Ralph Tarter, Ph.D., professor of psychiatry and neurology at the University of Pittsburgh School of Medicine. "As fitness goes, our metabolism slows, and with it, our ability to perform tasks requiring sustained strength and speed."

Lucky for us that we have a surefire defense against this downward decline:

lifelong physical activity. When you exercise, the body increases its output of growth hormone, a substance that helps maintain muscle mass, bone density and lean body composition. A study by Robert Mazzeo, Ph.D., a kinesiologist (he studies human motion) at the University of Colorado in Boulder, found that regularly active individuals had higher concentrations of growth hormone in their blood than people the same age who didn't exercise and sedentary people who were much younger.

"Even the elderly will see an increase in growth hormone levels from exercise, and with it will come increased strength, balance and speed," Dr. Mazzeo says.

The master control center for our ability to react to stimuli is the brain. In a split second, it processes information and then sends impulse signals to our muscles. "As we age, we see little change in the speed of these impulses," says Lawrence Z. Stern, M.D., director of the Muscular Dystrophy Association's Mucio F. Delgado Clinic for Neuromuscular Disorders at the University of Arizona Health Sciences Center in Tucson. "The greatest delays are in the processing of information that is necessary to formulate the messages that tell the muscles what to do."

Why? First, as we age, we lose brain cells that help us process new information. Also, we have much more information and experiences in our heads than we did when we were younger. This slows down our ability to make snap judgments. And we get lazy; it becomes easier to rely on old familiar ways than to deal with new ones.

## Reaction Time Reactivators

So how do you keep your mind sharp and your reactions quick?

**Use it.** "Maintain complex mental activities versus passive ones such as watching television," says Dr. Tarter. "Stay mentally engaged by exposing yourself to demanding tasks and new challenges every single day. When we constantly use the brain and push it to its full capacity, it stays faster, more alert and more efficient."

Check your vision. Before you can mentally or physically react, you must have an accurate picture of the world outside. For that, we must rely on our senses, vision in particular. "Seventy-five to 80 percent of reaction time is directly related to good visual skills," says Arthur Seiderman, O.D., an Elkins Park, Pennsylvania, visual consultant to many professional athletes and author of *20/20 Is Not Enough*. "That means more than just seeing objects clearly; it also means having the ability to detect, track and recognize fast-moving objects."

**Steer clear of alcohol and drugs.** Everybody knows that drunk drivers are slow to react behind the wheel, but even one or two drinks can be enough to send your reaction time plummeting, says Dr. Stern. And if you regularly drink alcoholic beverages or take any medication that affects the central nervous system, it could put your mind and body in a constant state of slo-mo.

# Setting Your Sights

An optometrist or ophthalmologist can put you on a program to improve the clarity and quality of your vision. In the meantime, Arthur Seiderman, O.D., an Elkins Park, Pennsylvania, visual consultant to many professional athletes and author of *20/20 Is Not Enough*, recommends these exercises.

**Have a ball.** Cut out a variety of letters, small shapes and colored pieces of paper, and tape them to a ball or beanbag. Then play a round of catch or bounce the ball off a wall, spotting and calling out one or more of the colors, shapes or objects before you catch it.

**Go for a spin.** Cut a piece of cardboard into the shape of a disc, paste different-size letters, numbers, words or figures on it, and put it on a turntable. Set the speed at 33⅓ rpm and call out the information on the disc for one to three minutes. When it gets easier, increase the speed to 45 rpm, then 78 rpm.

**Box to the beat.** Draw a large box with 16 squares on a chalkboard or piece of paper. Place the numbers 1 through 16 in the squares in random order. Turn on a musical metronome or other rhythm-making device, and point to each of the numbers in numerical order, keeping time with the beat. Try it again in backward order, then repeat.

**Flip some flash cards.** For this you'll need 50 3- by 5-inch cards. Draw a black dot in the center of each card, below the top edge. Write a different two-digit number on each side of the dot, about ½ inch from the dot. Mark another card with a different pair of two-digit numbers, each placed ¾ inch away from the dot. Continue marking each card, spacing the numbers at ¼-inch intervals until you reach the far corners; then work back toward the center dot.

Hold the stack of cards 14 to 16 inches in front of you. Then flip through the stack while focusing on the center dot and call out the numbers on the card. It should get increasingly difficult to identify the numbers as they are spaced farther from the center. Start slow, then build up your flipping speed.

**Don't smoke.** Tobacco saps speed in more ways than one, says Dr. Tarter. We all know the effect it has on our cardiovascular system. If our lungs and heart don't work efficiently, neither will our bones and muscles. Smoking also dramatically reduces the amount of oxygen in our bloodstream, and the brain needs a steady supply of fresh oxygen to stay in good working order.

**Catch some Zzzs.** A good night's sleep is nature's way of recharging our mental batteries. "Regular quality sleep every night is essential for the brain to stay alert and perform cognitive tasks at maximal levels," says Dr. Stern.

**Zap some aliens.** Video and computer games have been shown to dramatically improve mental and motor skills, says Dr. Tarter. "They are often used to help rehab patients develop speed, and even pilots these days practice on video simulators before they climb in the cockpit." If beeps, buzzes and explosions aren't your cup of tea, try some other fast-paced activity, such as Ping-Pong.

# RESPIRATORY DISEASES

## *Working toward Breathing Free*

You hike along a path that leads to a snow-covered peak in the Austrian Alps. Below is the Mozart-mad town of Salzburg; above is silent, glacier-cold rock and sky.

Drawing the crisp mountain air deep into your lungs, you hold it, exhale as long as you can, then repeat the process over and over again until every cell in your body is flooded with fresh, clean air.

If you had the flu, a cold or emphysema, you couldn't do this. You'd have to suck air on every hill as though you were 100 years old. You'd cough every time you took a deep breath. And you'd wheeze.

But if you keep your lungs healthy, you won't have to, says Robert Bethel, M.D., a staff physician at the National Jewish Center for Immunology and Respiratory Medicine in Denver.

Our lungs are made to last through any workout we hand them well into our seventies. Smoking, of course, can change that scenario, clogging up the lungs and making us gasp for air. Colds, flu, pneumonia and other infectious diseases can do the same, but only temporarily. Other diseases can also affect the lungs, but these are less common.

## Strengthening Your Natural Defenses

Every day, your respiratory system draws in approximately 9,500 quarts of air and mixes it with up to 10,600 quarts of blood pumped by the heart into the lungs. Your lungs send oxygen through arterial highways to support the rest of the body and to provide an exhaust system for gaseous metabolic garbage such as carbon dioxide.

Since your lungs are internal organs that draw in the microorganisms of the outside world with every breath, the strength of their natural defense system is

# TB: It's Back

Tuberculosis (TB), a bacterial lung infection that scientists thought they had virtually eliminated in the United States, is not only alive and well but also thriving.

While the disease had been declining since the late 1940s, the number of cases of TB increased nearly 16 percent in a six-year span between the late 1980s and early 1990s.

Cities have been hit the worst. By the early 1990s, TB had increased to approximately seven times the national average in Atlanta, six times in Newark, New Jersey, and five times in New York City, according to the Centers for Disease Control and Prevention in Atlanta.

The cause? Rampant spread of the bacteria that cause TB among those who have AIDS, those who are homeless and those who have newly emigrated to the United States—plus the development of drug-resistant strains of the bacteria.

TB is spread by airborne droplets in sneezes, coughs and just plain breathing. The bacteria are inhaled into the lungs. In those with strong immune systems, the bacteria are surrounded by a legion of bacterial fighters that render them harmless. In others, the bacteria settle into

particularly important in maintaining oxygen flow to and from the rest of your body. Fortunately for most of us, the lungs' defensive players, including mucus and hairlike filaments called cilia, can sweep pollens, dust, viruses and bacteria out of the airway.

Most of the time they do a great job. But sometimes they're undermined by irritants such as cigarette smoke or overwhelmed by invading microbes.

More than 14 million men and women suffer from chronic obstructive pulmonary disease, which includes both chronic bronchitis and emphysema. And in one year alone, 7 to 8 million men and women had asthma, 129 million had the flu, 4 million had pneumonia, and practically every one of us had some kind of cold virus.

How can you protect your lungs from the diseases and irritants that can slow you down? Here's what experts say.

**Keep your cilia sober.** Drinking interferes with the cleansing mechanisms that keep your lungs free of disease-causing germs, says Steven R. Mostow, M.D., chairman of the American Thoracic Society's Committee on the Prevention of Pneumonia and Influenza and professor of medicine at the University of

the lungs and multiply. With time, they may destroy extensive parts of the lungs and leave cavities. Eventually, the lungs look like Swiss cheese.

Today, ten million Americans carry the disease, many without the typical symptoms of cough, fatigue and weight loss.

"I think the general population is at risk," says Robert Bethel, M.D., a staff physician at the National Jewish Center for Immunology and Respiratory Medicine in Denver. "To a large extent, you can't control whether or not you're exposed to TB.

"Not that I want to be an alarmist," Dr. Bethel hastens to add. "But if you're on a bus, subway or airline with someone who has active TB and who is coughing, then the people around that person are exposed and vulnerable."

Fortunately, a complicated long-term drug regimen can usually fight TB into a dormant stage. But early treatment is important. If you think you've been exposed to TB, check with your doctor. A simple skin test or chest x-ray can usually determine whether or not you have the disease.

Colorado at Denver. "The respiratory system's cilia get drunk right along with the rest of you," he explains. If you're used to having one or two drinks on a daily basis, your cilia will be okay. But if you suddenly decide to drink more than you usually do, your cilia won't be able to do their job.

**Use ultrasound.** To keep your respiratory system in fighting trim, humidify your environment in winter with an ultrasonic humidifier, says Dr. Mostow. The increased moisture will help the cilia sweep out dust, viruses, bacteria and pollens.

**Work your lungs.** Don't just work your biceps. Get into an aerobic exercise program that works your heart and lungs, says Dr. Mostow. It will help keep your lungs functioning at peak efficiency. Walking, running and swimming for 20 minutes at least three times a week will certainly do the job, but check with your doctor before you start, so she can tailor your exercise prescription specifically to your needs.

**Smother smokes.** Smoking a cigarette or even being in a room where others are smoking can damage your lungs, says Dr. Bethel. The smoke may cause your body's natural defense system to release an enzyme that, in trying to attack the smoke's chemicals, literally digests the lung. Not only does this set the stage for future diseases, but breathing can be immediately impaired.

# Smothering Cold Symptoms

Colds, upper respiratory infections and bronchitis can be caused by any one of numerous microorganisms that can make you feel as though you lost the ability to breathe.

You get these diseases by inhaling somebody else's germs or touching someone that has a virus, then touching your eyes or nose, allowing the germs to enter your body.

Once the virus has invaded, it sets up shop in your throat and begins churning out baby viruses by the hundreds. These viruses spread through-out your body and trigger those beloved cold symptoms: a stuffy, drippy nose, sore throat, aches and pains and cough.

There's no way to cure a cold as yet, but here's how you can deal with its symptoms.

**Eat five-alarm chili and curry.** Hot peppers and spices such as curry and chili powder cause mucous membrane secretions. The extra fluid can thin out thick phlegm in your nasal passages and lubricate a sore, itchy throat.

**Steam and sip.** Sip chicken soup or linger in a steamy shower, suggests Thomas A. Gossel, Ph.D., dean of the College of Pharmacy and professor of pharmacology and toxicology at Ohio Northern University in Ada. The fluids you drink or inhale dilute the mucus in your nose and upper throat to help make breathing easier. Use decongestant sprays at bedtime for no more than five days to avoid inflaming tissues.

**Try the big D.** The D in many over-the-counter cough suppressants (such as Robitussin DM) is dextromethorphan. Doctors swear by it. Just make sure you follow package directions.

**Suck on zinc.** Zinc's ability to zap a cold has been suspected for years. And at least one study, at Dartmouth College in Hanover, New Hampshire, indicates that zinc tablets can cut the duration of a cold by 42 percent. But not any zinc tablet will do. You need those marked "zinc gluconate with glycine." They're fairly new on the market, so you may need to ask your druggist for help in tracking them down. If your druggist can't help, write the Quigley Corporation at 10 South Clinton Street, Doylestown, PA 18901.

**Numb your throat.** Suck on over-the-counter throat lozenges to numb and soothe your throat, suggests Dr. Gossel. Or aim a medicated spray at the back of your throat, hold your breath and squirt. Follow package directions for both lozenges and sprays.

**Purge pain.** Try aspirin, acetaminophen or ibuprofen to relieve the aches and pains of a cold, says Dr. Gossel.

**Fight malaise.** The too-tired-to-move feeling that usually accompanies a cold is often caused by dehydration, according to Dr. Gossel. Try drinking at least six glasses of water a day to prevent it.

**Chill out.** A study at Carnegie Mellon University in Pittsburgh indicates that the more stress you're under, the more likely you are to get a visit from any cold bug in the vicinity.

The researchers asked 394 men and women between the ages of 18 and 54 about any stress in their lives—recent bereavement, going on a diet, changing jobs, losing money, little sleep and arguing with family members—and then divided them into five groups. Each group received custom-made nose drops containing one of five viruses known to cause colds.

The result? Those who had the most stress in their lives were five times more likely to get colds than those who had the least.

## Coping with Emphysema and Bronchitis

One disease likely to send your respiratory system into an early retirement is chronic obstructive pulmonary disease. It includes chronic bronchitis, a condition in which the air sacs of the lungs are destroyed, and emphysema, a condition in which lung elasticity is lost and air is unable to flow freely in and out through the airway. It does not include the common bronchitis you might get with a cold—that's simply an irritation of the bronchial tubes that causes a few days of coughing and then goes away.

Both chronic bronchitis—roughly defined as a daily wet cough that lasts for three months or more—and emphysema are usually caused by smoking. Both have early symptoms of shortness of breath, limited ability to exert yourself, hacking up mucus and coughing, and both conditions are on the rise. The number of people who have these diseases has increased 41 percent in the last ten years, and chronic bronchitis and emphysema make up the largest number of respiratory illnesses (other than colds) in people between the ages of 30 and 45. Because more men than women smoke, men are nearly twice as likely as women to get emphysema, but women are rapidly catching up. When it comes to chronic bronchitis, women are more likely to get it. Emphysema and chronic bronchitis together kill approximately 75,000 people a year.

There's no cure for chronic bronchitis or emphysema, but the following strategies can lessen the shortness of breath that eventually comes from an obstructed airway and make life with the diseases a little easier.

**Avoid people who sneeze.** Any type of respiratory infection can make emphysema and chronic bronchitis worse, says Dr. Bethel. As much as possible, avoid crowded areas or people who have infections. See your doctor if an illness such as a cold or flu is aggravating your breathing problems.

**Get shot.** Prevent the complications of influenza and bacterial pneumonia by getting immunized against both flu and pneumonia, says Dr. Bethel.

**Learn to save your breath.** If you have emphysema, ask your doctor to recommend both an occupational therapist and a physical therapist in your local area.

"An occupational therapist can work with people who are short of breath and who are limited in their day-to-day activities," says Dr. Bethel. "The therapist can teach people more energy-efficient ways of doing those activities."

A physical therapist can develop an exercise program that will train your body to use its available oxygen more efficiently. The result will be that the little oxygen you have will go farther.

**Dilate your airway.** Your doctor may prescribe medications to dilate your airway to its fullest, says Dr. Bethel. Use them according to directions.

## Asthma: An Increasingly Deadly Disease

Asthma is different from chronic bronchitis and emphysema in that its obstruction of the airway is both intermittent and reversible.

During an asthma attack, the airway constricts, the airway walls thicken with inflammation, and mucus accumulates within the airway. The result is an obstructed airway that makes you feel as though you were choking to death. But after an attack, the airway usually returns to normal. Unfortunately, years of these attacks can lead to permanent airway damage.

If you've never had asthma before, breathe easy. Once you're past age 30, you're unlikely to develop it, says Harold S. Nelson, M.D., senior staff physician at the National Jewish Center for Immunology and Respiratory Medicine and a member of the National Asthma Education Expert Panel of the National Heart, Lung and Blood Institute.

"Asthma tends to run in families," says Dr. Bethel. "There may be a predisposition in some people, but we think that asthma is caused by an inflammation of the airway.

"All the mechanisms aren't clear," he adds. "Sometimes the inflammation is caused by allergens that people inhale. Sometimes it's workplace exposures. Exposure to a large number of agents—solder used in the electronics industry or fumes from the making of plastics—may sensitize the airway and make someone asthmatic. And many times people develop asthma, and it's not clear what caused it."

What is clear, doctors agree, is that asthma, which affects about 12 million Americans, is becoming more prevalent and more deadly every year. About 5,000 people die from it each year—and the death rate climbs with age.

What's behind the increase in asthma numbers and deaths is still a mystery, reports the American Lung Association. Any number of things can trigger an asthma attack, including allergies, cigarette smoke and other irritants, a viral infection in your respiratory system and heartburn, which can result in coughing and spasms in your lungs. Even strong emotions and hard exercise—especially in cold weather—can cause troubles, Dr. Nelson says.

New or recurring cases of asthma can start off feeling like regular respiratory tract infections, Dr. Nelson says. If you begin to develop wheezing, tightness in your chest or shortness of breath, see a doctor immediately.

If you're diagnosed with asthma, doctors can prescribe medication to ease the symptoms. Inhalers containing corticosteroids are the most effective way of reducing swelling and helping you breathe easier. Over-the-counter drugs rarely have much effect, Dr. Nelson says.

"This is not something you should treat by yourself," he says. "Asthma is much too serious for that." Here's what experts suggest to handle the disease.

**Fight pollution.** "There's evidence that living in polluted environments increases the incidence of lung diseases such as asthma," says Dr. Bethel. That's why you should try to avoid heavily polluted areas such as industrial districts and urban highways.

Air quality is frequently monitored by various agencies to see if it complies with federal and state standards. To find out how badly the area in which you live or work is polluted, call your state's environmental agency. The people there have the information at hand or can refer you to someone who does.

**Breathe through a scarf.** Breathing in cold, dry air can constrict the airway and induce wheezing, coughing and shortness of breath. The solution? Wear a scarf that you can draw up over your mouth and nose to breathe through during cold spells. And try to breathe mostly through your nose. Breathing through your nose warms and humidifies the air before it reaches the lungs.

**Head for the kitchen.** A review of what 9,000 adults eat every day revealed that higher vitamin C and niacin intakes were associated with fewer cases of wheezing. Good sources of vitamin C include black currants, guava, orange juice and red bell peppers. Good sources of niacin include chicken breast, water-packed tuna and swordfish.

**Use an early warning system.** The home peak-flow meter, a device that measures your breathing capacity, can help identify what's a normal flow and what's not, says Dr. Nelson. Since airflow sometimes drops a couple of hours or days before an attack, the peak-flow meter can give you an early warning that lets you ward off the attack with medication prescribed by your doctor.

Ask your doctor about where to get a peak-flow meter and how to use it.

**Take the right medication.** Prescription medications that treat asthma include anti-inflammatory drugs that suppress airway inflammation, such as steroids, as well as bronchodilators that dilate the airway itself.

But noting that some people use only bronchodilators, Dr. Nelson adds, "Anyone with more than the mildest occasional asthma needs to be on anti-inflammatory treatment rather than just bronchodilators. Together, they will decrease symptoms, probably decrease the number of acute episodes that would otherwise need hospital treatment, decrease the need for bronchodilators and, doctors hope, prevent the long-term development of irreversible obstruction."

# Surviving Flu and Pneumonia

Neither flu nor the most common forms of pneumonia are likely to damage your lungs, but they can make you so short of breath that you feel you can't even make it up a flight of stairs.

Flu, which generally causes fever, headache, sore throat, nasal congestion, muscle aches and a feeling of exhaustion, typically strikes between December and March. It's caused by one of two virus strains, A or B, that usually manage to infect anywhere from 33 to 52 percent of Americans each year. Because flu affects older folks so severely, it is the sixth leading cause of death in the United States.

Pneumonia, which is generally characterized by coughing, phlegm, fever, chills and chest pain, can be caused by a variety of infectious agents, including viruses, mycoplasma parasites and bacteria. It occurs in 80 percent of those who have AIDS. Called *Pneumocystis carinii* pneumonia, it is triggered by a parasite and is seen only rarely in people without AIDS.

Fortunately, both flu and the most deadly and common types of pneumonia can frequently be prevented or successfully be treated without permanently damaging your lungs. Here's how.

**Be alert for signs of danger.** Some types of pneumonia, such as staph or klebsiella, can seriously damage the lung, says Dr. Mostow, and "your lung is never the same afterward." So see your doctor quickly if you have a fever, breathlessness or a nagging cough that won't go away.

**Defend yourself against pneumonia.** The pneumonia vaccine doesn't prevent pneumonia, says Dr. Mostow, but it can prevent you from dying when pneumonia strikes. The vaccine is effective against 23 different types of bacterial germ—the kinds that are responsible for 90 percent of pneumonia deaths. You need to get it only once in your life.

**Protect against flu.** The flu vaccine is highly effective, says Dr. Mostow.

Anyone with chronic lung or heart disease, diabetes, impaired immunity, kidney disease, anemia or another blood problem should get the vaccine every year in the fall, as should anyone over age 65 and anyone who's involved in the care of patients.

Who should not get the shot? Since the vaccine is incubated in eggs, those who are allergic to eggs should avoid it. In general, if you can eat eggs, you can safely receive a flu shot.

**Visit your family physician.** If you forget to get your flu shot, there are two prescription antiviral drugs that can stop flu in its tracks, says Dr. Mostow. One is amantadine (Symmetrel), and the other is rimantadine (Flumadine). These two compounds are active against influenza A, the only flu virus that kills. Just one caveat: You must get them from your doctor within 48 hours of when you come down with the flu.

If you forget to get the pneumonia vaccine—or if you're unlucky enough to run into one of the pneumonias that's not in the vaccine—your doctor will prescribe an antibiotic that is specifically designed to kill the virus or bacteria that have attacked, says Dr. Mostow. If you have the form of pneumonia that affects those with AIDS, *P. carinii*, then your doctor will prescribe trimethoprim sulfate (Polytrim), a drug that won't cure it but will keep the disease under control.

# SEX PROBLEMS AND STDS

## *Most Can Be Prevented and Cured*

You've tried for years to have an orgasm to no avail. You've battled painful urinary tract infections and vaginal dryness.

Now you're worried about losing your sex appeal in a society that lusts after the beauty and bloom of youth. And all this talk about AIDS is making you wonder, for the first time, if your sexual practices might lead to a sexually transmitted disease.

And you thought sex was supposed to be fun.

It is, and it can be. But the reality is sexual difficulties and sexually transmitted diseases can strain your intimate relationships, destroy your self-esteem and, in the case of AIDS, kill you. At the very least, sexual problems can make you feel as if age is finally catching up with you—sapping your sex appeal and making sex seem as exciting as a church supper.

"In our culture, sex is viewed as very important and the territory of the young. So when a woman starts viewing herself as less sexually attractive or senses that something is going wrong in her sexual relationship, it can undermine her sense of self and make her feel like she's getting older," says Beth Alexander, M.D., sex counselor and associate chairperson in the Department of Family Practice at the Michigan State University College of Human Medicine in East Lansing.

Every year, about six million American women get sexually transmitted diseases. Untreated, these illnesses can lower sexual drive, trigger acute arthritis and some chronic diseases and disrupt the central nervous system. Some diseases cause dementia and even death.

"When a woman finds out she has a sexually transmitted disease, she can feel psychologically dirty. It affects her sexuality, often to the point that she loses all interest in sex," says Michael Brodman, M.D., professor of obstetrics and gynecology at the Mount Sinai School of Medicine of the City University of New York.

But fortunately, there are many ways that you can prevent sexual problems and sexually transmitted diseases from developing in the first place, doctors say. Even so, most sexual difficulties or diseases can be remedied, meaning you'll have a lifetime of active and fulfilling sex to look forward to.

# Heading Off the Problem

Many women have or will have sexual problems sometime during their lives, including painful intercourse, urinary tract infections and inhibited sexual desire, says Domeena Renshaw, M.D., director of the Sexual Dysfunction Clinic at Loyola University of Chicago Stritch School of Medicine.

Some of these problems are caused or complicated by ailments such as diabetes or heart disease and require medical attention. But doctors say most of us can head off the heartache of sexual disorders and improve our chances of having vigorous sex lives if we follow these basic guidelines.

**Stomp on your cigarettes.** "If you're in your thirties or forties and want to continue having a wonderful sex life until you're 70 or 80, you better stop smoking now," Dr. Alexander advises. Smoking constricts blood flow to the sexual organs and inhibits arousal in women.

**Stow the booze.** Sure, a glass or two of wine or beer can loosen sexual inhibitions, but more than that can hamper your ability to have an orgasm, says Dr. Alexander. Alcohol can also trigger hormonal changes that will decrease sexual desire.

**Ask about medications.** "A lot of drugs can affect your sexual response," Dr. Alexander says. Medications for high blood pressure, antidepressants such as fluoxetine hydrochloride (Prozac) and lithium (Lithotabs, for example), steroids, ulcer drugs and beta-blockers such as timolol (Timoptic, for example) are among the hundreds of drugs that can adversely affect sexual response. If you suspect a medication is interfering with your sex life, ask your doctor if the drug can be changed or the dosage reduced.

**Slow down, you're going too fast.** If you're constantly rushing around and working 50-plus hours a week, you may be heading for a sexual problem, Dr. Alexander says. "If you can change things that are stressful to you, do it, because lowering your stress and taking more time for yourself will improve your sexual performance," she says. Find ways to make sure you relax regularly—take an evening walk around the neighborhood or unwind with a good novel before tumbling into bed.

**Sleep on it.** Avoid having sex when you're tired; you're less likely to encounter a sexual frustration if you do. "You shouldn't feel like you're expending your last bit of energy to have sex at the end of a long day," says Shirley Zussman, Ed.D., a sex and marital therapist and co-director of the Association for Male Sexual Dysfunction in New York City. "I recommend that you put time aside for sex. That sounds unspontaneous, but in the long run it adds something to your relationship. Not only can sex happen that way, but you can do it with a certain zest."

**Give yourself a break.** Every woman, no matter how experienced she is in bed, will have an occasional sexual frustration. When it happens, you should avoid dwelling on it. Otherwise, you might be setting yourself up for a chronic sexual disorder, says Marty Klein, Ph.D., a licensed marriage counselor and sex therapist in Palo Alto, California, and author of *Ask Me Anything: A Sex Therapist Answers the Most Important Questions for the '90s.*

"If you believe it's going to happen to you at some point, when it does happen, it's no big deal," he says. "It's like getting a rash. Everyone gets rashes sometime in their lives. But if you believe that you never will, and then one day you do, you'll totally freak out. This could even set the stage for it happening again and again in the same circumstances."

## Difficulty Achieving Orgasm

Nature can have a warped sense of timing. Take orgasms, for instance. It takes women up to four times as long as men to reach climax, says Dr. Renshaw. It's little wonder, then, that only 20 to 30 percent of women regularly have orgasms and up to 10 percent say they've never climaxed during intercourse. Here are a couple of suggestions that can help.

**Do Kegel exercises.** These can help women achieve orgasms by increasing the body's awareness of sexual sensations, says Cynthia Mervis Watson, M.D., a family practitioner in Santa Monica, California, and author of *Love Potions.* Kegels strengthen the pubococcygeus (PC) muscles around the genital area. To find these muscles, try to stop your urine flow. Spread your legs apart so that your thighs don't touch. As you attempt to clamp off your urine flow, you'll feel like you're pulling upward with your pelvis and sense a tightening around your anus. That's how Kegel exercises are done. Once you master the technique, squeeze those muscles, hold, then release for three seconds at a time. Work up to a set of 30.

**Don't dwell on it.** Simply tell your lover that you're not going to try to have an orgasm for the next two weeks. Doing that should relieve any of the pressure you may feel to climax and allow you to enjoy sex more, says Dr. Klein. Of course, the more relaxed you are, the more likely it is that you will have an orgasm.

## Urinary Tract Infections: Flushing Out UTIs

During intercourse, the penis can drive bacteria up into the bladder and cause a urinary tract infection (UTI). One in five women has at least one encounter with this annoying disorder that causes frequent urges to urinate, a burning sensation during urination, pain above the pubic bone and occasionally blood in the urine. Here are some things you can do to prevent it.

**Don't hold it in after sex.** Urinating after intercourse will reduce your risk of a UTI, says Thomas Hooton, M.D., associate professor of medicine in the Division of Infectious Disease at the University of Washington School of Medicine in Seattle. "If you urinate right after sex, you'll flush any bacteria that could cause an infection in the bladder back out," he says.

**Wipe carefully.** "After urinating, wipe yourself from front to back, toward your rectum," Dr. Brodman says. Wiping the other way can drag bacteria from the rectum into the urethra and increase your chances of getting a UTI.

**Re-examine your birth control method.** If you have frequent, recurrent UTIs and use a diaphragm with a spermicide, consider switching to a different form of contraception. In studies at the University of Washington, urine samples taken after sex revealed that women who used diaphragms with spermicide had a much greater risk of having the *Escherichia coli* bacteria that cause UTI. The combination of spermicide and diaphragm apparently kills off good bacteria that protect the vagina and urinary tract from infection and encourages *E. coli* bacteria to flourish.

# Low Sexual Desire:
# Rekindling the Flames

When you first got together, you and your mate counted the hours between your sexual interludes. But gradually, as your passion cooled, hours turned into days, then weeks, and now you actually find yourself trying to avoid sex.

Up to 48 percent of American adults lose interest in sex at least temporarily at one time or another, researchers estimate. About 70 percent of people who seek treatment for low sexual desire are women. Depression, alcoholism and chronic diseases such as liver disease are some of the physical causes that can accelerate that process, Dr. Alexander says. But physical problems rarely inhibit sexual desire in women younger than 55.

"The problem isn't necessarily that one person is unhappy or uncomfortable with her own desire for sex. The problem is that she usually wants more or less of it than her partner," says Michael Seiler, Ph.D., assistant director of the Phoenix Institute in Chicago and author of *Inhibited Sexual Desire*. "If you want less sex than your partner, you can feel weird, abnormal and certainly older."

Here are a couple of ideas for rekindling the passion in your relationship.

**Talk about it.** If your lover wants sex four times a week and you feel like it four times a month, you should talk about your needs and reach a compromise. Otherwise the problem will intensify. "A couple needs to talk about their feelings," Dr. Seiler says. "If they can't connect emotionally, the likelihood of them getting together in other ways is remote."

If you feel that your partner is losing interest in sex, avoid saying things such as "This is a major problem" or "You have this bad hang-up," suggests Anthony Pietropinto, M.D., a psychiatrist in New York City and author of *Not Tonight, Dear: How to Reawaken Your Sexual Desire*. Instead, try saying "I've noticed that you haven't seemed too interested in sex lately; is there anything I can do?" The important thing is to keep the pressure off your partner.

**Dream on.** "Learning to fantasize and playing sexually in your mind can rekindle your sexual desire," Dr. Seiler says. To do it, take five minutes each day to conjure up any sexual image that excites you. It could be a movie star, your spouse or even a former lover. Make a mental note of it. Then when you're in a sexual situation, recall it and see if it arouses you.

## Headaches Before and After

A good romp in bed occasionally cures a headache, but more often sex actually triggers one, says George H. Sands, M.D., assistant professor of neurology at the Mount Sinai School of Medicine. Most common is the explosive type of headache that feels like a grenade has gone off in your head as you near orgasm. Any headache that occurs during sex should be checked out by a doctor, since it could be a symptom of a serious condition, such as a cerebral aneurysm.

## Coping with Vaginal Dryness

It ranges from an occasional dull ache to frequent severe pain that makes sex virtually impossible. Although painful intercourse can be caused by genital herpes, premenstrual syndrome, pelvic or vaginal infections, emdometriosis, pregnancy or recent childbirth, often the culprit is vaginal dryness. And vaginal dryness is a common complaint of women going through menopause. Here's how to fight it.

**Take it easy.** Ask your partner to slow down and take more time during foreplay. Keep in mind that as women age, there is often less lubrication.

**Rub it in.** You might consider using a water-soluble, over-the-counter vaginal lubricant such as Astroglide, says Lonnie Barbach, Ph.D., a sex therapist and psychologist in San Francisco and author of *The Pause: Positive Approaches to Menopause*. Some women prefer petroleum-based gels, but remember, you shouldn't use these products with latex condoms because the oils can weaken the latex and increase the chances of leaks.

## When Sex Is a No-Go

Take your finger and move it slowly toward your eye. Just when it seems you're about to touch your finger to your eyeball, your eyelid slams down to protect it.

That's basically the same reflex that causes vaginismus, an involuntary clamping down of the muscles surrounding the vagina that makes intercourse impossible.

About 2 in every 100 women have this condition, triggered by painful intercourse, extreme fear of pregnancy, feelings of guilt or shame about sex or other psychological causes.

Overcoming vaginismus often requires the help of a sex therapist or psychiatrist.

# Doing without STDs

If every American who has a sexually transmitted disease moved to Canada, it would more than double the population of our northern neighbor. About 40 million Americans have sexually transmitted diseases, or STDs. Each year there are 12 million new cases, 6 million of them women.

"We have a tremendous epidemic on our hands," says Peggy Clarke, president of the American Social Health Association in Research Triangle Park, North Carolina.

Most STDs can be cured, although the longer you go without treatment, the more likely you are to have lingering and possibly permanent physical and mental disabilities as a result of these diseases. You should also be aware that STDs are often symptomless and can hide in a body for years while the person unwittingly infects others.

Short of abstinence, having your lover wear latex condoms is your best insurance policy against acquiring an STD, Clarke says. If you have or have ever had a lesion, discharge or rash in the genital area, see your doctor.

The federal Centers for Disease Control and Prevention in Atlanta has identified more than 50 sexually transmitted organisms and syndromes. Here's a look at some of the more common ones.

*Genital herpes.* Nearly 31 million people—one in six Americans—have genital herpes. Herpes, caused by the virus herpes simplex type 2, is a lifelong infection that produces genital sores as often as once a month in some women. Other women never develop symptoms, although they are infectious. Acyclovir (Zovirax), an oral prescription drug, can ease the symptoms but won't cure the disease. Sores from herpes or any other STD also increase your risk of contracting AIDS, since the virus can easily enter the body through open blisters.

*Syphilis.* Known as the Great Imitator because its early symptoms mimic a horde of other diseases, syphilis often begins with a painless sore in the genital area and progresses in three stages that can last more than 30 years. It can make a woman's life miserable, because it can induce heart disease, brain damage and blindness. Untreated, it can also cause death. About 120,000 people get syphilis each year. Antibiotics can cure it but cannot reverse the damage it has caused.

*Gonorrhea.* Known since ancient times, gonorrhea today strikes about 1.5 million Americans annually. This bacterial menace can cause painful urination and discharge from the vagina within two to ten days of infection. Untreated, it can lead to infertility, arthritis, skin sores and heart or brain infections. Gonorrhea can be passed on to a baby during childbirth. Antibiotics can cure it.

*Chlamydia.* This condition has symptoms similar to gonorrhea, although it,

# AIDS: Fighting the Scourge

Many of us know at least one person who has AIDS or has died from it. But behind the grim numbers that tell us more than one million Americans have this fatal viral disease, there is a faint glimmer of hope.

"In the beginning, people were dying within months of their diagnoses. But we've learned so much more about the disease since then, and we now have long-term survivors who are very healthy for good periods of time," says Peggy Clarke, president of the American Social Health Association in Research Triangle Park, North Carolina.

Antiviral drugs such as zidovudine (AZT), didanosine (Videx) and zalcitabine (Hivid) can slow the progress of the disease, which gradually destroys the immune system, allowing life-threatening infections and cancers to invade the body at will.

But there is no cure for this deadly disease. So the best way to fight AIDS is to not get it in the first place. That means using a latex condom or having sex in a monogamous relationship in which both partners have been tested and found to be free of the human immunodeficiency virus (HIV) that causes AIDS. If you use intravenous drugs, don't share needles with others, as HIV may be transmitted through bodily fluids that remain in the needle.

---

too, can be symptomless. The most common curable STD in the United States, chlamydia infects about four million people annually. A leading cause of infertility among women, it can permanently damage the fallopian tubes. It can also be cured with antibiotics.

*Genital warts.* Nearly a million new cases of genital warts are reported each year. This STD is caused by the human papillomavirus, some types of which have been linked to cervical cancer. There is no cure, although the warts can be removed surgically or burned or frozen off. Recurrences are common.

*Hepatitis B.* This disease can lead to cirrhosis of the liver or liver cancer. Up to 200,000 cases are reported annually, despite the fact that vaccination can prevent it.

For more information about STDs or referrals to self-help groups in your area, phone the Centers for Disease Control National STD Hotline (1-800-227-8922) or write the American Social Health Association, a nonprofit organization that offers educational information on STDs, at P.O. Box 13827, Research Triangle Park, NC 27709.

# SKIN CANCER

## *The Dark Side of the Sun*

**R**emember summers on the patio with an aluminum foil reflector and nothing but an itsy-bitsy bikini between you and the sun? Or slathering baby oil all over yourself in hopes of getting a deep, dark tan?

Ouch. The truth is, just one bad burn in childhood doubles your risk of skin cancer as an adult. Add a few more decades of sun exposure—even if you've always tanned without burning—and your risk goes up even more, along with the cosmetic age of your skin, which will look older because of sun damage. Fair-skinned, light-eyed ancestors also boost your chances. And if a parent or grandparent has had a skin cancer removed, you may be next in line.

Like many women, you probably give a lot of attention to the appearance of your skin. If it looks good, you assume it's healthy. That's why skin cancer can be such a shock—it seems like an ambush from nowhere. (It can be 20 years between the initial damage and the cancer.) And many of us are being ambushed in our late forties or early fifties instead of in our seventies and later, the ages that used to supply the majority of victims. Researchers speculate that damage to the planet's ozone layer, which protects us from the worst of the sun's radiation, is one likely reason.

Fortunately, the skin cancers that occur most often—the forms known as basal cell and squamous cell—very rarely spread, though if they're stubborn, they can recur, says Thomas Griffin, M.D., a dermatologist with Graduate Hospital and clinical assistant professor of dermatology at the University of Pennsylvania School of Medicine, both in Philadelphia. They appear as small bumps on the skin, usually on sun-exposed areas including your back, which receives radiation right through light fabrics. They can be flesh-toned or brown to gray, and some have tiny ulcers at the center of the growth that bleed easily. Squamous cell cancers may also have a hard spot within the growth.

# Tanning Parlors: Fountains of Aging

Don't buy the hype that tanning under a sunlamp or on a tanning bed is somehow safer than the radiation you get from the sun. Or that a "base tan" you acquire in a tanning parlor will somehow protect you from deeper sun damage.

Both claims are dangerously false, says Vincent DeLeo, M.D., associate professor of dermatology at Columbia Presbyterian Medical Center in New York City.

"Tanning parlors and sunlamps are the most worthless things you can pay money for—and very damaging to the skin," he says. A report from the National Institutes of Health says that some tanning lamps generate over five times more ultraviolet radiation (UVA) than you'd get sitting for the same amount of time on a beach at the equator.

If you feel desperate for the golden look, use a self-tanning lotion, suggests Dr. DeLeo. But don't forget to use a sunscreen, too.

The shark of skin cancers is melanoma. It occurs much less frequently than other skin cancers, but it can be fatal. Once melanoma grows deeper than one millimeter into the skin, it has a higher risk of spreading to other organs. It may start from a mole, though it can also begin in a large, flat brown freckle or bleeding spot.

Although men have a higher rate of melanoma than women, it is increasing more rapidly in young women than in any other age group, says David J. Leffell, M.D., chief of dermatologic surgery at Yale University School of Medicine in New Haven, Connecticut. "We're not sure why, but it may be that women now in their thirties had enormous sun exposure in the 1960s when they were children," he says.

Yet doctors say skin cancer is cause for caution, not for alarm. In most cases, it's nearly 100 percent curable, as long as it's caught in time. And best of all, it's preventable.

## Reducing Your Odds

Even if you've spent quite a few summers in the sun, you can dramatically reduce your chances of developing skin cancer by controlling your exposure from now on. You also need to know how to detect cancer

# A Safe Tan in a Tube

Today's self-tanning lotions won't turn you the awful streaky orange that skin dyes did years ago, thank goodness. The new breeds of tan-in-a-bottle are easy to apply, look natural and won't harm your skin.

A self-tanner actually interacts with your skin to turn it a natural, golden-looking color, says Yveline Duchesne, international training director for New York City–based Clarins Cosmetics. The tan fades gradually as you shed your dead skin cells, usually within a few days.

The main active ingredient in self-tanning lotions is a chemical called dihydroxyacetone (DHA). DHA combines with certain amino acids and keratin on the very superficial cell layers of skin to produce the color.

With the new products, you can be attractively tanned without damage to your skin—if you continue to wear sunscreen. Most self-tanners have sunscreen with only a low sun protection factor (SPF), so it's best to also use your own sunscreen of SPF 15 or higher. The best timing? Since self-tanners take a few hours to develop, apply them the night before, Duchesne suggests. Then apply your sunscreen the next morning, at least an hour before going out.

Other tips for making the most of your self-tanner:

**Always allergy-test.** Before you try a self-tanner all over, apply the lotion to a small patch of skin and leave it on overnight to see if your skin is sensitive to DHA. (If it reacts, a bronzing gel or tinted sunscreen is your best bet for color.)

**Exfoliate before you apply.** DHA can take unevenly in areas where there's a buildup of dead cells. Be sure to include hands, elbows and knees.

**Start at the top.** Work down from your forehead, covering all exposed areas, but skip the eyebrows, where color can concentrate. Apply evenly, including your ears and under your jaw.

**Moisturize the rough spots.** Elbows and knees will look more natural if you moisturize first and apply self-tanner lightly.

**Wait for results.** How often you reapply, not how much, determines the depth of your tan. It takes from three to five hours for color to develop, so don't reapply until you've seen the full results.

**Let it dry.** Wait a half-hour before dressing or going to bed, since some tanners can stain fabric.

**Wash up.** Wash your hands after you apply your self-tanner, or you'll end up with tan palms.

on sun-exposed skin or in an abnormal mole before it grows to the danger point. Here are the top tactics for saving your skin.

**Screen it.** Wear a full-spectrum sunscreen that blocks both kinds of ultraviolet radiation (UVA and UVB)—and wear it every day, summer and winter, says Perry Robins, M.D., associate professor of dermatology at New York University in New York City, president of the Skin Cancer Foundation and author of *Sun Sense*. Check to be sure that your sunscreen has a sun protection factor (SPF) of at least 15.

**Spend noon indoors.** Try to limit your outdoor activities during the hours when the sun's rays are the strongest—from 10:00 A.M. to 2:00 P.M., says Dr. Griffin.

**Check for changes.** Examine your skin thoroughly twice a year, with a hand mirror or with help from a friend or spouse. Look for any kind of spot that changes, says Dr. Robins. The change can be in color, texture or size (the spot gets bigger), or the spot can begin to bleed, he says. If you have a family history of skin cancer or you've had severe sunburns, ask your dermatologist to "map" your body for potential trouble spots and to keep track of any changes with follow-up visits.

**Memorize the ABCDs.** This will help you monitor moles for signs of melanoma, says Vincent DeLeo, M.D., associate professor of dermatology at Columbia Presbyterian Medical Center in New York City:

- A is for asymmetry (no symmetrical shape).
- B is for border (an irregular border).
- C is for color change (a dark area arises within a mole, or a mole shows areas of lightening).
- D is for diameter (the mole gets larger or is larger than a pencil eraser).

If you have any of the ABCDs, get to a doctor immediately, says Dr. DeLeo.

# Early Detection, Early Cure

What happens when your early detection efforts pay off? You've called your dermatologist's attention to a growth, and she confirms that it must be removed.

For most cancers, local anesthetic is all that you'll need, and the removal won't leave a noticeable scar. Depending on the depth and nature of the growth, your doctor will use one or a combination of procedures. They include burning, scraping, freezing and cutting out the growth. Some shallow cancers can be treated with a topical chemotherapy cream.

For difficult or recurring cancers, a surgeon can remove malignant cells in very thin layers, leaving healthy skin untouched. Even melanoma has a potent new enemy—a melanoma cell vaccine that significantly increases survival rates.

# SMOKING

## *Clear the Air and Put Time on Your Side*

If you're among the millions of women who started smoking as teenagers because they wanted to look and feel older, you got your wish—and maybe more than you bargained for. Nothing ages your appearance, spirit and health more than America's most practiced and most dangerous vice.

Just ask Elizabeth Sherertz, M.D., a dermatologist and researcher at Bowman Gray School of Medicine of Wake Forest University in Winston-Salem, North Carolina. "We found that on average, smokers tend to look between five and ten years older than their actual ages because of the wrinkles caused by smoking," she says. "People who smoke are more likely to develop wrinkles, because smoking damages the elastic tissue that keeps skin tight and probably also enhances the sun's damaging effects to the skin."

Or ask Richard Jenks, Ph.D., a sociologist at Indiana University Southeast in New Albany who studies the effects of smoking on our emotional state, who found that once again, puffers suffer. "Smokers know that their habit is a sure road to health problems, and they're actually even more likely than nonsmokers or ex-smokers to describe it as dirty," he says. "But what my study found was that smokers tend to feel they have less control over their lives, and feel less satisfied with their lives, than nonsmokers."

Or ask any other researcher or doctor who has ever studied the effects that smoking has on our physical and emotional well-being. Study after study—and there have been hundreds of them—backs up what experts already know: If it doesn't kill you—and one in five people worldwide dies from smoking-related diseases each year—it will most certainly take years off your life. Says Margaret A. Chesney, Ph.D., a women's health and smoking researcher and professor at the University of California, San Francisco, School of Medicine, "If you want to radically slow down the aging process and live longer, stop smoking."

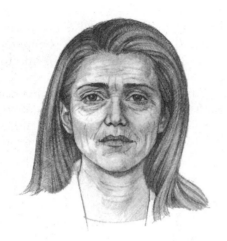

*Smoker—behold your future face. Note the wrinkles that radiate from the lips and the corners of the eyes. Note, too, the deeply lined cheeks and the crevices running up and down the lower jaw.*

# A Tough Battle for Women

But that's easier said than done—especially for many of us. "When the surgeon general's first report on smoking and health was published in the 1960s, twice as many men as women were smoking," says Douglas E. Jorenby, Ph.D., coordinator of clinical activities for the Center for Tobacco Research and Intervention at the University of Wisconsin Medical School in Madison. "Today, the smoking rate between men and women is almost even, and in the next few years, it will probably cross for the first time—and there will be more women smokers than men."

In real numbers, that translates to more than 24 percent of American women over age 18 who smoke, down from the 34 percent who smoked when the surgeon general's report came out in 1964. About 28 percent of American men smoke today—a drastic decrease from the 52 percent who smoked in 1964. The alarming bottom line is that because more kids are starting to smoke, the smoking rates will no longer be dropping. And lung cancer now kills more women each year than breast cancer.

Once women start smoking, statistics show we have a harder time quitting—both physically and psychologically. "There is evidence that equal numbers of men and women attempt to quit, but men succeed at about twice the rate," says Dr. Jorenby. "One reason is that women report more depression when they quit smoking, and we know from various studies that depression makes it more likely that you'll go back to smoking."

But, he adds, it seems as though women are less likely to want to quit. "Many women feel so overwhelmed by their families and jobs that a lot of them say cigarettes are their only refuge. And they're hesitant to give that up, even though they know quitting has a big benefit to their health."

Women, particularly those under age 25, have become a major target market for cigarette companies. "One of the big messages behind the advertising to women is that smoking helps you control your weight," says Dr. Jorenby. "In one cigarette advertisement I saw, there was a photo of a model who was already pretty skinny. But the photo was distorted to make her look even thinner—thinner than any human being can really be. The message, which is targeted to women in their teens and early twenties, is obvious: Smoking helps you to be thin and glamorous."

That message seems to be working. While the Centers for Disease Control and Prevention in Atlanta doesn't keep statistics on gender breakdown of young smokers, spokeswoman Suzie Gates of its Office on Smoking and Health says most of the 3,000 people who start the habit each day are females under age 25, and some are as young as 12.

## Smokers Aren't Thinner

Despite what Madison Avenue would have you believe, smokers aren't thinner. True, nicotine slightly curbs the appetite, meaning that smokers consume fewer meals. But when they eat, smokers are more likely than nonsmokers to gravitate toward foods that are higher in calories and fat, says Doris Abood, Ed.D., associate professor of health education at Florida State University in Tallahassee. In her study, which examined the smoking, eating, drinking and exercise habits of 1,820 people, she also found that smokers exercise less and consume more alcohol, which is notoriously high in calories. Dr. Abood and other researchers found that the more people smoke, the more bad habits they practice, and to a greater extent.

Still, regardless of these other habits, it's smoking itself that does the most

---

## No Weighty Move Here

For many women who want to quit smoking, the biggest fear is gaining weight.

Well, fret no more, because it's official: According to the Centers for Disease Control and Prevention in Atlanta, when you quit, the average weight gain is about five pounds. And the weight gain can be prevented through a careful diet and stress management. In fact, some people actually lose weight after they quit.

For many women, quitting smoking is part of an overall get-healthy program that includes regular exercise and improvements in diet, says Douglas E. Jorenby, Ph.D., coordinator of clinical activities for the Center for Tobacco Research and Intervention at the University of Wisconsin Medical School in Madison.

# In the Meantime, Take Your Vitamins

While they're no substitution for quitting, antioxidant vitamins have been shown to offer at least some protection against the harmful effects of smoking.

Jeffrey Blumberg, Ph.D., associate director of the U.S. Department of Agriculture Human Nutrition Research Center on Aging at Tufts University in Boston, recommends these vitamins to keep your immune system strong and offset some of the damage caused by tobacco.

*Vitamin C.* 250 to 1,000 milligrams daily. The Recommended Dietary Allowance (RDA) is 60 milligrams. Good food sources include citrus fruits, broccoli, cantaloupe, red peppers, kiwifruit and strawberries.

*Vitamin E.* 100 to 400 IU daily. The RDA is 12 IU or 8 milligrams alpha-tocopherol equivalents. Good food sources include cooking oils, wheat germ and mangoes.

*Beta-carotene.* 15 to 30 milligrams daily. There is no established RDA. Best sources are yellow-orange and dark green fruits and vegetables such as carrots, sweet potatoes and squash, as well as spinach and other green leafy vegetables.

---

damage, causing nearly 419,000 deaths a year. It also plays a leading role in scores of diseases, from cancer to colds, from heart disease to hip fractures. "The effects of smoking are distributed so much throughout the entire body that it has an impact on virtually any disease you can think of," says Dr. Jorenby.

## Why Smoking Kills

Cigarette smoke contains about 4,000 chemicals, including minute amounts of poisons such as arsenic, formaldehyde and DDT. With each puff, these poisons are inhaled through the lungs—which retain up to 90 percent of the compounds—and then passed through the bloodstream. Some of these poisons, such as carbon monoxide, are the so-called free radicals that rob blood cells of oxygen. Free radicals have been linked to a host of problems, ranging from wrinkles to cancer.

Meanwhile, the nicotine in tobacco smoke causes the adrenal glands to secrete hormones that increase blood pressure and heart rate, which makes your heart work harder—the primary reason why women who smoke are twice as likely as nonsmokers to have strokes and have nearly three times the risk of heart disease. Their risk goes up even more if they take oral contraceptives.

Smoking makes you more susceptible to infectious diseases such as colds and flu, since it damages the cilia, tiny hairlike bodies that trap and sweep out foreign substances from the lungs. Without the cilia to do their work, the tar from cigarettes clogs breathing passages, leading to emphysema and lung cancer. It also hobbles your ability to stay fit, sapping your body and mind of energizing oxygen. On the average, women smokers reach menopause at least one year earlier than nonsmokers, and menopause is associated with higher risk of early heart attack.

But even symptoms associated with smoking do their own damage. For instance, women who smoke have a higher rate of urinary incontinence because of the coughing caused by their habit. "Even if smoking is not a causal factor in a particular disease, it can certainly exacerbate it," says Dr. Jorenby. "For instance, we know that smoking doesn't cause diabetes, but people with diabetes who smoke have a much worse prognosis than those who don't."

Another case in point: A study by British researchers found that smokers with the human immunodeficiency virus develop full-blown AIDS twice as quickly as nonsmokers, although scientists aren't sure why.

# How to Quit—For Good

The good news is that some of this damage can be undone. Just one year after you quit smoking, your risk for heart disease is cut in half, and after three years, your risk becomes comparable to that of someone who never touched a cigarette. Your risks for other diseases, such as emphysema, bronchitis and cancer, also diminish. Plus you'll look and feel younger, with more energy and stamina and fewer wrinkles.

Sure, quitting is tough. Fewer than 10 percent of the 20 million smokers who try to quit each year actually succeed, says Rami Bachiman, director of community education for the American Lung Association of New York in New York City. There are various strategies to help you along—keeping your hands busy, chewing on carrot sticks, taking deep breaths of fresh air, drinking lots of water or even rewarding yourself with a present. But here's how you can increase your chances of quitting successfully and not relapsing during those crucial first few weeks.

**Log your progress.** The first thing you should do is set a deadline up to three weeks away for when you'll have your last smoke. But in the meantime, log each cigarette you smoke—where you smoke and under what circumstances, advises Don R. Powell, Ph.D., president of the American Institute for Preventive Medicine in Farmington Hills, Michigan, and a former smoker. This will help you identify situations that cause you to smoke and then find alternative behaviors other than smoking cigarettes.

**Delay the desire.** If you are quitting gradually, each time you get the urge to smoke, hold off lighting up for 5 minutes, suggests Dr. Powell. After a few

# Do Shortcuts Work?

Nicotine patches and gum and hypnosis may take some of the sting out of the withdrawal symptoms that come with quitting, but don't expect these aids to replace grit and determination.

Smokers who quit with the assistance of these tools are two to three times more likely to succeed than those doing it cold turkey. Although quitting cold turkey is the most popular method, it is also the least successful, having a success rate of only 5 percent. The smoker using nicotine gum or patches plus enrolling in a comprehensive behavioral smoking cessation program increases her chances of stopping and can anticipate a one-year success rate of 23 to 40 percent. Meanwhile, there's a 15 percent success rate using hypnosis.

There are some side effects to nicotine patches and gum, which are prescribed by a doctor usually to heavy smokers who simply can't quit or who have had severe withdrawal symptoms when they've tried.

The patch, an adhesive square that secretes nicotine through the skin and into the bloodstream to help ease the pain of withdrawal, can cause itchiness and minor burning. And smoking even one cigarette while wearing the patch can cause a heart attack.

The effectiveness of the gum, meanwhile, is washed away if you eat or drink anything—especially diuretics such as coffee and cola—within 15 minutes of chewing it. And although the gum isn't supposed to be used after four months from your last cigarette, 1 in 12 smokers continues using it for over a year after quitting.

The bottom line: If you've tried to quit and failed in the past, ask your doctor about these products. But, says psychologist Mitchell Nides, Ph.D., of the University of California, Los Angeles, you have to "learn" how to be a nonsmoker, and that's something that no pharmaceutical can do by itself.

days, extend the delay to 10 minutes. After another few days, extend it to 15 minutes, and so on. "You'll find that the actual urge to smoke at any given moment fades relatively quickly," he says.

**Seek support.** Whether you're quitting cold turkey or doing it gradually by slowing decreasing the number of cigarettes you smoke, you'll probably fare better if you have a lot of encouragement. "Since they have a harder time quitting, women need as much support as they can get," says Dr. Jorenby. "Having some kind of group support can make a big difference in how you do, whether it's from friends and family or some sort of group therapy." There are probably groups in your area offering free counseling and group therapy for women trying to quit. Contact the local chapter of the American Heart Association for more information.

**Drink orange juice.** The hardest part of quitting cold turkey, which is the most popular method, is getting through the symptoms of nicotine withdrawal, which last one to two weeks. But you'll get over the irritability, anxiety, confusion and trouble concentrating and sleeping that come with nicotine withdrawal a lot faster if you drink a lot of orange juice during that time.

That's because OJ makes your urine more acidic, which clears nicotine from your body faster, says Thomas Cooper, D.D.S., a nicotine dependency researcher and professor of oral health sciences at the University of Kentucky in Lexington. "Besides," adds Dr. Jorenby, "the citrus taste in your mouth makes the thought of having a cigarette pretty disgusting."

If you're quitting with the aid of doctor-prescribed nicotine gum or patches, however, avoid orange juice and other acidic drinks, because you want to keep nicotine in your system with these products.

**Imagine it's the flu.** "Before we had nicotine gum and patches, I used to tell people who were quitting smoking to imagine they were having the flu," says Dr. Jorenby. "A lot of withdrawal symptoms are similar to the flu: You fly off the handle easily, you have trouble concentrating, your stamina is down. And as with the flu, there's little you can do other than let it run its course. But you will get over it. As long as you don't relapse and have a cigarette, the withdrawal will be over and done within a week or two."

**Stay out of bars.** The greatest chance of relapsing occurs in bars, says Dr. Jorenby. "For many people, having a drink in one hand means having a cigarette in the other. I advise that anyone trying to quit stay out of bars for at least the first two weeks after they stop smoking." Instead, he advises, go to libraries, museums and other public places where smoking is prohibited. "People who quit smoking don't have to swear off going to bars, but we know from many studies that they are at much higher risk of going back to smoking unless they stay away for the first few weeks."

**Write a letter to a loved one.** When a nicotine fit hits, pick up a pen instead of a butt and write a letter to a loved one explaining why smoking is more important than your life, suggests Robert Van de Castle, Ph.D., professor emeritus of behavioral medicine at the University of Virginia Medical Center in Charlottesville. In the letter, try to explain why you continue a habit that you know will kill you rather than quit and live to see a child graduate from college or get married or to witness other important events. When Dr. Van de Castle's patients try this letter, he says, they feel so selfish that it often gives them the courage to put up with withdrawal symptoms and stay smoke-free.

# SNORING AND SLEEP APNEA

## The Nighttime Chain Saw Massacre

**Y**ou can't understand it. You seem to be getting plenty of sleep, but from the minute you rise, you're tired and sluggish. At work, you have trouble concentrating; even the simplest task seems like a major chore. And coming home tonight, you almost veered the car into a telephone pole because your mind was in the twilight zone.

Not only that, but a very worn-out face has been staring back at you from the mirror. Who is this woman with the frazzled, haggard features, the puffy, baggy eyes, the blank, world-weary expression?

Brace yourself. This woman is you.

You've just seen what a person looks like when she hasn't gotten a good night's sleep for many nights. One reason for the sorry state of your slumber may be that you've been snoring up a storm.

## Sawing Lumber in Your Slumber

While it's unusual for women to let 'er rip like a Black & Decker chain saw, and those of us who do rarely duplicate the ear-splitting force of a snoring man, that doesn't mean we can't produce our fair share of snorts and wheezes. Five percent of women between the ages of 30 and 35 snore; by age 60, that figure swells to 40 percent.

Doctors say most snoring is harmless. But heavy snoring can alter your physical and mental well-being. Severe nighttime breathing problems have been linked to heart disease and decreased mental acuity and have even been suspected as causes of sudden death while sleeping. And besides, snoring can really sap your youthful glow.

"At a minimum, it seems to take away your vigor," says Richard Millman, M.D., director of the Sleep Disorders Center of Rhode Island Hospital in Providence. "Many people come into our offices with obstructive sleep breathing problems who are in their forties, but they look, feel and act ten years older."

## When Your Airway Says No Way

We all know it when we hear it, but what exactly is that cacophony of nasty nighttime noises we call a snore? It's a partial obstruction of breathing that takes place in the airway running from the nose to the voice box.

If the muscles and tissues in this airway are flabby or toneless, they will cave in. "It's like sucking air through a soggy straw," says David N. F. Fairbanks, M.D., clinical professor of otolaryngology at the George Washington University School of Medicine and Health Sciences in Washington, D.C. "When you breathe, the airway narrows and partially collapses. The structures in the airway vibrate against each other."

Snoring usually is not a problem for women unless they are heavy, have low

---

## The Snore You Can't Ignore

Many of us would never suspect that we snore. We can't hear ourselves, after all.

And sometimes our partners don't want to tell us about it for fear of hurting our feelings.

Here's a way to find out if you've been grinding out the Zzzs: Tape-record the hours you sleep, advises David N. F. Fairbanks, M.D., clinical professor of otolaryngology at the George Washington University School of Medicine and Health Sciences in Washington, D.C. For many women, hearing is believing, and the sound of one's own snore is enough to convince them to try a self-help remedy or at least ask a doctor for some suggestions.

If you don't have anyone else in the house to inform you that you may be snoring, Dr. Fairbanks says to keep an eye out for these tip-offs: morning headaches and grogginess, frequent awakenings and gaspings at night, daytime sleepiness, a change in blood pressure, chest pains and dry mouth.

estrogen levels, have had a hysterectomy or have gone through menopause. While the connection between low estrogen levels and snoring is unclear, doctors do know that estrogen stimulates muscles, preventing them from relaxing.

"Sometime in their forties or fifties, women will begin to lose tone and develop fat in the throat area. Their tongues and larynxes and certain tissues may enlarge a bit as well. Eventually, their airways will collapse. Actually, the percentages of men and women who snore are the same by age 60, and snoring is a common occurrence," says Willard Moran, M.D., clinical professor of otolaryngology at the University of Oklahoma College of Medicine in Oklahoma City.

Snoring is three times more common in overweight people than in thin ones. People with short, thick necks may also do more than their share of sawing wood.

Other snore makers include bulky tongue or throat tissue, large tonsils or adenoids, tumors or cysts in the airway, a recessed jaw, an excessively large uvula (the soft lobe that hangs from the roof of the mouth), and obstructed nasal passages and nasal deformities.

Snoring is a progressive disorder. So a snore that's light or occasional now will probably become more intense as time passes.

## Apnea: An Exhausting Condition

When the airway is completely blocked, you may actually stop breathing for ten seconds to one minute. This condition is called sleep apnea, and people who have it wake up briefly every time their breathing ceases, which can be hundreds of times a night. Sleep apnea is most common in middle-aged men, but women can suffer from it, too.

"The brain, sensing a lack of oxygen, signals a loud snorting response that restores tone to the airway and restarts the breathing," says A. Jay Block, M.D., professor of medicine and anesthesiology and chief of the Pulmonary Division at the University of Florida College of Medicine in Gainesville.

Much of the time, people with apnea don't even realize they're waking up and falling asleep all through the night. But the process leaves them exhausted.

In addition, the oxygen levels in their blood may plunge well below normal, forcing the heart to pump harder and causing cardiovascular problems such as high blood pressure, irregular heart rhythms, heart failure, heart attack and stroke.

## Snore Stoppers

Snoring does not have to be a life sentence. Today, physicians specializing in sleep and breathing disorders can do wonders for cases of snoring and sleep apnea. But even the heaviest of snores may not need a doctor. The following tips may be all you need to quiet the storm once and for all.

**Stop smoking.** Smoking irritates the tissues of the nasal passages and upper airway, causing them to swell and obstruct airflow, says Dr. Fairbanks. So this gives you another good reason to kick the habit.

**Drop some pounds.** People who are overweight are more likely to snore, so trim the fat from your body by trimming the fat from your diet. Most doctors and researchers recommend that you limit your fat intake to 25 percent of the total calories in your diet.

**Open your nose.** People who breathe through their mouths are more likely to snore, says Dr. Block. Sometimes a cure can be as simple as clearing a chronically stuffed nose. Keep your nasal passages open with an over-the-counter nasal spray (such as Afrin) or saline solution—but follow the instructions carefully. Overuse of nasal spray can cause passages to clog even more. Very severe nasal blockages may require allergy treatments or surgery to correct a nasal deformity.

**Curb your alcohol.** Alcohol is a depressant that affects the central nervous system and causes the throat muscles to become relaxed and floppy, says Dr. Millman. Don't drink alcohol for four hours prior to going to bed.

**Stay off pills and medicines.** Tranquilizers and sleeping pills also act on the central nervous system to over-relax throat muscles and cause snoring, says Dr. Millman.

**Eat light.** Don't eat a large meal three hours before retiring, and steer clear of midnight snacks, says Dr. Moran. That's because the process of digestion causes muscles everywhere—including those in your throat—to relax.

**Back off.** According to Dr. Moran, sleeping on your back increases the likelihood of snoring, because the tongue drops back in the mouth, creating an obstruction. One way to make sure you don't roll over onto your back is to sew a pocket on the back of your pajamas and place a tennis ball inside. The ball will cause such discomfort when you lie on your back that you'll either wake up or unconsciously roll off your back.

**Hoist your head and shoulders.** Sleeping on an incline helps keep the airway open, says Dr. Millman. But don't prop your head with pillows; this will only kink the airway. Instead, place bricks under the bedposts at the head of the bed to raise it four to five inches.

**Whip your snore.** Wearing a neck brace or whiplash collar to bed will keep your chin extended, so your throat may stay open, says Dr. Fairbanks. To guard against a stiff neck the next morning, Dr. Fairbanks suggests using a foam collar rather than a plastic one. Foam cushions the neck better and is less restraining. But if you do have some morning kinks, gently stretching your neck muscles, giving yourself a gentle massage or taking a warm shower will help, he says.

**Pop in a dental appliance.** Many sleep disorder centers and orthodontists provide retaining devices that prevent the tongue from falling back into the throat. Some appliances accomplish this by actually holding the tongue in place; others pull the bottom jaw forward slightly. While these devices sound cumbersome, Dr. Millman says most patients experience little discomfort.

# STRESS

## *Control Is the Cure*

You can't get enough rest, and you can't get enough done. And your stomach is always wrapped up in a knot.

"Stress will do that to you," says Leah J. Dickstein, M.D., professor in the Department of Psychiatry and Behavioral Sciences at the University of Louisville School of Medicine in Kentucky and former president of the American Medical Women's Association. "It can really wear you out. And the real problem is that you could be paving the way for other troubles later on."

The American Institute of Stress in Yonkers, New York, estimates that 90 percent of all visits to doctors are for stress-related disorders. In women, stress has been linked to fatigue, hair loss, bad complexion, insomnia, disruption of the menstrual cycle, low libido and lack of orgasm, among others. There's even evidence that it can increase your risk of more serious problems such as high blood pressure and heart disease.

"Stress speeds up your entire system and produces conditions in younger people that are more commonly associated with growing old," says Allen J. Elkin, Ph.D., director of the Stress Management and Counseling Center in New York City. "Virtually no part of your body can escape the ravages of stress."

There are lots of ways we can reduce the stress in our lives. But before we can beat it, experts say we have to understand what stress is—and how it works.

## You Can't Always Run

Despite its bad reputation, stress is one of our bodies' best defense systems. When we sense danger—such as a car coming at us—our bodies release adrenaline and other chemicals that make us more alert, raise our blood pressure and increase our strength, speed and reaction time.

# Is Stress Adding Up?

Remember: Stress comes from within. Your attitudes about life have a lot to do with how much stress you feel. This quiz, from the book *Is It Worth Dying For?* by Robert S. Eliot, M.D., and Dennis L. Breo, tests your outlook and overall stress level. Read each statement, then score one point if you almost never feel that way, two points if you occasionally feel that way, three points if you frequently feel that way and four points if you almost always feel that way.

1. Things must be perfect.
2. I must do it myself.
3. I feel more isolated from my family or close friends.
4. I feel that people should listen better.
5. My life is running me.
6. I must not fail.
7. I cannot say no to new demands without feeling guilty.
8. I need to generate excitement constantly to avoid boredom.
9. I feel a lack of intimacy with people around me.
10. I am unable to relax.
11. I am unable to laugh at a joke about myself.
12. I avoid speaking my mind.

That's great if we're responding to a threat that requires physical action. Unfortunately, Dr. Dickstein says, our bodies don't recognize the difference between physical threats and mental ones. When we get nervous about meeting a deadline, for instance, we may produce the same stress chemicals as when we see that oncoming car. And if we don't burn off these chemicals through physical exertion, they can linger in the bloodstream and start causing problems.

Studies show that stress can reduce the power of our immune systems. A study in Britain exposed 266 people, most of them in their thirties, to a common cold virus and then tracked who became sick. The study showed that 28.6 percent of those with few signs of stress caught the cold. But the figure jumped to 42.4 percent for those who were under high stress.

The reason? Stress may inhibit the disease-fighting cells in our bloodstreams. "Everybody gets sick from time to time," Dr. Dickstein says. "But if you're under a lot of stress, a virus may get to you that you would have been able to fight off otherwise."

13. I feel under pressure to succeed all the time.
14. I automatically express negative attitudes.
15. I seem further behind at the end of the day than when I started.
16. I forget deadlines, appointments and personal possessions.
17. I am irritable and disappointed in the people around me.
18. Sex seems like more trouble than it's worth.
19. I consider myself exploited.
20. I wake up earlier and cannot sleep.
21. I feel unrested.
22. I feel dissatisfied with my personal life.
23. I feel dissatisfied with my work life.
24. I'm not where I want to be in life.
25. I avoid being alone.
26. I have trouble getting to sleep.
27. I have trouble waking up.
28. I can't seem to get out of bed.

Add up your marks. If you scored 29 or less, you show low stress. Totals of 30 to 58 show mild stress. If you scored 59 to 87, you show moderate stress. If you scored higher than 87, you may be under high stress.

Other studies show that women who have trouble coping with stress may be at risk of building up dangerous abdominal fat. A study at Yale University in New Haven, Connecticut, of 42 obese women found that those with abdominal fat—so-called apple-shaped women—secreted more stress hormones than those with pear-shaped bodies, who carry extra weight on their hips. And doctors know that apple-shaped people are more at risk of heart disease.

Until menopause, women have extra protection against heart problems. That's because of estrogen, which blocks the buildup of plaque in our arteries. But once we stop producing estrogen, our risk of heart attack rises to that of men. And that's when stress can really cause trouble. "Stress increases heart rate and blood pressure, therefore changing the inner lining of our blood vessels, making our blood more likely to clot," says Robert DiBianco, M.D., director of cardiology research at the Washington Adventist Hospital in Takoma Park, Maryland. "Stress may change the way cholesterol is handled by our blood vessels and, in doing so, may increase plaque formation."

# Is Work Wearing You Out?

Everyone feels pressure at work. But sometimes it gets out of hand, leaving you angry, tired and unproductive.

To check your stress level at work, take this quick quiz developed by Paul J. Rosch, M.D., president of the American Institute of Stress in Yonkers, New York. Score one point for each question you disagree with, two points for each one you agree with somewhat and three points for each question you agree with strongly.

1. I can't say what I really think at work.
2. I have a lot of responsibility but not much authority.
3. I could do a much better job if I had more time.
4. I seldom receive acknowledgement or appreciation.
5. I'm not proud of, or satisfied with, my job.
6. I am picked on or discriminated against at work.
7. My workplace is not particularly pleasant or safe.
8. My job interferes with my family obligations and personal needs.
9. I tend to argue more often with my superiors, co-workers or customers.
10. I feel I have little control over my life at work.

Here's how to score the quiz: 10 to 16 points means you handle stress well, 17 to 23 points means you're doing moderately well, and 24 to 30 points means you need to resolve problems that are causing excess stress.

Though we usually get a two- or three-decade reprieve from heart disease, younger women are already facing other troubles with stress. A study of 5,872 pregnant women in Denmark showed that women who are under moderate to high stress in the last trimester are 1.2 to 1.75 times more likely to give birth prematurely. Noise also stresses us out more than men. Studies show that women are irritated by sounds at half the volume that troubles men and can hear higher-frequency sounds better, according to Caroline Dow, Ph.D., assistant professor of communication at the University of Evansville in Evansville, Indiana.

A study that Dr. Dow helped conduct shows what noise can do. One hundred female college students were given a standardized test on a computer. Half had terminals that emitted high-pitched sounds, while the other half didn't.

The women with noisy computers scored 8.5 percent lower on the test. They worked faster and were more prone to mistakes—an indication, Dr. Dow says, that they were operating under stress.

Even society itself can stress us out. Now that women are building careers like men do, we face working-world stress like never before. In fact, our jobs cause the majority of our stress, Dr. Dickstein says. But it doesn't stop there. Women with careers must still cook, clean, look after children and be loving spouses. And that kind of double-barreled stress can be hard on your system. A Swedish study of men and women automobile plant managers between the ages of 30 and 50 showed that the blood pressure and levels of stress hormones went up for everyone during the workday. But when men went home, their blood pressure and stress readings dropped dramatically, while the women, with more left to do in the day, stayed higher.

"That study encapsulates everything," says women's health researcher Margaret A. Chesney, Ph.D., professor at the University of California, San Francisco, School of Medicine. "It's psychological proof that women are going home to second jobs. Men know that there's a distinction—that they're off duty at home. Women are not off duty. They're under more duress."

## Pull the Plug on Pressure

The key to beating stress? Creating a sense of control. We have to understand that some stress is inevitable. In fact, a little stress helps us accomplish tasks and meet goals, Dr. Dickstein says. But too much from the wrong sources—such as arguments with spouses or unrealistic expectations at work or at home—can make us feel helpless and unable to cope. And that's when stress does most of its dirty work.

Here are some tips to help you put stress in check.

**Work it out.** Nothing eases stress more than exercise, according to David S. Holmes, Ph.D., professor of psychology at the University of Kansas in Lawrence. "Regular aerobic workouts reduce stress more effectively than meditation, psychiatric intervention, biofeedback and conventional stress management," he says.

Exercise helps burn off all the stress-related chemicals in your system. During a workout, your body will also release mind-relaxing endorphins, Dr. Holmes says. And exercise strengthens your heart, too, further protecting you against the ravages of stress.

Research by Robert Thayer, Ph.D., professor of psychology at California State University, Long Beach, showed that 30 minutes of intense aerobic exercise immediately reduces body tension—and it does so even more effectively than moderate exercise such as walking.

**Don't be listless.** So many projects, so little time. To beat stress, you have to learn to prioritize, according to Lee Reinert, Ph.D., director and lecturer for the Brandywine Biobehavioral Center, a counseling center in Downingtown,

Pennsylvania. At the start of each day, pick the single most important task to complete, then finish it. If you're a person who makes to-do lists, never write one with more than five items. That way, you're more likely to get all the things done, and you'll feel a greater sense of accomplishment and control, Dr. Reinert says. Then you can go ahead and make a second five-item list. While you're at it, make a list of things that you can delegate to co-workers and family members. "Remember: You don't have to do everything by yourself," Dr. Reinert says. "You can find help and support from people around you."

**Just say no.** Sometimes you have to learn to draw the line. "Stressed-out people often can't assert themselves," says Joan Lerner, Ph.D., a counseling psychologist at the University of Pennsylvania Counseling Service in Philadelphia. "And so they swallow things. Instead of saying 'I don't want to do this' or 'I need some help,' they do it all themselves. Then they have even more to do."

Give your boss a choice. "Say 'I'd really like to take this on, but I can't do that without giving up something else,' " says Merrill Douglass, D.B.A., president of the Time Management Center in Marietta, Georgia, a company that trains individuals and corporations in the efficient use of time and energy, and co-author of *Manage Your Time, Manage Your Work, Manage Yourself.* " 'Which of these things would you like me to do?' " Most bosses can take the hint, Dr. Douglass says. The same strategy works at home, with your spouse, children, relatives and friends. If you have trouble saying no, start small. Tell your hubby to make his own sandwich. Or tell your daughter to find another ride home from volleyball practice.

**Pad your schedule.** "Realize that nearly everything will take longer than you anticipate," says Richard Swenson, M.D., author of *Margin: How to Create the Emotional, Physical, Financial and Time Reserves You Need.* By allotting yourself enough time to accomplish a task, you cut back on anxiety. In general, if meeting deadlines is a problem, always give yourself 20 percent more time than you think you need to do the task.

**Trade in the Jag for a Hyundai.** Living beyond your means can actually make you sick. A researcher at the University of Alabama in Tuscaloosa studied British census data on 8,000 households and found that families that tried to maintain lifestyles they couldn't afford were likely to have health problems.

**Sit up straight.** A good upright posture improves breathing and increases blood flow to the brain. We often slouch when stressed, which restricts breathing and blood flow and can magnify feelings of helplessness.

**Get a grip.** Keep a hand exerciser or a tennis ball in your desk at work and give it a few squeezes during tense times. "When stress shoots adrenaline into the bloodstream, that calls for muscle action," says Roger Cady, M.D., medical director of the Shealy Institute for Comprehensive Health Care in Springfield, Missouri. "Squeezing something provides a release that satisfies our bodies' fight-or-flee response."

# A Swift Solution

When you get wound too tight, often the first place you feel it is your neck. Try this four-way neck release recommended by former world-class track and field athlete Greg Herzog in his book *The 15-Minute Executive Stress Relief Program* (repeat each of the following exercises three times):

1. With your right hand, reach over your head and behind your left ear, grasping your neck with your fingers. Pull your head gently toward your right shoulder.

2. Do the same exercise, but this time use your left hand to pull your head toward your left shoulder.

3. Clasp your hands behind your head, with your elbows flared and your head bowed toward your chest. Relax in this position for 30 seconds. Then while pulling down with your hands, slowly push your head back until you are looking at the ceiling.

4. Place the palm of your left hand on your forehead, with the bottom of your palm at the bridge of your nose. Hold your right arm across your body so that you can rest your left elbow on your right wrist. Now push against your left palm with your forehead while keeping your right arm locked. Switch hands and repeat.

**Pop a bubble.** A study found that students were able to reduce their feelings of tension by popping two sheets of those plastic air capsules used in packaging. "Now we know why people hoard those things," says Kathleen Dillon, Ph.D., psychologist and professor at Western New England College in Springfield, Massachusetts, and the author of the study.

**Practice your snorkeling.** Want to really relax your muscles? Soak in a hot tub. To get the most relaxation from a hot bath, soak for 15 minutes in water that's just a few degrees warmer than your body temperature, or about 100° to 101°F. But be careful: Longer soaks in warmer water can actually lower your blood pressure too much.

**Tune out—have a potato.** If you want to unwind at the end of the day, eat a meal high in carbohydrates, says Judith Wurtman, Ph.D., a research scientist at the Massachusetts Institute of Technology in Cambridge and author of *Managing Your Mind and Mood with Food.* Carbohydrates trigger release of the brain neurotransmitter serotonin, which soothes you. Good sources of carbohydrates include rice, pasta, potatoes, breads, air-popped popcorn and low-cal cookies. Dr. Wurtman says just 1½ ounces of carbohydrates, the amount in a baked potato or a cup of spaghetti or white rice, is enough to relieve the anxiety of a stressful day.

**Try some fiber.** "Stress often goes right to the gut," says George Blackburn, M.D., Ph.D., associate professor of surgery at Harvard Medical School and chief of the Nutrition/Metabolism Laboratory at New England Deaconess Hospital, both in Boston. That means cramps and constipation. To avoid these problems, Dr. Blackburn suggests eating more fiber to keep your digestive system moving. You should build up gradually to at least 25 grams of fiber per day. That means eating more fruits, vegetables and grains. Try eating whole fruits instead of just juice at breakfast time, and try whole-grain cereals and fiber-fortified muffins.

**Have a laugh.** Humor is a proven stress reducer. Experts say a good laugh relaxes tense muscles, speeds more oxygen into your system and lowers your blood pressure. So tune into your favorite sitcom on television. Read a funny book. Call a friend and chuckle for a few minutes. It even helps to force a laugh once in a while. You'll find your stress melting away almost instantly.

**Hold your breath.** This technique should help you relax in 30 seconds. Take a deep breath and keep it in. Holding palm to palm, press your fingers together. Wait 5 seconds, then slowly exhale through your lips while letting your hands relax. Do this five or six times until you unwind.

**Take a ten-minute holiday.** Meditation is a great stress reliever, but sometimes it's hard to find the time or place for it. Dr. Reinert suggests taking a mini-vacation right at your desk or kitchen table instead. Just close your eyes, breathe deeply (from your stomach) and picture yourself lying on a beach in Mexico. Feel the warmth of the sun. Hear the waves. Smell the salt air. "Just put a little distance between yourself and your stress," Dr. Reinert says. "A few minutes a day can be a great help."

**Keep it down.** If you work, live or play in a high-noise area, consider wearing earplugs. Make sure the ones you buy reduce sound by at least 20 decibels, says Ernest Peterson, Ph.D., associate professor of otolaryngology at the University of Miami School of Medicine.

You can also use sounds to your advantage. Try listening to gentle music, with flutes or other soft-sounding instruments, says Emmett Miller, M.D., a nationally known stress expert and medical director of the Cancer Support and Education Center in Menlo Park, California. He also suggests taking walks in quiet places and listening to leaves rustle or streams babble. Recordings of ocean waves or gentle rainstorms also help, he says.

# STROKE

## *It's Not Too Early for Prevention*

**O**f all the thieves of youth, stroke is the swiftest and most tragic. In an instant, a vital, vibrant woman can lose her ability to speak, to move freely—even to think as clearly as she did just seconds before.

And despite its reputation as an older person's problem—an older man's problem at that—stroke doesn't discriminate. More than 8,000 American women between the ages of 30 and 44 suffer strokes each year. Nearly one in every three strokes is fatal. And the aging effects on those who survive can be brutal. Survivors could suffer brain damage affecting speech, memory, thought patterns and behavior. Sometimes there is temporary—or permanent—paralysis.

The good news is that you can significantly cut your risk of stroke. "We're beginning to realize that stroke is not an inevitable process," says Michael Walker, M.D., director for the Division of Stroke and Trauma at the National Institute of Neurological Disorders and Stroke in Bethesda, Maryland. "It's preventable, and it is treatable."

It may mean eating more fruits and vegetables, exercising a few times a week and staying vigilant about your blood pressure. But when you weigh the options, it's not a bad trade-off.

## The Risk for Women

Stroke is a sudden severe illness that attacks the brain. There are two basic types. Ischemic strokes, which account for about 80 percent of all strokes, happen when blood flow to a part of the brain is cut off, causing brain cells to die from lack of oxygen. This frequently occurs due to hardening and clogging in your carotid arteries, which feed blood from your neck to your head. Ischemic strokes can also be caused by atrial fibrillation, an irregular heartbeat that leads to clots that may travel through your body and lodge in the brain's arteries.

Hemorrhagic strokes account for the remaining 20 percent. These strokes are caused by bleeding from ruptures in either a blood vessel on the surface of your brain or an artery in the brain itself. These strokes can be even more deadly than ischemic strokes, with a mortality rate of close to 50 percent.

Women ages 30 to 44 are about half as likely to have strokes as men in the same age group, according to figures from the American Heart Association. Black women are at greater risk than white women of dying from stroke. Family history of stroke can play a role, too, though just how much remains unclear. And the risk of stroke goes up as a woman ages. American Heart Association statistics show that the incidence of stroke more than doubles each decade for a woman after she reaches age 55.

Younger women have some protection against stroke because their bodies produce large amounts of estrogen. That helps keep cholesterol levels lower and checks the onset of atherosclerosis, or hardening of the arteries. After menopause, though, the rate of stroke rises quickly. By age 65, women and men have about the same incidence of stroke.

Pregnancy can cause a slight increase in stroke risk, though the odds are still quite low. There are a few reasons for this increased risk, says Harold Adams, Jr., M.D., professor of neurology at the University of Iowa Hospital and Clinic in Iowa City. A woman's blood clots differently during pregnancy. And her blood pressure also tends to be a bit higher. Studies also show that certain forms of birth control pills may slightly increase stroke risk, too—especially for smokers older than 35 or for women with high blood pressure.

Of course, you have no say over age or gender. But Dr. Adams says there are many risks you can definitely control.

High blood pressure, for example. Also known as hypertension, it's the single most important risk factor for stroke. "About half of all strokes are caused by high blood pressure," says Edward S. Cooper, M.D., past president of the American Heart Association.

High blood pressure causes stroke by speeding up atherosclerosis and damaging smaller blood vessels. And in Dr. Cooper's words, it can cause tiny blood vessels in your brain to "blow out like an overinflated tire."

Smoking also puts you at increased risk for stroke by accelerating clogging of the carotid arteries, says Jack P. Whisnant, M.D., chief investigator for a study of carotid artery disease at the Mayo Clinic in Rochester, Minnesota. Women who smoke are over 2.5 times more likely to suffer strokes than non-smokers, according to a Harvard Nurses' Health Study that tracked 117,000 female registered nurses between the ages of 30 and 55 at entry to the study. The more women in the study smoked, the greater their risk. Compared with nonsmokers, women who smoked 1 to 14 cigarettes per day had twice the risk of stroke, while women who smoked 35 to 44 cigarettes per day—about two packs—had a fourfold increase in risk. Those who smoked more than 45 cigarettes per day were 5.4 times more likely to suffer strokes.

Women with diabetes are also at increased risk for stroke. And obese women and those with high blood cholesterol levels may be at higher risk of developing atherosclerosis and thus having strokes.

# An Intervention Strategy

Strokes are still shrouded in mystery. They seem to strike without warning. Sometimes it's hard to tell when you're even in danger.

But early prevention can be the key to improving your chances of avoiding stroke. "The process leading to a stroke begins in your forties, even earlier, so now is the time to intervene," says David G. Sherman, M.D., head of neurology at the University of Texas Health Science Center at San Antonio.

To help lower your risk, try these tips.

**Ease the pressure.** Many people don't even know they have high blood pressure, because it has few outward signs. That's why the American Heart Association recommends having your blood pressure checked by a doctor or another health care professional at least once a year if your blood pressure is 130/85 or higher. If your blood pressure is lower, get it checked every two years. Many cases of high blood pressure begin developing between ages 35 and 45.

Research shows that controlling high blood pressure can cut your risk of stroke by as much as 40 percent. Any reading above 140/90 is considered high.

Your doctor will be able to prescribe treatments for high blood pressure, from dietary changes to getting more exercise to drug therapy. Follow the advice like your life depends on it. It might.

"Controlling hypertension is absolutely vital in stroke prevention," Dr. Adams says.

**Kick the habit.** The Nurses' Health Study showed that women who stopped smoking cut their stroke risk substantially. In fact, the risk of stroke dropped to normal levels for women two to four years after they quit.

"Don't just cut back on cigarettes," Dr. Adams says. "There's no such thing as moderate smoking. You have to stop altogether, all the way, right now."

**Go low with the Pill.** For years, doctors warned women about birth control pills and increased stroke risk. But with the low-dose estrogen pills now in use, Dr. Adams says the risk of stroke is lower.

"We're seeing more and more evidence that low-dose estrogen oral contraceptives are safer," he says. "Low-dose estrogen is probably safe."

There are two caveats, however. Smoking and the Pill are a dangerous mix—especially for women over age 35. And high blood pressure, combined with the Pill, can also increase stroke risk. "If you have those risk factors, birth control pills are not advisable," Dr. Adams says.

**Check your neck.** Ask your doctor to listen for a bruit, a whooshing sound in the carotid arteries in your neck. This is caused by partial blockage and turbulence in the crucial blood vessels that feed oxygen to the brain.

# Stroke Warning Signs

Quick action can mean the difference between tragedy and recovery when it comes to stroke. Heed these warning signs, says the American Heart Association:

- Sudden weakness or numbness in the face, arm or leg on one side of the body
- Loss of speech, or trouble talking or understanding speech
- Sudden dimness or loss of vision, particularly in only one eye
- Sudden severe headache with no known cause
- Unexplained dizziness, unsteadiness or sudden falls, especially along with any of the previous symptoms

If you notice any of these symptoms, get help immediately by calling 911 or the emergency phone number for your area. A study of response times showed that people with stroke signs who called this emergency number got to the hospital two to three times faster than those who called their doctors or tried to transport themselves to the hospital. And with stroke, minutes matter.

What seems like a stroke may actually turn out to be a transient ischemic attack (TIA). These are sometimes called temporary strokes, since the symptoms quickly disappear. But you shouldn't ignore a TIA, since it is the single most important warning of impending stroke, according to Harold Adams, Jr., M.D., professor of neurology at the University of Iowa Hospital and Clinic in Iowa City.

"This is especially important if you have atherosclerosis causing blocked blood vessels elsewhere in your body," says Patricia Grady, Ph.D., acting director of the National Institute of Neurological Disorders and Stroke.

Also, make sure the doctor checks your heart. Treating atrial fibrillation can reduce stroke risk by up to 80 percent.

**Get some exercise.** Physical inactivity may be a risk factor for stroke, but a total exercise time of at least 20 minutes a day, three times a week, could reduce your risk for stroke. Walking, tennis, bicycling, stair climbing, aerobics and even gardening and Ping-Pong can be potential stroke busters.

A British study showed that the sooner you start exercising, the better. Women who started exercising between ages 15 and 25 had a 63 percent reduction in their risk for stroke. Even if you're a little late getting started, you can still benefit from exercise: The study showed that people who began exercising between ages 25 and 40 reduced their risk by 57 percent and that people who started exercising between ages 40 and 55 cut their risk by 37 percent.

"Exercise has so many benefits," Dr. Adams says. "If you're not exercising, you could be robbing yourself of years later on."

**Crunch some carrots.** The same Nurses' Health Study that looked at smoking also discovered a link between the nutrient beta-carotene and stroke.

"We found a 22 percent reduction in the risk of heart attack and a 40 percent reduction in stroke for those women with high intakes of fruits and vegetables rich in beta-carotene compared with those with low intakes," says JoAnn E. Manson, M.D., co-principal investigator of the cardiovascular component of the Nurses' Health Study who is co-director of women's health at Brigham and Women's Hospital and associate professor of medicine at Harvard Medical School, both in Boston.

Just one large carrot, which has 15 milligrams of beta-carotene, provides the amount of the nutrient that was associated with the lowest risk in the study. Other foods that worked were sweet potatoes, mangoes, apricots and spinach. Beta-carotene can be found in most dark green and orange fruits and vegetables.

**Pass the potassium.** Researchers at the University of California, San Diego, have found that adding a single daily serving of potassium-rich food to your diet could cut your risk of fatal stroke by as much as 40 percent. The reason for the benefit isn't completely clear. Although potassium is known to help lower blood pressure, the amount of potassium the test subjects ate had little direct effect on their blood pressure readings. Studies at the University of Mississippi Medical Center in Jackson showed that potassium may help prevent the formation of blood clots, one of the primary factors in heart attack and stroke.

If you're looking for a high-powered potassium boost, eat a baked potato every day. Potatoes are one of the richest sources of potassium. Other foods rich in potassium include dried apricots, lima beans, Swiss chard, bananas, skim milk, roasted chestnuts, okra and oranges.

**Know about aspirin.** Aspirin might help ward off ischemic stroke by thinning potential blood clots, Dr. Adams says. But unless you already have a risk factor, such as atherosclerosis or a prior stroke, it may not do you much good. In fact, research shows that aspirin might be linked to a slightly higher incidence of hemorrhagic stroke.

Just how much aspirin you should take also remains debatable. Some studies have found benefits with an 81-milligram daily dose (a children's aspirin). Others tout a 325-milligram daily dose (a regular-strength adult aspirin). And now some researchers say that as many as three regular aspirin tablets daily may be necessary. The bottom line: See your doctor before you start an aspirin regimen for stroke prevention.

**Keep it in balance.** What's good for your heart is good for your brain. Keeping your cholesterol in check can slow atherosclerosis and ward off ischemic stroke. So eat a low-fat diet. The current recommendation from most doctors and researchers is to limit fat to no more than 25 percent of your total calories.

"Along with exercise and quitting smoking, what you eat is key to preventing stroke," Dr. Adams says. "What we're talking about is a good diet that will help lessen the risk of hardening of the arteries." This diet doesn't need to be extreme, he says. It does need to be well balanced and low in fat.

**Toast your health—in moderation.** Excess drinking means increased stroke risk. Numerous studies show that having more than four drinks a day greatly increases your chances of having a hemorrhagic stroke.

But some studies show a link between moderate alcohol intake and a slightly reduced risk of ischemic stroke, at least among whites.

"There may be something about alcohol that helps in small levels. It may prevent both heart attack and stroke. I'm not telling my patients to drink for their health," Dr. Adams says. "If you're not drinking now, I don't recommend starting. If you do have more than a couple of drinks a day, the potential complications of alcohol are probably going to hurt you in the long run. The key to alcohol use is moderation."

# TELEVISION

## *Pandora's Electronic Box*

Karen Dykeman's social life was crammed into a 19-inch box in her living room. She had breakfast with Regis Philbin, lunch with Phil Donahue, dinner with Dan Rather and a midnight snack with Johnny Carson.

"My life revolved around television virtually from first thing in the morning to late at night," says the 35-year-old switchboard operator in Seven Lakes, North Carolina. "Thank God, I've gotten away from that. In the two years since I gave up watching television, I've lost 60 pounds, gotten involved in a community theater group, gone back to college, started dating and just had a great time. I have a real life now. I definitely feel more vigorous and feel like I think more clearly."

Karen's energetic lifestyle since she kicked her TV habit comes as no shock to doctors who have long suspected that television's magnetic appeal saps us of our youth in many ways.

"There's absolutely no question that large amounts of TV viewing can make you feel old and weary before your time," says Kurt V. Gold, M.D., a physical medicine and rehabilitation physician at Immanuel Medical Center in Omaha, Nebraska, who has studied the effects of TV viewing on children. "Just think about what happens when you watch television. You're sitting passively, not using your muscles much. After you've watched a long program, you feel stiff, tired and mentally drained.

"Over the long run, that can lessen your ability to think and perform physical tasks. If you watch a lot of television, you're simply not doing something that is going to refresh your body. As a result, your muscles sag, and your mind stagnates. It's common sense. If you don't use it, you lose it."

## A Pox on Your Fitness

But the danger of television isn't confined to losing muscle tone or abusing brain cells. Some researchers also believe there is a definite link between heavy

TV viewing and that dreaded middle-age bulge. In one study of 4,771 working women whose average age was 35, Larry A. Tucker, Ph.D., professor and director of health promotion at Brigham Young University in Provo, Utah, discovered that those who spent more than three to four hours a day watching television had twice the risk of being obese as women who watched less than one hour daily.

A study of 800 adults, published in the journal *American Dietetic Association*, found that the risk of obesity may be even greater than that. In this study, the incidence of obesity among those watching an hour or less of television a day was 4.5 percent, but prevalence shot up to 19.2 percent among those watching four or more hours a day.

Further evidence of the connection between TV viewing and fading fitness comes from another study at Brigham Young University. In this study of 9,000 adults, researchers concluded that people who watched television for less than one hour a day were the most fit. Compared with them, viewers with three- to four-hour habits were 41 percent less fit, and those who did regular four-hour-plus marathons of TV viewing were 50 percent less fit.

"Excessive TV viewing may not be the start of physical decline, but it can be a part of it," says Dr. Tucker. "People who watch a lot of television tend to be less physically active, eat more high-fat snack foods and be more obese. Other research has shown that people who watch a lot of television are more likely to be smokers. So there are a lot of negative health consequences that may be associated with watching lots of television."

In a study of 11,947 adults, Dr. Tucker found that people who watched three to four hours of television a day had twice the risk of developing high cholesterol levels as people who watched less than an hour a day. Even those who watched two or three hours a day were 1.5 times more likely to have high cholesterol. Excessive blood cholesterol is a risk factor for cardiovascular disease.

# This Is No Pick-Me-Up

But how many women have the time to watch that much television every day? A lot. In fact, the average American woman watches more than 30 hours of television a week or more than 4 hours daily, according to a report from Nielsen Media Research. That means a lot of women could be facing high risk of developing unflattering stomachs, heart disease and other chronic ailments normally associated with aging.

TV viewing may also dull your mind. Researchers found that two years after television was introduced into a Canadian village in 1973, the average resident's time in front of a television increased from 0 to 22 hours a week. That increase in viewing drastically curtailed residents' participation in community social activities and sports. Researchers also found that residents who watched a lot of television did not solve puzzle problems as well as residents who watched less television. In addition, after television came to the village, residents gave up trying to solve these problems much more quickly than before its arrival, says

# Are You a Victim of Television?

Check each question that you answer yes.

1. Do you watch more than two hours a day of television?
2. Do you stop talking with others while you view television?
3. Do you become unhappy or irritated if you have to turn off the television to do something else?
4. Do you occasionally feel extremely tired during a regular day's schedule?
5. Do you frequently eat junk food or unhealthy snack food when you sit down to watch television?
6. Do you frequently experience insomnia and use television as a means of distracting yourself during your sleeplessness?
7. On a pleasant day, are you more likely to stay indoors and watch television than to go do something outside?
8. Is it difficult for you to share or communicate your feelings and experiences with others?
9. Are you actively involved in less than two hobbies, clubs or sports at least four hours a week?
10. Do you frequently turn on the television and search the stations without having a specific program in mind to watch?

## Adding Your Score

For every odd-numbered question that you answered yes, give yourself two points. These factors were determined by experts to be indicators of too much TV watching.

For every even-numbered question that you answered yes, give yourself one point. These factors, in conjunction with poor viewing habits, signal potential trouble.

Tally your score and use the following scale as a rating guide.

**3 or less.** No problem.

**4 to 6.** Potential trouble brewing.

**7 to 9.** Yes, you're probably watching too much television.

**10 or more.** Whoa! Your brain is becoming fused to your set's circuitry.

Tannis MacBeth Williams, Ph.D., professor of psychology at the University of British Columbia in Vancouver.

Don't count on television to perk you up, either. In fact, research has shown that watching television for long periods leaves people in worse moods than they were in before they started watching. Irritability, difficulty relating to others and boredom may also be linked to excessive TV viewing.

"I wouldn't say that television is a total waste of one's leisure time. There are some good programs that inform and entertain us," Dr. Tucker says. "However, there is a tendency to overindulge in television, and that is wasteful and, to some extent, unhealthy."

Here are a few ways you can control your television rather than having it control you.

**Set boundaries.** Put a limit on the amount of time you will watch each week and stick to it. "You need to set limits, or your viewing can easily get out of control," Dr. Tucker says.

**Have an off-night.** Make the television off-limits one night a week. See what creative things you and your family can find to do, Dr. Tucker says.

**Be your own guide.** Browse through a programming schedule and mark one or two programs an evening that you want to watch. Turn on the set when the show begins and turn it off immediately after it ends, Dr. Tucker says. This will discourage you from getting hooked on the next program.

**Put a camera on yourself.** Before you turn on the television to watch a program, take a moment to visualize yourself walking over to the set and turning it off once the show is over. "That will program it into your brain that the television will actually go off at that time, and you will find something else to do," says Jane M. Healy, Ph.D., an educational psychologist in Vail, Colorado, and author of *Endangered Minds: Why Our Children Don't Think and What We Can Do about It.*

**Reward yourself for not watching.** For every hour that you don't watch television when you normally would, give yourself a point. After you've accumulated 10 or 20 points, treat yourself with tickets to a play, an evening at a comedy club or a dinner out with your family or friends, suggests Leonard Jason, Ph.D., professor of clinical and community psychology at DePaul University in Chicago.

**Say what?** Try turning on the set but turning off the sound, says Dr. Healy. More than likely, you'll quickly find something else to do with your time. "Much of the enticement of television comes from the sound track," says Dr. Healy.

**Move it out of sight.** Try putting your television in an unusual place, such as a cluttered room with no chairs, so you have to make an effort to watch it. "I've been remodeling my house, and I've put a bunch of furniture in front of my set, so I can't get to it very easily," Dr. Gold says. "You know what's nice? I've been working on my yard and spending time with my family instead of the television."

**Get out of the house.** Take a stroll, or go to the pool and have a leisurely swim. Get out into the real world. "If you watch three hours of television, do you usually feel invigorated? Probably not. If you go out for a 15-minute walk, you'll get a chance to talk to your neighbors and get some fresh air. I'd bet you'd come home feeling energized and ready to do anything but watch television," says C. Noel Bairey Merz, M.D., medical director of the Preventive and Rehabilitative Cardiac Center at Cedars-Sinai Medical Center in Los Angeles.

**Call on me.** "Arrange to have a friend phone you at the end of your favorite program. That might be all the incentive you need to break your habit, because once you get pulled away from the set, it's going to be easier not to go back to it," Dr. Healy says.

**Get a hobby.** "Find something that interests you, whether it be sketching, photography, caring for pets or going to school," says Karen Dykeman. "I got involved in things such as theater that made me feel important, needed and useful. If you find something useful in your life, you can break the TV habit really quickly."

**Don't get cable.** The fewer viewing options you have, the more likely you'll find something else to do with your time, Dr. Gold says.

# THYROID DISORDERS

## *Keeping Your Regulator Fit*

For most of our lives, the thyroid functions like a silent partner in a company, working behind the scenes to keep our bodies up and running. Small and butterfly-shaped, it rests unassumingly at the base of the throat, producing hormones that regulate the body's metabolism, temperature and heart rate. When it's functioning properly, we hardly know it's there.

But this unpretentious gland often makes its presence known in a big way. Like the ice maker in your freezer, it can go on the fritz, either pumping out hormones at a frantic pace or reducing its production to barely a trickle.

When this happens, the over- or underactive thyroid can dramatically rev up or slow down your body's metabolic activity. At the same time, these metabolic changes can produce a wide range of unpleasant symptoms that can take a devastating toll on the way you look and feel. Untreated, a malfunctioning thyroid can eventually trigger heart problems—and can even lead to coma or death.

As bad as all that sounds, it really isn't. "With early detection and proper treatment, almost all the problems of an abnormal thyroid can be corrected, and the symptoms, reversed," says Brian Tulloch, M.D., clinical associate professor at the University of Texas Medical School at Houston. "And most patients go on to live normal, functional, productive lives."

## The Underactive Thyroid

As your thyroid loses steam and cuts back its hormone production, your body gradually shows all kinds of signs that it's running on empty: fatigue, chills, dry skin, coarse hair, heavy periods, swelling and puffiness around the face and eyes, to name a few. It can also affect your mental functioning, leading to poor concentration, forgetfulness and depression. Your sex drive and your fertility can sputter and stall. This condition is called hypothyroidism.

The problem with hypothyroidism is that many of the symptoms associated with it are so common that you might not even suspect your ailing gland is the culprit. "It's easy to overlook an underactive thyroid, because the symptoms are similar to those associated with other common illnesses and mimic many of the physical changes we associate with normal aging," says Lawrence Wood, M.D., president and medical director of the Thyroid Foundation of America and a thyroidologist at Massachusetts General Hospital in Boston. "Many patients—and even some doctors—just take these symptoms to mean that the body is getting older, so quite often, the problem goes unreported or is undiagnosed."

Generations ago, thyroid enlargement, or goiter, was common in America due to a lack of iodine in the diet. Today, however, iodine deficiency is not a problem in the typical American diet; the most common cause of hypothyroidism is Hashimoto's disease, a disorder of the body's autoimmune system.

Because hypothyroidism slows down the way the body burns calories, many overweight women wishfully try to blame their weight gains on a sluggish thyroid. But it's not to blame. "Obesity and major weight gains are rarely related to an underactive thyroid," says Dr. Tulloch. "Most thyroid-related weight gains amount to only a few pounds, and that's due mostly to water retention."

While doctors can't usually make an underactive thyroid active again, they can easily treat and control it. "All we have to do is restore the right balance of thyroid hormone in the system by replacing what isn't being produced," says Martin I. Surks, M.D., head of the Division of Endocrinology and Metabolism at the Montefiore Medical Center in New York City. Women with sluggish thyroids take little tablets containing a synthetic version of the hormone thyroxine. The drawback: They must take them every day for the rest of their lives.

## The Overactive Thyroid

Now imagine the thyroid acting in reverse, pumping out too much hormone. These excess hormones push the body's metabolism into overdrive, producing a unique combination of hyper-symptoms that includes rapid heartbeat, weight loss, weakness, nervousness, irritability and tremors.

Not surprisingly, this is called hyperthyroidism. Its most common cause is Graves' disease, the autoimmune disorder that struck both former President George Bush and Barbara Bush. The former first lady, you may remember, was bothered by rapid weight loss, bulging eyeballs and vision problems—classic Graves' symptoms. Her husband became aware of his Graves' disease after a scare from an irregular heartbeat.

When treating an overactive thyroid, physicians have several options. The simplest and most prescribed is to use radioactive iodine to reduce the number of overproductive thyroid cells. Doctors can also prescribe drugs that block the production of thyroid hormone or that block the effects of the hormone on the body. And as a last resort, doctors may surgically remove all or part of an overactive thyroid. But since surgery and radioactive iodine can cause women to later develop hypothyroidism, a lifetime of thyroxine tablets is often necessary.

## Who's at Risk

Several key factors can put a woman at risk for developing thyroid disorders. The most important is just being a woman. "Women are about five times more likely than men to develop problems with their thyroids," says Dr. Surks. "Many thyroid disorders also manifest themselves during or following pregnancy or after menopause."

Graves' disease and other causes of overactive thyroid are most common in the 20- to 40-year-old age group, but they can occur in older people, too. By age 50, at least one woman in ten has signs of an underactive thyroid. And 17 percent of women over 60 suffer from some form of hypothyroidism.

Genetics also plays a role. If your family has a history of thyroid disease or autoimmune diseases such as diabetes and rheumatoid arthritis, you're a candidate for thyroid problems as you get older. Another fact to consider: According to a Dutch study, cigarette smoking appears to be a significant factor that produces Graves' disease in predisposed people. These findings imply that kicking the habit may prevent the development of the disease if it runs in your family.

Other risk factors: having had radiation treatments around the head and neck as a child, the use of certain medications such as lithium or going through a particularly stressful experience such as losing a loved one.

## What Women Should Do

With the exception of eating a balanced diet and not smoking, there's not much you can do to prevent thyroid disease. "It's important to detect thyroid disease early, before it fouls up your body, your emotions or your life," says Dr. Wood.

Have your doctor check out any symptoms or abnormalities that may suggest hypo- or hyperthyroidism. According to Dr. Wood, any woman over age 50, especially if she's in a risk group, should make a thyroid test part of her annual physical exam. "Regular exams become increasingly important as you get older, because many of the symptoms of thyroid disease become less obvious and harder to detect on your own," he says.

Checking for thyroid function usually requires only a blood test. If a lump or nodule is present, a doctor may take a sample of thyroid tissue for examination in a relatively painless procedure called a fine needle aspiration biopsy.

While treatments with thyroid hormone are almost always safe, studies have shown that too much replacement thyroid hormone may increase a woman's risk for osteoporosis, the bone-weakening disorder that can lead to fractures of the hip and vertebrae. That's why it's important to get an annual checkup that includes a thyroid-stimulating hormone test, take the dose of thyroid hormone that's right for you and maintain an appropriate program of nutrition and exercise.

# TYPE A PERSONALITY

## *This "A" Is for Aging*

You have never liked losing—not at the office, not on the tennis court, not even when your daughter gets lucky and beats you at Chutes and Ladders. And you don't like wasting time, either—especially when it's because of something you can't control, such as a slow-moving driver on the freeway or a slow-talking co-worker. With all the hurdles life puts in your path, it's no wonder you can't hold your temper anymore.

Whoa! Time out! These are some of the classic signs of Type A behavior. If you're running your motor at 150 miles per hour, 24 hours a day, it may be time to re-examine some goals and habits and your outlook on life. Because if you don't, you could be setting yourself up for problems—from headache to heart disease—that will erode your body's youthful edge.

"Type A behavior is very hard on your system," says C. David Jenkins, Ph.D., professor of preventive medicine and community health at the University of Texas Medical Branch at Galveston. "You're putting yourself under a lot of needless pressure. And believe me, that will take its toll in the long run, in ways you may not expect."

## Anxious, Angry—And at Risk

The American Heart Association lists six characteristics of Type A women. They love competition, attempt to achieve many poorly defined goals, have a strong need for recognition and advancement, are always in a hurry, show intense concentration and alertness and are prone to anger.

Fewer than half of the women in America are Type A, Dr. Jenkins says. But the figure is creeping higher, he says, as more women enter the workplace and take on higher-stress jobs. If you're a saleswoman, newspaper reporter or air traffic controller or in another high-pressure job, the odds are that you were drawn to your field by Type A tendencies. In fact, even if you weren't Type A to start with, Dr. Jenkins says that the demands of these jobs can push you in that direction.

The key problem with Type A behavior is stress. Hard-driving women put themselves under constant strain, and their bodies react in pressure-packed ways. Studies show that Type A women are more likely to grind their teeth, which can lead to jaw pain, headaches and dental troubles. Because of stress, they also may suffer from chronic muscle fatigue and soreness in their necks and shoulders.

A study of 72 female college students in Ohio showed that Type A women may also face more anxiety and depression than other women—while at the same time receiving less support from friends and family. Researchers speculate that this may happen because society tends to shun and isolate competitive, hard-driving women, even as it encourages men with the same traits.

Scientists are even exploring a possible link between cancer and Type A behavior. There's no concrete evidence on this one. But a continuing study of 3,154 American men shows that Type A behavior might predispose people to develop cancer. Scientists think that this may happen because stress represses the immune system, making the body less able to fight off disease.

Then there's heart disease. Estrogen gives women extra protection against heart disease, at least until menopause. But after that, Type A behavior can hurt. A study at Harvard Medical School in Boston of about 500 men and women—most of the women past menopause—showed that the Type A's had a 50 percent higher risk of suffering heart attacks than their mellower Type B counterparts.

Dr. Jenkins says the process probably works like this: Every time you lay on the horn at an intersection or argue with your boss, your body produces a stress hormone called noradrenaline. This spunks up your body, making you more alert and raising your blood pressure temporarily. Dr. Jenkins says it can also cause minor damage to the lining of your blood vessels. As your body repairs the blood vessels, they pick up cholesterol flowing in your bloodstream. Over time, this patchwork can lead to a buildup of cholesterol in your arteries—setting you up for blockages and heart attacks.

# A-mazing Solutions

You can't really "cure" Type A personality, Dr. Jenkins says. Not that you'd want to; there's really nothing wrong with a touch of assertiveness and a sturdy work ethic. But you may want to change some daily habits and attitudes to help lower your risk of Type A health trouble. Here are a few suggestions to get started.

**Aim lower.** Sure, you want to succeed at everything. But there are only 24 hours in a day—and sometimes something has to give. So be a little more choosy. "I think setting realistic goals is the most important thing a Type A person can do," says Lee Reinert, Ph.D., director and lecturer for the Brandy-wine Biobehavioral Center, a counseling center in Downingtown, Pennsylvania. "Goals make you focus on what's important, instead of whatever crisis is facing you at the moment."

At the start of each week, make a list of things you feel you absolutely must do. Each time you write something down, ask yourself what would happen if you didn't do it. If you can't come up with a legitimate concern, scratch that item off the list. Now comes the tough part: Cut the final list by five items. You may try delegating a few of the items to your spouse, children or co-workers. "What's left is a more achievable set of tasks," Dr. Reinert says. "You'll get a greater sense of accomplishment this way, and you won't be chasing after brush-fires that keep popping up."

**Try aerobics.** You'll sweat the stress a little less if you work out regularly. Aerobic exercise relieves stress and can ward off its long-term consequences, says David S. Holmes, Ph.D., professor of psychology at the University of Kansas in Lawrence.

One word of caution, however: Don't overdo it. Because they tend to over-train, Type A women get injured more during exercise, reports *Sports Medicine Digest*. In fact, Type A women lose twice as much training time as others to in-jury. "Get a good workout. Raise your heart rate, but don't try to win at all costs. Don't keep trying to beat your own record," Dr. Jenkins says.

**Account for your anger.** Keeping journals helps women discover the roots of their aggressiveness and anger, Dr. Reinert says. "A lot of times, you're not really mad at what's going on right now. You're upset about more of a core issue—maybe an unhappy family relationship," she says. Writing down your thoughts and feelings may help you discover what's really angering you. It can also help you detect patterns. Maybe you always get mad when you're waiting in line. Or when Marla in accounting won't let you get a word in at the staff meeting. If you anticipate these moments, you can either find ways to avoid them or ask yourself whether they're really important enough to blow your stack over.

**Make amends.** Is that little old lady in the slow-moving Buick really trying to make you mad? Was she awake deep into the night plotting ways to make you late? Or is she just a little old lady who needs to use a little extra caution to drive these days? In his book *Anger Kills*, Redford B. Williams, M.D., director of the Behaviorial Medicine Research Center and professor of psychi-atry at Duke University Medical Center in Durham, North Carolina, suggests putting yourself in the other person's shoes. When you look at the world from the perspective of the people who anger you, you'll probably be a little less cynical about them—and a little less Type A in the process. Dr. Williams also suggests doing some volunteer work as a way to relieve hostility and gain em-pathy for other people.

**Come up for air.** Type A women typically schedule their days to the mil-lisecond. That leaves no margin for error—and sets you up for extra stress when things go wrong. So try to give yourself a 10 percent pad. If you work a ten-hour day, leave at least one hour free to deal with the unexpected. If that sounds like an awfully big block of time, Dr. Reinert suggests setting aside five or six minutes per hour instead.

These cooldown periods can help you organize your thoughts and create new plans of attack. They can also spark creativity, making the rest of the workday more productive. "If you don't have a little downtime, you're not giving yourself a chance to absorb all the information that's flying at you," Dr. Reinert says. "You'll be more creative and efficient if you just take time to process."

**Pay attention to your body.** Find another 10 or 15 minutes a day to check in with your body. Sit on a comfortable chair in a quiet room, close your eyes, and breathe deeply. Tense, then release, the muscles in your feet. Then do your calves. Work up your body, paying special attention to the areas that feel tight or are throbbing (especially your shoulders and neck). "This is a great stress reducer," Dr. Reinert says. "It lets your body relax. And it shows you how needlessly tense you become during the day."

# ULCERS

## *Taming the Fire Within*

If you have an ulcer, think twice before casting the blame on the usual suspects. Many of the one in ten people who have or will develop one think that ulcers are the result of either too much pressure at work or too much spicy food.

But in reality, researchers say, those excuses may have bigger holes in them than the one that's formed in your belly. In fact, research shows that ulcers are more common among the unemployed. And there's no evidence that spicy food plays any role in their formation.

"It's often not what people think, but there are many causes of ulcers, and age seems to play a role in most of them," says Jorge Herrera, M.D., associate professor of medicine at the University of South Alabama College of Medicine in Mobile. That seems only fitting, since ulcers seem to age a woman before her time, causing pain that can hamper physical activity and command a lot of attention. Most women seem to handle ulcers by treating their jobs and pressures with kid gloves and by adopting Grandma's diet of applesauce, cottage cheese and other bland foods.

## How We Set Ourselves Up

Ulcers form when digestive juices—acids, really—start burning through the delicate pink lining of your digestive organs. This is usually the result of a deterioration in a protective layer that covers the lining of the stomach and duodenum, the top part of the small intestine.

There are two major types: Gastric ulcers, which show up more frequently in women and usually after age 50, occur in the stomach, and symptoms include a burning or "hungry" feeling in the stomach or under the breastbone, a vague uneasiness of the stomach and even chronic nausea. Duodenal ulcers, which are more common among men and tend to strike between ages 20 and 40, hit lower, in the upper portion of the small intestine. With duodenal ulcers, pain is often relieved after eating; with gastric ulcers, it's not. Either type of ulcer can lead to stools that are black or maroon and foul-smelling and to vomiting what appears to be coffee-ground material.

"The biggest cause of gastric ulcers is taking certain medications," says Dr. Herrera. "These ulcers are more common in women, particularly as they get older, because many of these medications are for conditions that usually occur as you age, such as arthritis drugs and other painkillers."

But even young women may be setting themselves up for gastric ulcers. "Probably the worst offenders, simply because they're the most frequently used, are aspirin and other nonsteroidal anti-inflammatory drugs available over the counter," says Dr. Herrera. "If you take any of these drugs for more than three months at a time, as many women do, you increase your risk of ulcers significantly."

These drugs do their dirty work by inhibiting the production of mucus and protective acid-neutralizing agents; aspirin can also weaken the stomach lining and cause bleeding. "In fact, many patients don't even realize they have ulcers because of the painkillers in the drugs they take," he adds. "Sometimes they come into the office for problems with bleeding or their stools, and only then do they realize they have ulcers."

Duodenal ulcers often result from smoking, which causes the production of excessive amounts of digestive acids. But studies show that at least 95 percent of patients with duodenal ulcers also harbor common bacteria called *Helicobacter pylori*, says William B. Ruderman, M.D., chairman of the Department of Gastroenterology at the Cleveland Clinic Florida in Fort Lauderdale. The bacteria are spread from person to person, like other infectious diseases, and can be cured with antibiotics. "These bacteria are more common as you age," says Dr. Ruderman. "For one thing, exposure to these bacteria increases over time. And your body's defenses may get impaired over time." In fact, as many as one in five people with these bacteria comes down with duodenal ulcers.

# How We Can Escape the Trap

If you think you have an ulcer, see your doctor. A doctor can prescribe drugs that reduce acid secretions and ease pain as well as antibiotics for *H. pylori*. In the meantime, here's what you can do to prevent ulcers or to lessen their severity.

**Choose Tylenol.** For headaches and other minor aches and pains, take acetaminophen, which is in products such as Tylenol, rather than ibuprofen, commonly sold as Advil and Nuprin. Ibuprofen is an anti-inflammatory, and products containing it can cause ulcers, says Dr. Herrera. "Sure, they have painkilling ingredients, but so do other medications that won't lead to ulcers. So if you have a headache or other minor problem that requires a painkiller, take Tylenol."

And stay away from aspirin, since it can do even more damage than ibuprofen. Aspirin can weaken the stomach lining and cause bleeding.

**Stop smoking.** Cigarettes do double damage to the ulcer-prone. "Smoking can lead to ulcers because it increases acid production several-fold, especially if you smoke after dinner or before bed," says Dr. Herrera. "That's because acid production is usually worse at night."

Once you have ulcers, the acid created by smoking makes it hard to get rid of them. "It keeps ulcers from healing and makes it more likely that they will come back," adds Mark H. Ebell, M.D., assistant professor in the Department of Family Medicine at Wayne State University in Detroit.

**Mellow out.** People who view their lives as being too stressful are up to three times more likely to develop ulcers than those who learn to roll with life's punches, says Robert Anda, M.D., of the National Center for Chronic Disease Prevention and Health Promotion in Atlanta. But since we're all under stress, why do some of us get ulcers and others don't?

"It's how you interpret stress," says Dr. Anda. When you feel the weight of the world is on your shoulders and perceive stressful events as negative, you're a prime candidate for ulcers, because this perception results in the production of more stomach acids. On the other hand, women who acknowledge they have stress but view it as a fact of everyday life and don't let it overwhelm them are less likely to get ulcers.

Many women who react negatively to stress find it helps to talk about their problems with good friends, to do regular meditation or relaxation exercises or even to start regular exercise programs, says Howard Mertz, M.D., assistant professor of medicine at the University of California, Los Angeles, UCLA School of Medicine.

**Reassess your bland diet.** While there's no proof that eating a bland diet will help, there is evidence that drinking one may hurt. In fact, the old remedy of drinking milk for an ulcer may actually do more harm than good, says Richard W. McCallum, M.D., professor of medicine and chief of gastroenterology at the University of Virginia School of Medicine in Charlottesville. That's because while milk may initially have a neutralizing effect on these acids, after 30 minutes or so, you get a "rebound effect" in which the calcium and protein from the milk actually stimulate acid production.

# UNWANTED HAIR

## Hair, Hair, Go Away

You may not have noticed it when you were young, when a little peach fuzz on smooth, childish skin didn't matter a bit. But now that you're older, you may find the hair is more profuse or suddenly darker. You may remember a loving aunt whose smile carried a pronounced shadow—but surely, you haven't reached her age already!

Perhaps you have. Or maybe the unwanted hair has simply come on sooner. In any case, it makes you feel aged and unattractive, as though your body is sabotaging your beauty. It's a common problem for a lot of women, though a lot of us would rather die than admit it.

Often it's genetically based, doctors say. If your family tree has Mediterranean roots, you may develop a dark, downy crop on your upper lip or below the "sideburn" hairline. Sometimes just a few stubborn whiskerlike hairs will appear, often on the chin.

But the most common cause of excess hair growth as women get older is the hormonal changes of menopause, says Victor Newcomer, M.D., professor of dermatology at the University of California, Los Angeles, UCLA School of Medicine. "Most women have a little down on the upper lip after puberty, and in brunettes, it can be very heavy. But after menopause, it really kicks in with coarse, fibrous hairs." That's because the effects of the male hormone androgen (which every woman has) become more pronounced when levels of the female hormone estrogen drop. The androgen then is free to stimulate more hair growth, he says.

If excess facial or body hair isn't common among the women in your family, you may want to ask your doctor whether any medications you are taking could be causing the problem, says Seth L. Matarasso, M.D., assistant professor of dermatology at the University of California, San Francisco, School of Medicine. Sometimes blood pressure medicine, steroids for arthritis, diuretics (water pills) or birth control pills can stimulate hair growth, he says.

## Electrolysis: The Permanent Solution—Eventually

There's one way to remove hair permanently, and that's professional electrolysis. This method is appropriate for hair on any area of the body, from the upper lip to the nipple area to the toes—anything but eyelashes, nose and ears—although it's painful and time-consuming. Here's what you'll experience in a licensed electrolysist's office at fees that range from $15 to $100, depending on the length of the session.

The electrolysist cleans your skin with alcohol, guides a sterile electric needle into the hair follicle and turns on the current. The current will destroy the hair follicle, but sometimes it takes multiple sessions. And some women find the treatments simply too painful to tolerate. What motivates many of them to endure the process is that if you persist with the treatments, the hair will eventually stop growing back.

For a small area of unwanted hair, it might be worth it, says Seth L. Matarasso, M.D., assistant professor of dermatology at the University of California, San Francisco, School of Medicine. But there are risks involved. There is some possibility of pigment change in your skin, slight scarring or folliculitis, an inflammation of the hair follicles, he says. And though it's highly unlikely with the sterilization techniques used by

If hair growth of more than a few hairs appears suddenly, Dr. Matarasso says, see your doctor for endocrinological tests. Although it's very rare, unusual hair growth in women may indicate a thyroid or hormonal problem.

And though leg and arm hair is normal, it's very unusual to have any hair growth on the cheeks or forehead. Hair in these areas could result from several causes, including disease in the ovaries or in the pituitary or adrenal glands, says Dr. Newcomer. Some rare liver diseases may also stimulate hair growth on the cheeks or forehead, he says.

Or your problem may simply be that you're annoyed by persistent facial or body hair that you've had since puberty. Whether the hair is age-related or not, there are several ways to deal with it.

## Gentle and Not-So-Gentle Methods

So how do you get the excess fleece to flee? Here are some suggestions.

**Bleach away.** With hair that's dark but not too heavy, try a facial hair

most professional electrolysists, there is the potential to spread disease, including hepatitis, he says.

Your best protections against infection are to be sure your electrolysist uses a new needle each time and to ask her to wear latex gloves, says Victor Newcomer, M.D., professor of dermatology at the University of California, Los Angeles, UCLA School of Medicine.

If you've wondered whether the home electrolysis units you see in mail order catalogs work just as well as salon equipment, experts are skeptical.

"Some of these units are supposed to work painlessly with radio waves and destroy the hair follicle at the base," says Carole Walderman, a cosmetologist and esthetician and president of Von Lee International School of Aesthetics and Makeup in Baltimore. "But hair is not a conductor of electricity, so how could this method destroy the hair root?"

Even when the galvanic current from regular electrolysis machines cauterizes the follicles directly, Walderman says, you still get up to 90 percent regrowth, which is why repeated treatments are necessary to permanently remove the hair.

bleach that you can buy at your pharmacy, says Dr. Newcomer. Bleaching may make the hair less noticeable, so there's no need to remove it.

But if the hair growth bothers you or you feel you would look better and smoother-skinned without it, here are some other temporary solutions.

**Shave away the hair.** It's one of the earliest grooming myths that women pass along to each other, but shaving does not cause hair to grow back thicker, says Dr. Matarasso. It's easy to be confused, because the growing-in hairs may look darker, he says. All hairs begin to cycle at the same time, and when they reach the surface of the skin all at once, the stubs appear thick and feel rough, he says. But there's not really more or thicker hair growing back.

The choice between an electric razor and a blade is up to you; whatever feels best, Dr. Matarasso says. They shave the same, although you use an electric razor on dry skin. If you use a blade, soak it in water for a few minutes first, then let your favorite shaving cream or gel sit on the skin for a moment or two before you shave, he says. It will soften the hair and give you smoother results. And if you're thinking of shaving a part of your face, there's no harm in that. But if facial growth is profuse, check with your doctor first to rule out medical causes.

**Use tweezers.** For just a few recurring hairs, one of the simplest removal methods is tweezing, with the aid of a magnifying mirror if you need it, says Dr. Newcomer. Some benefits of tweezing are that it is effective and you can do it in privacy. But even though tweezed hair follicles will eventually give up the ghost, it can take many years for that kind of permanent result, he says.

**Try a depilatory.** Chemical lotions such as Neet and Nair are perfectly fine to use, says Dr. Matarasso, as long as you patch-test a small area first to make sure you're not allergic to the product. "The chemicals aren't bad, but they can be abrasive," he says. They work by dissolving hair at or just below the skin line, so results last for up to two weeks, says Dr. Matarasso.

Depilatories are simple and painless to use, but some have nasty odors. You apply the thick lotion to the skin, wait for up to 15 minutes and then rinse off with warm water. You want to avoid using it near your eyes or pubic area.

If you use a depilatory on your face, apply only a little at first. Don't leave it on too long, or you'll wind up with a rash, says Dr. Newcomer. "If you're an oily-skinned brunette, you can tolerate it longer. But thin-skinned blondes have less tolerance" to the chemicals, he says. The texture of the hair also makes a difference in how depilatories work. Big, coarse hair takes longer to dissolve, and fine hair comes off easier, he says.

**Consider waxing, at least once.** You've probably heard hair waxing compared to Band-Aid removal, but it's a little more challenging than that. The delightful side of waxing (and the reason so many women grin and bear it) is that you'll have hair-free skin for about six weeks afterward. And the new growth is soft and silky at first.

Waxing is appropriate for any area of the body—face, arms, legs and even the bikini area. But be very careful near the groin, Dr. Newcomer says. "The wax can get tangled up in the pubic area, and you can't get it off," he says.

How does it work? At a salon, heated wax is applied to your skin with a wooden spatula. When the wax hardens, the technician yanks off the strips, lifting away the hair. You'll be treated to a soothing lotion afterward, but some women find the process quite painful. You can buy do-it-yourself waxing kits for face or body at a pharmacy, but, as Dr. Newcomer says, "it takes a brave soul to pull off that strip."

Is the pain of pulled hair a little too intense? "Go see your dermatologist about an hour before you wax, and have him numb your skin with a local anesthetic," says Dr. Matarasso. "You'll hardly feel a thing."

If you'd like to try waxing and you happen to use the anti-wrinkling cream tretinoin (Retin-A) or any skin lotion containing glycolic acid, be sure to stop using it a few days before waxing, says Dr. Matarasso. These preparations are exfoliants and actually remove the outer two layers of skin, making the skin much more sensitive, he says. "If you wax on top of denuded skin, you'll give yourself a rip-roaring wound," he says. "You can take off a significant amount of the skin."

Also keep in mind that you have to wait until hair grows back to ¼ inch long before you can have it waxed again. This could be a problem in summer, when you might want to go bare-legged.

**Avoid the mitts and electric coils.** Don't use the pumicelike hair removal mitts sold in many salons and pharmacies, says Dr. Matarasso. "They really are quite abrasive and can injure your skin," he says. The mitts "just mechanically break off the hair, like another crude razor," says Dr. Newcomer.

The vibrating coils work by lifting up many hairs at once and pulling them out from their roots. Unlike waxing, which pulls out hair quickly against the direction of growth, the coils yank hair in every direction. "It's mechanized or group tweezing," says Dr. Matarasso. "Some women who use it are very stoic. The vast majority of people find this method too painful, and it doesn't leave you hair-free that much longer than shaving or a depilatory."

# VARICOSE VEINS

## *You Don't Have to Live with Them*

What woman doesn't hate varicose veins, whether they're small and spidery or bulgy blue ropes? Varicose veins creep up the legs of over half of us after age 40, and they're a potent reminder of aging. All of a sudden, wearing shorts or a swimsuit isn't an automatic choice anymore.

What we call spider veins doctors call venous telangiectasia. They are actually dilated veins, often found on the upper calves and thighs. Both spider veins and varicose veins, which are usually found on the legs, are veins that are larger than they should be.

Although many women find spider veins just a cosmetic annoyance, larger varicose veins can be truly uncomfortable. Sometimes they cause a feeling of heaviness, tiredness and chronic aching in the calves. They can trigger night cramps and restless legs that disturb sleep and leave you dragging and worn out. Swollen veins often become itchy and sore. And although it's rare, varicose veins may indicate a clot in a deeper leg vein.

## For Women Mostly

Where do they come from? Your genes, for starters. You can inherit the tendency to form varicose veins from either side of the family.

But the fact is that varicose veins are up to six times more common in women than in men, which leads scientists to believe that female hormones play a strong role in their formation.

One theory suggests that when a woman is pregnant, her greater blood volume increases vein pressure. At the same time, her higher levels of the hormone progesterone may help dilate veins. Add to this the weight of the uterus pressing on pelvic veins, which, in turn, transmits more pressure to leg veins. It's the blueprint for varicose veins.

Menstruation can also cause pressure on your veins because of the increase in blood volume just before you menstruate. It's why your legs may feel achy right before your period.

Lifestyle factors can also aggravate vein problems. If you smoke, varicose veins are much more likely to creep up on you, because smoking affects blood flow by interfering with the regulation of fibrin, a blood-clotting protein. Although being heavy doesn't cause varicose veins directly, being 20 percent over your ideal weight can coax out varicose veins in those who have hereditary tendencies toward them. Lifting very heavy weights and running on hard surfaces may also hasten the appearance of varicose veins.

Sometimes the underlying problem is physiological. People with varicose veins have an inherited weakness in the valves inside the leg veins. These veins normally prevent blood from leaking back down as it flows up to the heart. If a valve leaks, gravity forces blood into lower veins when you stand up. Once this process is repeated enough times, vein walls can become permanently stretched.

"Whenever you're standing or sitting with your legs below the heart, gravity's working against you," explains Malcolm O. Perry, M.D., professor and chief of vascular surgery at Texas Tech University Health Sciences Center in Lubbock.

## Fallout from a Low-Fiber Diet

There's one thing doctors know for sure about varicose veins: They are not a natural part of aging. In fact, Glenn Geelhoed, M.D., professor of surgery and international medical education at George Washington University Medical Center in Washington, D.C., has studied varicose veins in populations around the world and has found that in some Third World cultures, varicose veins are all but nonexistent, even in women who have borne children. He has also found that when these people move to countries such as the United States and adopt our habits—mainly, a low-fiber diet and a sedentary lifestyle—they start to develop varicose veins.

Too little fiber produces constipation and straining on the toilet, and that may be where diet affects vein health most. Western populations on low-fiber diets pass smaller and harder stools than do Third World people, who have few varicose veins, Dr. Geelhoed notes. And when you strain in vain, that increases pressure in rectal veins, which in turn passes on more pressure to leg veins.

In fact, the famed Framingham Heart Study, which followed the lifestyles of residents of this Massachusetts town for over 40 years, found that the risk factors for varicose veins are the same as for heart disease—particularly being over-

# Removing the Webs

Some women call them spider veins—those visible red lines that usually crop up on the legs, especially the thighs, and seem to resemble the fragile patterns of a spider's web.

How do you get rid of them? If they're big enough, usually conventional sclerotherapy is the best bet, says Arthur Bertolino, M.D., associate clinical professor of dermatology at New York University Medical Center in New York City and a dermatologist in Ridgewood, New Jersey.

"The optimal size for treatment is at least as large as the line you'd write on a piece of paper with an ordinary ballpoint pen," he says. "If they're too small, you can't put a needle in."

If you have just a few tiny spiders, consider a cover-up makeup with a greenish base, which conceals red tones, Dr. Bertolino suggests.

But for more than a few on the face or legs, sclerotherapy is usually very successful, he says. A tiny needle is inserted into the vein, and a solution is injected. You can actually see the red network disappear as the clear solution enters the vein, he says.

weight and sedentary. The Framingham study also showed that compared with women without varicose veins, those with vein problems were more often obese, were less active, had higher blood pressure and were older at the onset of menopause.

## They're Not Inevitable

If varicose veins run in the family but haven't yet turned up on you, there are many things you can do to help forestall them.

**Shed some weight.** If you are significantly overweight, a gradual, healthy weight loss plan can be your veins' biggest ally, says Alan Kanter, M.D., medical director of the Vein Center of Orange County in Irvine, California. Extra pounds put unnecessary pressure on your legs.

**Fiber up your diet.** Make sure your diet is high in fiber to keep bowels healthy and stools soft. This will prevent straining due to constipation, Dr. Kanter says. Fiber is found in abundance in fruits, vegetables and whole grains.

**Drink water.** Another way to soften stools is to be sure you're well hydrated by drinking at least eight glasses of water a day, says Dr. Kanter.

**Don't smoke.** Or if you do, stop, says Dr. Geelhoed. Smoking increases

Side effects? Occasionally, the solution will cause a temporary muscle cramp near the ankle or the back of the lower calf, which your doctor can massage away in a minute or two. Rarely, a skin ulcer may result from fluid that escapes a leaky vessel, or new spider veins called mats may form, he says. There may also be a brownish discoloration of the skin, which almost always fades completely on its own but can often be removed using a copper vapor laser.

The pulsed-dye laser is also used by some physicians to remove dilated facial capillaries, says David Green, M.D., a dermatologist at the Varicose Vein Center in Bethesda, Maryland. The light waves emitted by the laser are absorbed by hemoglobin molecules in the blood. "This vaporizes the hemoglobin, which turns the light energy into heat energy and 'fizzles' the vessel wall," he says.

"Current lasers are not great on veins or capillaries below the waist," Dr. Green says. "But they're great on those above the neck, particularly on the nose and cheeks."

your risk of developing underlying vein disease, which can contribute to varicose veins, he says.

**Lift weights wisely.** Weight-lifting exercise will help with weight control, but you need to do it right to avoid encouraging a vein problem, says Dr. Kanter. Use smaller weights and do more repetitions rather than straining with heavy weights, he says. Ask a trainer to set up a program for you.

**Jog on gentle ground.** Plan your running route along soft surfaces such as dirt, grass or cinder track whenever possible, Dr. Kanter suggests. The impact of running on pavement can aggravate vein swelling.

**Keep moving on the job.** Don't sit for two or three hours straight while you work, says Dr. Perry. Be sure to get up and move around often to keep blood circulating. The Framingham study found that women who spent eight or more hours a day in sedentary activities, sitting or standing, had a much higher incidence of varicose veins.

## Home Treatment for the Ones You Have

If you already have a few varicose veins developing, here's how to keep them under control.

**Sleep on a slope.** Put six- by six-inch blocks under the foot of your bed and leave them there, says Dr. Perry. This keeps blood from pooling in your legs at night. You can quickly adapt to the tilt.

**Wear support hose.** For a few small veins, choose high-quality support hose from a good clothing store and wear them regularly, says Dr. Perry. Support hose are available in knee-high, stocking and panty-hose styles. The slight compression will help keep the veins down, he says. For more or larger veins, you may need to use gradient compression stockings, available over the counter in most drugstores.

**Try gradient stockings.** If the veins you have are fairly large, even good-quality support hose aren't enough, says Dr. Perry. Ask your doctor to prescribe custom-fitted gradient compression stockings instead. "They're hot and heavy, but they help," he says. Most women opt to wear them under pants for work and save the more sheer support hose for special occasions.

# The Big Cover-Up

There are two basic medical treatments available for varicose veins: sclerotherapy (injection) and surgical removal (stripping).

The latest advance in both sclerotherapy and vein surgery is the use of sound wave technology, called duplex ultrasound imaging. The ultrasound equipment is used to locate deeper problem veins and to guide injections precisely, says Dr. Kanter. And ultrasound is both painless and safe.

Sclerotherapy involves injecting a solution into a vein, causing the vein's walls to be absorbed by the body. No anesthesia is needed, and "you can be up and about your business right afterward," says David Green, M.D., a dermatologist at the Varicose Vein Center in Bethesda, Maryland. A few weeks to months later, the vein shrivels to an invisible thread of scar tissue under the skin.

If you have had large varicose veins treated with sclerotherapy, you will need to wear gradient compression stockings for up to six weeks afterward, Dr. Green says.

The cost usually ranges from around $100 to several hundred dollars, depending on the number of injections needed. Multiple treatments may be required if you have many affected veins.

Who's a candidate? Virtually anyone, as long as you are not pregnant and have no history of blood clotting disorders, Dr. Green says. But although the procedure is simple and effective, there are potential side effects. If the solution escapes the vein, it can cause an ulcer on the skin. And in up to 20 percent of patients, a brown line appears on the skin, following the course of the vein. In greater than 90 percent of these patients, the discoloration fades completely over months or a year or two, Dr. Green says.

Lasers can remove the discoloration when wielded by a physician skilled in using the copper vapor laser. One Australian study showed that 11 of 16 patients treated with copper vapor laser therapy for discoloration caused by sclerotherapy had significant improvement after three months.

Surgical stripping is sometimes recommended for severe varicose veins. Although some patients can undergo the surgery with local anesthesia, most surgeons prefer a light general anesthesia, Dr. Perry says. Many patients have the surgery as outpatients, going home late the same day. Compression stockings are worn for several weeks to months afterward.

Even though the affected veins are completely removed, there is no risk to your circulation, because other vessels can easily compensate for the loss of the superficial veins, Dr. Perry says.

While some scarring usually results from surgery, often long lengths of vein can be removed through several tiny incisions.

What are the advantages of surgery? Many vein specialists say that even large varicose veins can be effectively treated with sclerotherapy. But some vascular surgeons point out that there is a high rate of recurrence with the injection treatment, and multiple visits are often required if you have many affected veins. However, when ultrasound imaging is used to help guide the surgery, preliminary results show a higher success rate in fewer visits.

# VISION CHANGES

## *Set Your Sights High*

**Y**ou've booked the corner table at Chez Chic, and it's time to wow the clients from out of town. The sommelier hands you the wine list. You sigh nonchalantly, make a joke about bad California Chablis and open the list with a practiced touch of disdain.

Uh-oh. You can't read it. Your eyes won't focus on the fine print. So much for being nonchalant. You straighten your arms, hold the list a yard from your face and start to squint.

Just like that, you've gone from deal maker to dear old grandma, sitting there reading a large-print version of *The Old Farmer's Almanac*. What's next—knitting needles, a rocking chair?

It's a fact of life that sooner or later, your vision is going to fade a bit. Nine in ten women between ages 40 and 64 wear glasses or contact lenses to make reading and other close work a little easier.

But don't despair. You may be able to slow the process with regular eye exams, a healthful diet and maybe even some do-it-yourself eye exercises. More importantly, you can take steps now to deal with serious vision problems such as glaucoma, cataracts and macular degeneration that could lead to greatly reduced sight or even blindness.

## Up Close and Blurry

Remember all the ladybugs in Mom's old flower garden? You'd pick them up gently and let them crawl on your fingers, holding them right up to your nose and counting the little black dots on their backs.

Try that now. Odds are you couldn't tell a ladybug from a breath mint until it was seven or eight inches from your face. That's because the lenses in your eyes begin to stiffen with age. And the less they bend, the harder it is to focus on something close.

The condition is a form of farsightedness called presbyopia, and it's as inevitable as rain at a picnic. "There's really no way around it," says Richard Bensinger, M.D., a Seattle-area ophthalmologist and spokesman for the American Academy of Ophthalmology. "It's easy to correct, but it means you're probably going to have to wear glasses or contact lenses."

If you do end up needing corrective lenses, the choice between glasses and contact lenses is usually up to you. "In most cases, it's just a matter of preference," Dr. Bensinger says. "Some people like glasses, which they can take off when they don't want them. And some like contact lenses, which allow them to see well without showing people that they need glasses."

Even if you eventually need bifocals, which help correct your vision both near and far, you don't have to advertise it to the world. Doctors have developed blended lenses that eliminate the telltale line across the center of each lens. You could also try bifocal contact lenses, which allow you to change focus as your eyes move up and down. Dr. Bensinger says they can be much more expensive than standard contacts, however, and warns that not everyone can adjust to them.

Your eye doctor might also prescribe so-called monovision contact lenses. You put a distance vision contact in your dominant eye (usually the right) and the reading contact in your other eye. "It's not as hard to adjust to as it sounds," Dr. Bensinger says. "You don't have to consciously adjust to it every time you change your focus." Monovision lenses are made like regular contacts and are less expensive than bifocal contacts, he says.

In addition to presbyopia, spots and floaters may appear more often as you

---

## Common Eye Myths

**Reading in dim light can damage your eyes.** Myth. Low light can cause eye fatigue but will not harm your eyes.

**Watching television hurts your eyes.** Myth. There's no evidence that sitting too close to the television or watching for long periods causes any problems.

**Too much reading wears out your eyes.** Myth. Again, reading can make your eyes tired, but there's no evidence that it will hurt them in the long run.

**Eating lots of carrots improves your vision.** Semi-myth. You need vitamin A to see, but just a small amount—less than a carrot's worth a day. A healthful diet, with or without carrots, gives you all the vitamin A you need.

get older. These are little specks or dots that pop up occasionally in your field of vision, then disappear after an hour or a day or more. Dr. Bensinger says they're caused when parts of the clear vitreous fluid that fills your eye get a little stringy or lumpy.

"Usually, it's nothing serious," Dr. Bensinger says. "The spots just drift down out of your vision, and that's it. But if you suddenly see lots of spots or flashes of lights in your eyes, that could be a sign that something more serious is wrong, and you should see a doctor immediately."

And if you live in especially dusty or windy areas, you may be at risk of developing pterygiums, which are fleshy, benign growths around the eyes. These can start growing in your mid-twenties, usually on the sides of your eyes closest to your nose. Dr. Bensinger says they're just a cosmetic problem unless they grow large enough to block your sight. Pterygiums are easily removed with minor surgery.

## Taking the Long View

Barring accidental injury, your eyes will probably serve you well right up to your mid-sixties. You may need a new set of reading glasses every few years, but you probably won't notice any serious deterioration of vision.

Still, experts warn that you should never take your eyes for granted. Most serious eye diseases are painless and show no symptoms for years. If you don't get your eyes examined on a regular basis, you may not know how bad things have gotten until it's too late to help. Here are some diseases to watch out for.

*Glaucoma.* This progressive disease causes 12 percent of all blindness in America. It is marked by increased fluid pressure in the eye, which, over the years, can cause irreversible damage to the nerves that send vision impulses to your brain.

Doctors don't know what causes most kinds of glaucoma, and they don't know how to cure it. Vision lost to glaucoma cannot be restored, but when detected early enough, glaucoma can be controlled. Eyedrops or oral tablets can sometimes help lower the pressure in the eye. If that fails, laser surgery may help unclog the eye's natural drains, allowing fluid to escape and lowering pressure. And if that doesn't work, eye surgeons can create an artificial drain to carry away the fluid.

An estimated three million Americans have glaucoma, and half of them don't even know it. Another five to ten million people have the eye pressure buildup that precedes the disease, and far fewer than half of them know it. The best advice for dealing with glaucoma? Find out if you have it—now. "The earlier this disease is picked up, the better able we'll be to control it," says Carl Kupfer, M.D., director of the National Eye Institute in Bethesda, Maryland. That means regular eye exams, especially if you're at high risk for glaucoma.

*Cataracts.* Although they usually don't become a problem until you near retirement age, cataracts often start forming much earlier in life, especially if you have ever had an eye injury or have undergone such procedures as radiation

# Are You at Risk for Glaucoma?

Yes. Everyone is at risk, but some more so than others. To find out where you stand, answer the following questions from Prevent Blindness America.

1. Do any immediate family members have glaucoma?
2. Are you over age 40?
3. Are you African-American?
4. Do you take steroid medication?
5. Have you had an eye injury or eye surgery?
6. Do you have diabetes?

If you answered yes to any of the questions, schedule an eye exam to discuss glaucoma with your doctor. If you answered yes to two or more, you are at higher risk and probably need to see an eye specialist on a yearly basis.

---

treatments, chemotherapy or an organ transplant.

Over the years, the once-clear lens in each eye may turn yellow because of protein buildup. In time, the lens may become milky white and translucent, clouding vision to the point where you need an artificial lens implant. This plastic replacement lens does not flex to focus light, as the original lens did. But with corrective glasses, your vision can be restored quite well. "While we can't yet cure cataracts, we can certainly provide patients with good sight," Dr. Bensinger says.

Cataracts, like glaucoma, may have a hereditary link. So if anyone in your family has had cataracts, you may be at higher risk and should have your eyes examined more often than the standard every three years.

*Macular degeneration.* This insidious eye disease robs you of your fine visual skills. "In more advanced cases, you would be able to tell that someone was standing in front of you, but you couldn't tell who," Dr. Bensinger says. "You could see there was a bus coming down the street, but you couldn't tell which one, because you couldn't read the sign."

The cause remains unknown, but the condition somehow causes deterioration of the macula, the central part of the retina that's responsible for sharp focus. Unfortunately, there's little hope right now for restoring sight lost to macular degeneration, though laser surgery may help stabilize sight for a time. There is some hopeful news, though: Because macular degeneration strikes people who are over age 60 almost exclusively, you can start now—perhaps with

# Eye-robics: Exercises for Your Eyes

You work out every week to flatten your stomach, tighten your thighs and firm up your arms. So why not take a few minutes to work out your eyes?

Not all experts think that exercises aid your eyes. But a growing number of vision therapists believe a few daily exercises can help keep your eyes younger.

"The logic behind vision therapy," says Steven Ritter, O.D., of the State University of New York College of Optometry in New York City, "is that if you can harm your visual system with close-up tasks, you should be able to rehabilitate it."

Vision therapists can prescribe as many as 280 different exercises. No single set can cure everybody's vision problems. But you can't go wrong with any of these.

**Do the fine-print sprint.** If you work at a computer terminal for hours at a time, try this: Tack a page of newsprint to a wall about eight feet from where you ordinarily sit. Interrupt your work every ten minutes or so and look up at the newspaper. Bring the print into focus. Then look back at the computer screen. Do this repeatedly for 30 seconds, about six times an hour. It could help eliminate the blurriness many people experience at the end of the workday.

**Hit the wall.** If you play handball, racquetball, squash or tennis, this two-person exercise may come in handy. Stand three to five feet from a blank wall. Ask your partner to stand behind you and toss a tennis ball against the wall. When the ball caroms off the wall, try to catch it. This exercise can help improve your hand/eye coordination.

**Read your thumb.** Hold your thumb at arm's length. Move it in circles, X's and crosses, closer and farther away. Follow it with your eyes. As you do so, keep as much of the room as possible in your field of vi-

the help of an improved diet—to ward it off before it starts.

*Diabetic retinopathy.* It primarily strikes people with diabetes and is the leading cause of blindness in people ages 20 to 50. Loss of vision begins to occur when blood vessels in the back of the eye leak, blurring vision and sometimes denying nutrients to the eye.

"If you have diabetes," Dr. Bensinger says, "I cannot urge you strongly

sion. Continue the exercise with one eye closed. Repeat with the other eye. This can improve your peripheral vision.

**Track the flashlight.** This amusing exercise can improve your ability to track an object visually. It requires a partner and two flashlights. Stand in a darkened room facing a wall. Have your partner shine a flashlight on the wall and wave the disk of light in sweeping motions. Try to eclipse the circle of light with light from your flashlight while balancing a book on your head. This forces you to track the light with your eyes instead of moving your head.

**Call the ball.** Write letters or numbers on a softball or styrofoam ball, then screw a hook into the top of it and hang it from the ceiling with string. The smaller the characters, the more difficult the exercise. Give the ball a push in any direction. Try to call out the numbers or letters you see. This exercise helps you keep a moving target in focus.

**Bead a string.** This exercise trains both eyes to converge on a target. It also trains your brain to not switch off one eye's vision. String three colored beads on a string six feet long. Fasten one end of the string to a wall at eye height, and hold the other end of the string to your nose. Slide one bead close to the wall, place the second bead four feet from your nose, and place the third bead 16 inches from your nose.

Look at the farthest bead. You will see two strings forming a V converging at the bead. Shift both eyes to the middle bead. Notice the X where the two strings seem to converge upon it. Shift both eyes to the nearest bead, and observe a similar X. Shift quickly from one bead to another, always observing the V or the X. If both eyes are working as a team, you should always see two strings crossing when you're focused on a bead. If your eyes aren't working together, you'll see different patterns or just one string.

enough to have your eyes checked regularly. It can literally save your sight."

Laser treatments can help slow the damage from leaking vessels. But again, help is available only if you get your eyes examined regularly. "Early detection of diabetic retinopathy is even more of a success story than testing for glaucoma," Dr. Kupfer says. If caught early, there's a 95 percent chance you can keep your sight for at least five years, Dr. Kupfer says.

# Test Your Vision at Home

More than ten million Americans over age 25 suffer some loss of sight. Many don't even know it. These simple tests could help you discover whether your vision needs some attention.

Remember: The tests are not a substitute for a professional eye examination. They can only serve as a warning to see an eye doctor.

These tests were prepared by Prevent Blindness America. For more information, write or call 500 East Remington Road, Schaumburg, IL 60173; 1-800-331-2020.

Vision Test 1: Distance vision (opposite page). *If possible, have someone help you with this test. Don't take it if you're tired. And if you have glasses or contacts, be sure you're wearing them. (1) Position the chart ten feet away from you, against a bare wall or door. Make sure the room is well lit and avoid glare from windows. (2) Lightly cover your left eye with a piece of paper. Keeping both eyes open, tell your assistant (or write down) where the opening is in each C on the chart. Start with the largest C and work down the page. Repeat with your right eye covered. (3) If you don't get all the C's correct on the next-to-bottom line, repeat the test another day.*

Nearly half of all blindness can be prevented. Everyone should have periodic eye examinations.

Vision Test 2: Near vision. *Wear your contacts or glasses only if you use them to read. (1) Sit in a well-lit room away from window glare. (2) Keeping both eyes open, hold the near-vision test about 14 inches from your eyes. (3) Read the test sentence or write it down as it looks to you. (4) Write down where the openings are for each C. If you didn't get them all right, take the test another day.*

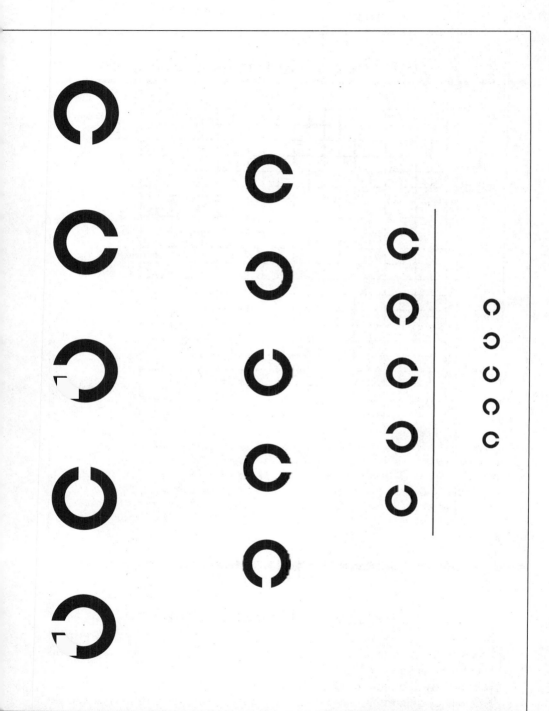

## Test Your Vision at Home—Continued

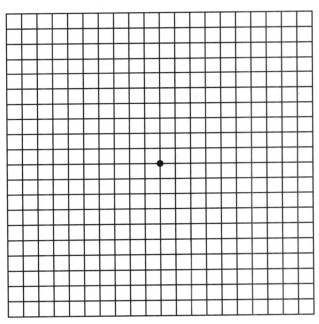

Vision Test 3: Macular degeneration. *For this test, wear your glasses or contact lenses only if they're for reading. (1) Have someone hold the grid against a bare wall or door in a well-lit room without glare from windows. Make sure the center dot on the grid is at eye level. (2) Stand 14 inches from the grid. Look at the dot in the center of the grid and cover your left eye with a piece of paper. You should see all four corners of the grid. If the grid looks distorted or you see any blank spots or wavy lines, make a mental note of it. Repeat with your right eye covered.*

## Focusing on Prevention

You can't change your genes, so there's not much you can do about the biggest vision risk factor of all—heredity. Still, here's some advice to give you the best chance of staying 20/20 into the twenty-first century.

**Get your eyes checked.** Doctors just can't say this enough.

"Regular eye examinations are by far the most important thing you can do to help preserve your vision," Dr. Bensinger says.

If you are between ages 30 and 50 and have no previous eye problems, the American Academy of Ophthalmology suggests seeing an ophthalmologist every three years. If you have a family history of glaucoma or diabetes or are already wearing glasses or contact lenses, your doctor may suggest more frequent visits.

The academy suggests an immediate visit to the doctor for any of the following:

- Sudden vision changes in one or both eyes
- Unexplainable redness
- Seeing a number of spots or floaters or showers of sparks in the corners of your eyes
- Eye pain that won't go away
- Accidental contact with chemicals, especially lye

**Hide behind some shades.** Sunglasses that block both UVA and UVB rays and visible blue light may help decrease the risk of cataracts, Dr. Bensinger says. Wraparound glasses that cover the sides of your eyes are a good idea, since they shield your eyes completely. And try to wear a hat with a visor to block direct sunlight from your eyes. "Exposure to sunlight drops the age at which you may develop cataracts," Dr. Bensinger says. "So if you're going to be outside, it makes sense to cut that sunlight as much as possible."

**Stop smoking.** Cancer. Wrinkles. Stinky clothes. Yellow teeth. Emphysema. If you really need another reason to quit, here it is: Cigarette smoking might cause cataracts. A Harvard Medical School study of 120,000 nurses showed that women who smoke 35 or more cigarettes a day have a 63 percent greater risk of developing cataracts.

The reason isn't known, but researchers speculate that smoking may reduce antioxidant levels in your blood, promoting cataract growth.

**Try some see-food.** The links between diet and vision are still weak. But there's growing evidence that a substance called glutathione may help control the spread of macular degeneration. It's found in fresh green, red and yellow vegetables. Canned or frozen vegetables lose all their glutathione in processing.

Zinc may help, too. Though there's no hard evidence yet, Dr. Bensinger says taking multivitamin supplements containing zinc "is probably not a bad idea, as long as you're not spending too much money on fancy brands."

Antioxidants—vitamins A, C and E plus beta-carotene—showed promise as cataract fighters in the Harvard Nurses' Health Study. A report in the *American Journal of Clinical Nutrition* claimed that people who eat 3½ servings of fruits and vegetables every day have a lower risk of cataracts, too.

"Eating a healthy diet may delay the usual aging of the lens and so delay cataracts," says Paul F. Jacques, Sc.D., an epidemiologist with the U.S. Department of Agriculture Human Nutrition Research Center on Aging at Tufts University in Boston.

# WORRY

## *Don't Agonize—Energize*

You watch your little boy board the school bus every morning. Are the brakes okay? Will he be warm enough? Is he eating his lunch?

Off to work. Did that proposal make it to Dallas on time? The economy's so bad; are you going to be laid off? What will you do without a job?

Back home in time for the evening news. The ozone layer is disappearing. War, hunger and violence are everywhere.

Life provides plenty to worry about. And sometimes it can become too much to handle. Maybe you're suffering from constant tension headaches or feeling tired all the time. Maybe worrying leaves your stomach in knots. Just a few years ago, you felt flush with youthful hope and optimism, ready to solve the planet's problems. But now you may be starting to feel powerless, worn out, unable to deal with even the smallest dilemmas.

"Worries are like a straitjacket," says Mary McClure Goulding, co-author of *Not to Worry! How to Free Yourself from Unnecessary Anxiety and Channel Your Worries into Positive Action.* "You feel like you can't do anything, and so you don't. It's a totally unproductive way to spend the best years of your life. And it's something you need to change—and can change—starting immediately."

## The Fearful Facts

We all worry. The average person (men worry, too) spends about 5 percent of each waking day—about 48 minutes—worrying about one thing or another. Surveys show that the most common sources of worry for Americans are family and relationships, jobs and school, health and finances.

For as many as 6 percent of women, worrying becomes chronic. It can even evolve into a clinical condition called generalized anxiety disorder. People with this disorder worry about multiple problems at the same time, including things they have little or no control over, such as the weather or nuclear war. And they worry excessively. Chronic worriers report spending an average of 50 percent of each day worrying, and some report as much as 100 percent, says psychologist Jennifer L. Abel, Ph.D., associate director of the Stress and Anxiety Disorders Clinic at Pennsylvania State University in University Park. Chronic worry typically begins in a woman's twenties or thirties.

There's no evidence that worrying directly causes disease, says Timothy Brown, Psy.D., associate director of the Phobia and Anxiety Disorders Clinic at the State University of New York at Albany. Worry can lead to poor sleep in many cases, with resulting fatigue, restlessness and irritability. But it's the psychological toll that's usually most devastating. "Worriers can't concentrate, get headaches and may not be able to effectively confront and resolve their problems," he says.

Worriers almost always come from fretting families, Goulding says. You may have learned to worry by watching your mother, father, grandfather or an aunt. Worriers may have low self-esteem, Goulding says, and have often been taught to repress feelings—especially happy ones.

All of which leads to a central problem: a feeling of helplessness. "You don't feel in control of your life," says Susan Jeffers, Ph.D., a psychologist and author of *Feel the Fear and Do It Anyway*. "You think everything is going to go wrong. That makes it hard to overcome even simple problems without great effort and anxiety."

A study of 24 American college students bears this out. When asked what would happen if they didn't get good grades, a group of non-worriers typically talked about ending up with bad jobs and earning less money. The chronic worriers talked about those same concerns. But then they took their worries much further. Some worried about becoming drug addicts. Others worried they would be in constant physical pain. And still others said they would die—or even end up in hell.

"At that point, you have to ask yourself whether worrying is worth the effort," Dr. Jeffers says. "You have to decide whether you're going to spend the rest of your life worrying about things or whether you're going to do something about it. It's a difficult decision, but hopefully, you'll choose the latter."

# Winning over Worry

It takes years to build a world of worries. You may need a while to tear it all down. But time is on your side. A study of both young and elderly worriers showed that we tend to worry less as we grow older. The oldest of the 163 people studied by professors at the University of Massachusetts at Amherst were less anxious about social and financial problems and no more worried about health issues.

But why wait for things to get better? If you're ready to start banishing worry right now, here's some expert advice.

**Think it through.** Go ahead and fret a little. It's better than trying to suppress all the anxiety. "Give up trying to stop those unhappy thoughts," says

# Calm the Worrier Within

Call her Fretful Fanny. She's the unhappy little doomsayer in your head who won't stop talking about things that can and will go wrong.

It's time to quiet her for good.

"You have to silence that voice of self-harassment," says Mary Mc-Clure Goulding, co-author of *Not to Worry! How to Free Yourself from Unnecessary Anxiety and Channel Your Worries into Positive Action*. "If you listen to it, you'll always keep worrying."

Become aware of the voice. Sit in a quiet place and listen to your thoughts. When you start hearing negative thoughts, consciously replace them with positive ones. Affirmations—simple positive statements that you repeat frequently—might work. Try phrases such as "There is nothing to fear," "I'm in control of my life," "I'll handle it," "Everything is working out perfectly."

"Repetition is the key. At first, you don't even need to believe what you're telling yourself," says Susan Jeffers, Ph.D., a psychologist and author of *Feel the Fear and Do It Anyway*. "Just talking positively changes our energy and helps us move forward."

Goulding suggests being more direct with your inner critic. Stand up, put your hands on your hips and yell at Fanny: "Just shut up! I'm not listening to you anymore!" Curse, swear, do whatever feels good. "Drive that voice away," she says. "And then you can fill your mind with happier thoughts instead."

Daniel Wegner, Ph.D., professor of psychology at the University of Virginia in Charlottesville. "My research shows that the more you try to suppress unwanted thoughts, the more likely you are to become obsessed with them. That's particularly true when you're under a lot of pressure, stress or mental overload. So just when you're trying to avoid unhappy thoughts, you'll actually get sadder than if you'd confront those unhappy thoughts head-on."

Dr. Jeffers likes to point out that 99 percent of what we worry about never happens. "Feel the fear. That's part of being human," she says. "But go out and do things anyway, knowing that most of your fears are unfounded."

**Take your time.** It's one thing to think about your problems. It's another to let them dominate your thoughts. Dr. Wegner says research on chronic worriers shows that if they spend time at night actively worrying about their problems, the degree of worrying in their lives goes down overall. "There's something boring, after all, about thoughts you spend an hour a night thinking about," he says.

Michael Vasey, Ph.D., assistant professor of psychology at Ohio State University in Columbus, suggests setting aside 30 minutes a day, always at the same place and time, to worry. "Focus on your worry for the entire period, and try to think of solutions to the problem," he says. If you're worried that you'll be fired, imagine the scenario—the firing and the consequences—and don't let the image drift away.

You'll probably be even more anxious at first. But things will improve. "If you practice focusing on worries and thinking of solutions for 30 minutes each day for several weeks, your anxiety will start to taper off," Dr. Vasey says. "You'll get better at generating solutions or realize it's not worth worrying about."

**Write a new ending.** People who worry can be amazingly creative, Goulding says. They turn any harmless scenario into a disaster by imagining the worst. Try putting that creativity to good use by turning your fears into fantasies. If you worry about a school bus crash, try picturing your little boy grabbing the wheel and steering everyone to safety. Then imagine the parade the town will hold for him. Maybe he'll even get the key to the city.

You're disarming your worries this way, Goulding says. By putting a happy or silly ending on a worry, you're allowing yourself a chance to be positive, she says. And that's a major step toward beating worry.

**Tally your troubles.** List all your worries. Are you afraid that it's going to rain on the family reunion this weekend? You can't control that, so Goulding suggests that you file it under the heading "Beyond My Skills." Do you worry that other people find you unattractive, even when you really know you're not? That goes on the "Creative Fiction" list.

What's the sense of worrying about things in these categories? "There isn't any," Goulding says. "Why worry about the weather? Why worry about things that aren't true?" Once you expose these thoughts as worthless worries, she says, it's easier to dismiss them.

**Take action.** Some worries are more legitimate. Are you concerned about your health? Well, list all the things you could do to improve things. Maybe you could start walking every day. Or eat better. Then decide which ones you're going to do. The secret is doing, doing, doing. "When you're actively working on a solution, worry is less likely to be a problem," Dr. Jeffers says. "You'll begin to feel like you're the creator of your life, not a victim of it."

**Find a friend.** Tell someone special about your fears. "When you talk about your worries, it deflates those worries. They can't be suppressed. That cat's out of the bag. And thank goodness, it is just a cat and not some horrible monster," Dr. Wegner says.

Just be careful that your friend doesn't unintentionally make things worse. Out of kindness, she may tell you it's okay to worry or say "Gee, I understand why you're so worried." Goulding says that might help reinforce your need to worry. If you decide to share your thoughts, make sure the other person agrees to be honest with you and helps you find positive, constructive ways to deal with your worries.

# WRINKLES

## *Draw the Line on Early Lines*

Frowning with concentration, you're all business when you put on your makeup. You squint gently as you glide on a touch of eyeshadow. You raise your eyebrows as you stroke on mascara and a sweep of blush. Then you pucker for lipstick. Nice. You reward yourself with a smile in the mirror.

Then it hits you. The frown is still there, along with the squint and the smile lines.

Wrinkles—already? Character is great, and you've always admired women who age with grace, but these lines feel premature—like a message from the future delivered too soon. You're just not ready for wrinkles.

Suddenly, you feel old. And maybe less attractive. You worry that a big smile will show your big wrinkles. You keep your eyes wide open, to erase those crow's-feet.

## The Roots of the Ruts

Doctors say that the inevitable wrinkles from genetics and gravity really shouldn't arrive until you near your sixties. But they come a lot earlier—in the late twenties and thirties—for many of us. Here's why.

During the 1920s, French designer Coco Chanel came back from the tropics bronzed and glowing—and the centuries-old tradition of keeping skin in the shade was lost in the glare of the news. Fashion-conscious women everywhere began to bask in the sun. In search of elegant tans, they started a new tradition: of sunburns and tanning booths—and skin cancer and early wrinkles. Even in naturally dark skin, sun damage causes 80 to 90 percent of the visible signs of aging, including wrinkles, doctors say.

The number-two cause of wrinkles is smoking, which speeds your skin's aging by up to ten years. Smoking reduces blood flow to the skin, blunting its ability to repair damage. It also sets off enzymes that attack the tissues of your skin the way meat tenderizer weakens the fibers of meat. And because skin gets a "memory" when it's folded in the same place over and over again, the mechanics of smoking cause wrinkles, too. Constant puckering to draw on a cigarette forms lip creases, and squinting against the smoke carves crow's-feet.

Some lines will form simply because we express emotion—with a ready smile or worried frown. The way you sleep can leave a wrinkle memory in your skin, too, especially if you snooze facedown.

But what can you do if you already have years of wrinkle-promoting habits behind you? Can the damage be undone? Yes, it can. You can prevent most new wrinkles from forming and remove the worst of the old ones with help from your doctor.

# A New Wrinkle on Prevention

If you're determined to fight wrinkles, even if it means abandoning bronze for a paler, healthier beauty, here's where to begin.

**Put up a chemical parasol.** Sunscreen is your number-one weapon against further sun damage, says Albert M. Kligman, M.D., professor of dermatology at the University of Pennsylvania School of Medicine in Philadelphia. Use a full-spectrum sunscreen that blocks both kinds of ultraviolet radiation (UVA and UVB), and use it every day, year-round, Dr. Kligman says. After you cleanse your skin in the morning, leave it slightly damp and apply pea-size dabs of sunscreen on your cheeks and forehead, working it into the skin all over your face. Don't forget the backs of your hands, neck and décolletage.

You need to use a sunscreen of SPF 15 or higher. *SPF* stands for sun protection factor, and SPF 15, which most doctors recommend, means that you can stay out in the sun 15 times longer than you normally could before burning. Remember, too, that although daily use of SPF 15 sunscreen will protect you adequately while you dash in and out of buildings, for long hours in the outdoors you'll need to use higher-SPF products and reapply frequently.

Doctors disagree on how high to go with SPF numbers, however. Some say that numbers over 25 may give a false sense of security. While higher numbers do screen out the burning UVB rays, they may let in more UVA radiation. The UVA rays penetrate deeper into skin and cause most age-related changes such as wrinkles, says Melvin L. Elson, M.D., medical director of the Dermatology Center in Nashville.

Joseph Bark, M.D., a dermatologist in Lexington, Kentucky, and author of *Retin-A and Other Youth Miracles*, disagrees. He says research shows that skin will burn somewhat even with SPF 15 sunscreens, and he recommends using the highest SPF you can find, even for everyday use.

And read the sunscreen's contents. "The best of the broad-spectrum sunscreens contain titanium dioxide—fine particles that stay in your skin and resist washing or rubbing off," says Dr. Kligman. An example is Sundown.

**Don't rely on cosmetics.** Your favorite cosmetic counter may offer foundations and moisturizers that contain low-SPF sunscreens, but these are too weak for real protection, Dr. Kligman says.

**Protect your eye area.** While you exercise, you don't want sunscreen to sting your eyes when you sweat. Try this workout tip from Dr. Elson. "Take a wax-based sunscreen made for lips and apply it around and over your eyes. It won't run," he says. You should also protect your eyes with a good pair of shades, preferably the wraparound kind. Make sure they shield UV radiation.

**Dress for the sun.** Innovative clothing manufacturers have come out with basic collections of shirts, swimsuits and casual wear that are specially knit to prevent the sun's radiation from reaching your skin.

**Dump that nasty habit.** Yeah, yeah, you've been told before that smoking isn't cool anymore. Now you have one more reason to quit.

**Feed your face.** For general skin health, eat a balanced diet full of fruits, whole grains and vegetables. You may also want to try supplements that have been proven to reduce sun damage to skin, says Karen Burke, M.D., Ph.D., a dermatologist in private practice in New York City. She recommends daily supplements of 100 micrograms of selenium (best taken as l-selenomethionine) plus 400 IU of vitamin E. Use the d-alpha tocopheryl acetate, d-alpha tocopheryl acid succinate or d-alpha tocopherol form of vitamin E—not the "dl tocopherols" form, which is far less active. You should have no side effects from these safe doses, Dr. Burke says. Although research has not been designed specifically to link these nutrients with wrinkle repair, they may help, she adds.

**Take your measure in the mirror.** Set a small hand mirror beside your telephone for a few days and watch yourself in conversation. You may have a few face-wrinkling habits you're not aware of, such as frowning or squinting while you mull something over. The mirror will help you learn to relax the facial muscles you're working overtime and to reduce expression lines.

**No aerobics for your face.** Although facial exercises have been touted in many beauty books, most of them actually increase wrinkling, says Dr. Burke. When you grimace or contort your face through exercises, you wind up working the same muscles that caused wrinkles in the first place, she says.

**Sleep on your back.** "It's the best position for a younger-looking, unlined face," says Gary Monheit, M.D., assistant professor of dermatology at the University of Alabama School of Medicine/University of Alabama in Birmingham. If you've been burrowing into your pillow face-first for years, lying on your back every night with a pillow under your knees may help you to change the habit.

# The ABCs of Wrinkle Repair

Now that you're committed to preventing new wrinkles, are you stuck with those you've already acquired? Not at all. There are many new developments in dermatology and plastic surgery that can remove your wrinkles. They range from prescription peeling lotions and creams to surface repairs and surgery.

But remember this: "You can't go out and get an unlimited amount of plastic surgery. Do as little as possible to get the maximum amount of improvement possible," says plastic surgeon Geoffrey Tobias, M.D., of Mount Sinai School of Medicine of the City University of New York. "You're never going to be 21 years old again or take 20 years off your face. But if two or three wrinkles bother you, take care of them. You'll look and feel better."

Consider this.

**Smooth them with Retin-A.** Tretinoin (Retin-A), derived from vitamin A, has earned its reputation as an excellent wrinkle smoother, particularly for the fine lines caused by years of indulging in the sun. But be warned: Retin-A cream is available only by prescription. The legions of similar-sounding ingredients in many cosmetics and lotions are only that: sound-alikes. See your dermatologist. (For tips on using Retin-A, see page 607.)

**Try AHA lotions.** Your dermatologist has a gentle new approach to wrinkle reduction, says Dr. Elson. Highly concentrated lotions made from alpha hydroxy acids (AHAs), derived from wine, milk, apples, lemons or sugarcane, will gradually peel off the top layers of dead skin. "Over time, they will make crow's-feet and fine wrinkles less visible," says Dr. Elson. Some of the most popular lotions contain glycolic acid from sugarcane, which has small molecules that are easy for skin to absorb. Low-concentration AHAs are also available at your drugstore or cosmetics counter in some cleansers and moisturizers such as Avon's Anew Alpha Hydrox Skin Treatment System and Eucerin Plus Alphahydroxy Moisturing Lotion, but these are less effective than the higher-strength products your dermatologist can provide.

So far, AHAs offer the only real competition for Retin-A's wrinkle-fighting ability. AHA lotions give less dramatic results than Retin-A, but they are also less likely to irritate your skin.

**Peel away the lines.** Though the name may sound drastic, chemical peeling can be a fairly gentle procedure, says Sorrel S. Resnik, M.D., clinical professor of dermatology and cutaneous surgery at the University of Miami School of Medicine. The dermatologist wipes your face with acetone, a strong cleansing solvent, and then applies acid to your skin with a swab. The skin turns white and stings briefly as the acetone penetrates; then several layers of skin (and fine wrinkles) peel off a day or two later. Many doctors offer a series of three to six light acid peels at intervals of several weeks, for results that are only a little less effective than a medium or deep peel. With the series, you'll have less discomfort and a quicker healing time, usually only a few days. Trichloroacetic acid has a good record for safety and effectiveness, and glycolic acid, which is less penetrating, is also popular.

Very deep peels can be dangerous, says Dr. Resnik, and are usually offered only to people with extremely weathered, leathery skin. The chemical most often used for deep peels is phenol, which may cause cardiac or kidney problems. Phenol must be applied in the operating room because it requires close heart monitoring.

# Resetting the Clock with Retin-A

Retin-A is not just for acne.

"I don't know how to treat a patient for wrinkles without a prescription for Retin-A," says Melvin L. Elson, M.D., medical director of the Dermatology Center in Nashville. "Retin-A cream works by changing the skin to make it normal and smoother." It increases blood flow in the skin to give it a youthful, pink tone again and also attracts collagen-making cells closer to the surface of the skin, which tend to fill in wrinkles.

The effects of tretinoin (Retin-A) on wrinkles were discovered by Albert M. Kligman, M.D., professor of dermatology at the University of Pennsylvania School of Medicine in Philadelphia. Many of his patients who were using Retin-A for severe acne pointed out their noticeably smoother, firmer skin. Since then, Retin-A's anti-aging effects have been proven in numerous studies, and Dr. Kligman recommends using it early in life to get a head start on wrinkle prevention.

"If you have a lot of wrinkles and you're young, even in your twenties, don't wait until you are 40 or 50 and have deep wrinkles and a lot of blotches," he says. "If you're a light-skinned person who had a normal childhood in America, you should start Retin-A early and get into a program that will last you the rest of your life."

Retin-A for wrinkles is sold in gel and cream forms in various strengths, and you and your dermatologist may need to experiment to find out which is right for you. At first, your skin may become irritated and flaky, but within a month or two, it should adapt. If you have very sensitive skin, try applying it once every third day and then every second day once your skin adjusts, or start with the lower strength (.025 percent cream) and increase gradually to higher concentrations, Dr. Kligman suggests. A less irritating form of Retin-A, called Renova, is awaiting approval of the Food and Drug Administration.

If you're committed to wrinkle fighting with Retin-A, you need to know that it's a lifelong relationship. If you stop using the drug, your fine wrinkles will return. And because Retin-A increases your skin's sensitivity to the sun, a daily regimen of sunscreen with a high SPF (sun protection factor) is vital.

**Ask about fillers.** Plumping up the skin beneath a wrinkle is an alternative to peeling off wrinkles from the surface, says Dr. Monheit. Dermatologists use several substances as wrinkle fillers, but the best known is cattle-derived collagen. Collagen is a fibrous tissue that forms a supporting network just under the surface of the skin. The doctor injects the collagen into your wrinkle, and a lump appears above the skin surface. When the lump fades (in as little as six hours), the wrinkle will have been smoothed away.

The problems with collagen? It's temporary—results last from 4 to 15 months, Dr. Monheit says. And some people may be allergic to this form of collagen, so the doctor must first perform an allergy test.

If you do prove allergic to cattle collagen, ask about a newer method called autogenous tissue implant, says Dr. Elson. A patch of skin harvested from another part of your body is sent out to a company that processes your own collagen from the skin. The processor then returns to your doctor a syringe filled with the collagen for an injection.

A wrinkle filler called Fibrel may last up to five years, says Dr. Monheit. Fibrel is a gelatin-based material that is mixed with your own blood serum and injected beneath a wrinkle. Your body responds by making its own collagen, which, in turn, fills out the wrinkle. Drawbacks? Fibrel injections hurt more than collagen shots, and the procedure is more time-consuming, Dr. Monheit says.

"The best filler would be something natural from your own body," says Michael Sachs, M.D., a plastic surgeon in private practice in New York City. A technique for wrinkle filling that's still in the experimental stage is called fat transfer, or microlipoinjection. The doctor extracts a tiny amount of fat from another part of your body, such as your belly or buttock, and injects it beneath the wrinkle. There's no danger of an allergic reaction, since this is you being injected into you. However, results are short-lived. Researchers aren't sure why, but the fat cells just don't seem to last long in their new location.

Surgical thread can plump up a wrinkle, too, says Dr. Sachs. "The surgeon places a protein-based thread directly under the wrinkle line, where it stimulates local cells to produce their own collagen. In about six months or so, the thread dissolves, and the remaining collagen will fill out the wrinkle for two to five years." Dr. Sachs developed this procedure. Check with your doctor about its availability.

**Scrape them away.** A procedure called dermabrasion, which is often used to remove acne scars, can also be very effective on wrinkles around the mouth but not on areas where the skin is very thin, such as around the eyes, Dr. Sachs says. A special instrument called a dermabrader literally sands away the top layer of skin, leaving a scab that will heal within about ten days, he says. A drawback is that dermabrasion often removes pigment from the skin, adds Dr. Resnik. So if you choose this method of wrinkle removal, you'll need to always wear makeup on the treated areas.

## When You're Thinking of Surgery

There's a wide range of surgical options for wrinkle removal, says Dr. Tobias. Some surgeries will lift and tighten facial skin, smoothing wrinkles in the process. Other procedures remove wrinkly bags and pouches or fill out wrinkle folds in the skin. Here are two options.

**Smooth the eye area.** Over the years, eyelids may crease into heavy folds that make you look tired all the time. With a traditional blepharoplasty, or eye-lift operation, a surgeon trims and removes this excess skin for a firmer, younger-looking eye area. Or you may have wrinkly bags above or beneath the eyes that are composed primarily of fat. A new procedure invented by Dr. Sachs, called fat-melting blepharoplasty, can help. A surgeon inserts a heated probe through a tiny incision at the corner of the eye and vaporizes the water content of the fat, which literally melts away the pouches. Recovery times can vary from a few days to a week or more, depending on the procedure used, Dr. Sachs says.

**Get rid of gaunt.** One of the natural processes of aging is the gradual loss of bone along the jaw and of soft tissue beneath the cheeks. Solid silicone implants can fill out the aging hollows and wrinkle folds that result, says Dr. Tobias. Solid silicone implants have not been associated with the difficulties that have been seen with liquid silicone implants, he adds. Working from incisions within the mouth, a surgeon can insert these forms under cheeks and along the jowl line.

# Part III
## *Boost Your Youthfulness*

# ADVENTURE

## *Reach for Your Outer Limits*

For her summer vacation, Anne Bancroft went to Antarctica, where a balmy day is about –23°F. Then she and three other women spent 67 days pulling 200-pound sleds for 660 miles into headwinds up to 50 miles per hour to reach the South Pole.

Why?

"A trip like this rejuvenates you," says Bancroft, a 38-year-old motivational speaker and polar explorer from St. Paul, Minnesota, who was the first woman to trek across the ice to both poles. "You're in the best shape of your life and there's something wonderful about that. You get the feeling when you get back home and get back into the craziness of life that you're going to live a lot longer because you did have an adventure like that. It makes you feel strong and good."

No, you don't have to cross miles of barren ice like Bancroft did to feel younger, but doctors do say that if you're truly looking for a Fountain of Youth, try tossing more adventure into your life.

"Absolutely, adventure and risk taking can make you feel and think like a person who is years younger. It's believed that when you do thrill-seeking adventures, there's a release of certain chemicals in the brain that are truly uplifting to mood," says Bernard Vittone, M.D., a psychiatrist and director of the National Center for the Treatment of Phobias, Anxiety and Depression in Washington, D.C.

But other experts suspect that adventure does more than just jump-start your emotions.

"Any time you are re-energized in a vibrant way as through an adventure, there are very positive physiological effects, including increased blood and oxygen flow to the tissues in your body. That, along with the emotional effects of rediscovering your life's energy, can make some people literally look younger," says Mark Weaver, Ph.D., a psychologist with the Experiential Learning Institute in Oklahoma City.

# Learn, Grow and Feel Younger

Remember the mixture of anxiety and absolute exhilaration the first time you rode a bicycle, plunged into the deep end of the neighborhood pool or went to summer camp? It's that awe of overcoming your own natural fear of the unknown that makes adventure such a vital part of learning, growing and keeping yourself feeling young, Dr. Weaver says.

"The importance of adventure isn't so much that you climbed a mountain, rafted on an unfamiliar river or even started your own small business. The key point is to achieve something new and to discover how you can reach beyond your comfort zone and stretch yourself as a human being," Dr. Weaver says. "If you don't stretch yourself, you'll spend a lifetime trapped within the conventions of how you're used to living your life."

So why do some women feel the urge to explore the Amazon rain forest while others spend their evenings clipping coupons? Some adventurousness is learned from your parents. "If you have parents who are always amplifying the danger of a situation, you'll learn to view situations as more threatening," Dr. Vittone says. "On the other hand, if you have parents who encourage adventure, you're going to develop a higher threshold of excitement."

But biology plays a role, too. "We all react differently to different types of stimulation," Dr. Vittone says. "There are certain anxiety centers in the brain that are tripped off more easily in some people than in others. So everyone has their own threshold of adventure or risk-taking behavior that they feel comfortable doing."

As we age, these anxiety centers in our brains become more sensitive, and we gradually lose our ability to distinguish between the negative sort of anxiety that is associated with work, stress and tension and the more positive types of anxiety that are a natural and exciting part of experiencing something new, Dr. Vittone says. As a result, we become more fearful and begin avoiding anxiety-producing situations, including relatively safe activities such as hiking.

"The problem is that people start viewing all those feelings of anxiety in the same negative way, instead of realizing that some anxiety can be positive," Dr. Vittone says. "It's that lumping of those positive and negative feelings together that makes people gravitate toward wanting to feel safe and comfortable all the time." It's why some women are content to sit back and let their kids (or their husbands) have all the fun.

# Consequences of Playing It Safe

Unfortunately, that overwhelming desire for safety and comfort causes many of us to develop what some experts call stagnant spirits.

"Trying to escape risk is like trying to escape living. You really can't grow as a person without some sense of adventure in your life," says Jasper S. Hunt, Jr., Ph.D., professor of experiential education and leadership studies, director of adventure education programs in the Department of Educational Leadership at

Mankato State University in Mankato, Minnesota, and a leader of wilderness-survival outings for Outward Bound, an adventure-travel club. "So either you live adventurously or you die emotionally. The choice is yours."

Fortunately, you don't have to climb Mount Everest, become a mud wrestler or take up hang gliding to get adventure into your life.

"Since we're all different, there's going to be a range of adventures that people are going to find thrilling," Dr. Vittone says. "For some people, just driving to a new town and exploring may do it. For others, it may take parachuting. Even a change in your routine can be an adventure. Finding a new way home from work or going to a different health spa could do it. Whatever you do, it's that feeling of a thrill that you're looking for."

Here are some ways to get more thrills into your day.

**Let your mind wander.** "Every adventure starts with curiosity," says Andrea Shrednick, Ph.D., a clinical psychologist in private practice in Los Angeles. "Allow your mind to wander free. Imagine if you had a week all to yourself. Where would you go? What would you do? What would it look like? What would it smell like? What types of foods would you eat? If you allow yourself to daydream like that, it will whet your appetite for the real thing."

**Know your limits.** Take an honest look at your skills and abilities and see if they realistically match up with the adventure you have in mind. "A person who doesn't take a careful inventory of their skills and capabilities is a fool," Dr. Hunt says. "That's being reckless, and recklessness is not virtuous."

**Be prepared.** "Every adventure, no matter how small, is a step-by-step process," Bancroft says. "We always know what we're facing before we get started on an expedition. You can't control Mother Nature, but before you start you can test your gear, get yourself in shape and do all the other things that make your chances of a successful trip far greater."

**Take small steps.** Keep your adventures simple at first, then gradually increase the difficulty as your competence and confidence grow. If you want to learn to climb, for example, join your local hiking club and build up your expertise before deciding to tackle Mount McKinley, Dr. Hunt says.

**Winning isn't the only thing.** Don't push yourself into a dangerous situation. You're only asking for trouble that way. "If you look at mountaineers, the ones who are still alive to tell about their adventures don't try to conquer the mountain at all costs. They do their homework and know when it's unsafe and time to back off. That's a good lesson for all of us to learn," Bancroft says.

**Share your dreams.** "If you're facing a scary challenge, tell someone about it," Bancroft advises. "I don't think any of us are very successful strictly by ourselves. We all need pats on the back and encouragement from others to fulfill our dreams."

**Have some laughs.** "For me, the best tool in my bag of tricks for getting through hard struggles is not taking myself too seriously," Bancroft says. "I don't think I could do any of this without a sense of humor. You tend to lose sight of the purpose of the adventure if you don't have fun."

# How Do You Define Risk?

Do you still enjoy rock concerts? If you held a sales job, would you want to be paid on commission or on a straight salary? Do you get bored easily, or is routine salve to your soul? Answer these and the other questions in this quiz to help determine what kind of risk taker you are.

There are no right or wrong answers. Circle only one number per question. Answer all questions. If no answer feels exactly right to you, pick the one that's closest. To determine your score, total all numbers circled and see the scoring key at the end of the quiz.

1. During the past ten years, how often have you changed residence?
    1. 10 times or more
    2. 5 to 9 times
    3. 2 to 4 times
    4. 0 to 1 time
2. Which adjective best describes your behavior before age 12?
    1. hyperactive
    2. mischievous
    3. basically well behaved
    4. very well behaved
3. In the average week, how many hours of television do you watch?
    1. 0 to 5 hours
    2. 6 to 10 hours
    3. 11 to 20 hours
    4. more than 20 hours
4. How often do you tape shut already-sealed envelopes before mailing them?
    1. almost never
    2. seldom
    3. often
    4. regularly
5. For a sales job, how would you prefer to be paid?
    1. straight commission
    2. mostly commission with a substantial draw
    3. a substantial draw with some commission
    4. straight salary

6. In highway driving, how often do you drive faster than 65 miles per hour?
    1. regularly
    2. often
    3. seldom
    4. almost never
7. If you were living on the East Coast a century ago, do you think you would have joined a wagon train headed west?
    1. definitely
    2. probably
    3. probably not
    4. definitely not
8. Suppose you had equal competence at any one of the following activities. Which would appeal to you most?
    1. skydiving
    2. mountain climbing
    3. producing a play
    4. building a house
9. Which opportunity sounds more appealing to you?
    1. starting your own business
    2. purchasing a successful business
10. Which statement describes you better?
    1. I get bored easily.
    2. When necessary, I can tolerate routine.
11. What kinds of risks would you say are the hardest for you to take?
    1. commitment risks (long-term involvement with a person, activity or career)
    2. emotional risks (in relationships or showing my feelings)
    3. financial risks (of losing money)
    4. physical risks (of life and limb)

Assume that you are equally capable of all of the activities listed below. For each set, pick the one that you would most enjoy. (If neither activity appeals to you, pick the one that's least unappealing.)

12. 1. driving a dune buggy
    2. hiking in the desert

*(continued)*

# How Do You Define Risk?—Continued

13. 1. skiing down a steep slope
    2. ski touring through woods
14. 1. scuba diving
    2. snorkeling

Circle the number of the word that best describes your reaction to the following activities.

15. Building a cabinet
    1. tedious
    2. satisfying
16. Climbing rocks
    1. exhilarating
    2. scary
17. Attending a rock concert
    1. arousing
    2. jarring
18. Teaching school
    1. boring
    2. challenging

19. With a report due at work in two weeks, what would you be most
likely to do?
  1. start working on it the day before it's due, then stay up most of
     the night completing it
  2. work hard on the report for a day or two before it's due
  3. start working on it during the second week
  4. budget time throughout the two weeks to produce the report
20. In general, whose company do you prefer?
  1. people you've recently met
  2. professional colleagues, co-workers or fellow members of a club
     or church

## Scoring

Add up all the numbers you circled.

**30 or below.** Suggests a high need for excitement and a low tolerance for boredom. You're more likely than other women to take physical risks and avoid long-term commitments.

**31 or above.** Suggests you find it hard to take physical and financial
risks, but easy to take long-term risks, such as deciding to raise a family
or committing yourself to a career.

# AEROBICS

## Take a Sip from the Fountain of Youth

What do you think of when you hear the word "aerobics"? Chances are it's aerobics class, the one you faithfully attend two or three days a week—whenever you have time.

Aerobics classes are one of the most popular activities at health clubs these days, particularly among women. So much so that "aerobics" has become kind of a buzzword for fitness.

And that's fitting. Aerobics classes rev up your heart, usually last from 20 minutes to an hour and work your major muscle groups, improving your cardio-vascular system and getting you fit.

But the term *aerobics* extends well beyond your gym classes. A whole range of exercises—biking, running, walking and swimming, for example—are aerobic. And they can do more than make you feel fit. They can make you feel younger, both today and in the years to come. In fact, when it comes to age erasers, aerobic exercise is right at the head of the list. Its benefits are long ranging.

Aerobic exercise helps combat aging by preventing heart disease, maintaining bone and muscle strength and keeping your mind sharp. It may also play a role in fending off diabetes and certain forms of cancer. And it can help take the edge off daily stress by boosting your mood and energy level. Premenstrual syndrome (PMS) and menopausal symptoms are often reduced with exercise.

"The cliché is that if ever there were a Fountain of Youth, this is it," says William Simpson, M.D., professor of family medicine in the Department of Family Medicine at the Medical University of South Carolina in Charleston. The person who regularly engages in aerobic exercise along with resistance training really has the optimal physical preparation for aging, he says.

# A Friend of the Heart

A major benefit of aerobic exercise is its effect on your heart and cardio-vascular system. Evidence shows that aerobic exercise helps decrease the risk of cardiovascular disease, the number-one killer of both men and women in the United States, says Alan Mikesky, Ph.D., an exercise physiologist and professor at Indiana University School of Physical Education in Indianapolis. And that's the main reason aerobic exercise should be a priority, he says.

The amount of protection exercise offers against heart disease in women isn't known, says Dr. Simpson. That's because studies over the last two decades have concentrated on men. "There really haven't been large studies with females yet," he says. But researchers suspect that women reap the same benefits as men.

Research shows that aerobic exercise can decrease the risk of a first heart attack in men. In a study of 16,936 Harvard alumni ages 35 to 74, men who were less active were at 64 percent higher risk for a first heart attack than more active men.

Compelling data also indicate that sedentary men have a 30 to 40 percent greater risk of death from coronary heart disease than men who burn over 1,000 calories a week exercising—the equivalent of walking ten miles (about 40 minutes a day, three to four times a week).

# Pump It Up So the Pressure Goes Down

Aerobic exercise can help lower your risk of heart disease by strengthening the heart and making it more efficient. When you exercise, your muscles require more fuel—oxygen, that is. So your heart pumps harder in order to push more blood—the vehicle that transports oxygen—to the outlying muscles. When the heart works harder like this on a regular basis, it grows stronger and more efficient, says Dr. Simpson. "You get a stronger pump working."

Exercise also helps improve the quality of circulation. "Exercise tends to dilate vessels so that the heart can pump more easily to supply blood to the rest of the body," says Dr. Simpson. The result is that resting blood pressure declines. "The heart doesn't have to work as hard against resistance."

Aerobic exercise also helps increase your metabolic rate—the rate at which your body burns calories. At heart-pumping levels, exercise burns enough calories to reduce body fat, thus leading to weight loss.

Keeping trim not only helps you feel better but it can also help keep down blood pressure, a major risk factor for heart disease. Studies indicate that blood pressure can also be reduced by exercising at least three times a week. And in one study of 641 women ages 50 to 89 conducted at the University of California, San Diego, blood pressure was significantly lower in active women compared with sedentary women.

# Clobber That Cholesterol

Exercise may also help to decrease your risk of heart disease by keeping your cholesterol under control. Studies show that exercise increases HDL (high-density lipoprotein) cholesterol, the good cholesterol that helps sweep LDL (low-density lipoprotein) cholesterol, the bad cholesterol, from the arteries. High-intensity exercise has been shown to increase HDL levels 5 to 15 percent.

Research indicates that aerobic exercise increases HDL cholesterol levels in women as well as in men. When women engage in regular exercise—say, the recommended 30 minutes of exercise three times a week at a minimum of 50 percent of maximum heart rate (220 minus your age)—elevated cholesterol levels tend to decline.

The good news for women is that they may not have to work as hard as men to get the same results. For women, moderate levels of exercise appear to be effective in raising HDL. Men, on the other hand, seem to require more strenuous exercise.

# A Good Way to Bone Up

Aerobic exercise is effective in helping to maintain bone strength as well. Weight-bearing exercise places stress on the bone, and that stress helps maintain or increase bone strength. This is important particularly in postmenopausal women, who experience rapid bone loss at the rate of 2 to 4 percent per year.

The decline in bone density that occurs with aging, known as osteoporosis, is responsible for 1.3 million bone fractures per year. One-third of women older than 65 get spinal fractures and 15 percent fracture their hips.

Aerobic exercises that are particularly effective are weight-bearing ones such as walking and running. Even riding a bicycle, either stationary or moving, can be effective. Just increase the resistance against which you are pedaling, says Sydney Bonnick, M.D., director of osteoporosis services at Texas Woman's University in Denton. "That strengthens the muscles of the upper hips and thighs so they pull on the bone, which is a good stimulus to bone growth," she says. Unfortunately, a popular exercise for older women, swimming, is not weight-bearing and appears to be less effective.

# A Matter of Memory Maintenance

Did you know that exercise can keep you younger by fending off the decline of your mental fitness? Well it can, according to Joanne Stevenson, R.N., Ph.D., professor of nursing at Ohio State University College of Nursing in Columbus who specializes in how exercise affects memory in the elderly.

Long-term memory—the ability to remember distant events—doesn't generally deteriorate with aging. But short-term memory—the ability to remember recent events—does. Part of the reason for this, says Dr. Stevenson, is that as we get older, brain cells don't receive the same level of nutrients and oxygen that they used to. Aerobic exercise can decelerate that. It also helps increase the number of brain chemicals called neurotransmitters so that messages can be carried more quickly across brain cells, she says. "Exercise, by maintaining a high nutrient level and high oxygenation level, sort of wards off the process of aging."

Aging can also affect what researchers call fluid intelligence—your ability to conceptualize. This type of memory requires more oxygen to the brain than any other mental chore. "Real quick thinking and real quick gaining of ideas—getting the whole gestalt—slows down through middle adulthood and into old age," says Dr. Stevenson. "Aerobic exercise would slow down this slow-down," she says, and enable people to maintain mental flexibility and quickness for a longer period of time.

## Disease Deterrence

Exercise may also play a role in fending off diabetes and cancer.

Type II diabetes, a disease in which the body produces less insulin and becomes insulin resistant, affects 10 to 12 million adults age 20 or over. Preliminary evidence suggests that exercise helps increase insulin sensitivity and resistance to the disease.

In one study of 87,253 women ages 34 to 59 conducted at the Channing Laboratory of Harvard Medical School and Brigham and Women's Hospital, both in Boston, women who exercised vigorously at least once a week reduced their risk of diabetes.

In another study of 5,990 male alumni of the University of Pennsylvania in Philadelphia, the incidence of diabetes declined as physical activity went up. For every additional 500 calories burned through activity, the risk of diabetes went down by 6%. The study indicates that increasing physical activity may help prevent or delay diabetes and that vigorous activities may have a greater impact than more moderate ones.

Physical activity may play a role in deterring cancer, particularly colon cancer. In a study of 17,148 Harvard alumni, those who were highly active lowered their risk of colon cancer by 15 percent compared with inactive alumni. Researchers suspect that exercise may protect against colon cancer probably by reducing the amount of time that potential cancer-causing agents take to move through the intestinal system.

## The Immediate Return

Aerobic exercise can make you feel younger today by boosting your self-esteem and improving your mental attitude. Regular exercise produces several rewards—muscle strength, gains in your aerobic fitness level, feelings of control over your environment and positive feedback from friends you exercise with—that can make you feel better about yourself.

One study of 26 college athletes found that a 30-minute session of riding a special exercise cycle reduced anxiety significantly and that the effect continued for as long as an hour after the exercise session.

Aerobic exercise can also help fight fatigue. "Despite what people sometimes feel, an exercise program tends to increase energy levels rather than decrease them," says Dr. Simpson. If people stop and pay attention to how they feel after exercise, they will recognize that they feel more alert and more energetic, and that those feelings can carry over several hours after the exercise session, he says.

Exercise probably helps reduce anxiety and fatigue by boosting endorphin levels, the body's natural mood elevators. Women who exercise regularly also find that exercise helps decrease PMS symptoms such as anxiety, irritability and depression as well as the feelings of depression that can accompany menopause.

Endorphins may also serve as the body's natural painkillers. That might be why regular physical activity, which triggers endorphin release, can help reduce premenstrual cramping.

With all these benefits it should come as no surprise that aerobic exercise may help you live longer. In a study of 3,120 adult women conducted by the Cooper Institute for Aerobics Research in Dallas, the higher their level of physical fitness, the lower their death rates.

A follow-up to a Harvard study found that by the time they were 80 years old, men who had gotten adequate exercise between the ages of 35 and 79 lived one to two years longer than men who didn't get regular exercise.

## What the Doctors Recommend

The general guidelines for aerobic exercise have been to get 30 minutes of continuous aerobic exercise that gets your heart rate up to between 50 percent and 90 percent of your maximum heart rate at least three times a week. How high you need to raise your heart rate to reap anti-aging benefits depends on your age, sex and current fitness level. Generally speaking, women who have a low fitness level should aim for an exercise intensity between 50 and 65 percent of their maximum heart rate. Women of average fitness status should aim for between 70 and 75 percent of their maximum heart rate and women in excellent shape should aim for between 80 and 90 percent of their maximum heart rate.

Statistics show that only 22 percent of Americans get the recommended 30 minutes three times a week. So if getting that much exercise is out of the question for you, try instead to accumulate 30 minutes of exercise over the course of the day—say by walking 10 minutes before work, 10 minutes at lunch and 10 minutes after you get home. There is growing evidence to suggest it is the cumulative amount of activity, not the amount done at any one time, that can reap long-term health benefits.

## Getting to It

It's one thing to know you should exercise, but it's another thing to get going and stick with it. Here are some tips to help you out.

**Get physical.** A physical checkup, that is. If you're just starting an exercise program, see your doctor. She'll check to see if you've ever smoked or whether you

# Coach's Corner:
# Keep a Handle on That Heart Rate

Let's say you haven't been exercising and are just starting out on a program. How will you know if you're working hard enough? One way to tell is to take your heart rate.

Begin by aiming for 50 to 65 percent of your maximum heart rate. Take your age and subtract it from 220. That figure is your maximum heart rate. Take 50 percent and 65 percent of that to get your target heart rate range.

So if you're 40, here's how to figure your heart rate range: 220 minus 40 is 180; 50 percent of 180 is 90, and 65 percent of 180 is 117. This means you're aiming for between 90 and 117 beats per minute. To assess if you're exercising at that rate, you can take your pulse for 15 seconds and multiply the number of beats by 4.

If the number you come up with is less than your target heart rate, in this case 90, you need to work a little harder. If it's 90, you're working hard enough to improve your fitness level. If your number is over 117, slow down a bit; chances are you're working at a pace that's too fast for your fitness level, and you probably won't be able to maintain that intensity for the designated 30 minutes. You can also get your blood pressure too high.

Another way to measure whether you're working hard enough is the RPE (rating of perceived exertion) scale. It's a 10-point scale ranging from 0 to 10. If you were exercising at an intensity that felt very light for you, you would be a 1 on the scale, whereas if you exercised at a level that was very heavy, you'd give yourself a 10. If you felt your exercise level was moderate, you'd get a rating of 3.

---

have a family history of heart disease, high blood pressure, high cholesterol, premature death or heart attack, says Dr. Simpson. During the physical exam your doctor will assess your blood pressure and check to see if you have had any previous injuries to your muscles or bones that could be exacerbated by exercise, he says. If you haven't exercised in the past, are over 35 and have risk factors for heart disease, your doctor may recommend a stress electrocardiogram or a treadmill test.

**Get some guidance.** When you first start out on your exercise program, it's very important to get supervision from someone who knows about exercise, says Janet P. Wallace, Ph.D., associate professor of kinesiology at Indiana University at Bloomington. On your own you'll tend to overdo it, so find a trainer to keep you at the right pace. Ask candidates if they have certification from the American College of Sports Medicine, the American Council on Exercise, the Aerobics and Fitness Association of America or the National Strength and Conditioning Association. Working with a trainer may also keep you on the exercise bandwagon, says Dr. Stevenson. This is because if you actually make an appointment to work out, you're less likely to forgo exercise for a few hours on the sofa at home.

**Make it a priority.** Instead of looking at exercise as a leisure activity, look at it as a necessity, says Dr. Mikesky. In other words, make an appointment with yourself to get exercise, and decide that it can't be canceled, postponed or rescheduled. Respect that appointment just like you would any other.

**Warm up.** It's important to warm up and stretch before plunging headlong into your workout session. Warming up increases circulation to the muscles, makes them more pliable and helps prevent injury, says Mark Taranta, a physical therapist and director of the Physical Therapy Practice in Philadelphia. Try walking, jogging slowly or riding an exercise bike at a slow pace for a few minutes until you get a light sweat going. Then stretch for eight to ten minutes.

**Make it fun.** People are more successful getting into a regular exercise program when they choose an activity they enjoy, says Dr. Wallace. If it's boring or too hard, you won't stick with it, so try different things until you find a type of exercise you really like.

**Mix it up.** "Aerobic activities are not the most exciting activities," says Dr. Wallace, so try combining them with another activity that you like. If you enjoy racquetball or tennis (anaerobic activities), try walking for 15 minutes before or after. Or combine different types of aerobic activities. "If you're at the health club with a lot of aerobic equipment, move from one to the next," she says. Spending ten minutes on each one will be less boring. So try the stair climber, then the bike and then the treadmill.

**Couple up.** Consider going to the gym with your partner, says Dr. Wallace. A study of 16 married couples at her institution found that the dropout rate for individuals who went to the gym with their spouses was much lower (6 percent) compared with those who went to the gym on their own (42 percent). You don't necessarily have to work out together; just plan on going there together, says Dr. Wallace.

**Get in a group.** If you really have trouble exercising on your own, aim for a group activity. Join an aerobics class or a running group. Start your own walking club with friends from work. Exercising with others will help you stick with it, says Dr. Stevenson, because you'll have to answer for yourself. If you miss a class one week, the next week someone will be asking where you were, she says.

**Give yourself a break.** Getting in a regular exercise routine can take some time, so allow yourself to slip up here and there. Take it a week at a time, says Dr. Wallace. "If you blow it one day or one week, you still have next week," she says.

# AFFIRMATIONS

## Phrases That Sing Your Praises

Some days, everyone's a critic. Like our husbands ("That dress looks awful"). And our daughters ("This meat loaf tastes awful"). Not to mention our bosses ("This proposal sounds awful"). Geez. Is it too much to ask for a little compliment once in a while?

Well, instead of waiting for someone else, why not say something nice about yourself to yourself—an affirmation? They're short, positive phrases about you, your life and your world. And experts say that repeating them daily can build self-esteem, give you a booster shot of vitality and help you see things in a more optimistic light.

"There's so much negativity around that it tends to pull you down after a while," says Susan Jeffers, Ph.D., a psychologist in Tesuque, New Mexico, and author of *Feel the Fear and Do It Anyway*. "Affirmations can help you live a happier life and diminish the negative clutter that clouds your sense of purpose. They're extraordinarily powerful little pick-me-ups."

## The Power of Positive Talk

Stop and listen to yourself think for a few minutes. If you're like most women, the chatter inside your head is overwhelmingly negative. "Anytime someone pays you a compliment, you immediately drown it out in a chorus of boos," Dr. Jeffers says. "For some reason, the chatterbox in our minds just doesn't want us to accept the fact that we have something on the ball."

Affirmations can counteract that powerful negative inner voice and eventually reduce it to a whisper. The more positive things we say—about our successes, our feelings and our ambitions—the less time we have for negative thoughts. Even if you don't believe what you're saying at first, Dr. Jeffers says the optimistic messages will eventually seep into your subconscious and become just as powerful as the negative thoughts once were.

## Winning Words

Want to be strong, aggressive and successful? Start talking like it! "So much of what we say to other people is full of pain words—phrases like 'I can't' or 'I should,' says Susan Jeffers, Ph.D., a psychologist in Tesuque, New Mexico, and author of *Feel the Fear and Do It Anyway*. "If we replace these pain words with power words, it really changes our attitude and outlook. Power words are like affirmations you can build into everyday speech, and use all the time."

Pay attention to what you say for a few days, suggests Dr. Jeffers. If you hear yourself repeating pain phrases like the ones in the left column, try replacing them with the power phrases on the right.

| Pain Phrases | Power Phrases |
| --- | --- |
| I can't. | I won't. |
| I should. | I could. |
| I hope. | I know. |
| If only. | Next time. |
| It's not my fault. | I'm responsible. |
| It's a problem. | It's an opportunity. |
| What will I do? | I can handle it. |
| Life's a struggle. | Life's an adventure. |

Sure, it sounds a little far-fetched. How can repeating a phrase like "I am successful in all I do" really make you successful?

"The power of suggestion is very strong," says Douglas Bloch, a Portland, Oregon–based counselor and lecturer and author of *Words That Heal: Affirmations and Meditations for Daily Living*. "When you say something out loud and repeat it, it makes that thought concrete. You start to believe it and begin taking action accordingly." In other words, if you say you're a successful businesswoman, you'll probably start acting with more confidence, drive and desire. And success is likely to follow.

Lest you doubt optimism's strength, consider this study. Researchers at the University of Pennsylvania in Philadelphia reviewed campaign speeches from all major candidates for President of the United States from 1948 to 1984. The result? The politicians who consistently delivered the most positive, action-based speeches on the campaign trail won nine of the ten elections. Candidates who wrung their hands and ruminated about issues—are you listening, Jimmy Carter?—were swamped.

"It's attitude," Dr. Jeffers says. "When we tell ourselves that we'll fail, that it's going to be a struggle, we set ourselves up for failure. But when we tell ourselves we'll handle whatever happens in our lives, we gain inner strength. And we set ourselves up for success."

Affirmations also are surefire stress busters. "You should have a list of affirmations ready that you can start repeating when you feel stressed," suggests Emmett Miller, M.D., a nationally known stress expert and medical director of the Cancer Support and Education Center in Menlo Park, California. "They don't have to be complicated. Just thinking to yourself 'I can handle this' or 'I know more about this than anyone here' will work. It pulls you away from the animal reflex to stress—the quick breathing, the cold hands—and toward the reasoned response—the intellect, the part of you that can really handle it."

## Patting Yourself on the Back

Before you start using affirmations, you must have two things. The first is patience. "It may take a while to overcome all the negativity you've built up," Dr. Jeffers says. "Some of the effects of affirmations are immediate; you'll start feeling a little more optimistic right away. But only with repetition can you

---

### Saying Yes to Yourself

Affirmations usually work best if you tailor them for your needs. But if you're just getting started, experts suggest you first try a few of these phrases:

I am alive with possibility.
I can handle it.
I feel myself growing stronger.
It is all happening perfectly.
There is nothing to fear.
I am confident and self-assured.
I deserve to be happy.
I forgive myself and others.
I accept myself as I am.
My prayers are always answered.

build a positive framework of inner thoughts that will last your whole life."

The second thing you need, of course, are affirmations. Here are some hints about how to create and use them.

**Keep it personal.** Affirmations are for you and you alone. So examine your life for areas that could use improvement. Do you want to be more confident? Would you like to be less angry? Do you want to get along better with your co-workers? Pick one or two goals to start with, Dr. Jeffers says, and write down the rest to address later.

**Make it short and sweet.** Maybe you've decided that one of your goals is to stop worrying so much. Put your thoughts in positive form, state your affirmation in one sentence and always form it in the present tense to make it more immediate. "I let go and trust" or "It's all working out perfectly" may work for you. Try saying your affirmations a few times to see if they click. "You can feel the tension releasing immediately if they're working," Dr. Jeffers says.

Pick affirmations that state the positive, says Dr. Jeffers. These are better than phrases that negate a negative. For example, say "I am creating a successful career" instead of "I am not going to ruin my career."

**Be realistic.** Affirmations are tools to help you achieve goals. They are not magic incantations, so don't ask for too much too fast. "There's a fine line between positive thinking and wishful thinking," Bloch says. You'll probably have the most success if you choose affirmations that deal with emotions, confidence and self-esteem. Try to avoid affirmations that deal solely with material wealth. "It's probably not going to work if you keep repeating 'I am now driving a beautiful red sports car. I am now driving a beautiful red sports car,'" says Bloch.

That doesn't mean you won't eventually get your dream car. If you use affirmations correctly, Bloch says they can help. An affirmation such as "I am confident and successful" could lead to another one, like "I am now ready to find a high-powered job" and maybe even to a real-life conversation along the lines of "I'll take that sports car now, Mr. Salesman, and make it red."

**Repeat, repeat, repeat.** Say your affirmations daily. Dr. Jeffers suggests at least 20 to 30 repetitions per day. And make sure you say them out loud. "There's something about hearing them that makes them more powerful," Dr. Jeffers says. It's a good idea to set aside a regular time to say them, then add more whenever necessary.

If you feel the need to say affirmations in a public setting, it's okay to say them to yourself, according to Dr. Jeffers.

**Play it again—and again.** In addition to your daily oral repetitions, try putting your affirmations on tape. Dr. Jeffers suggests playing them as you drift off to sleep and right after you wake up. "Those are times when you're particularly likely to absorb the message," she says. Other good times: during a workout, when you're walking the dog and while you're cooking dinner. If you don't like the sound of your unaccompanied voice, play some soothing background music while you record your affirmations.

**Surprise yourself.** Hide reminders in unexpected places. Write your affirmations on random days in your date book. Put them on a book marker in a favorite novel. Tape them underneath your bathroom sink so you find them when you're cleaning. "Seeing your affirmations in odd places at odd times is a great way to reinforce the message," Dr. Jeffers says. "It's a jolt of positive energy."

**Explore the spiritual.** Affirmations work best when you tap into a higher power, Bloch says. "We derive strength from the feeling that we are not alone. It's comforting and freeing to ask for spiritual guidance," he says.

Try an affirmation like "I am truly blessed" or "Wherever I am, God is." You could even use Bible verses as affirmations: "The Lord is my shepherd; I shall not want." If religious references make you uncomfortable, try looking inward toward what Dr. Jeffers calls your higher self. She suggests affirmations like "I trust in myself" or "I am one with the universe." She explains, "You don't have to believe there's a god. You just have to believe that you can reach a higher plane in your life through reflection and trust."

**Don't stop.** Affirmations are a long-term commitment. Keep using them even when things are going well. "Otherwise, you may find yourself falling back into habits that pull you down," Dr. Jeffers says. "There can be a lot of negativity in the world, but the proper use of affirmations helps us see the opportunity for growth in all things."

# ALCOHOLIC BEVERAGES

## *One a Day Can Help Keep You Young*

**Y**ou've rarely overindulged, seldom had a hangover and never worn a lamp shade on your head. But you do sip a soothing glass of wine at the end of each day, and despite all that you've heard about the benefits of moderate drinking, you wonder if you're doing the right thing.

Well, drink up—in moderation, doctors say—because a glass of alcohol a day may be just the tonic to relieve stress, help you think more clearly, fend off heart disease and promote longevity.

"If you take a look at mortality studies, the people who live the longest drink a glass or two of alcohol a day. So if someone can control her alcohol consumption, then a glass of wine, a can of beer or a mixed drink a day can extend her life," says Eric Rimm, Sc.D., a nutritional epidemiologist at the Harvard University School of Public Health in Boston.

In fact, death rates for women who savor a drink a day are 16 percent lower than for those women who either drink more or nothing at all, Dr. Rimm says.

## To Your Health

Most of us have heard about the French studies that concluded that drinking moderate amounts of red wine lowers heart disease risk. But other studies have shown that a 12-ounce beer, a cocktail made with 1½ ounces (or one shot) of liquor or a 5-ounce glass of white wine are about equally protective of the heart.

In Oakland, California, for example, researchers at Kaiser Permanente Medical Center followed 72,008 women for seven years. While they concluded that white and red wines were most protective—they reduced heart disease by 30 percent—

researchers also found that beer and liquor were only slightly less protective.

"It doesn't matter what you drink. If you look at the studies, they show it could be hard liquor, wine or beer," says William P. Castelli, M.D., director of the Framingham Heart Study in Massachusetts, which has followed more than 5,200 people since 1948.

# The Effect on Heart Disease

Overall, worldwide studies have consistently found a 20 to 40 percent drop in heart disease risk among moderate drinkers. That's about the same reduction in risk as lowering cholesterol or blood pressure or doing regular aerobic exercise, says Michael Criqui, M.D., professor of epidemiology at the University of California, San Diego, School of Medicine.

Women, for example, who had three to nine drinks a week were 40 percent less likely to develop heart disease than nondrinkers in a study of 87,526 nurses ages 34 to 59 at the Harvard Medical School in Boston.

Another large study by the National Center for Health Statistics followed 3,718 women for 13 years. Women who reported drinking up to two drinks a day were almost 40 percent less likely to develop heart disease.

Small amounts of alcohol may combat heart disease by increasing the amount of HDL (high-density lipoprotein) cholesterol in your blood stream, Dr. Criqui says. HDL, the good cholesterol, helps sweep LDL (low-density lipoprotein) cholesterol, the bad kind that can clog and damage arteries to the heart, out of the bloodstream. Dr. Criqui also suspects that alcohol can help prevent blood clots that can lead to heart attacks and some kinds of stroke.

In a British study comparing 172 women who had strokes and 172 women who hadn't, researchers found that the women who abstained from alcohol were nearly 2½ times more likely to have a stroke than moderate drinkers. But moderation is the key. Other studies have found that people who drink heavily have an increased risk of stroke.

Alcohol may also raise estrogen levels in postmenopausal women, says Judith S. Gavaler, Ph.D., chief of women's research at Baptist Medical Center and a member of the Oklahoma Medical Research Foundation, both in Oklahoma City. In a study of 128 women, Dr. Gavaler found that those who had three to six drinks a week had levels of natural estrogen that were 10 to 20 percent higher than women who didn't drink. Higher estrogen levels can help prevent heart disease and osteoporosis in women who have passed menopause.

In moderate amounts, alcohol also helps inhibitions melt and tension float away, says Frederic C. Blow, Ph.D., research director of the Alcohol Research Center at the University of Michigan in Ann Arbor. By decreasing sexual inhibitions, alcohol can help people relax, therefore making sex more enjoyable.

# What Drink Does for Your Mind

In addition, one drink can help keep your mind sharp, says Joe Christian, M.D., Ph.D., chairman of the Department of Medical and Molecular Genetics at the Indiana University School of Medicine in Indianapolis.

In a 20-year study of 4,000 male twins, Dr. Christian found that men who continued to drink one or two alcoholic beverages a day had better learning and reasoning skills in their sixties and seventies than those who drank less or more. Although his study didn't include women, he suspects that moderate amounts of alcohol improve blood circulation to the brain and probably have the same affect on women.

But if one drink a day is good, why aren't four drinks a day better? "Alcohol is clearly the most mixed of mixed blessings," Dr. Criqui says. "At one or two drinks a day, we don't see most of the complications of alcohol. However, the medical problems as well as the personal and social problems of heavy drinking are well known. There are terrible family problems, broken homes and spousal and child abuse. All of that is associated with heavy alcohol use."

In addition, the risks of stroke, heart disease, liver disease and alcoholism all rise with more than a couple of drinks a day. And the risk of breast cancer may rise with more than one. A study of 34 women between the ages of 21 and 44 at the National Cancer Institute found that just two drinks a day between days 12 and 15 of a woman's menstrual cycle can elevate estrogen levels anywhere from 21 to 31 percent. Elevated levels of estrogen are thought to increase the risk of breast cancer. Scientists aren't sure how much extra estrogen is enough to trigger disease, so they prefer that you err on the side of caution: Drink no more than one a day.

If you do drink, here are some ways to moderate your alcohol use.

**Don't binge.** A drink a day means exactly that. "The best evidence is the drinking has to be done in small amounts spread over several days," Dr. Criqui says. "Drinking seven drinks on Friday night and seven more on Saturday can dramatically increase your blood pressure and actually increase your potential for blood clots."

**Set a limit.** If you know how much you're going to drink before you take your first sip, it will be easier to stick to that limit, even if you're pressured by friends to have more, says William R. Miller, Ph.D., research director at the University of New Mexico Center on Alcoholism, Substance Abuse and Addiction in Albuquerque.

Women should not drink more than one a day, advises Sheila Blume, M.D., medical director of alcoholism, chemical dependency and compulsive gambling programs at South Oaks Hospital in Amityville, New York. Women get drunk on less alcohol than men because they weigh less, have less body water to dilute the alcohol and have less of an enzyme in their stomachs that helps metabolize the booze.

**Make it last.** If you drink slowly, you'll give your liver a chance to metabolize the alcohol so it won't build up in your body. Make your daily drink last more than an hour, says Dr. Blume.

**Chow down.** Eating will slow the rate at which alcohol is absorbed into your bloodstream. But avoid salty foods such as peanuts and pretzels that will make you thirsty and tempt you to drink more, Dr. Miller says.

**Do something.** Dance, play billiards or video games or talk to someone, Dr. Miller suggests. You'll probably drink less if you do.

**Dilute your drink.** Start out with a regular drink, but when it's half gone, add water or club soda to it. Every time your glass is half empty, add more water or club soda, Dr. Blume says.

**Drink water.** "If you're thirsty, your body wants water, not alcohol," Dr. Miller says. "All this nonsense about alcohol being a thirst quencher isn't true. It actually makes you thirstier. So if you drink a big glass of water first, you're more likely to drink alcohol in moderation."

**Try grape juice.** Grape juice, like red wines, contains resveratrol, a chemical produced in the grapes' skin to fight off fungus. Researchers suspect that the chemical lowers the risk of atherosclerosis. So instead of sipping on wine after your one-drink-a-day is gone, try drinking grape juice.

**Protect your baby.** Birth defects are more common if a pregnant woman continues to drink, Dr. Blume says. "One drink during the course of nine months isn't going to hurt the baby, but because we don't know what a safe level of alcohol consumption is for pregnant women—it's probably different for each individual—the safest course is not to drink," she says.

**Call a cab.** Alcohol is involved in nearly half of the fatal automotive accidents in the United States. If you weigh 150 pounds, for example, and have four drinks before you get behind the wheel, you're 4 times more likely to get into an accident than if you were sober, says Steve Creel, a California Highway Patrol Public Affairs officer. If you have ten drinks, your risk is 65 times greater. Even if you don't drink enough to be legally intoxicated, you can be arrested for drunk driving if the police believe you are endangering yourself or other motorists, Creel says. So if you drink, have a designated driver or get a taxi ride home.

# ALTRUISM

## *You Get a Lot by Giving*

**W**hat if research showed that one medicine could improve your overall health, reduce stress, relieve depression and decrease your awareness of pain? Would you be interested?

That research is in. A national survey of 3,000 Americans who tried this medicine showed that more than 95 percent of those who took it regularly said they experienced heightened physical sensations—a "helper's high"—which for many led to the effects just described. The amazing prescription is altruism—helping other people—and it works.

The research also shows that there's a particular kind of altruism that, over time, boosts your health and happiness the most. It's not when you write a check for charity and not when you take care of your own family and friends (even though these bring fulfillment, too.) The altruism that keeps you happier, healthier and feeling younger is when you have one-on-one contact with a stranger. Then the benefits bloom for both of you.

Why? Helping a stranger in need begins to break down the sense of "them" versus "us"—and that empathy is the key to experiencing the lasting euphoria and youthful energy that altruism brings, says Allan Luks, an attorney who heads New York City's Big Brother/Big Sister organization and who led the national volunteer survey, which he describes in his book *The Healing Power of Doing Good*.

More than 20 volunteer organizations across the country participated in the survey, and three-quarters of the more than 3,000 volunteers were female. They were asked questions about the type and frequency of helping activities they participated in, the state of their health and their perceptions of the physical and emotional effects of helping.

The volunteers' responses suggest that people who are altruistic more frequently report better health and increased happiness, says Howard F. Andrews, Ph.D., epidemiologist and senior staff associate in neurology at the Columbia

University College of Physicians and Surgeons in New York City. Dr. Andrews analyzed the data from Luks's research and concluded that those who help others often report significantly better health, including less depression, less pain and even fewer visits to doctors.

Problems and pain don't vanish completely when you volunteer, Luks says, but they can be alleviated to a great degree when you focus outside yourself. Helping someone else helps you leave your worries behind.

## An Antidote to Loneliness

Many people experience physical and emotional problems more often as they age, Luks says, and altruism offers real relief for some of these ills. It's a particularly effective remedy to loneliness and a sense of isolation, and it reduces stress levels that can eventually trigger illness, he says.

"By helping others—focusing intently on these people and getting good feelings back—the good feelings literally replace your negative feelings," Luks says. "You hold that person's hand, they smile at you, they hug you—these good feelings are buffering and reducing the negative stress in your life. What an incredible antidote to loneliness and isolation."

## Keeping Your Spirit Young

"A miserly spirit is a dying spirit. My advice is to give. It's the only way of life that makes sense," says Millard Fuller, president and founder of Habitat for Humanity International in Americus, Georgia, the organization of volunteers who build houses for people in need. "Every physical possession will ultimately be taken away from every person anyway," Fuller says. "The only thing that cannot be taken is that which has been given away."

Want to feel that kind of ageless spirit? Here's how to get started.

**Check out the possibilities.** If you're at a loss about where to begin, think of what you care about and head for the phone book, says Luks. "If you're concerned about a certain health problem or social cause, you'll often find a local nonprofit group in the telephone book," he says. "And many communities have a volunteer action center of some sort."

**Find the right fit.** You can also start by simply visualizing yourself in situations to see what feels like a good fit, Luks suggests. "Just imagine yourself— 'here's me helping a baby' or 'here I am tutoring for literacy' " he says. "Then when you call an organization in the area you've chosen, say 'Do you use volunteers? I'm thinking about volunteering. And can you send me some literature?' They'll be glad to hear from you."

**Give personally.** Meeting and spending time with the person you're helping will have a much greater impact on you than if you limit your helping to less personal tasks, such as collecting clothes or canned goods for the poor, says Luks. Of the volunteers he surveyed, only 5 percent of those who had one-to-one contact with the person they were helping did not report a feeling of euphoria. But people who never encountered those they helped were three times less likely to experience that youthful, buoyant feeling.

**Help through a group.** It's even more effective to help strangers in the company of kindred spirits, such as through involvement with a supportive organization of volunteers. Dr. Andrews's analysis of Luks's data suggests that people who helped strangers through a group rather than on their own made significantly fewer visits to the doctor and reported more positive effects and lasting good feelings from helping.

**Make it a habit.** Those warm holiday feelings inspire a desire in many of us to help people in need. But people who help frequently year-round will continue to experience the good feelings altruism brings the giver, Luks's national survey showed. So make your volunteer activity a regular routine to reap its fullest benefits, Luks says.

**Use your talents.** When you use your own particular skills and knowledge to help others, the experience is even more satisfying, Luks says. He cites surveys that asked people who were already volunteering why they continued, and one of the frequent reasons given was that they were able to use their skills to do something useful. Using your own talents to help or support someone else gives you a particularly strong sense of usefulness, which in turn reduces stress, he says. If you're a lawyer, help at a free law clinic. If you can teach, you can tutor. If you can grow a vegetable, you can feed the hungry. The opportunities are limitless, Luks says.

**Take a volunteer vacation.** You can use your time off not only to rejuvenate your own spirit, but also to help other people or rescue the environment. Habitat for Humanity International, for instance, will connect you with a nearby group working on housing for the poor, Fuller says. You can write to them at 121 Habitat Street, Americus, GA 31709-3498, for more information.

Or you could help to conserve endangered species, environments or cultures as a member of the EarthCorps. EarthCorps volunteers join Earthwatch expeditions and assist scientists on research expeditions all over the globe. "You can help on one of 165 projects in 58 countries and 25 states," says Mary Blue Magruder, Earthwatch's director of public affairs. Write to Earthwatch at P.O. Box 403 R.P., Watertown, MA 02272, for details.

# The Healthy Helper

Though nothing beats the selfless experience of helping other people, you have to keep your own needs in mind, too, Luks says. Here are his tips on how to avoid disappointment and "volunteer burnout."

**Go at your own pace.** Start gradually and volunteer at a pace that's right for you, Luks says. If it starts to feel like a weary obligation, you're doing too much or you're in the wrong volunteer activity.

**Don't fix everything.** If you try to rescue the whole world, you'll set yourself up for disappointment, Luks says. Don't take on total responsibility for even one person or blame yourself for circumstances you can't control.

**Do it together.** A good way to deal with "beginner's nerves" and take the first step to getting involved is to pursue a volunteer activity as a family or with a friend, Luks says. You will strengthen your relationships as you each receive the emotional and health benefits of helping, he says.

**Feel free to change your mind.** If one situation or project isn't bringing you satisfaction and well-being, it's perfectly okay to look for another, Luks says. Nobody is indispensable, and you need to find the helping activity that's right for you. You'll know it's the right fit when you feel more energetic after a volunteering session than you did when you started.

# ANTIOXIDANTS

## *The Best Defense Is a Good Offense*

You buy a lovely two-story house. You paint it, decorate it and make it special. But right under your very nose, or more specifically, under the woodwork, a colony of termites has moved in.

So while you're enjoying your domestic bliss, these hidden invaders are slowly but surely making mincemeat of your happy home. When you finally realize it, the damage has been done. Your floorboards are cracking, your foundation is collapsing and your house is leaning like the Tower of Pisa. Time to call an exterminator—and a contractor.

In real life, your aging body is besieged not by voracious creepy-crawlies but by harmful, unbalanced molecules called free radicals. These marauding substances roam your body looking for healthy cells. Once they find something to latch on to and destroy, they multiply, causing a domino effect of destruction.

So where's your body's exterminator? It could be in your refrigerator. Or in your medicine cabinet. Certain nutrients have shown the ability to stop these free radicals dead in their tracks. These age-erasing nutrients—vitamins C and E and beta-carotene—are called antioxidants.

## Oxygen: The Root of the Problem

It's one of the great ironies. Oxygen—the glorious stuff that fills our lungs and keeps us alive—is involved in a process that can seriously hurt us.

To get the energy they need, the body's cells use oxygen to burn fuels such as glucose (blood sugar) and, in the process, some oxygen molecules may lose an electron. Such a molecule is now a free radical, hell-bent on replacing its lost electron by raiding the other molecules making up the cell.

By swiping an electron, this larcenous free radical transforms the unsuspecting molecule into a new free radical. "Soon a chain reaction of electron

420

theft begins that can produce widespread damage to the chemistry and function of the cell," says Denham Harman, M.D., Ph.D., professor emeritus of medicine and biochemistry at the University of Nebraska College of Medicine in Omaha. "This biochemical oxidation process is not far removed from that which turns a shiny piece of metal into rust."

Wrinkled skin, shrinking muscles and weak bones—some of the signs of growing old that a woman most fears—could be due in part to this destructive oxidation process, the sum of millions of continuous free radical reactions. But of even greater concern to researchers is the notion that these free radicals are causing some of aging's most insidious diseases.

For example, atherosclerosis (hardening of the arteries), the leading cause of heart disease and stroke, is caused by the build-up of LDL (low-density lipoprotein) cholesterol, the so-called bad cholesterol. But it probably isn't until free radicals oxidize the LDL cholesterol that it assumes its potentially deadly form, according to Balz Frei, Ph.D., associate professor of medicine and biochemistry at the Boston University Medical Center.

If we could stop or slow down the free radical chain reaction before it starts, then LDL cholesterol may never go "bad" in the first place, says Dr. Frei. Or DNA, the genetic material within our cells, may never mutate to lead to the formation of cancer. Or tissues in the eye may be more resistant to cataracts. In other words, it would be possible to slow the aging process, extend life expectancy and improve the quality of life.

## Antioxidants to the Rescue

Your body isn't entirely helpless when free radicals go on the warpath. In fact, it actually starts producing certain enzymes to combat the invading free radicals. The problem is that it just doesn't produce enough to stop them all. It needs outside help—fast.

Enter dietary antioxidants—nutritional "scavengers" that patrol our bodies for free radicals, squelching the offending particles. "Because of their unique molecular structures, antioxidants can give up one or more of their electrons to free radicals without becoming harmful themselves," Dr. Frei says. "They actually render the free radical harmless and head off the destructive chain reaction before damage can occur or spread out."

Most researchers have focused their attentions on three antioxidant nutrients: vitamin C, vitamin E and beta-carotene, a substance the body converts to vitamin A. Study after study has shown that high dosages of each of these nutrients results in low instances of many chronic diseases.

In his research, Dr. Frei has found that vitamins C and E can protect LDLs from oxidative damage. "These studies suggest that antioxidant nutrients, vitamin C in particular, are capable of preventing heart disease or at least slowing down its progression," he says.

Scientists have also noticed a relationship between antioxidants and the in-

# A Word about Vitamin A

Besides being an antioxidant protector, beta-carotene is a great source of another important nutrient, vitamin A. The body converts beta-carotene into vitamin A on an as-needed basis.

But be aware that vitamin A and beta-carotene are not the same thing. Vitamin A will not give you the same antioxidant protection as beta-carotene, and too much vitamin A can be highly toxic.

For this reason nutritionists recommend that you don't go beyond the daily Recommended Dietary Allowances (RDAs) for vitamin A (800 micrograms retinol equivalents or 4,000 IU) and avoid all single vitamin A supplements or supplements containing more than 100% of the RDA for vitamin A unless prescribed by a doctor. "We get all the vitamin A we need from meats and vegetables or from foods containing beta-carotene," says Jeffrey Blumberg, Ph.D., professor of nutrition and associate director of the U.S. Department of Agriculture Human Nutrition Research Center on Aging at Tufts University in Boston.

Excessive doses of beta-carotene are not nearly as dangerous as those of vitamin A, says Dr. Blumberg. He says it is almost impossible to consume toxic levels of beta-carotene, but too much can produce an unusual side effect: It can make your skin turn orange.

---

cidence of cataracts. A study by Canadian researchers suggested that dietary supplementation of vitamins C and E can reduce your risk of cataracts by at least 50 percent.

Paul F. Jacques, Sc.D., an epidemiologist at the U.S. Department of Agriculture (USDA) Human Nutrition Research Center on Aging at Tufts University in Boston, observed that the risk of developing cataracts was five times higher in those with "lower levels of all types of carotene, including beta-carotene" in their blood.

Dr. Jacques has also studied the role of the antioxidant vitamin C in fighting high blood pressure. According to his research, rates of high blood pressure are approximately two times higher in those with a low intake of vitamin C in their diets (less than the Recommended Dietary Allowance, or RDA, of 60 milligrams).

There is also a growing body of evidence that antioxidants may be our best source of cancer protection as well. Researchers at the Harvard School of Dental Medicine have shown in recent experiments on hamsters that a mixture of beta-carotene, vitamin E and vitamin C produced significant protection against oral cancer.

And the research doesn't stop there. Cancer epidemiologist Gladys Block, Ph.D., professor of public health nutrition at the University of California, Berkeley, has reviewed 180 studies comparing the effect of fruits and vegetables and their antioxidant nutrients on various cancers. "One-hundred fifty-six of these studies have shown a statistically significant reduced risk of cancer at virtually all cancer sites," she says.

Among Dr. Block's findings are that a low intake of vitamin C doubles your risk of developing oral, esophageal and stomach cancer. Vitamin E and beta-carotene may be protective against lung and stomach cancer. She also notes that dietary vitamin C found in fruits and vegetables may be as strong a protective factor against breast cancer as saturated fat is a harmful one, and that there is evidence that vitamins C and E and beta-carotene may have a protective effect against cervical cancer.

## How Much Does a Woman Need?

The National Research Council's Food and Nutrition Board has established the RDAs as guidelines for how much of each nutrient we need to consume each day to meet our basic health needs and prevent deficiency diseases. For women ages 25 to 50, the daily numbers are 60 milligrams of vitamin C, 8 milligrams alpha-tocopherol equivalents (or 12 IU) of vitamin E, and 800 micrograms retinol equivalents (or 4,000 IU) of vitamin A or 4.8 milligrams of beta-carotene.

A balanced diet consisting of a wide variety of fruits and vegetables is the best way to guarantee that you meet your antioxidant RDAs every day. "Four to five servings of fruits and vegetables per day should easily provide you with most, if not all, of the RDAs for the antioxidants as well as other important vitamins and minerals," says Diane Grabowski, R.D., nutrition educator at the Pritikin Longevity Center in Santa Monica, California.

That's fine for basic health, but in order to achieve the kind of disease-fighting results seen in scientific studies, you need to surpass the current RDAs. Even the healthiest of diets falls short in supplying the same amount of antioxidants used in laboratory experiments.

That's where vitamin supplements can play a role. A supplement can ensure maximum antioxidant protection as well as correct any deficiencies in your diet. But popping a vitamin tablet alone isn't the answer. "These nutrients are not 'magic bullets' and work best in conjunction with other healthy nutritional practices such as eating low-fat, high-fiber meals," says Jeffrey Blumberg, Ph.D., professor of nutrition and associate director of the USDA Human Nutrition Research Center on Aging at Tufts.

More research is being conducted to determine the exact form and amount of the antioxidants needed for optimal health and disease protection. Until

# A GARDENFUL OF DELIGHTS

Much of your antioxidant protection can come from the foods you already love to eat. "A good rule of thumb is to eat from a rainbow of colorful fruits and vegetables," says Diane Grabowski, R.D., nutrition educator at the Pritikin Longevity Center in Santa Monica, California. "In general, the darker green or more vibrantly colorful fruits and vegetables have the richest antioxidant content."

Here are some of the very best sources available.

## Sources of Vitamin C

| Food | Portion | Vitamin C (mg.) |
| --- | --- | --- |
| Orange juice, fresh | 1 cup | 124.0 |
| Broccoli, fresh, boiled | 1 cup | 116.0 |
| Brussels sprouts, fresh, cooked | 1 cup | 97.0 |
| Red bell peppers, raw | ½ cup | 95.0 |
| Cranberry juice cocktail | 1 cup | 90.0 |
| Cantaloupe, cubed | 1 cup | 68.0 |

## Sources of Vitamin E

| Food | Portion | Vitamin E (IU) |
| --- | --- | --- |
| Sunflower seeds, dried | ¼ cup | 26.8 |
| Sweet potatoes, boiled | 1 cup | 22.3 |
| Kale, fresh, boiled | 1 cup | 14.9 |
| Yams, boiled or baked | 1 cup | 8.9 |
| Spinach, boiled | 1 cup | 5.9 |

## Sources of Beta-Carotene

| Food | Portion | Beta-Carotene (mg.) |
| --- | --- | --- |
| Sweet potato, baked | 1 | 14.9 |
| Carrot, raw | 1 | 12.2 |
| Spinach, boiled | ½ cup | 4.4 |
| Butternut squash, baked | ½ cup | 4.3 |
| Fresh tuna, cooked, dry heat | 3 oz. | 3.9 |
| Cantaloupe, cubed | 1 cup | 3.1 |
| Beet greens, boiled | ½ cup | 2.2 |

then, most researchers believe we can best protect ourselves with a combination of diet and supplements. Dr. Blumberg suggests that you try to get all or as many of your RDAs as possible of each antioxidant from the food you eat. For added protection, he suggests that you take daily supplements containing between 100 and 400 IU of vitamin E, between 500 and 1,000 milligrams of vitamin C and between 6 and 30 milligrams of beta-carotene.

## Maximizing Your Defenses

Here's how women can best put antioxidants to work and prevent the harmful effects of free radicals.

**Eat fewer calories.** Digestion requires oxygen—lots of it. The more calories we consume, the more oxygen is required and the greater our chances for free radical formation. Cutting back on the amount we eat can trim our risk of oxidative damage, says Dr. Harman. That doesn't mean you should starve yourself or do anything to reduce your intake of the essential nutrients, he warns. Instead, focus on trimming those nonessential calories from your diet like desserts, candy and soda.

**Get some air.** Free radicals are also generated in the environment by industrial chemicals, heavy metals, fumes, car exhaust, air conditioning and other airborne pollutants. While we can't escape all these man-made contaminants, anything that limits our exposure to them is beneficial, says Dr. Harman. For example, if you work in a factory or an office, you can take a walk at lunchtime to briefly get away from impurities that may be circulating around your workplace. Open windows. Or use a commercial air-purifying device.

**Dowse the cigs.** Cigarette smoke contributes huge amounts of free radicals with every puff. Antioxidants can prevent much of the oxidative damage caused by smoking, says Dr. Frei. But if you avoid the habit in the first place, those antioxidants will be available to fight free radicals elsewhere in the body.

**Lose the booze.** The occasional cocktail isn't going to cause any harm and may actually lower your risk of heart disease, but frequent alcohol consumption can increase the number of free radicals in the body, says Dr. Frei. Not only that, but people with alcoholism show reduced levels of antioxidants in their systems. According to a study at the King's College School of Medicine and Dentistry in London, alcoholic patients showed significantly lower levels of vitamin E and beta-carotene, which coincided respectively with higher incidences of cirrhosis and liver damage.

**Don't overdo your workouts.** When it comes to exercise, remember the adage "train, don't strain." As beneficial as exercise is to our health, the extra oxygen we take in whenever we work out subjects muscles and other tissues to additional oxidative damage. Pushing the body beyond its limits can lead to an overproduction of free radicals and that can have a devastating effect on the way you look and feel. "This may be why athletes who overtrain find that their performance suffers or they become sick," says Robert R. Jenkins, Ph.D., professor of biology at Ithaca College in New York.

Does this mean you shouldn't exercise? No! Most doctors and scientists believe that any oxidative damage is minimal with normal exercise and offset by the added benefits that exercise provides. According to a British study of endurance runners, regular, nonexhaustive exercise enhances the levels of some antioxidant enzymes in the blood. And a study conducted at the Washington University School of Medicine in St. Louis found that high doses of vitamin C, vitamin E and beta-carotene, while not preventing the body from undergoing any exercise-induced oxidative stress, do seem to lower the signs of oxidative damage in the body.

Regular, moderate exercise seems to strike the perfect balance, says Dr. Harman. And no matter what, keep up your intake of antioxidant vitamins.

# ASPIRIN

## *It's Available, It's Versatile— And It Works*

Every week you see the same screaming headlines in those supermarket tabloids: "Amazing New Pill Restores Youth and Vitality!" "Wonder Drug Whips Cancer!" "Powerful Tablet Prevents Heart Attacks!"

Unfortunately, erasing the signs of aging isn't as easy as popping a pill. No matter what the papers say, there's no substitute for a healthy diet, moderate exercise and stress-free, smoke-free living.

But if you're looking for a real-life drug that might help you stay young by working to prevent heart attacks, cancer, gallstones, migraine headaches and other ailments, you may already have it in your medicine cabinet.

It's aspirin, the world's most unassuming super-tablet.

## The Heart of the Matter

Doctors have been backing aspirin for nearly 2,000 years. Hippocrates himself told his Greek friends to chew on willow bark whenever they had pain or fever. Turns out that the bark contained salicylic acid, an unrefined form of aspirin.

You probably already know that aspirin can relieve minor pain, common headaches, arthritis symptoms and low-grade fevers. It works by inhibiting the body's production of prostaglandins, chemicals that help deliver pain messages from the site of an injury to the brain.

But there's an important side effect, too. Prostaglandins aid in blood clotting, so aspirin use reduces clotting. And while that can be a problem in some instances, evidence is growing that this may help prevent heart attacks by reducing clots in the coronary arteries that feed the heart.

A Harvard Nurses' Health Study that tracked more than 121,000 nurses for 15 years, found that women who took one to six aspirin tablets per week cut their risk of heart attack by 30 percent.

Aspirin isn't for everyone, says the co-principal investigator of the study's cardiovascular component, JoAnn E. Manson, M.D., associate professor of medicine at Harvard Medical School and co-director of women's health at Brigham and Women's Hospital, both in Boston. "Aspirin is likely to benefit post-menopausal women at high risk of cardiovascular disease." But for the rest of us, she says, the picture is not so clear.

"Under any circumstances, aspirin therapy should be undertaken only under a physician's supervision," says Dr. Manson.

Aspirin's anti-aging powers may reach even farther than your heart. Aspirin could help you ward off some forms of stroke by reducing blood clots. Experts warn, however, that aspirin therapy could put you at slightly higher risk for hemorrhagic strokes, which are caused by ruptured blood vessels. See your doctor before you start taking aspirin for stroke prevention. The landmark Physicians' Health Study showed that men who took aspirin every other day had a significantly reduced need for surgery to repair other blocked blood vessels in the body.

And aspirin might boost your chances of avoiding colon cancer. In one study of more than 600,000 people, those who took aspirin 16 or more times a month had a 50 percent lower risk of developing such cancer. Clark W. Heath, Jr., M.D., vice president for epidemiology and statistics at the American Cancer Society, says that's because aspirin appears to slow down the development of adenomas—polyps that are probably precursors to colon cancer.

On the headache front: The Physicians' Health Study also found that those who took aspirin every other day developed 20 percent fewer migraine headaches. Researchers are now trying to see if the same results hold true for women, according to Seymour Diamond, M.D., director of the Diamond Headache Clinic in Chicago and executive director of the National Headache Foundation. He also points out, however, that aspirin does little to stop migraines that are already under way.

People at risk of developing gallstones may benefit from aspirin, too. A British study of 75 patients predisposed to stone formation found that the 12 regular aspirin users in the group got no stones, while 20 of the 63 nonusers did.

## Helpful—But Not Harmless

So where's the catch? Well, aspirin is a drug, and like most drugs, it has side effects that may outweigh its benefits for some women.

For starters, aspirin can irritate the lining of your stomach. If that happens, you may feel a burning sensation, though usually the damage is not serious. In rare cases, aspirin use can trigger intense abdominal pain, ulcers or even gastrointestinal bleeding.

# Painkillers: Choose Your Weapon Wisely

Aspirin is not your only choice for minor aches and pains anymore, and it may not be your best. Other over-the-counter drugs can handle many of aspirin's smaller chores without causing side effects like upset stomach or ringing ears.

Every nonprescription painkiller relies on one or more of three drugs: aspirin; ibuprofen, which is found in brands like Advil, Nuprin and Motrin; and acetaminophen, found in Tylenol, Panadol and some Anacin products. The choice among them isn't that difficult when you know what each one does best.

*Headaches.* For everyday tension headaches, each of the three pain relievers can do the job, says Frederick Freitag, D.O., a member of the board of the National Headache Foundation.

*Minor aches and fever.* All three take care of this, but you might want to consider acetaminophen here because it's easier on your stomach lining than the others.

*Toothaches.* Ibuprofen is your best bet here. It out-performed aspirin and acetaminophen in a study reported in *American Pharmacy.*

*Sore muscles.* Ibuprofen and aspirin get the edge here because they are anti-inflammatory agents that help reduce swelling of sore or bruised muscles. Ibuprofen is less irritating than aspirin to most people's stomachs.

*Sprains and tendinitis.* Again, aspirin and ibuprofen get the nod because they help cut swelling.

*Menstrual cramps.* Ibuprofen is the drug of choice. Best results will occur if it's started three days in advance of menses.

There's also a possibility that aspirin could increase your risk of stroke triggered by bleeding into the brain, says Julie Buring, Sc.D., principal investigator of the Women's Health Study and associate professor of ambulatory care and prevention at Harvard Medical School. On the other hand, aspirin may decrease the risk of the most common form of stroke, which is caused not by bleeding but by blood clots in the head.

Aspirin also can cause tinnitus, or ringing in the ears. The condition is usually temporary, and aspirin will cause no permanent damage to your ears. If aspirin makes your ears ring, doctors suggest trying a product containing acetaminophen.

# Tablet Tips

If you think aspirin may help boost your chances of avoiding heart disease or other problems, just remember:

**Don't play doctor.** Aspirin therapy carries risks. Talk to your physician about whether or not it's right for you. "You should consult your doctor before taking aspirin for a sustained period of time," says James E. Muller, M.D., co-director of the Institute for Prevention of Cardiovascular Disease at New England Deaconess Hospital in Boston.

**Easy dose it.** If a little aspirin works wonders, why not take a lot? Simple: Test results show that taking megadoses of aspirin does no more good than taking smaller doses.

Most research has focused on those who take a 325-milligram tablet—the size of a regular-strength aspirin—every other day. The landmark Physicians' Health Study found that an aspirin every other day helped cut heart attack risk.

A Dutch study showed that smaller doses—perhaps one-tenth the size of a regular tablet—may provide essentially the same results. "This study adds more weight to the view that doses of aspirin currently used for prevention may be higher than need be," says Dr. Muller.

Your doctor should be able to set a proper dosage for you, Dr. Muller says. He also warns not to cut down on your dosage if a doctor has already prescribed aspirin.

**Avoid a gut reaction.** Try to take aspirin with a meal because you'll be less likely to feel stomach pain or nausea. If you're between meals, try swallowing aspirin with a full eight-ounce glass of water instead.

**Bypass your belly.** Some regular-dose and low-dose aspirins have special coatings that let them pass through your stomach and digest in your small intestine instead, which is a little easier on your digestive system. Look for brands that are buffered or "enteric-coated."

**Focus on healthy living.** No matter how powerful aspirin proves to be, it won't solve all your problems. It may help prevent a heart attack, but so do a healthy diet and regular workouts.

"You should do everything you can to reduce the risk factors such as high cholesterol, smoking, overweight and lack of exercise," says Alexander Leaf, M.D., founder of the Cardiovascular Health Center at Massachusetts General Hospital in Boston.

# BREAKFAST

## *A Meal You Don't Want to Miss*

The day is young and you can be, too—if you eat breakfast. Scientific studies show that a good morning meal can help protect your heart and keep you trim.

Let's start by talking about your losing battle—that seemingly never-ending quest to be thin—and how breakfast can make you a winner.

Breakfast appears to act as a wake-up call for your body's metabolism, stimulating it to burn more calories. A study conducted by Wayne Callaway, M.D., associate professor of medicine at George Washington University in Washington, D.C., found that breakfast eaters had metabolic rates 3 to 4 percent above average, while breakfast skippers had sluggish rates, 4 to 5 percent below average. That means that in the course of a year, breakfast skippers will "conserve" 10 to 15 pounds of body fat, explains Dr. Callaway.

Eating breakfast can also help you to control your hunger, and when you do get hungry, to choose the right low-fat foods. A study at Vanderbilt University in Nashville led by David Schlundt, Ph.D., clinical psychologist and assistant professor of psychology, found that breakfast eaters chose fewer high-fat foods and more healthy high-carbohydrate foods and more successfully fought off their cravings for late-day, unhealthy snacks than did non–breakfast eaters.

Shifts in brain chemistry throughout the day make us more likely to crave fats as the hour gets later, explains Dr. Callaway. Most of us wake up craving carbohydrates rather than fats. "It's as if we are biologically programmed to eat a healthy breakfast," he says.

A healthy, high-carbohydrate, low-fat breakfast will address more than your midlife battle of the bulge. It can also address another weighty matter—circulatory disease, the national epidemic of clogged arteries that leads to millions of disabling and deadly heart attacks and strokes.

One cause of circulatory disease is blood clots, sticky plugs that block arteries. The clots are formed from platelets, the tiny disk-shaped parts of blood

# CHOOSING THE RIGHT CEREAL

It's not all that hard to pick out the most nutritious cereal. You want a cereal with plenty of vitamins, minerals and fiber, but not a lot of fat, calories, sugar or sodium. Look for adult choices on the top shelf in most supermarket cereal aisles and check out the healthy options below. The levels of nutrients are for single servings. See the side of the box for how much cereal constitutes one serving.

| Cereals | Fiber (g.) | Calories | Fat (g.) | Sugar (g.) | Sodium (mg.) |
|---|---|---|---|---|---|
| All-Bran (original) | 10 | 80 | 1 | 5 | 280 |
| Cheerios (original) | 3 | 110 | 2 | 1 | 280 |
| Common Sense Oat Bran | 4 | 110 | 1 | 6 | 270 |
| Cracklin' Oat Bran | 6 | 230 | 8 | 18 | 180 |
| Fiber One | 14 | 60 | 1 | 0 | 140 |
| Frosted Mini-Wheats | 6 | 190 | 1 | 12 | 0 |
| Grape-Nuts | 5 | 200 | 0 | 7 | 350 |
| Healthy Valley Organic Amaranth Flakes | 4 | 100 | 0 | 8 | 10 |

that are responsible for normal clotting (like when you cut yourself) but can go into overdrive and become more like Krazy Glue than Scotch tape.

Researchers at the Memorial University of Newfoundland in St. John's looked at the effect of breakfast on platelets. They found that morning levels of the factor that makes platelets sticky were much higher in people who didn't eat breakfast. Scientists already know that most heart attacks and strokes occur in the morning. Does that mean that skipping breakfast can make your heart skip a lot more than a beat?

"It is definitely prudent and important to have breakfast every morning," says George Fodor, M.D., a professor of clinical epidemiology at Memorial University who led the study.

Breakfast might also help your heart by lowering cholesterol. Researchers at St. Joseph's University in Philadelphia looked at the breakfast habits of

| Cereals | Fiber (g.) | Calories | Fat (g.) | Sugar (g.) | Sodium (mg.) |
|---|---|---|---|---|---|
| Kellogg's Complete Bran Flakes | 5 | 100 | 0.5 | 6 | 230 |
| Kellogg's Corn Flakes | 1 | 110 | 0 | 2 | 330 |
| Kenmei Rice Bran | 1 | 110 | 1 | 4 | 250 |
| Multi Bran Chex | 7 | 220 | 2 | 11 | 320 |
| Nabisco 100% Bran | 8 | 80 | 0.5 | 7 | 120 |
| Nut & Honey Crunch | 0 | 120 | 2 | 10 | 200 |
| Oat Bran O's | 3 | 110 | 0 | 7 | 10 |
| Product 19 | 1 | 110 | 0 | 3 | 330 |
| Quaker Oat Bran High Oat Fiber | 6 | 150 | 3 | 1 | 0 |
| Raisin Nut Bran | 5 | 210 | 4.5 | 15 | 260 |
| Rice Chex | 0 | 120 | 0 | 2 | 230 |
| Rice Krispies | 1 | 110 | 0 | 3 | 360 |
| Special K | 1 | 110 | 0 | 3 | 250 |
| Total (original) | 3 | 100 | 0.5 | 5 | 200 |
| 100% Whole Grain Wheat Chex | 5 | 190 | 1 | 5 | 390 |
| Wheaties | 3 | 110 | 1 | 4 | 210 |

12,000 people and found that those who ate cereal—any cereal—for breakfast had the lowest cholesterol levels. Guess who had the highest? The folks who didn't eat breakfast.

"We've known that one of the worst things you can do for proper nutrient intake is skip breakfast. But now we have new evidence that people who eat a breakfast including cereal have lower cholesterol," says John Stanton, Ph.D., the study's author and director of the Food, Nutrition and Health Research Institute at St. Joseph's.

Breakfast may also help protect you from developing gallstones, says James E. Everhart, M.D., a researcher with the Division of Digestive Diseases and Nutrition at the National Institute of Diabetes and Digestive and Kidney Diseases. People who skip breakfast are essentially undergoing a short-term fast, and fasting has been shown to increase the risk of gallbladder disease.

# Rise and Dine

Okay, you're convinced—eating breakfast can tone your body, inside and out. But maybe breakfast feels like a blind date with Count Chocula. Maybe you just can't get used to the idea of a hearty meal so early in the day. Or maybe you like breakfast—the eggs and bacon variety that turns your arteries into a cholesterol junkyard. Well, here are some easy, healthy ways to say good morning to yourself.

**Just do it.** You can get your body used to eating a healthy breakfast even if you've never eaten it in your life, says John Foreyt, Ph.D., director of the Nutrition Research Clinic at Baylor College of Medicine in Houston. "Eat breakfast, lunch and dinner for a week even if you have no appetite," he says. Within a week or so it will start to feel like an old habit.

**Don't nibble at night.** Snacking at night will make you less hungry in the morning, says Robert Klesges, Ph.D., professor of psychology and preventive medicine at Memphis State University. And that, he says, starts a vicious circle: You have no appetite for breakfast, which makes you hungrier in the evening, which makes you snack more at night.

**Make cereal a habit.** No matter what you eat for breakfast, make part of the meal cereal, says Dr. Stanton. Choose a brand that's low in fat and high in fiber and add some fresh sliced fruit for extra flavor and nutrients.

**Eat cakes for breakfast.** Pancakes, that is. "Pancakes are high in energy-boosting carbohydrates and low in fat if you make them without a lot of oil," says Dr. Schlundt.

You can make enough for a week and freeze a single layer on a foil-lined tray. Then stack them and wrap them tightly with wax paper or plastic wrap. On a hectic weekday morning, just stick two in a toaster oven; that's all it takes for a great breakfast.

**Be a smooth operator.** Smoothies are delicious, nutrition-packed breakfast drinks that only take a minute or so to make. Take one cut-up piece of fruit, one cup of nonfat yogurt (any flavor), a quarter-cup of orange juice and a few ice cubes. Whip it all up in a blender and pour it into a glass—or even into your car mug.

**Don't bring home the bacon.** "Nobody needs to eat meat at breakfast," says Dr. Schlundt. "Eat bread, cereal, juice or fruit, plus skim milk or low-fat yogurt," he suggests. "With these foods, it's really easy to feel full in the morning, and their carbohydrates are a great source of energy."

# BREAST CARE

## *Keeping Your Breasts Firm and Healthy*

You turn to the right and look at your breasts sideways in the mirror. You turn back to the front, lift your arms over your head and check again. Then you turn to the left and check one more time.

What are you looking for?

Two things: the sags and stretch marks that suggest you're beginning to age—and which you intend to fight with every trick in the book—and any lumps, bumps, dimples, discharge, droops, wrinkles or differences in size, shape or color that may signal the presence of cancer.

While none of us wants to see the signs of aging, what we fear most is breast cancer. And for good reason—it's the most common type of cancer that women get.

Most breast cancer is found by women themselves, not by the doctor or a mammogram. They notice that something doesn't look or feel right. Yet 80 percent of women say that they don't do breast self-examinations, or BSEs, on a regular basis. Some say they feel uncomfortable touching themselves and others simply can't face the possibility that breast cancer could happen to them.

These feelings reflect the fact that our breasts act as physical markers for our transitions from one stage of life to another: They emerge as we begin to menstruate, bloom as we begin an active sexual life, ripen into fullness as we prepare to give birth and eventually wither or sag.

Yet the very reasons that may make us reluctant to examine our breasts are also the most compelling reasons that we should.

Breast cancer is a major health threat to any woman who has passed her 30th birthday, says Sondra Lynne Carter, M.D., a gynecologist in private practice in New York City who treats patients with breast problems. And the threat escalates with every year.

Where you had a 1 in 21,441 chance of having breast cancer at age 25, by age 30 it's 1 in 2,426. By age 35 it's 1 in 622. By age 45 it's 1 in 96 and by age 80 it's 1 in 10.

Since the majority of breast cancer actually occurs after age 45, many women may tend to think of breast cancer and saggy breasts in the same way: "It's something to worry about when I'm old." That's wrong. Both may be most likely to occur after age 45, experts agree. But preventing both needs to start with good breast care in the decades before.

## The Breast Self-Exam

Good breast care begins with learning when and how to do a breast self-exam.

Doctors agree that a self-exam should be done the first week after your period every month. Your goal is twofold: one, to become so familiar with the normal ridges, lumps and bumps in your breasts that anything out of the ordinary will be very apparent and, two, to detect any lump (about a half-inch in size, for example) that suddenly appears, stays in the same place and remains for one or two cycles.

What's the best way to do a self-exam? Any way you feel comfortable, doctors say. Some women prefer to do it standing in the shower when their breasts are slippery with soap. Others prefer to do it standing in front of a mirror. Still others prefer to do it lying on their backs.

Here's how doctors suggest you make a breast exam as accurate as possible.

**Stretch first.** What's important is that before you start, stretch your arms over your head and look in the mirror to see if there are any obvious changes in your breasts. Look for something major: a dimpling you've never noticed before or a nipple that has suddenly inverted, developed eczema or has a discharge that isn't a result of being squeezed. Put your hands on your hips, push your shoulders back and look for changes again. Then push your shoulders forward, contracting your chest muscles. Any dimpling should be obvious in this position.

**Choose a search strategy.** There are several different ways to do the breast exam itself: You can use the nipple as a focal point and feel for lumps along imaginary lines radiating out from the nipple all the way up to the collarbone and down to the brassiere line; you can use the nipple as a center and keep circling it with your fingers in ever-larger circles; or you can simply imagine a grid placed over your breast and examine it in up-to-the-collarbone and down-to-the-bra-line strips.

Whichever method you choose, put the hand on the side you want to examine behind your head before you start. This shifts any breast tissue that's under your armpit over to the chest wall where you can check it thoroughly.

## The Anti-Cancer Lifestyle

Good breast care also means adopting a lifestyle that reduces your risk of cancer. No one has figured out exactly why, but women who adopt lifestyle

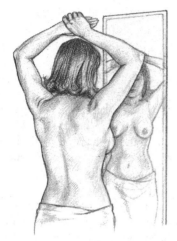

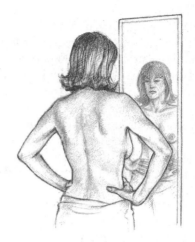

*Put your arms over your head and look for any dimpling, nipple discharge or other changes in appearance.*

*Put your hands on your hips, push your shoulders first back, then forward, and look for any changes in your breasts that occurred since your last self-examination.*

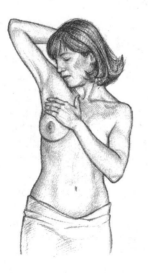

*Place your right hand behind your head. With the finger pads of your left hand, examine your entire right breast from collarbone to bra line and into your armpit. Repeat the process on your left breast with your left hand behind your head. See the opposite page for a description of the different search strategies.*

strategies that reduce the amount of estrogen circulating throughout their bodies may significantly reduce their risk of developing breast cancer. And that includes women who have a family history of the disease.

Which strategies are best? Here's what doctors suggest.

**Lower the fat.** A study at Tufts University School of Medicine in Boston compared estrogen levels in a group of women who ate a diet that got 40 percent of its calories from fat with a group of women who got only 21 percent of their calories from fat.

The result? Pre-menopausal women in the higher-fat group had blood levels of estrogen that were 30 to 75 percent higher than their lower-fat eating sisters. In the postmenopausal group, women who ate the higher-fat diet had estrogen levels that were 300 percent higher.

**Eat plant fiber.** Animal studies indicate that the substances in plants—phytoestrogens—may be able to prevent the estrogens circulating in your body from causing breast cancer. Good sources of phytoestrogens include soy products, alfalfa sprouts, apples, barley, oats and peas.

**Nosh on veggies.** In a Harvard Nurses' Health Study, which studied nearly 90,000 women in Boston, researchers found that those who reported eating two or three servings of vegetables a day had a 17 percent reduced risk of breast cancer compared with those who ate less than one full serving per day.

No one's willing to bet the ranch on an explanation, but many scientists suspect that it may have something to do with the presence of vitamins A and C, antioxidants believed to block cancer-causing substances produced by the body's normal metabolic process.

**Avoid mid-cycle drinking.** A study at the National Cancer Institute found that just two mixed drinks a day between days 12 and 15 of a woman's menstrual cycle will elevate estrogen levels anywhere from 21 to 31 percent.

# Beating Breast Sag

Although good breast care primarily means keeping your breasts healthy, for some women it also means keeping your breasts smooth and firm.

There are two ways to sag when we pass our thirties, doctors say: When large breasts sag, the nipples do a swan dive and head toward your waist; when small breasts sag, the nipples gracefully sink back toward your chest.

One way you look like a cow that needs milking. The other way you look like a boy. It may not be what God, nature and Victoria's Secret intended, but sag can be the reality of the post-30 breast.

"Somewhere between the ages of 30 and 40, the elastic tissue in the breast begins to degenerate," explains Albert M. Kligman, M.D., professor of dermatology at the University of Pennsylvania School of Medicine in Philadelphia. The breast fibers, which act like rubber bands and provide that resilient bounce as you walk, will still stretch. But they don't snap back quite as well. The result is saggy breasts with a few stretch marks thrown in for good measure.

Adding to the problem, hormonal changes—both during pregnancy and as you reach menopause—make breasts sag more.

During pregnancy, the hormones estrogen and progesterone, which are secreted by the ovary and the placenta, stimulate development of the 15 to 20 lobes of milk-secreting glands embedded in the breast's fatty tissue. These changes are permanent. And although the glands may be empty after they're no longer needed to produce milk, they will still add bulk and firmness to the breast.

---

# Getting a Lift

You stand up straight and pull your shoulders back, and they sag. You stand up straight, pull your shoulders back and suck in your gut, and they still sag.

What's sagging are your breasts. The score is: woman 1, gravity 2.

But does that mean you're ready to have a breast lift? Only you can answer that question based on discussions with your doctor. But here is some information on your options.

"There are basically two kinds of lifting procedures we do in this country," says Robert L. Cucin, M.D., clinical instructor of plastic surgery at Cornell University Medical College in New York City.

"For smaller degrees of sagging, we can do what's called a doughnut mastopexy. You take some skin out from around the nipple's areola, then tuck the skin underneath where it gives you a modest degree of lift and tightening."

When sagging is more severe, American surgeons tend to use the inverted T, or anchor, mastopexy, says Dr. Cucin. The surgeon cuts around the nipple, straight down from the nipple to the bra line, then along the bra line in both directions for several inches. Excess skin and fat are removed, the nipple is repositioned and the remaining skin is drawn tight to support the breast. Scars will be about nine inches long, and the amount of sensation left in your nipple depends on how much it's moved during the procedure.

---

Once menopause arrives, however, the drop in estrogen and progesterone signal the breast that its milk ducts and lobes can retire. As a result, the breast shrinks, adds fat and begins to sag over and above the demands of gravity.

Fortunately there are several ways to prevent, and sometimes reverse, both sag and stretch marks.

**Think weights.** "There's no way I know of to build up the breast's fatty tissue," says Dr. Carter. "But you can build up the pectoralis muscles underlying the fatty tissues so that you get the same effect."

To prevent or reduce sag, get a couple of two-pound weights—no heavier—and work those muscles five times a week, says Dr. Carter.

With a weight in each hand, extend your arms sideways and do 15 small, backward circles about a foot in diameter. Widen the circles slightly and do another 15; widen them again and repeat. Slowly work your way up to 50 circles for each repetition.

**Roll your shoulders.** Put your weights aside and with your arms hanging at your sides, roll your shoulders backward, down and forward in a circular motion 15 to 20 times, says Dr. Carter. Do it five days a week.

**Hit the deck.** "Start off trying to do 10 push-ups and work your way up to 20," says Dr. Carter. It may take up to six months, she adds. But you're more likely to do them regularly if you add one push-up at a time. Just get on your hands and knees, raise your feet six inches off the floor, and lower your upper body down to within an inch of the floor. Do these five days a week as well.

**Get some support.** Wearing a bra is a good way to prevent sagging, says Dr. Kligman. In fact, he suggests that any female over the age of 15 do so.

Get a style that has great support and allows minimal bounce, says Dr. Kligman. And wear it all day, not just when you work out.

**Shrink the stretch marks.** If you've just had a baby and the stretch marks on the top and sides of your breasts are red and inflamed, you can treat them with daily applications of tretinoin (Retin-A), says Dr. Kligman. Talk to your doctor about getting a prescription for the drug. Not only does Retin-A tighten the stretched skin but there's some evidence that it also builds a new superstructure under the skin to help firm it.

**Talk to your doctor about HRT.** Hormone replacement therapy, or HRT, can halt breast sagging that occurs after menopause by helping to keep breast fibers from further degenerating, doctors say. It won't turn back the clock to your twenties, but it will keep your breasts from sagging more.

# CALCIUM

## *A Crucial Bone Builder, and More*

**M**any women defy aging by spending time and energy shaping their bodies—reducing a curve here, building a muscle there. But what about the bones beneath those muscles and curves? Your bones give you stature and support. They are living organs full of blood vessels, constantly manufacturing new cells to give strength to your frame.

If you want an upright, sturdy frame for years to come, it's important to understand that your bones need nourishment. The nutrient that gives youth and strength to your bones, and, more importantly, wards off the bone-thinning effects of osteoporosis, is calcium. And if your bones could speak, they'd probably ask for more.

If you're like most women, you already know that the easiest way to get your calcium is by drinking milk and eating other dairy products. But, if you're like most women, you're not getting enough. You may drink milk only as a dollop in your coffee. Or perhaps you're swearing off dairy products like cheese because you're watching your fat intake.

If you're counting on calcium from vegetables, you may be getting less than you think. The calcium in dark leafy vegetables such as spinach and kale may not always find its way to your bones, says Clifford Rosen, M.D., director of the Maine Center for Osteoporosis Research and Education in Bangor. "Because people absorb calcium from vegetables in variable ways, you won't know whether you are absorbing it efficiently, even though you may be taking in generous amounts," he says.

Sometimes the stresses of busy lives and a culture that pressures women to be thin encourage us to eat sporadically or diet repeatedly over the years. That kind of on-the-run nutrition can leave you seriously deficient in calcium.

# You Can't Do without It

Calcium is a mineral you need to survive. When your body calls on its daily dose of calcium and can't find it in food, it plucks it from your bones. As you get older, this feeding off bone eventually causes your bones to become porous and brittle. Unfortunately, your bones may not let you know it until it's too late—when you fall and break one. This bone loss is called osteoporosis, and it's especially cruel to older women.

The female hormone estrogen to a great degree helps protect your bones from calcium theft. But once menopause hits and estrogen wanes, your bones are left vulnerable. Couple this loss with low calcium intake, and bone depletion accelerates.

Calcium can also help lower your cholesterol. In one study, researchers found that when people with cholesterol levels in the high range of 240 to 260 took in an extra 1,800 milligrams of calcium a day, they reduced their total cholesterol by 6 percent, reports the study's conductor, Margo Denke, M.D., assistant professor of medicine at the Center for Human Nutrition at the University of Texas Southwestern Medical Center at Dallas and a member of the nutrition committee of the American Heart Association. Even better, LDL (low-density lipoprotein) cholesterol—the bad cholesterol that causes all the damage to coronary arteries—dropped by 11 percent. Although the study was conducted on men, Dr. Denke feels the result would be similar for women.

# Getting Our Share

Because calcium is so important, our need for it changes throughout life. A child with growing bones has a recommended dietary allowance (RDA) of 1,200 milligrams. After the age of 24, when bone growth has stopped, the RDA is only 800 milligrams.

But many doctors believe that women should be getting much more. Many researchers say 1,000 to 1,500 milligrams daily is the safe and optimum level for bone protection. And some, including Dr. Denke, say that 2,000 milligrams a day is needed to achieve a cholesterol-lowering effect.

Studies show that 85 percent of all women don't get even the RDA for calcium. It's estimated that the average calcium intake for American women between the ages of 35 and 50 is 530 milligrams a day. Here's what you can do to boost that number.

**Don't go a day without dairy.** How important is dairy? "Calcium is most available to your body when it comes from milk and milk products," says Richard J. Wood, Ph.D., chief of the Mineral Bioavailability Laboratory at the U.S. Department of Agriculture Human Nutrition Research Center on Aging at Tufts University in Boston.

To avoid the fat and calories, only reach for low-fat options. Your favorite supermarket offers low-fat versions of the full array of dairy products: milk,

# YOUR BEST SOURCES OF CALCIUM

Calcium is available in many foods, but dairy products are the leaders of the pack. Here's a rundown of some excellent food sources.

| Food | Portion | Calcium (mg.) |
| --- | --- | --- |
| Nonfat yogurt | 1 cup | 452 |
| Low-fat yogurt | 1 cup | 414 |
| Skim milk | 8 oz. | 351 |
| Part-skim ricotta cheese | ½ cup | 337 |
| Low-fat fruit-flavored yogurt | 1 cup | 314 |
| Low-fat milk 1% | 8 oz. | 300 |
| Low-fat milk 2% | 8 oz. | 296 |
| Whole milk | 8 oz. | 290 |
| Buttermilk | 8 oz. | 285 |
| Chocolate milk | 8 oz. | 280 |
| Whole-milk yogurt | 1 cup | 274 |
| Swiss cheese | 1 oz. | 269 |
| Whole-milk ricotta cheese | ½ cup | 256 |
| Provolone cheese | 1 oz. | 211 |
| Monterey Jack cheese | 1 oz. | 209 |
| Broccoli, cooked | 3½ oz. | 205 |
| Cheddar cheese | 1 oz. | 202 |
| Muenster cheese | 1 oz. | 200 |
| Pink salmon, canned, with bones | 3 oz. | 181 |
| Sardines, drained, with bones | 2 sardines (about 1 oz. total) | 92 |

cheeses, sour cream, cream cheese and yogurt, just to name a few. And don't turn up your nose until you've tried it.

Dairy products also give you the most calcium per spoonful. An eight-ounce cup of plain low-fat yogurt offers 414 milligrams. Skim milk boasts 351 milligrams per eight-ounce serving. A half-cup of part-skim ricotta cheese, which you might find in a healthy portion of lasagna, has 337 milligrams.

**Add nondairy sources.** If you have difficulty digesting dairy products or simply do not enjoy them, broccoli is a good choice as a calcium source. Just

3½ ounces of cooked broccoli will give you 205 milligrams of calcium—much more than other vegetables.

Also try tofu, a mild, versatile soy product you'll find in the produce section of your grocery store. It's loaded with calcium. But some tofu brands have more calcium than others, depending on the ingredient used to form the curds. A half-cup of tofu made with nigari (magnesium chloride) contains 258 milligrams of calcium. But the same amount of tofu made with calcium sulfate contains a full 860 milligrams of calcium. Check the curding agent on the label.

**Don't forget the fish.** Since calcium makes its home in your bones, it only makes sense that bony fish are a good source of calcium. Canned pink salmon with bones contains 181 milligrams of calcium per three-ounce serving, and two sardines (about 1 ounce total) contain 92 milligrams.

**Fortify with vitamin D.** "No matter how much calcium you include in your diet, your bones won't retrieve it without the help of vitamin D," says Michael F. Holick, M.D., Ph.D., director the Vitamin D, Skin and Bone Research Laboratory at Boston University Medical Center. Fortunately, for most women, getting enough vitamin D isn't a problem. Casual, everyday exposure to sunlight—just 15 minutes will do—will meet your body's daily requirements for vitamin D, says Dr. Holick. How? Sunlight triggers the production of vitamin D in your skin, he says.

Also, vitamin D comes in an array of fortified foods we eat every day, like milk, cereals and breads. Doctors advise against taking vitamin D supplements, however, because too much can be toxic.

**Dump the Popeye diet.** Spinach contains plenty of calcium but it also contains compounds called oxalates, which bind with the mineral and render much of it unavailable to your body. Although you should enjoy spinach for the other good nutrients it has to offer, don't overdo it, says Paul R. Thomas, Ed.D., R.D., staff scientist with the Food and Nutrition Board of the National Academy of Sciences in Washington, D.C. "Eating spinach salad four to five times a week is fine; just don't depend on it as your major source of calcium," he says.

## Supplement Your Diet

Most doctors will tell you that a well-rounded diet consisting of lean meats and fish and plenty of fruits, whole grains, vegetables and low-fat dairy products will provide you with all the vitamins and minerals you need to maintain good health. But they may also tell you that eating a well-rounded diet is no guarantee that you're getting all the calcium you need, especially if you're a woman over 30. So your best protection may be calcium supplements.

"If you prefer to get your calcium from supplements, choose those made with calcium citrate," says Dr. Denke. All forms of calcium can sometimes interfere with iron absorption or cause kidney stones. Calcium citrate is the supplement that is least likely to promote kidney stone formation.

If you do choose calcium carbonate, it's best to take it with meals, says Dr. Rosen. The acid your body produces when you eat will break down the calcium carbonate and allow it to be absorbed.

Calcium carbonate is found in antacid tablets, and many women opt to chew them as a source of calcium. But you need to be cautious. Some antacid brands, such as Gelusil, Maalox and Mylanta, are not recommended as calcium sources because they also contain aluminum, which can prevent adequate mineralization in bone. Your best bets, says Dr. Rosen, are Tums and Rolaids—both aluminum-free.

How much should you take? "If you drink three eight-ounce glasses of milk a day, then one 500-milligram calcium supplement would be plenty," says Dr. Rosen. "If you can get to 1,500 milligrams either through diet or a combination of diet and supplements, then you're okay."

# CAREER CHANGE

## *It's Never Too Late*

**W**hen you think of television news reporters, visions may come to mind of power parties, exotic overseas assignments and exclusive interviews with the rich, the famous and the criminal. But the reality is often different.

"I was a reporter for ten years and after covering the Christmas shopping story every December and the local Fourth of July parade every summer, I got bored," says Shirley Brice, former reporter for KTVK, the ABC affiliate in Phoenix.

If you look for Brice today, you won't find her in front of a camera. Instead, you'll probably spot her behind the counter at Cornlockie's cookies in Springfield, Virginia. "I always wanted to run a business that was innovative, had potential and afforded me a great deal of control," she says. "I got this idea of starting a low-fat gourmet cookie store and then used my reporting skills to research the possible competition. When I found out that no one else was doing anything like this, I jumped in with both feet. And I love it."

Yesterday's career woman often launched into a chosen profession and stuck with it through thick and thin. While this arrangement had something going for it in the way of security, it often became something of a straitjacket, never allowing for room to grow or change, never providing for new excitement.

Some women today find themselves in the same grind, sticking to careers they've outgrown, feeling trapped, bored, tired . . . and old.

"If you are stuck in a poorly fitting job and feel trapped there, it can have a tremendously negative impact on your spirit, motivation and health," says Beverly Potter, Ph.D., lecturer, consultant and author of *Finding a Path with a Heart: How to Go from Burnout to Bliss*. "You actually start feeling fatigued, heavy and down. Your immune system is affected. Your level of general interest is affected. Everything slides."

Luckily, there's a way out of this pit and many women today are taking it.

# Moving On, Moving Up

It's quite normal today for a woman to have four or five separate careers in her lifetime, says Patti Hulvershorn, director of Ability Potentials, a career counseling and aptitude measurement service in Alexandria, Virginia. "I don't mean job changes; I mean complete changes of careers," she adds.

And why not? People change. People grow. "A job that made you quite happy eight years ago may no longer answer your needs," says Hulvershorn. "In fact, I see people getting the career-change itch about once every ten years. It first happens between the ages of 28 and 30, then again between 38 and 40 and again between 48 and 50. Careers are part of growth, and you occasionally have to shed one like a skin to grow another that's more accommodating."

For many women whose careers have always come second to a husband's, a change in later life might be a big one. You may have stayed for years at a low-paying and unchallenging position to make sure you could always be home by 5:30 P.M. to start dinner. Now you're ready for a change.

But before you rush out to trade in that tired old job for something new and invigorating, there's a lot of planning and self-examination that needs doing. After all, you don't want to give up the security of a steady paycheck before you have a solid game plan.

# Change the Career or Just the Job?

Some women have made complete career changes when a better alternative may have been to keep the career but change the job. It's sort of like killing a fly by hitting it with the living room couch.

"It's classic," says Dr. Potter. "A schoolteacher stuck in a poor district becomes frustrated with the lack of educational funds, teaching materials and administrative support. So she quits and becomes a real estate agent. Fine, except that she loved teaching and the only real problem was the environment, not the career."

Before chucking your current career, make a list of everything you like and dislike about it. "If you find yourself writing down that you don't like your boss, hate the hours or can't stand the geographic location, you've got a situational problem, not a career problem," says Hulvershorn. "A change of job, not of career, is what you want." But if your problems stem from the nature of the work itself, then read on.

# Making the Big Jump

Okay. You've been a lawyer for ten years and you are sick of it. You are bored, tired and as cranky as an 80-year-old woman who just watched a baseball come through her picture window. No amount of fiddling with your current career is going to make you happy. It's time to burst out. But where do you start?

"The first thing to do is make sure you are not just running away from a career you don't like," says Dr. Potter. "Rather than being motivated by escape, you should be motivated by the idea of moving toward something positive—a goal, a dream, something you want. Otherwise, you may end up in a new career hating the very same things you hated in your former career."

**Take a good long look at what you like.** "What do you like to read when you don't have to read anything?" asks Hulvershorn. "What is your subject matter of choice when you read? What has been a continuing interest that you've maintained since you were young or an interest that went by the wayside because you were too busy to keep up with it?"

You're looking for experiences that give you either a great deal of pleasure or satisfaction. "Think of college and high school courses you loved," continues Hulvershorn. "And along those lines, papers you had to write in school that you thoroughly enjoyed researching or hobbies that always intrigued you. Note the magazines you always pick up first at the dentist's office. Are they technical, financial or intellectual? What part of the newspaper do you read first? All these things can give you clues as to what really interests you."

**Dig even deeper.** It's not enough to say that you love pottery or that you want to travel around and find great pottery to sell in your own little shop. "You have to know what it is specifically about the idea that you really like," says Hulvershorn.

The problem is that often only one facet of an idea is what truly excites us, while the rest of what's involved in the job may be downright annoying. "Let's say you love the woods, so you decide to become a forest ranger," says Dr. Potter. "Sure enough, you get to see plenty of woods . . . but what you didn't count on was spending even more time dealing with the government bureaucracy of the National Forest Service. You may even have quit your last job to escape bureaucracy."

One way to avoid all this is to make a list of simple values that you want to incorporate into your next career. Don't write down something specific such as you want to be a tap dancer or a farmer. Write down that you want to entertain people or make things grow. Do you want to work at home, outside or in a posh corporate environment? Do you want to make big bucks or is helping others more important than helping yourself?

Then make a list of everything you don't want. No corporate politics, no time clock, no paperwork, no computers and so on.

"Put all your values, dislikes, interests and skills together, and it could be that they point in a single direction toward a career that you might be uniquely suited for," says Dr. Potter.

**Find a hook.** "When you've found what you like, you've then got to find a hook," says Charles Cates, Ph.D., general manager of EnterChange, a national outplacement firm with corporate headquarters in Atlanta. "Something you've done in another area, be it volunteer work or professional, that will allow you to swing from your former career to the one you want."

According to Dr. Cates, most people approach career change a little starry-eyed and don't consider the fact that companies hire you for what you've done

# Moving from the Home to the Workforce

Ever since you were married, your husband has been the one bringing home the bacon, while you stayed home with the kids. Is it too late now for a successful outside career? Not by a long shot, says Beverly Potter, Ph.D., lecturer, consultant and author of *Finding a Path with a Heart: How to Go from Burnout to Bliss.*

"In this day and age where everyone works, the housewife has become something of an anomaly with negative connotations," says Dr. Potter. "But just because you don't have a business card, it doesn't mean you don't have a job, and it doesn't mean you can't get tired of that job."

According to Dr. Potter, housewives typically have two problems that they need to overcome in making a successful transition from the home to the workforce. "Many times it's easy for the housewife to think that she has no marketable skills, but this is typically a combination of low self-esteem and a lack of self-examination," says Dr. Potter.

So the first step is to look at the home like a business and ask yourself what you do to run it properly. "A wife and mother teaches the children, balances the finances, plans, budgets and acquires food, clothes and other necessities for the family and performs many other tasks as well," says Dr. Potter.

The second step is to apply those tasks to a business situation. "No one will deny the fact that the job market is tight for those without prior experience," notes Dr. Potter. "So one way to make the transition a little easier is to volunteer. You might not get paid initially, but you will be building workplace experience. You'll have a title and you'll make contacts." From there you can then move into the professional world with confidence.

in the past and what you can do for them in the future. They really don't care how keen you are to embark on a new career. "You have to be able to make a case for yourself. You have to show them that despite your past career path, you are well suited for this new career."

And that means experience. "Get it any way you can," says Dr. Cates. "It may mean a low-paying apprenticeship in your off-hours; it may mean volunteer work . . . but you need to build a portfolio of experience."

**Explore opportunities in your company.** "Whenever you work at a company for a period of time, you begin to build a power base," says Dr. Potter. "And I don't mean power in the sense of lording it over others. I mean power as the ability to accomplish and influence through your network of relationships and understanding of how things are done at your company. A power base is very valuable and not something to be thrown away lightly by leaving your company."

What Dr. Potter suggests, if possible, is a lateral move within your present organization, such as a move to another department or to a different position. "That way you keep your power base and can expand on it by gaining knowledge of other areas of the company. In turn, this makes it easier for you to explore new possibilities, and it also makes you more valuable to the company and more likely to get challenging assignments."

**Reshape your job.** If you can't make a lateral leap, look for ways to expand your current position in the direction of your interests. "I tell people to look for unassigned problems," says Dr. Potter. "These are problems that don't belong to anyone. They are opportunities and, by solving them, they act as vehicles to get you where you want to go."

Dr. Potter remembers one woman in particular who dreamed of being a counselor or running her own import-export business. "But she was a chemist and a well-paid one at that. To become a counselor would have meant leaving her job, training, struggling . . . things she wasn't really prepared to do."

What she did instead was talk to her supervisor about making a presentation to the other chemists, working with them on their flagging job satisfaction as one chemist to another. Her supervisor agreed and one presentation led to another. She still had her regular job, but the job counseling side began to expand. "Now she travels all over the world to make these presentations at her company's overseas divisions," says Dr. Potter. "She's doing the counseling she wanted, doing the traveling she dreamed of doing with her import business and the company is paying for her learning curve." All from calling dibs on an unassigned problem.

**Leave your company but take small steps.** You're tired of being a secretary for a plumbing supply company. And, having inventoried all your hopes, dreams, values and dislikes, you now know that you want to edit romance novels. Go for it, but slowly. "Changing careers in a competitive job market is not an easy thing to do," notes Hulvershorn. "Anything you can do to make your current skills work for you in gaining access to a new career is a big plus."

A good way to make a small step in the right direction is by changing industries without changing job functions. Become a secretary for a publishing company, suggests Hulvershorn. "It's easier to get things accomplished, make connections and learn the industry from the inside rather than by looking at want ads."

From secretary you might move to proofreader, then associate editor and maybe someone would then give you a crack as editor.

**Go back to school any way you can.** When people come to Hulvershorn for a career makeover, it often requires that they go back to school. A lucky few can afford to hit the classroom full-time. Most cannot and many end up viewing the need for additional school as an insurmountable stumbling block on their road to a new career.

"But, what many people don't realize is that due to the increase in career changes, most universities are moving toward more flexible programs to accommodate professionals who haven't the time for the standard route," says Hulvershorn.

"The first thing I try and get my clients to do is cut down on their hours or at least work out a flextime deal with their bosses. Maybe they go to school Tuesdays and Thursdays and put in makeup time in the office on Saturdays."

Some schools offer weekend programs where you head for the campus Friday night and come home on Sunday night. Others have correspondence courses. "There's always a way to do it no matter how impossible it may seem at first," says Hulvershorn. "The important thing is to take the first step, and then you'll be surprised when you realize what you can do."

**Think tangentially.** "Large or small, the company you currently work for does not operate in a vacuum," notes Dr. Cates. "It has suppliers and it has clients. The question you need to ask yourself is whether any of the companies currently doing business with your office has anything to offer with respect to your interests."

The advantages to this kind of thinking are many. "First, you speak the same language as these other companies, making it easier to find a possible position with them," says Dr. Cates. "Second, while they may or may not be personally familiar with you, they at least know your company, making you more than just an outsider from off the street."

**Speak the lingo.** Sometimes, the ability to show pertinent experience may be no more difficult than presenting what you've already done in a new light. Every industry has its own language, and if you want to change careers, you'll need to take your past experience and rephrase it in a manner that seems pertinent to the new job. "For example, a high school teacher who wants to become an in-house corporate training director might describe past experience in terms of group motivation and training plans rather than lessons and curriculum," suggests Dr. Cates.

# Be Ready for New Opportunities

With so many people changing careers, Hulvershorn advises getting used to the idea that you, too, may be career hopping someday. So be prepared for it. Here are a few tips.

**Encourage your activities outside the office.** "A hobby at 30 can become a full-blown career at 50," says Hulvershorn. "One of my clients was a stockbroker who happened to have a little farm on the side. That same person is now a full-time organic farmer. My advice is to constantly be growing through your outside interests in an active way that later can become something more."

**Network like there's no tomorrow.** "Those most successful in making career changes are those who maintain an elaborate network of people they know outside the industry," says Dr. Cates. "Cultivate contacts in the community, at the PTA or at your kid's sports league. That's how you get referred and that's how you hear about opportunities an outsider would never know about."

**Create a slush fund.** Career change can sometimes be an expensive proposition. Tuition, downtime without pay, business start-up costs and relocation expenses can all be major roadblocks if you don't have ready cash. "I always tell people, especially young lawyers, to never live on their entire income," says Hulvershorn. If you spend all your money and save none of it, you are basically denying yourself the freedom to explore new possibilities.

Hulvershorn suggests that people try not to expand their lifestyle expenses every time they get a raise. "Instead, put that money into an interest-bearing account that will buy you the freedom you'll need five years down the road when it's time for a change.

**Be prepared.** "Keep your resumé constantly up-to-date," says Dr. Cates. "And keep an eye on the want ads. This not only makes it easier to make the leap when the time is right, it also gets you into a career-change mind-set."

**Never think it's too late.** "People are always asking me if it's too late to make a career change," says Hulvershorn. Her reply is simple: "You're still breathing aren't you?"

# CHANGE AND ADAPTABILITY

## Dare to Be Different

Imagine if you went out to dinner with your friends every Wednesday night at the same restaurant, ate the same food and talked about the same things. Then suppose you went home and watched the same old TV programs while you painted your nails the same color you've worn for years. Pretty boring, huh?

Sure, most of us don't get that deeply entrenched in ruts, but more than a few women could use a booster shot of spontaneity and a splash of change in their lives, doctors say. For as much as we like routine, occasionally altering course can prevent us from feeling like life is passing us by.

"Staying flexible will keep you from falling into too many ruts," says William Rakowski, Ph.D., of the Center for Gerontology and Health Care Research in the Department of Community Health at Brown University in Providence, Rhode Island. "Leaving room in your life for new things certainly keeps a spark burning within you that helps keep you creative and motivated."

"On the other hand, it's far too easy to say to yourself that you can't change your life because you're getting old," says Dr. Rakowski. "What you're really telling yourself when you say something like that is the future is locked into place, and there's nothing you can do to change it. That could be a warning sign that you're giving up too much control of your life. Don't let stuffiness get the better of you."

## Why We Resist

If you look at your daily life, it's probably very structured. "Most people have their alarms set at a certain time. They take the same route to work, see the same people, watch the same TV programs or listen to the same radio stations day after day," says John Putzier, a Pittsburgh management consultant

453

who conducts seminars nationwide on the importance of change and adaptability. "That's not necessarily bad because routine is comfortable, and most people do like feeling comfortable in their lives. But as a result, it makes it more difficult for them to adapt to change as they get older."

To illustrate his point, Putzier often asks his seminar participants to trade seats with another person in the room. "They don't want to do it. You can't believe the resistance that people have to doing something that simple. In a matter of 30 minutes, they've established their turf. They literally think 'This is my seat and I'm not going to give it up,'" Putzier says. "I ask them, 'If you can't handle this, how do you think you're going to react when somebody comes in and changes your job or expects you to do something in your life differently?'"

Lack of self-esteem—all too common for women to begin with—is one of the major roadblocks to change, says Sidney B. Simon, Ed.D., counselor and professor emeritus of psychological education at University of Massachusetts–Amherst and author of *Getting Unstuck: Breaking Through Your Barriers to Change*. A woman, for example, may not believe that she is good enough to have what she really wants or she may think she doesn't have the skills or willpower to change.

Other women's resolve withers away because they don't get support from family or friends, or they are perfectionists who avoid making a change because they are waiting for an ideal moment or situation that never will occur, Dr. Simon says.

But fear of losing control—which can be experienced by loss of finances, status or respect—is, by far, the most common reason that women resist change. "Fear can be paralyzing. It keeps us stuck in our old ways," says Susan Olson, Ph.D., director of psychological services at the Southwest Bariatric Nutrition Center in Tempe, Arizona. "As we age, we begin to realize that life is bigger than we are, and we don't have control over a lot of things. So we start to treasure our little routines and convince ourselves that we are safe within those limits."

## Overcoming the Barriers

"That old saying isn't true; an old dog *can* be taught new tricks, but you have to want to learn," Dr. Olson says. "We can change our thoughts. We can change our actions. We can change our relationships. We don't have to be stuck within our boundaries if they no longer serve us."

"Change doesn't occur overnight," Dr. Olson says. "But if you're persistent, you can learn plenty of ways to limber up your mental flexibility." Here's how.

**Have a few laughs.** Take a moment each day to laugh at yourself and the world around you, Dr. Olson suggests. Laughter will help you enjoy your day and open up creative ways of seeing the world.

**Break the rules.** "Most of us have learned that if you have some free time, you should be doing something productive. But ask yourself 'Who wrote that rule in the first place?'" Dr. Olson says. "So if you've cleaned your house every

Wednesday night for the past 15 years, why not skip it one night and do something frivolous like going to an amusement park?"

**Be a leader of the pack.** Break away from the crowd and wear a new outfit. Who knows, you might start a fashion trend. Go to a different type of movie than you've ever seen. "The point is, don't be a follower," Dr. Olson says. "Make your life a unique piece of art."

**Make the stars shine on you.** "Make a schedule of your daily activities and put a star next to activities you like and a check by activities you don't enjoy. Is there a balance? If not, maybe it's time to make some changes so you get some fun and excitement into your life," Dr. Olson says.

**Know what friends are for.** If you're trying to change an attitude or break a habit, tell a friend or relative about it. Ask them to point out any time you fall into your old patterns, says Rebecca Curtis, Ph.D., professor of psychology at Adelphi University in Garden City, New York, and author of *How People Change.*

**Do it his way for a day.** "Many fights in relationships are over toilet paper and toothpaste," Dr. Olson says. "Why not relax your standards for a day and try it the other person's way. You might find out they had a better idea after all."

**Walk a mile in their shoes.** "If you have difficulty understanding another person's point of view, close your eyes and imagine that you're that person," Dr. Curtis says. "If you work with a selfish man, for instance, try to imagine what it's like to be him." While this won't excuse his behavior, "once we start letting these feelings into our consciousness, we realize that we're all human, we all have insecurities and we all have the potential to express them in many different ways," Dr. Curtis says.

**Stop, look, listen.** When you feel that you're making a judgment, stop and ask yourself if you've considered all viewpoints. Do you really have enough information to make a reasonable conclusion, or are you making a decision based on your biases? "Listen to at least one other person who has a different viewpoint of the situation than you do. You might discover she has a point," says Dorothy Booth, Ph.D., assistant professor in the School of Nursing at the University of Michigan in Ann Arbor.

**Tune in.** Reprogram your car radio with new stations that you don't regularly listen to. Listen to the new stations—and none of the old ones—for a minimum of three weeks. "It's a mundane thing, but it teaches you to always be on the lookout for ways to break away from your habits and become comfortable with change. Get into the habit of not getting into habits," Putzier says.

**Plan to act.** No change is long-lasting unless you have a plan, Dr. Simon says. So on a sheet of paper, draw a four-column chart. Label the four sections "Do," "Get," "Be" and "Act." In the "Do" column, write down a goal like "I want to accept changes in my job." Under "Get," jot down the benefits of achieving that goal, such as "less stress" or "my boss will appreciate my cooperation." In the next column, write down a one-word description of how you'll have to be to reach your goal. In this case, "open-minded." In the last column, list the actions you'll have to take, such as "I need to write a computer program to keep track of the new information my supervisor wants me to gather now." Writing down your plan will make it more likely that you'll follow through on it. "That list is so important that I'd laminate it and carry it in my wallet instead of money," Dr. Simon says.

**Never say "can't."** Every time you say you can't do something, write it down. Then beside it, write down the same statement, but this time change "I can't" to "I won't."

" 'I can't' is a crippling statement. It takes control out of your hands. 'I won't' makes you realize you're making a choice," Dr. Olson says. "So if you say 'I can't go back to school,' try changing that to 'I won't go back to school because I'm too old.' Suddenly that empowers you—who really says you're too old?—and you might decide to enroll in some night classes."

**Forget perfection.** Many women who are rigid avoid making decisions because they fear making a wrong choice. "In their minds, a decision is all good or all bad," Dr. Olson says. If you feel that way, try making a small decision that doesn't feel perfect, like buying a magazine you've never read before. Chances are the world won't end if you don't like it. Try on the habit of congratulating yourself each time you make a "shades of gray" decision. This will help keep you focused away from perfection.

# CONFIDENCE AND SELF-ESTEEM

## Being Your Own Best Friend

**W**hen you picture yourself in your mind's eye, what do you see? Perhaps you see someone who is energetic, intelligent and successful, someone you'd want to be best friends with. Or maybe you see a woman somewhat battered by years, a woman whose most noticeable attributes are tiny creases around her eyes and dimples on her thighs.

It's amazing how just a few wrinkles or a little cellulite can shatter a woman's self-esteem—her appreciation and acceptance of her inner worth. A few minor signs of aging can also smash a woman's confidence—the faith she has in her abilities and talents. "Our culture places an extremely high premium on youth," says Bonnie Jacobson, Ph.D., director of the Institute for Psychological Change in New York City. "If you use youth as the only benchmark of how good you are, you will inevitably experience feelings of worthlessness and doubt as you show more signs of aging."

But this doesn't have to happen to you. Confidence and self-esteem really aren't matters of age or appearance, but of attitude. For some women, confidence and self-esteem only get stronger as they age, regardless of a few wrinkles, gray hairs or a dress size that has gone up over the years. And how fortunate these women are.

Confidence and self-esteem produce some very youth-engendering results. A confident, self-assured woman—despite whatever signs of aging she may show—looks, feels and carries herself like a much younger woman. She almost beams with inner strength and energy, says Thomas Tutko, Ph.D., professor of psychology at San Jose State University in California. The self-assured woman is also more likely to respect her body by eating right, getting exercise and avoiding harmful things like cigarettes, drugs and booze.

Confidence and self-esteem also do wonders for your mind. They provide a buffer against anxiety. They relieve feelings of guilt, hopelessness and inadequacy. They give us the courage to fulfill our dreams. And they give us a willingness to try new things, meet new challenges and widen our worlds, says Dr. Tutko.

Best of all, confidence and self-esteem are self-perpetuating; the benefits we derive from them tend to boomerang and bolster what we've got. In general, the stronger our feelings of confidence and self-esteem, the more satisfied we are with life. And that gives us the power not only to survive but also to embrace life.

# Why Do We Hate Math?

For years you've felt that you're just no good at math. Join the club, because many women feel that way, says Sylvia Beyer, Ph.D., assistant professor of psychology at the University of Wisconsin-Parkside in Kenosha.

Are women genetically inferior mathematicians? Not really, says Dr. Beyer. But over the years women have been conditioned, she says, to underestimate their abilities and to have lower expectations for themselves in math and in other traditionally male-oriented fields.

In her research Dr. Beyer has looked at mathematics test scores and performance expectations of both men and women. She has found that women tend to have lower performance expectations going into a math test than men. And afterward, women are much more likely to think they did worse on the test than they really did.

These findings may shed light on why few women attempt to pursue traditionally male-dominated subjects or careers, even if they have the skills to succeed. "Because they have been brought up to think that they aren't supposed to be good in a subject like math, many women will minimize their accomplishments even if they are successful," says Dr. Beyer. "They'll say that their performance was a fluke or come up with some other excuse. The danger of this type of thinking is that it could prevent some very talented women from ever pursuing an interest or a career in an area where they may have great potential or find a great deal of happiness."

The answer? Realize that you've been needlessly lowering your expectations all these years and know that there's probably no reason that you can't excel in mathematics, engineering, auto mechanics—or whatever you like.

# Messages from Within

It's hard to talk of confidence and self-esteem except as a package deal. "A person with high self-esteem has a good picture of herself, and that invariably inspires confidence," says Dr. Tutko. "Likewise, a strong belief in your abilities, and the positive attitude that comes with it, will boost your feelings of self-esteem."

Where do these feelings come from?

According to a study by Robert A. Josephs, Ph.D., and his associates at the University of Texas at Austin, men and women derive their confidence and self-esteem from different places. While a man's feelings of self-worth are more tied up with his achievements, a woman's are more likely linked to her interpersonal roles—how she sees herself as a wife, mother, daughter and friend.

It all goes back to our childhood years. "Boys are much more encouraged to learn skills and how to do things. Girls, on the other hand, are generally encouraged to develop pleasing personalities and to be pretty," says psychologist Nathaniel Branden, Ph.D., head of the Branden Institute for Self-Esteem in Beverly Hills and author of *The Six Pillars of Self-Esteem*. "The problem is that neither prettiness nor personality suggests any kind of competence or provides personal fulfillment and thus does not produce any real lasting sense of confidence or self-esteem."

# Hold Your Head Up

If you feel that your confidence and self-esteem could use a boost, that's probably a sign that they could. Here's what the experts recommend.

**Shape up.** Can working out improve your self-esteem? Yes, indeed. In one study at the State University of New York College at Brockport, 57 people were divided up into two groups: One group lifted weights for 16 weeks, while the other group completed a physical education theory course. Guess which group wound up with the lifted spirits?

Merrill J. Melnick, Ph.D., the sports sociologist who led the study, explains why the exercise group fared so much better: "You may see yourself as inferior if you're unhappy with your physical self." By building a little muscle and losing a little fat, he says, you can improve your feelings about your body and about yourself.

**Gag your internal critic.** Women with low self-esteem tend to hear a little voice in their heads. It says "You can't," "You're weak" and "You're worthless." Whenever your critical inner voice begins putting you down, silence it immediately, says Dr. Jacobson. Be aware of the times it's most likely to appear, such as when you're feeling down. Acknowledge that it's trying to hurt you. Then counter its arguments with assertions to the contrary. Tell yourself over and over that you are strong, capable and worthy until the voice goes away. The same rules apply for external critics, too. "You have to take away the power of other people by learning to accept yourself on your own terms," she says.

**Take a personal inventory.** "Instead of dwelling on our shortcomings, we need to draw satisfaction from the things we have and can do well," says Stanley Teitelbaum, Ph.D., a clinical psychologist in private practice in New York City. To do this, list all your achievements, activities, positive traits and strengths on one side of a piece of paper. Then list your weaknesses, negative traits and things you wish you could change about yourself on the other side. You may be surprised to learn just how many pluses you have in your favor. And this alone can make you feel remarkably good about yourself. Then, for long-term confidence and self-esteem, accentuate the positives and eliminate the negatives.

**Set up a hierarchy of goals.** Setting up unrealistic goals for yourself is sure to lead to failure, which can take a toll on your self-esteem. "Reaching for a goal is great, but you must learn to crawl before you can walk," says Dr. Tutko. Suppose you have a goal of bowling a 300 game. A worthy goal, but somewhat unrealistic if your average is, say, 58. Instead of shooting for your ultimate goal, concentrate on reaching plateaus: 100, 150, 200, 250, then 300. "Find success on one level first, then try to transfer it up to the next," he says.

**Specialize in something.** Are you a jack-of-all-trades and master of none? Are you involved with so many tasks that you can't give adequate attention to any? Spreading yourself too thin only sets you up for disappointment, says Dr. Tutko. Find two or three things in life that you really enjoy—be it playing the clarinet, working with computers or cross-country skiing—and focus most of your energies on them. It's better to be successful at a few things than to fail at many.

**Pursue what you love.** The easiest way to lose faith in yourself is to get trapped doing something that you dislike or that others tell you you're supposed to do, says Dr. Tutko. Rather than wallow in a career or activity that makes you miserable or that you attempt halfheartedly, seek out those things that really turn you on and pursue them with gusto. You're more likely to do them well, which will have a positive effect on your psyche.

**Be of service.** Lending your time and talents to help your community or people in need boosts confidence and self-esteem in many ways, says Dr. Jacobson. Foremost, it gives you a wonderful feeling of accomplishment and reinforces your belief that you are useful and worthwhile.

**Seek out positive people.** The last thing you need in your life when your self-confidence is flagging are people who criticize or find fault with you. Instead, you should surround yourself with people who look for the good in you. Invariably, those are people who themselves have high levels of confidence and self-esteem. "People with high self-esteem and confidence aren't quick to judge or put down others," says Dr. Jacobson. "They have a lot of love and encouragement to give, and their attitudes toward life can rub off on you."

**Reward yourself.** Stroke your confidence and self-esteem by doing something nice for yourself whenever you do something well, says Dr. Tutko. Congratulate yourself or treat yourself to a little gift. This reinforces your faith in yourself and gives the value of your accomplishment more weight.

**Act your age.** "Some people mistakenly believe that if they purchase all

# How Confident Are You?

Do you think highly of yourself, or do you see yourself as over-the-hill and going headlong into the valley of antiquity? It seems like a simple question, but it's not, says Thomas Tutko, Ph.D., professor of psychology at San Jose State University in California. Many women are vaguely aware that they have some kind of problem in their lives, but they can't quite put a handle on it.

Here are some signs that will tell you whether you have a problem with self-esteem.

- You are obsessed with your faults, foibles and mistakes and criticize yourself for them.
- You often let others put you down.
- You frequently try new hairdos, clothes, diets or gimmicks to make you more attractive or acceptable to others.
- You value the judgments and opinions of others more than your own.
- You frequently compare yourself and your accomplishments with others.
- You feel devastated by negative criticism.
- You become easily disillusioned.

Here are the warning signs of low self-confidence.

- Your daily routine rarely changes.
- You shy away from new challenges and uncomfortable situations.
- You rarely try things a second time.
- You always choose the safe over the risky.
- You measure success solely in terms of winning or acquiring.
- You can't express your inner wants and desires.
- You make up excuses for not doing things or to rationalize why things are the way they are.

the external trappings of youth, it will enhance the way they feel about themselves," says Dr. Teitelbaum. The truth is, you won't become a teenager again by mashing yourself into a napkin-size bikini. You'll probably look silly.

**Be *your* best, not *the* best.** Competitive sports are a great way to enhance your confidence and self-esteem. But if you consider beating opponents and winning trophies the only measure of success, your confidence and self-esteem are already on shaky ground. "Playing sports can be fantastic, but only if you do it for the sheer love of it and for the exploration of being the best you possibly can," says Dr. Tutko.

**Don't fear failure.** View failure not as an evil but as an opportunity for a new success, says Daniel Wegner, Ph.D., professor of psychology at the University of Virginia in Charlottesville. "Life is a trial-and-error process, and we don't make any progress if we don't take chances in the face of failure," he says. "In the grand scheme of things, most of the actual 'failures' we will experience are not nearly as harmful as the damage we do to ourselves when we obsess and worry about our failures yet to come."

**Deflate your worries.** Silencing your inner critic isn't always easy. Sometimes you can just slam the door on her; other times she puts up a fight. Sometimes the more you try to suppress unwanted thoughts and anxieties, the more likely you are to become obsessed by them, says Dr. Wegner. Instead of wasting energy suppressing unhappy thoughts, try giving in to them for a little bit. Schedule daily 30-minute "worry sessions" to get them out of your system; then get on with enjoying life.

**Get your kicks.** Did you ever consider learning a martial art? As a professor of psychology and director of the martial arts program at Wake Forest University in Winston-Salem, North Carolina, Charles L. Richman, Ph.D., strongly endorses the attitude-enhancing effects of martial arts. Like other sports, they will build you up and improve your body image, which by itself can improve your self-esteem, he says. Martial arts also tend to emphasize discipline and control. "When you combine this disciplined thinking with the mastering of new skills and the realization that you can defend yourself from physical attack, you experience an amazing transformation in both confidence and self-esteem," says Dr. Richman. Check your Yellow Pages or newspaper for schools in your area.

# COSMETIC DENTISTRY

## Something to Smile About

You've always been ready with a quip and a grin, and people respond to your warmth. But lately, even when you feel like smiling, you catch yourself covering your mouth with your hand. You're just not happy about what the years have done to your teeth.

If your teeth aren't what they once were, don't despair. Cosmetic dentistry can often take years off your smile. A cosmetic dentist can remove the stains that reveal lifetime habits of coffee and cigarettes. If you've lost teeth along the way, the dentist can replace them. She can also fix chips and cracks and build up surfaces to counteract the wear that comes from decades of gnawing steak or chomping ice.

It's all about looking young, fit and healthy instead of down in the mouth. And today's cosmetic dentistry doesn't mean a jaw full of teeth that look like Chiclets. Results can be so natural that no one will ever know your secret.

## Getting Back the Gleam

By the time you reach your mid-thirties, that pearly smile has probably lost some of its gleam. Teeth tend to yellow over the years as tiny cracks in the enamel soak up stains from coffee, tea, wine, tobacco and food dyes. Fortunately, these age-related stains bleach away very well, says Stephen Sylvan, D.M.D., associate professor of dentistry at the State University of New York at Stony Brook and a dentist in New York City.

Your dentist can offer two good bleaching alternatives.

At-home bleaching takes commitment, but it's a simple process. Your dentist sends you home with a custom-fitted mold of your teeth and a bottle of buffered peroxide gel. You fill the mold with the gel and wear it for three hours daily (usually after dinner or overnight) for two weeks. The cost of the procedure ranges from $150 to $500 for either your uppers or your lowers. (Many people bleach just the uppers, since they show most when you smile.)

If you want faster results, or dislike wearing the mold, you can ask your dentist for an in-office power bleaching. Your dentist can place a rubber dam over your teeth to protect the gums and apply a stronger peroxide solution that is activated by five to ten minutes under a high-intensity light. After two to four sessions a few weeks apart, at a cost of around $200 per visit, your teeth will look years younger, says Dr. Sylvan. The treatment itself is painless, but some people experience slight tooth sensitivity for a few days afterward.

Dr. Sylvan points out that there are also over-the-counter bleaching products available, but he doesn't recommend them. They can be too abrasive on teeth and too harsh on gums, and their effectiveness is questionable, he says.

## Take Cover—Quickly

Severe stains—like those you get from taking the antibiotic tetracycline (such as Achromycin) as a kid—may be too tough for bleaching to tackle. That's where veneers come in. Ultra-thin porcelain veneers can cover even the worst of stains as well as fix up chipped and poorly spaced teeth.

Veneers are eggshell-thin pieces of porcelain, but hardly delicate. They are carved, colored and custom-shaped to the tooth they'll cover and then are attached by a process called bonding. The underside of the veneer and surface of the tooth are "etched"—painted with a mild acid that microscopically roughens the surface. Then, the surfaces are fused with a type of resin that hardens under a high-intensity light. The process doesn't hurt and can often be accomplished without the need for anesthetic.

"The bonding of the veneer is so strong that the porcelain becomes an integral part of the tooth," says George Freedman, D.D.S., director of the programs in postgraduate esthetic dentistry at Case Western Reserve University in Cleveland and Baylor College of Dentistry in Dallas.

Making the veneer look natural is an art, says Dr. Freedman. "We can create a whole variety of true-to-life shades and even do a gradient of natural-looking colors on a single tooth. You really can't tell a veneer from a natural tooth, even close up."

Veneers can also be made slightly longer or wider than a tooth to fill in small gaps or improve a lousy smile. Prices for veneers range greatly—from $350 to $2,500—depending on the area of the country you live in or the severity of your dental problem. But they can last more than ten years, depending on how well you take care of them.

## Going for the Heavy Guns

A veneer may not be able to correct severely decayed, misshapen or badly positioned teeth, but a crown or a bridge can. Where a veneer is a very thin covering, a crown (or cap) is thicker and heavier and requires grinding down the tooth it will be attached to. A crown is made of porcelain, metal or a combination of the two and then cemented onto a tooth. A bridge is two or more connected crowns.

You and your dentist will need to decide between all porcelain or porcelain over metal. Porcelain usually looks more natural when there's no metal behind it, but you may need the metal base for back teeth, where the pressure from chewing is greater, says Irwin Smigel, D.D.S., president of the American Society for Dental Aesthetics.

And some new porcelains are so good that they look convincing even over metal. "It used to be that the metal backing always made the crown look artificial," says Barry G. Dale, D.M.D., a cosmetic and general dentist in Englewood, New Jersey. "But the new porcelains provide close-to-lifelike quality."

What's the procedure like? Your dentist first gives you a local anesthetic. Then he grinds down about 1½ millimeters of your tooth (otherwise, you'd have something fatter than the original tooth, which would look out of place and

## Lifelike Dentures That Don't Budge

You need a partial or complete denture to fill in your missing teeth, but you gag at the thought. You'd feel like your grandmother. Then how about new, natural-looking teeth that are permanently attached to your jaw?

It's possible with dental implants. "Implants, because they're fixed in your mouth, are akin to having your own teeth," says Albert Guckes, D.D.S., deputy clinical director of the National Institute of Dental Research.

Here's how they work.

A tiny metal cylinder—made of lightweight titanium, the same metal used for replacement hips—is surgically placed into your jawbone. Then a thin metal post is screwed into the cylinder. This part of the procedure, usually done under local anesthesia, will leave your mouth sore and swollen for about a week.

The next part of the procedure takes place about six months later. By then, bone has grown tightly around the metal cylinder. It's in rock solid. Your new artificial tooth is mounted onto the metal post.

For each implant post you'll pay between $750 and $1,500. Then you ante up for the replacement teeth—usually an additional $1,000 each. That's a lot of loot. But given that implants can last up to 20 years, you may consider them a worthwhile investment, Dr. Guckes says.

could irritate the gum). During a second visit he cements the custom-shaped crown or crowns into place.

Crowns cost between $450 and $1,000 each. They generally last 10 to 15 years.

How will your mouth feel after a crown is in place? "It's a foreign body, so it's natural that the bite may feel a little strange," Dr. Smigel says. But if after a week you're still experiencing discomfort, check back with your dentist to have the fit adjusted.

# Shopping for a Dentist

Needless to say, any cosmetic procedure is only going to be as good as the dentist who does it. You might ask a friend who has undergone cosmetic dental procedures for her recommendations.

Or you could contact the American Society for Dental Aesthetics (ASDA).

## Are You Big Enough for Braces?

Braces aren't just kid stuff anymore. "They are appropriate for people of almost any age," says Mervin W. Graham, D.D.S., an orthodontist in private practice in Denver whose oldest patient with braces is 65.

But at any age, braces work the same way. Here's how, according to Dr. Graham: The braces' tightened wires and rubber band elastics push on your teeth. Bone on one side of a tooth's root breaks down, allowing the tooth to move. And bone builds up on the other side of the tooth, assuring that it will fit snugly into its new home.

The process starts with a fitting, after which you'll need to visit your orthodontist for regular adjustments. Your teeth will be somewhat sore for a few days after each visit. Depending on how much your teeth are misaligned, the time you'll need to wear your braces can vary from one to several years.

The price of braces will depend on the severity of the correction, but generally ranges from $1,800 to $4,500.

If you decide to make the investment, don't worry—nobody will call you Metalmouth. When you were a kid, braces used to mean good-size stainless steel straps and bands around each tooth. But these days, you can be fitted with tiny brackets made of steel or even nearly invisible tooth-colored porcelain, says Dr. Graham.

"Dentists applying for membership present before-and-after cases before the society's board," says Diana Okula, ASDA secretary. "And they're judged not only on how good the results are functionally but also on how the results look."

Write to the ASDA at 635 Madison Avenue, New York, NY 10022. Enclose a self-addressed, stamped envelope, and they'll send you a list of recommended dentists in your area.

# COSMETIC SURGERY

## *A High-Tech Answer to Aging*

Is it still a secret rite of the Beautiful People? Hardly. Any woman may consider a surgical solution to unwanted signs of aging. And a lot of them are—at earlier ages than you might expect.

"We have a youth-oriented, physically fit society," says Alan Matarasso, M.D., a plastic surgeon at the Manhattan Eye, Ear and Throat Hospital. "Every time you see a cola commercial with a 12-year-old girl dressed up to look like an adult, that subtly increases the pressure on all of us."

Many women are fascinated by the idea of turning back the clock surgically, Dr. Matarasso says. "Anyone who's ever looked in the mirror and been concerned about getting older will consider it at some point."

"All the same, we should never take it lightly," Dr. Matarasso says. "For certain people, cosmetic surgery wouldn't be right."

If you're more than just curious, it's important to recognize first what cosmetic surgery will *not* do. It won't turn you into a supermodel or make you the life of the party. It may make you look younger, but you'll need realistic expectations of the outcome, as well as money, since most health insurance plans cover only part of the bill.

And be sure you're not opting for the scalpel when a more conservative treatment might do. The fine lines and blotchy texture caused by moderate sun damage can be treated very effectively in a dermatologist's office. She may offer you light chemical peels, dermabrasion, wrinkle-filling injections or a prescription for the popular wrinkle-eraser, tretinoin (Retin-A). (For tips on these approaches, see Wrinkles, page 384.)

But you may be distressed by more significant changes in your appearance. Heredity, serious sun worship, repeated lose-and-gain-it-back diets or just the years of yielding to gravity may have caused deep wrinkles, a pouchy jawline, a sagging neck or baggy eyelids. In these cases, you may wonder about cosmetic surgery.

Surgical techniques have been refined and simplified over the years, and most cosmetic procedures involve a lot less trauma than they used to. Sometimes a local anesthetic is all that's needed, or tranquilizers plus a local to put you in "twilight sleep"—a sort of dozy fog you hardly remember afterward. Recovery times are shorter than they used to be, but they vary widely depending on the individual, the procedure and the surgeon. Any discomfort is easily handled with analgesics, surgeons say.

## Resculpting the Face

Forget the tight masks of Hollywood fame. Today's cosmetic surgery can offer very natural-looking, subtle corrections for many age-related changes. Here's what it can do.

**Lift a weary brow.** When your forehead muscles slump, you can look tired all over. A forehead lift will smooth a slouching brow and ease deep crow's-feet and frown lines, says Dr. Matarasso. "This procedure is virtually painless," he says. "All stitches are hidden in the hairline, and though you may have swelling along the cheeks and some bruising, you could go back to work in 48 hours."

**Banish baggy eyes.** You're not feeling tired, but bags under the eyes or sagging lids may make you look that way. Eye surgery called blepharoplasty offers the most dramatic change of all cosmetic surgery procedures, says Michael Sachs, M.D., a plastic surgeon in private practice in New York City. Though the under-eye work is usually done with a scalpel, he has developed a simpler method called fat-melting blepharoplasty. Using a heated probe and a tiny incision, the surgeon vaporizes the water content of the fatty pouches, melting away eye bags instantly. Saggy upper lids can be partially corrected with the fat-melting technique, Dr. Sachs says, but excess skin on upper lids must still be surgically trimmed.

**Shape the nose.** Nowadays most nose repairs (rhinoplasties) are done without fracturing the bone, Dr. Matarasso says. The results of today's rhinoplasties are much more natural than the piggy-looking, scooped-out, turned-up and pinched-in look common in the sixties. Some of the changes of aging, such as the nose drooping toward the upper lip or thickening at the tip, are corrected with delicate sculpting of the cartilage from incisions inside the nose, he says.

**Smooth a sagging jawline.** Where bone has thinned along the jawline, the overlying skin may begin to sag. A solid silicone implant can be inserted from a small incision within the mouth, says Geoffrey Tobias, M.D., a plastic surgeon at Mount Sinai School of Medicine of the City University of New York. The implant firms the jaw profile, giving skin a less jowly drape and a smoother line. "These implants are solid and do *not* contain the liquid silicone that caused problems in the past," Dr. Tobias says. "The solid implants don't budge."

**Find the fallen apples.** Solid silicone implants may also be used to fill out hollow cheeks. Whether you exercise fanatically or are just naturally on the slim side, you may have discovered that the "apples" of your cheeks are vanishing as you age, leaving gaunt hollows. If these mid-face depressions make you feel haggard rather than fit and lean, consider the implants, Dr. Tobias says.

**Lift the face.** Ever tugged your facial skin up and back to see what a face-lift might do? You looked younger in the mirror, sure, but also sort of stiff. A stretched-looking face-lift used to be the norm, but techniques have changed, with gratifyingly natural results. "In the past, they'd tighten only the skin, which gave that masklike look," says Dr. Matarasso. "Now face-lifts are customized to each person's anatomy. Sometimes we hardly pull the skin and just work underneath, removing fat and tightening the layers of muscle to give a youthful jawline."

**Firm the neck.** A lower face-lift concentrates on a sagging neck or double chin, says Dr. Matarasso. The surgeon removes excess skin, tightens cords of muscle and removes fat to resculpt the chin into a firmer shape. "Stitches are hidden behind the ear," he says. "Some people just have the neck lift, and some do both the neck and face."

## What about the Rest of You?

If you're a mother, you may have special body concerns as you age, says Dr. Matarasso. Though many bodies droop with age, the sag is especially noticeable after childbirth. Both breasts and abdomen are stretched by pregnancy, and in some women the skin stays lax afterwards. The glandular structure of the breasts loses volume, and they may sink considerably. And that rounded belly? Women lack a muscle fascia, or covering, in the lower abdomen. The stresses of pregnancy increase this weakness tremendously, Dr. Matarasso says, producing a hard-to-flatten bulge. Here's what can be done.

**Restore youthful breasts.** Plastic surgeons define a youthful breast as one with the nipple "at or above the lower breast crease when viewed from the side," Dr. Matarasso says. During a breast lift, incisions are made in the crease beneath the breast and around the outer edge of the nipple. The surgeon tightens the gland and removes excess skin during the procedure, which is generally performed on a outpatient basis, he says. You'll be asleep with the same kinds of anesthetic gases used during some dental procedures, he says.

If your quest is breast enlargement, the path is paved with painful questions in the aftermath of the serious debates over liquid silicone implants. While experts continue to evaluate silicone's safety, saline implants are still available.

**Flatten the abdomen.** Popularly called the tummy tuck, there are really four types of abdomen-flattening surgeries, Dr. Matarasso says. A fat-suctioning technique called liposuction actually removes stubborn pockets of fat. A mini-abdominoplasty uses liposuction along with a pubic-hairline incision (the same often used for Caesarean births) to tighten muscles and remove a wedge of ex-

# Choosing a Cosmetic Surgeon

First, ask around. Often a tip from a friend who's satisfied with her own cosmetic surgery will lead you to a good surgeon. But be sure to go beyond word of mouth and check any doctor's credentials. Find a surgeon who is certified by the American Society of Plastic and Reconstructive Surgeons by writing the organization at 444 East Algonquin Road, Arlington Heights, IL 60005. Or, call a county or state medical society or nearby teaching hospital and ask for referrals. Also, don't hesitate to ask for telephone numbers of other women who have already undergone the procedure you're thinking about.

Help yourself to make the decision by asking yourself if your expectations are realistic, says Michael Sachs, M.D., a plastic surgeon in private practice in New York City. "Cosmetic surgery can improve your appearance and help you make the most of your assets, but it won't cure an ailing relationship or promise you a promotion," he says.

Then, when you go for your first appointment, start with these basic questions, he suggests.

*What's my problem?* Can the doctor pinpoint exactly what is making you look older than you'd like?

*How will this procedure help?* Exactly what is involved in the procedure the doctor is recommending? What steps will be followed, and how long will it take? What kind of anesthesia and pain relief will be offered?

*Will I have a noticeable scar?* Will there be any visible scars left after the healing process is over?

*How risky is it?* What could go wrong? How likely are any complications?

*What will I look like afterward?* Can the doctor give you a realistic idea of what this surgery will do for you?

*What's it going to cost?* Will your insurance pay for part of it? How much will the total bill be?

If you have lingering questions, don't hesitate to ask for a second appointment, says Dr. Matarasso. "And watch out for slick promoters," he says. "Chances are, they're not out for your benefit."

---

cess skin. A modified abdominoplasty uses a bikini-line incision to correct pouching or fullness above and below the navel. And if the entire abdomen is to be treated, the surgeon will extend the bikini line incision several inches at both ends. (For tips on liposuction, see "Is Liposuction for You," page 97.)

# CREATIVITY

## *Keeping Mind and Body in Tune*

Painting with watercolors is creative. So is writing a symphony, directing a play, or sculpting a fountain.

But creativity is not limited to the arts. Planting a garden is creative, as is designing a computer program, developing a new recipe, planning a meal, mapping genes or building a gingerbread house with a bunch of kids.

Simply put, creativity is defined as the act of making, inventing or producing. And it's something we all do.

"I call everyday creativity mindfulness—when we focus on the process of inventing as opposed to the outcome. This everyday creativity or mindfulness is actually good for one's health and well-being," explains Ellen J. Langer, Ph.D., professor of psychology at Harvard University in Cambridge, Massachusetts, and author of *Mindfulness*.

It's so essential to our existence that the newness, surprise and variety provided by our creativity actually fuels our will to live. Dr. Langer's research with the elderly has shown that when the elderly are encouraged to be creative or mindful, as she says, they actually live longer and happier lives. "When we don't keep our minds active, the mind and body gradually turn themselves off," says Dr. Langer.

In other words, when we stop creating, we stop living.

Fortunately, the capacity to create remains intact all our lives, although the actual number of certain types of products we might create—the paintings, gardens or sculptures—may decline as we get older.

"Creative productivity generally peaks at age 30 for math, science, poetry and anything that requires abstract thinking," says Carolyn Adams-Price, Ph.D., assistant professor of psychology at Mississippi State University in Starkville. "For history, philosophy, writing and anything that requires a lot of knowledge, it generally peaks at 60."

472

# Killers of the Creative Spirit

Some days creativity flows through your body and out into the world without effort. Other days it's as though the flow is blocked by an impenetrable wall.

"Creativity is a fragile commodity that can be suppressed or impaired much easier than it can be turned on," says Teresa Amabile, Ph.D., professor of psychology at Brandeis University in Waltham, Massachusetts.

But, she says, you can prevent interfering with its flow by avoiding these creativity killers.

• Naysayers. Critics and skeptics can limit your scope of thought and shatter your creative progress.
• Material motivation. Most creative motivation comes from within, but extrinsic motivators—like money, fame, awards and acceptance— can severely dampen our creative powers.
• Keeping score. The pressure of having to score points, meet certain standards or live up to others' expectations can seriously stifle your creative abilities.
• Creating in a crowd. How creative could you be if you knew your teacher, boss or the whole world was looking over your shoulder every minute? Dr. Amabile's research has shown that such environments can stifle creativity. Try to work in a setting that will put some distance between you and a pair of penetrating eyes.
• Too little time. Clocks, schedules and deadlines can hinder the evolution of a great idea. Try working at a comfortable, even pace.
• Drugs and alcohol. There is no good scientific evidence that creativity can be chemically enhanced. In the long run, these substances have the potential to destroy your creative abilities far more than they could possibly enhance them.

But it's only the number of creative products that declines, not the ability to create or the quality of what's produced, emphasizes Dr. Adams-Price.

## A History of Suppression

Until the last half of the twentieth century, the education and training that would allow women to express their creativity was often discouraged by cultural stereotypes that defined and limited a woman's role in the world.

Virginia Woolf, for instance, imagined William Shakespeare to have had an equally creative sister, Judith, who was sent to mend stockings or fix dinner while Will was sent to school to study literature and drama.

Historically, men have had a distinct advantage over women when it comes to getting help in developing their creativity.

Studies show that, more often than not, society has been quicker to provide men with educational possibilities and admission to professional societies and other specialized training to stimulate their creativity. Studies show, too, that teachers have more readily tended to reinforce creative behavior in boys while expecting girls to be well behaved and eager to follow the rules. Experts have also suggested that our culture's encouragement of a boy's natural assertiveness, dominance, ego and risk taking—in everything from football to physics—helps young men to develop the drive, single-mindedness and persistence necessary to pursue their own creative visions in a culture often hostile to creativity.

## Tapping Your Powers of Imagination

Today, women are well represented in art galleries, theaters, dance ensembles, medical schools, businesses and other institutions. In fact, the numbers of women in art and ballet schools now exceed the numbers of men.

How can you liberate the creativity hidden within you? Whether you're intent on creating a public work of art or a private expression of your inner self, all it takes to get started is an idea and a desire to explore. Here's how to begin.

**Identify a problem.** Ask yourself: "What could the world really use right now? Creative alternatives to nursing homes for the elderly? Ways to capitalize on the talent of retired individuals?" Often, the first step merely requires identifying a problem, says Dr. Langer. From there your ideas can branch off in hundreds of different directions.

A great way to come up with good ideas is to think up many ideas without judging them. Then simply choose the good ones, says Dr. Langer.

Scribble out an idea on a sheet of paper. Then, drawing inspiration from the first idea, jot down as many related ideas as possible. Compile a list of ideas, go through it carefully and pull out the ones you like best. Discard the others.

"Sometimes a great idea is merely taking an older idea and turning it on its head," says Gabriele Rico, Ph.D., professor of English and creative arts at San Jose State University in California and author of *Pain and Possibility*. For example, ice cream was once served on top of a flat waffle. But some innovative thinker chose to fold that waffle into a funnel, and voilà! The world had its first waffle cone.

**Jot down your ideas and dreams.** Great ideas can materialize and vanish in an instant, so many creative women keep a log or diary to record ideas that come to them throughout the day, says Dr. Rico. All you need is a small notebook that fits in your pocket or briefcase or even under your pillow, since dreams can be rich in creativity, too.

## Creativity and Madness

Isadora Duncan danced in the moonlight with fairies. Vincent van Gogh cut off his ear. Sylvia Plath committed suicide.

Does this mean that highly creative people are more likely to be mad than the rest of us?

It's an intriguing question. But despite the best efforts of science, the answer is still not clear.

In a study of more than 1,000 men and women conducted at the University of Kentucky in Lexington, researcher Arnold M. Ludwig, M.D., found that poets, writers, artists, musicians and others in creative professions were more likely to exhibit a tendency toward madness than others in supposedly less creative professions—people who were public officials, in business and were military officers.

Those in the theater demonstrated higher rates of alcohol and drug abuse, manic episodes, anxiety disorders and suicide attempts. Writers were more inclined toward depression and alcohol. Artists had more alcohol-related problems, depression, anxiety and adjustment difficulties. Musicians and composers were more likely to be depressed. Poets were more prone to alcohol and drug abuse, depression, mania, suicide and psychosis in general.

The tendency toward madness in creative people seems clear until you consider a couple of points, as Dr. Ludwig does in his study. First, the demands on those in the more creative professions may be more likely to aggravate already existing problems. If you were genetically predisposed to depression, for example, a career in the theater might push you over the edge into depression, while a career as a banker might not.

A second point is that since our culture expects its writers and artists to be weird and its military officers and bankers to be stable, professions such as music and art may simply attract people who are predisposed to excess, while professions such as banking and the military attract people who are more likely to be stable.

"The mind makes some of its most unique connections and associations while you are asleep," says Dr. Rico. So start the day off by scribbling what you remember of your dreams on a note pad.

**Reconsider failures.** Mistakes and unexpected results can yield the biggest rewards of all, says Dr. Langer. For example, a new glue developed by the 3M Company was thought to be a failure because it wasn't sticky enough. But when that glue was applied to a sheet of paper, it became one of the most innovative office products of all time: Post-it Notes. So the next time you have an apparent "bomb" on your hands, don't be so quick to condemn it. Instead, turn it around and look at it from another direction.

**Challenge orthodox thinking.** "One of our society's drawbacks is that it encourages inhibition and blind conformity," says Dr. Langer. "We become afraid to look at the world from different perspectives to challenge established ideas." To enhance our creativity, we must be willing to unlearn many of the conventions we've spent a lifetime learning.

A creative person should not be afraid to challenge ideas or to think in directions others may consider unorthodox.

**Learn.** If you've chosen to express your creativity in a particular medium such as paint or song, learn as much about the medium as possible, says Dr. Rico. Start slowly, practice in your medium regularly and identify your strengths and weaknesses. As your familiarity and skill increase, your ability to manipulate your chosen medium to express your creativity will expand.

**Find a role model.** You can draw a great deal of inspiration by emulating the work and techniques of some of the creative giants in your area of interest, says Dr. Rico. But don't be a copycat. Imitation is not creativity. Instead, turn to your role model to get yourself thinking in ways you never considered. Or take themes they have explored and approach them from another angle.

**Explore yourself.** The creative woman must be willing to delve into a wide range of deep-seated emotions, experiences and memories. "Older people often use their personal experience as a source of creativity," says Dr. Adams-Price.

**Explore the world.** Most of us draw inspiration and creative energy from the things around us: the sight of a sunset, the aroma of a flower, the sound of a train whistle, the touch of moss. "The more things we know, feel and experience about our world, the more creative we will be," says Dr. Rico.

# FIBER

## Staying Young Inside and Out

It's hard to admit sometimes, but it's starting to look like Mom really did know best. Okay, so maybe that haircut she forced you to get in the sixth grade wasn't exactly cool. But just about everything else she made you do was right on the money. Like when she had you start your day with oatmeal. And when she filled a corner of your dinner plate with cooked carrots and told you to have an apple instead of a brownie for dessert.

Today, science has proven what Mom always said: There's something special about fruits, vegetables and grains that really does a woman's body good. She called it roughage. Nutritionists call it dietary fiber, and it's one of the simplest and most potent weapons we have in our age-erasing arsenal.

Fiber is a front-line warrior in the battle against heart disease, breast and other cancers, atherosclerosis, high cholesterol, high blood pressure, constipation, digestive problems, diabetes and even overweight. Get enough fiber and your body will be healthier and run like a well-oiled machine.

But most women don't get enough fiber. The recommended intake is 25 grams of fiber every day. "Most Americans, however, only consume about one-third of that total," says Diane Grabowski, R.D., nutrition educator at the Pritikin Longevity Center in Santa Monica, California.

## Nature's Cure

Fiber is a complex mixture of indigestible substances that makes up the structural material of plants. It has very few calories and provides little food energy to the body. When we ingest it, it passes through our system without being broken down.

Fiber works its magic by carrying the bad stuff—like cholesterol, bile acids and other toxins—out of our system. And it comes in two basic forms: soluble, which dissolves in water, and insoluble, which doesn't. Most plant foods contain both types of fiber, though certain foods are richer in one or the other.

The coarser, insoluble fibers really live up to the word *roughage*. "They literally scour you out," says David Jenkins, M.D., Ph.D., director of the Clinical Nutrition and Risk Factor Modification Center at St. Michael's Hospital, University of Toronto. "Once inside the body they absorb water, making stools softer, bulkier and easier to pass. This keeps food moving through the intestinal tract."

It also makes a natural remedy for such ills as constipation, irritable bowel syndrome, diverticulosis and hemorrhoids.

Soluble fibers act differently. Inside the body they become gummy and sticky. As they move through the digestive tract, they pick up bile acids and other toxins, then haul them out of the body.

## Squaring Off against Disease

Fiber plays a vital role in the offensive against heart disease and atherosclerosis. Studies have shown that a diet high in soluble fiber reduces blood levels of low-density lipoprotein (LDL) cholesterol, the so-called bad cholesterol. A study by Dr. Jenkins found that high intakes of soluble fiber continued to lower cholesterol even after dietary reductions of fat and cholesterol had been achieved.

"Cholesterol builds up in our blood and clogs arteries if it is not excreted as bile acids from our digestive tract," says Dr. Jenkins. "When soluble fiber carries these substances out of the body, it draws cholesterol out of the bloodstream to be converted into more bile, which we continue to flush out of the body—as long as we regularly consume soluble fiber."

Other studies have shown that fiber is effective at lowering blood pressure, thereby reducing your risk of heart attack and stroke.

That's not all fiber can do. Insoluble fiber is believed by doctors to be a key in preventing breast cancer, the most common cancer among women. How? By reducing estrogen levels. High levels of estrogen raise your risk of breast cancer.

A high-fiber diet also appears to lower your risk for colon and rectal cancer. It does this by diluting the concentration of bile acids and other carcinogens and moving stools quickly through the intestines, decreasing the time the colon wall is in contact with carcinogens. Also, fiber increases the acidity of the colon, making it less hospitable to cancer-causing toxins.

Fiber can also help you better manage diabetes by controlling blood sugar and thus reducing the need for insulin. Fiber delays the emptying of the stomach, causing the sugars in your food to be absorbed more gradually.

A fiber-filled diet makes weight loss a lot easier, too, because it fills you up—meaning you're going to eat a lot less of those fat-laden foods that put on the pounds. Fibrous foods provide robust mouthfuls that must be chewed thoroughly, slowing down your eating time. And they tend to have fewer calories in every bite.

# Bran: Where to Find a Lot of It

One sure-fire way to get a heap of fiber into your diet is by eating bran, the coarse outer layers of oats, wheat, rice and corn that contain the highest concentrations of fiber.

Consider oat bran, the bran that has received the most public attention in recent years. "What sets oat bran apart from other brans is that it is extremely high in a fiber called beta-glucan," says bran researcher Michael H. Davidson, M.D., medical director of the Chicago Center for Clinical Research at Rush Presbyterian-St. Luke's Hospital. "Beta glucan appears to be far more effective than other soluble fibers in lowering blood cholesterol levels."

How effective? Just two ounces of oat bran per day (a medium-size bowl) is enough to lower your LDL cholesterol 10 to 15 percent. The catch is that you have to eat oat bran daily; otherwise your cholesterol levels will creep back up.

Wheat bran is jam-packed with insoluble fiber, so it's the bran of choice for people with digestive problems. This is probably the most common bran, found in most bran breakfast cereals and all whole-wheat products.

Rice, oat and corn bran are high in both soluble and insoluble fiber.

Unless your physician says otherwise, the best bran plan for most women is to get a smattering of each. This way you'll get a healthy dose of soluble and insoluble fiber, not to mention some variety in your diet.

Getting your fill of bran is as easy as eating a bran breakfast cereal, a bran muffin or a whole-grain bread. But make sure you're always getting the goodness of the bran. "Refined grain products like white rice, white bread and most flour have had the fiber-rich bran removed in the milling process," says Grabowski. "Instant oatmeal, for example, has a lot less fiber than whole oats or pure oat bran."

# Adding Fiber to Your Life

Making the commitment to a high-fiber diet is relatively easy. Here are some tips.

**Ease into it.** As great as fiber is, too much too fast can have some nasty side effects including gas, bloating, diarrhea and cramps, says Dr. Jenkins. Start off your first week by increasing your intake by about five grams a day. Then take about a month to work up to the recommended level. From there, if your doctor says it's okay and if you feel no ill effects, you can increase your intake even more.

**Don't dry out.** We all know a high-fiber diet helps constipation, but if you don't get enough water, it can actually have an opposite effect and clog you up, says Dr. Jenkins. Drink eight to ten glasses of water a day to prevent constipation.

**Vary your sources.** Doctors aren't certain what ratio of soluble to insoluble you should use when choosing your daily 25 grams of fiber, says Dr. Jenkins, so it's probably wise to get an even dose of both. The best way to do that is to eat a wide variety of fiber-rich foods throughout the day.

*(continued on page 482)*

# GETTING ENOUGH:
# IT'S EASIER THAN YOU THINK

Does 25 grams of fiber a day seem impossible to consume? Not if you know where to get it. Here's some help.

| Food | Portion | Fiber (g.) |
|------|---------|------------|
| **BREADS AND BREAD PRODUCTS** | | |
| Whole-wheat | 1 slice | 2.1 |
| Pumpernickel | 1 slice | 1.9 |
| English muffin | 1 | 1.6 |
| Rye | 1 slice | 1.6 |
| Bagel | 1 | 1.2 |
| Waffle | 1 | 0.8 |
| White | 1 slice | 0.5 |
| | | |
| **FRUITS** | | |
| Strawberries, fresh | 1 cup | 3.9 |
| Dates | 5 medium | 3.5 |
| Orange | 1 | 3.1 |
| Apple, unpeeled | 1 | 3.0 |
| Applesauce | ½ cup | 1.9 |
| Pineapple, canned | 1 cup | 1.9 |
| Banana | 1 | 1.8 |
| Prunes | 3 medium | 1.8 |
| Cantaloupe, cubed | 1 cup | 1.3 |
| Grapes | 1 cup | 1.1 |
| Orange juice | ½ cup | 0.1 |
| | | |
| **VEGETABLES** | | |
| Brussels sprouts, cooked | ½ cup | 3.4 |
| Peas, frozen | ½ cup | 2.4 |
| Carrot, raw, 7½-inch | 1 | 2.3 |
| Broccoli, cooked | ½ cup | 2.0 |
| Green beans, frozen | ½ cup | 1.8 |
| Mushrooms, cooked | ½ cup | 1.7 |
| Tomato | 1 medium | 1.6 |
| Beets, canned | ½ cup | 1.4 |
| Iceberg lettuce, shredded | 1 cup | 1.4 |

| Food | Portion | Fiber (g.) |
|---|---|---|
| Corn, canned | ½ cup | 1.2 |
| Celery, chopped | ½ cup | 1.0 |
| **BEANS AND LEGUMES** | | |
| Black-eyed peas, boiled | ½ cup | 8.3 |
| Red kidney beans, canned | ½ cup | 7.9 |
| Chick-peas, canned | ½ cup | 7.0 |
| Pork and beans, canned | ½ can | 6.9 |
| Lentils, dried, cooked | ½ cup | 5.2 |
| Pinto beans, boiled | ½ cup | 3.4 |
| **BREAKFAST CEREALS** | | |
| All-Bran with Extra Fiber | ½ cup | 15.0 |
| Fiber One | ½ cup | 14.0 |
| Bran Buds | ⅓ cup | 11.0 |
| All-Bran (original) | ½ cup | 10.0 |
| Raisin Bran | 1 cup | 7.0 |
| Fiberwise | ⅔ cup | 5.0 |
| Grape-Nuts | ½ cup | 5.0 |
| Common Sense Oat Bran | ¾ cup | 4.0 |
| Cheerios (original) | 1 cup | 3.0 |
| Frosted Bran | ⅔ cup | 3.0 |
| Nutri-Grain Wheat | ⅔ cup | 3.0 |
| Spoon Size Shredded Wheat | ⅔ cup | 3.0 |
| Total (original) | ¾ cup | 3.0 |
| Wheaties | 1 cup | 3.0 |
| Puffed Rice | 1 cup | 1.2 |
| Product 19 | 1 cup | 1.0 |
| Special K | 1 cup | 1.0 |
| Rice Krispies | 1¼ cups | 1.0 |

**Go for the green.** Brans and grains are not your only source for fiber. "Don't forget your fresh fruits and vegetables," advises Grabowski. Legumes, beans, peas, salads and fruits can add a whole lot of the much-needed fiber to your diet. For some extra fiber, select fruits that have edible seeds, such as strawberries and kiwis, suggests Grabowski.

**Add a few sprinkles.** "Fiber is easy to obtain in your diet if you include whole foods such as whole-wheat bread, beans, peas and fresh fruits and vegetables," says Grabowski. But for additional fiber, pick up a box of oat bran at the grocery store and sprinkle it on yogurt, ice cream, fruit, breakfast cereal and salads. Use it in place of bread crumbs in meat loaf or stuffings or as a thickener for soups, stews and sauces. Or substitute oat bran for white flour in baked goods.

**Read labels carefully.** Don't assume that a product with the words "fiber," "bran" or "oats" in its title necessarily has the fiber content you're looking for. Always check the nutritional information on the box or bag to see just how much fiber is available in each serving. "Also, look for the word 'whole' to precede 'grain' on the ingredient list," suggests Grabowski. "This way you know nothing has been removed and you are sure to get the full benefit of the bran."

**Avoid fiber pills.** Fiber pills and drink mixes are a quick way to get more fiber, but most professionals don't recommend them, says Grabowski. They're expensive, and it takes several pills and drinks to equal the fiber content of a piece of fruit. Your best bet is to meet your fiber requirements by eating foods that are naturally rich in fiber.

**Go whole.** Slight changes in the way you eat can infuse your diet with fiber, says Grabowski. Instead of your morning glass of orange juice, try eating a whole piece of fruit, since almost all the fiber gets left behind in the juicing process. Serve whole brown rice instead of white. And if you like meat and potatoes, substitute a baked potato with the skin in place of mashed spuds.

**High fiber alone won't do.** You might think that eating fiber means you can eat more fat since fiber will cart the bad stuff out of your body. Not so. "A high-fiber diet doesn't somehow neutralize or balance out other unhealthy eating habits," says Dr. Davidson. "Eating an extra candy bar or cheeseburger only makes it harder for fiber to do its job. Fiber will only work when used in conjunction with a low-fat, low-cholesterol diet and plenty of exercise."

# FLUIDS

## *Go with the Flow*

There you are. A candlelit dinner for two. He reaches into the ice bucket, pulls out a carafe and fills your long-stemmed glass with . . . water.

What's all this? Just a colorless, no-cal liquid that packs a hefty age-erasing punch. Water is very much a part of us. Present in every cell and tissue, it plays a vital role in almost every biological process from digestion to respiration to circulation. It transports nutrients throughout the body and carries harmful toxins and waste products out of the body. It regulates our body temperature. And it lubricates our joints and organs.

Because water does so much, the body needs a constant fresh supply. "Water needs to continuously flow in, through and out the body," says Diane Grabowski, R.D., a nutrition educator with the Pritikin Longevity Center in Santa Monica, California. "A minimum of two to three quarts are eliminated daily in our urine, sweat and breath, all of which must be replaced."

That's just to meet our minimal health needs. Getting plenty of water is essential for a woman to maintain everything from youthful skin to strong muscles. "Consistently meeting your daily fluid needs makes all the organs in your body function better," says Grabowski. "It's a key ingredient if you want to look, feel and perform at your very best."

## Draining Your Assets

Unless you're a camel, your body can go only about three days without water before calling it quits. But don't think that dehydration occurs only when you're as dry as a bone. You can be technically dehydrated even if your internal fluid levels dip just a bit below normal.

Ordinarily, this is no problem, because your sense of thirst will holler, "I need some water . . . NOW!" But sometimes your thirst-detecting powers can't keep pace with other factors, such as hot weather, high altitude, exercise—or age. And yes, our sensitivity to thirst begins to diminish as we get older.

When you become dehydrated, you lose water and valuable electrolytes—essential minerals in water like potassium and sodium. This can leave you feeling especially tapped out. "When your body gets even a little low on fluids, physical performance and brain power can hit the skids," says Miriam E. Nelson, Ph.D., a research scientist and exercise physiologist in the Human Physiology Laboratory at the U.S. Department of Agriculture Human Nutrition Research Center on Aging at Tufts University in Boston. "Long before you experience the sensation of thirst, your body can produce symptoms like fatigue, dizziness, headache and flushed skin. All of these conditions are caused by an increase in body temperature."

Frequent or long-term dehydration can really leave you high and dry, causing an irregular heartbeat, an unsteady gait, difficulty swallowing and shortness of breath. Extreme cases of dehydration can produce shriveled skin and lips.

# Dehydration Alert

Dehydration can sneak up on you. You could be dangerously dry and not even know it. Keep an eye out for these danger signals.

## Early Signs
- Dizziness, fatigue
- Weakness, headache
- Flushed skin
- Dry mouth
- Loss of appetite

## Advanced Signs
- Blurred vision, hearing loss
- Difficulty swallowing
- Dry, hot skin
- Rapid pulse, shortness of breath
- Unsteady gait
- Extremely frequent urination (especially if you haven't been drinking fluids and the urine is cloudy and deep yellow)

# Fill 'Er Up

The faucet isn't your only source of water, though. Experts recommend that we need to consume six to eight eight-ounce glasses of liquid a day. This can mean six to eight glasses of water, juice, broths or other beverages.

"Heavier people require more, so a good rule is to try to drink about one-half ounce for each pound of body weight," says Grabowski. If you weigh 160 pounds, that means ten eight-ounce glasses per day. You'll also need more if you're dieting, living in a hot or dry environment or suffering sick with fever, vomiting or diarrhea, all of which can rob your body of its fluids.

Water is everywhere, so it's fairly simple to keep up your fluid intake. Here are some tips to get you started.

**Greet the day with a glass.** As you slept, your poor body went for hours without water. So pour yourself a glass after you wake up, says Grabowski. Don't rely on your morning coffee. Though stimulating, it can be dehydrating because it's a diuretic.

**Keep it up.** Don't try to guzzle your entire daily intake at once. You'll feel like you're bursting at the seams and, because your body can't take such a fluid overload, you'll excrete more, says Grabowski. Instead, take frequent water breaks—about one every hour or two—so you're constantly hydrated. Drink even more if it's hot or humid or if your eyes, mouth or skin feel dry.

**Eat regularly.** Much of your daily fluid intake comes during meals. Eat plenty of water-rich foods such as fruits and vegetables and always have water or another beverage with your meal, says Grabowski.

**Skip alcohol and caffeine.** Booze, beer, coffee, tea and colas are diuretics—that is, they encourage fluid excretion. These beverages may quench your thirst initially, but they ultimately draw fluids out of your body, says Grabowski.

**Avoid water-sapping foods.** Salty foods can dry you out, says Grabowski. If you must have them, limit your intake and make sure you drink plenty of fluids.

**Watch those laxatives.** Using laxatives frequently can draw an enormous amount of water from the body and disrupt the normal function of your digestive and elimination systems. These shouldn't be taken regularly unless you're under a doctor's care, Grabowski says.

**Don't toss the pulp.** Home juicing machines provide a great means for getting your daily fluids, says Grabowski. But some of these gadgets completely separate the juice from the fruit or vegetable pulp, the part that contains the greatest concentration of fiber as well as additional nutrients and water. Put some of that pulp into your glass.

# Managing Exercise and Fluids

A woman can sweat away two quarts an hour when she exercises or plays sports, especially if it's extremely hot and humid, says Dr. Nelson. That's why active women need to pay attention to their fluid needs. Keep these tips in mind.

**Drink before, during and after.** Drink 8 to 20 ounces of water an hour before your workout, says Dr. Nelson. "Body size and the temperature of where you will be exercising affect the amount of water that you should drink. The larger you are and the hotter it will be, the more you need," says Dr. Nelson. However, don't overdose on water; this will result in poor performance, warns Dr. Nelson. Symptoms of too much water intake include an uncomfortable bloated feeling and stomach cramps. As you exercise try to drink up to ½ to ¾ cup of water every ten minutes. Afterward, drink as much as you need to stave your thirst.

**Hop on a scale.** How much should you drink after exercise? If you weigh yourself before and after you exercise, you'll find out how much water you lose. For every half pound you lose, drink eight fluid ounces, says Dr. Nelson.

**Go beyond thirst.** Even if your immediate thirst feels quenched, your body's fluid reserves may not be adequately refilled, says Dr. Nelson. Play it safe and take a few additional slurps. A few minutes later drink some more, and so on, for about an hour afterward.

**Cool it.** Cool water will lower your body temperature faster than warmer water. It's also dispersed much faster to the parched tissues of the body, Dr. Nelson says.

**Adjust to your environment.** If you come out of an air-conditioned building on a hot day and immediately try jogging five miles, the shock to your system will draw more water from your body than if you slowly accustom yourself to the outdoor heat, Dr. Nelson says.

**Block the sun.** Direct sunlight on a hot summer day will dry you like a prune, says Dr. Nelson. If you exercise in the heat and sun, wear a hat and light, loose-fitting clothing that breathes and lets in cool air. "If you feel dizzy or disoriented, stop exercising immediately," warns Dr. Nelson. Find some shade and fluids to help cool your body temperature.

**Ease into it.** If you haven't been exercising, don't try to take on an advanced exercise program. Because you'll have to exert yourself more, you'll sweat more than someone who is in better shape. To avoid dehydration risk, start your workout program slowly, get used to exercising and gradually increase the intensity. This will go a long way in helping your body to regulate its fluids and body temperature, says Dr. Nelson.

**Use sport drinks sparingly.** Sport drinks, which are rich in the electrolytes we lose when we exercise, are often touted for their replenishing abilities, and many of them do make excellent fluid sources. But you certainly don't need a sports drink for every workout. "After a workout or if you need a pick-me-up during a game, they can be a big help, but they are no more effective than water, which is what your body is really thirsty for," says Dr. Nelson. The only time these drinks have an advantage over water is if you have just come off an extremely draining workout, such as a marathon or two hours of tennis in the hot sun. Then you may need an immediate electrolyte boost.

# FORGIVENESS

## *Good Therapy for Body and Soul*

**W**e've all been victims of life's injustices. There's the boyfriend who breaks your heart. The boss who fires you. The thug who takes your purse. You get mad—and most of the time, you get over it.

But when you can't let go of the grudges, you stand to lose a lot more than just your temper. Your hurt and anger may gnaw at you, disrupting your productivity and performance at work, your relationships and even your happiness. If you're not careful, you can do some serious damage to yourself.

"There's no question that holding on to grievances and unforgiving thoughts can age you," says Gerald G. Jampolsky, M.D., founder of the Center for Attitudinal Healing in Tiburón, California, and the author of nine books on relationships including *Love is Letting Go of Fear* and *Good-Bye to Guilt: Releasing Fear through Forgiveness*. "Besides the depression and anxiety it causes, it can also lead to wrinkles, heart disease, depression and a host of other physical problems that take the zip and zest out of your life. The good news is, when you forgive you can wipe the slate clean, and sometimes maybe even reverse some of the damage done."

## You Don't Have to Roll Over

But to do that, you have to realize what forgiveness isn't. It's not being a doormat or turning the other cheek so it can get slapped. You don't have to "play nice" with the subject of your rage or even allow the people who make you mad back into your life.

"Forgiveness doesn't mean that you should pretend the situation didn't happen," says Robert Enright, Ph.D., educational psychologist and professor of human development at the University of Wisconsin–Madison. "It means that you're accepting what happened, trying to accept the one who hurt you and acknowledging your hurt, but making a decision to *not* allow it to destroy your life."

Adds Redford B. Williams, M.D., director of the Behavioral Medicine Research Center and a professor of psychiatry at Duke University Medical Center in Durham, North Carolina. "It doesn't mean that you should forgive and forget. It's okay to remember; it just shouldn't control your thinking. Once you give up the notion of revenge, you make a conscious decision to save yourself from thinking about your hurt all the time. And when you do that, you will feel better, emotionally and physically."

## Just What the Doctor Ordered

In research with S. T. Tina Huang, Ph.D., associate professor of psychology at the National Chung-Cheng University in Chia-i, Taiwan, Dr. Enright found that the longer people hold on to their resentment, the more it tends to affect their blood pressure readings. "We found in the people we studied, whenever they were recalling stories of deep hurt, there were spiked increases in blood pressure in those who didn't have this outpouring of forgiveness," Dr. Enright says.

But those people who learned to forgive experienced a drop in blood pressure. And that's significant, since experts believe that a long-term grudge can cause the same damage to a woman's heart as it does to a man's. Men, by the way, have higher rates of heart disease and, coincidently, have a harder time learning to forgive.

"Everything bad that unresolved anger does to men, it also does to women," says Dr. Williams, author of *Anger Kills*. "And the 'badness' occurs in women at the same rate as in men. But the damage isn't just to your heart. People prone to traits associated with an unwillingness to forgive are at a higher risk of dying from all causes."

Including cancer. Research shows that a tendency to hold resentment and a marked inability to forgive have been linked with an increased risk of cancer, says O. Carl Simonton, M.D., director of Simon Cancer Counseling Center in Pacific Palisades, California, and co-author of *Getting Well Again*. Other researchers say that the stress associated with holding a grudge is also linked to higher rates of headache, backache, ulcers and wrinkles and even colds, flu and other infectious diseases.

The emotional tolls of failing to forgive can also age you. "We found that those with the lowest tolerance for forgiveness also had the lowest levels of self-esteem and the highest levels of anxiety and depression," says Dr. Enright. "But when they learn to forgive, their self-esteem increases while their depression and anxiety decrease. And I guess you could say that people with high self-esteem tend to take better care of themselves, so they feel better," he says. It's even possible that you'll look and act younger.

# How to Foster Forgiveness

So how do you learn to forgive? After all, isn't that sending a message that you're over your pain or even that you're condoning the behavior? Doesn't forgiveness say that you're a sucker?

"Not if you realize that there's a difference between forgiveness and reconciliation," says Dr. Enright. "Let's say that when you were growing up, one of your parents was somewhat emotionally distant from you. Perhaps your father was working all the time or didn't spend a lot time with you. With forgiveness, you try to understand the situation from his point of view: Perhaps he's worked so hard to be a good provider. In forgiveness, you do what *you* can to build on that relationship. In reconciliation, you *both* try to build that relationship. You may not even address your feelings but instead try to mend that relationship and build from it now."

And luckily, both get easier as we mature. "In one study, college students in particular were less likely to forgive than their parents and had more anxiety relative to their problem than their parents," says Dr. Enright. In adulthood, we're statistically most willing to forgive. Experts say that by practicing forgiveness now regardless of age, you could help keep your youthful outlook and health well into your golden years. And here's how.

**Think of today.** Kids live for the present, neither dwelling on the past nor worrying about the future. And that's good advice for women trying to come to grips with their hurt. "When you're four years old and a friend takes your toy, you swear you'll hate that kid forever and never play with him again. Meanwhile, ten minutes later, you're out playing together like nothing happened," says Dr. Jampolsky.

"It's important to have peace of mind as our only goal and to recognize that the attachment to anger doesn't really bring peace," says Dr. Jampolsky. "The people who feel less burdened by age are those who are in their eighties and nineties with what I call celestial amnesia; they live for the present."

**Choose to be happy, not right.** It's important to ask ourselves if we want to be happy or right, and it's important not to make others wrong and ourselves right. "The first step in forgiveness is willingness to forgive," says Dr. Jampolsky. "When we recognize that holding on to unforgiving thoughts is really a decision to suffer, it makes it easier for us to have a desire to forgive, let go and heal the past. When we forgive, the other person doesn't have to change at all. It's just a matter of changing our own thoughts and attitudes. To forgive does not mean you have to agree with the behavior," he says.

**Keep it to yourself.** Do you feel embarrassed or stupid saying "I forgive you"? Then keep it to yourself. You don't have to offer forgiveness directly to people who hurt you, says Sidney B. Simon, Ed.D., a counselor and professor emeritus of psychological education at the University of Massachusetts–Amherst, who with his wife, Suzanne Simon, wrote a book called *Forgiveness: How to Make Peace with Your Past and Get On with Your Life*. You can simply try to see things from their perspective.

**Ask what's really bugging you.** Sometimes the source of your resentment can be deep in your emotional well, hidden even from you—until you catch your panty hose on a table edge and all hell breaks loose. "When we get uptight about the smaller things that happen each day, we are really getting upset about something deeper that we might never have forgiven," says Dr. Simon. So ask yourself about the root of your anger and try to come to grips with it. If you can't do this on your own, perhaps a therapist can help you.

**Don't be a victim again.** Resentment often results from your being a victim—of a crime, broken heart or some other situation where you felt power-less. Sometimes the inability to forgive ourselves stems from feelings that we didn't do enough to stop the terrible deed. But by taking action after the fact, many women find it easier to forgive themselves. Take action against unfair treatment: If your car mechanic is patronizing you, tell him to stop it or he'll lose your business. If your husband is cheating on you, make your feelings known. If you've been the victim of a crime, press charges.

**Put it on paper.** Maybe you feel anger and resentment but aren't sure why. Or maybe you know why but you can't bring yourself to forgive the scoundrel. Either way, get it down on paper, says James Pennebaker, Ph.D., professor of psychology at Southern Methodist University in Dallas and author of *Opening Up: The Healing Power of Confiding in Others*. Simply write down your feelings— *how* you feel rather than just reporting that you feel bad. By doing this daily, for about 20 minutes a day, keeping a "kvetching diary" can help you vent your feelings while focusing your resentment, so you'll be better able to forgive.

# FRIENDSHIPS

## *They're Good for Life*

Lynn was so happy to be getting away from the city for a week with her friend Teresa that she hugged her when they met up at the bus stop. They started talking on the two-hour trip to the beach, and it seemed like they didn't stop for the whole vacation.

Walking to the farmers' market to buy vegetables, they discussed their marriages. Out for a run, Lynn talked about how she and Peter had lately made an effort to improve their sex life. Lying on the beach, Teresa said she no longer felt useful in her job—and Lynn knew just what she meant. The feelings just poured out of both of them. Somehow, when Lynn and Teresa got together there was always this cleansing fountain of emotion.

Peter was home when Lynn returned. He had just spent a week fishing at a remote lake with Robert, Teresa's husband.

"How was the fishing?" Lynn asked.

"Wonderful," he said. "Did you and Teresa have a good time?"

"Gosh, we talked for hours and hours. It seemed like we'd never stop. I told her every secret I'd ever had. She's such a wonderful friend. Did you and Robert talk about personal things?"

Peter had to think about it for a moment. "Not really," he said.

This story reflects the fact that men tend to "do" things together while women tend to "share" things, notably their feelings and needs. But while they might have different ways of going about it, men and women get the same thing from their friendships: longer, more healthful lives.

## What They Do for You

"Friendship has a profound effect on your physical well-being," says Eugene Kennedy, Ph.D., professor of psychology at Loyola University of Chicago.

# Make Yourself Likable

Likability is a talent. And like any talent, it can be honed, says Arthur Wassmer, Ph.D., a psychologist in private practice in Kirkland, Washington, and author of *Making Contact*. Here are several tips that will make you liked by all but the most miserable people when you meet them.

- Break the ice with questions like "Where are you from?" or "Are you enjoying the party?"
- Be an active listener.
- Ask questions.
- Reveal your feelings and experiences.
- Pay a compliment.

"Having good relationships improves health and lifts depressions. You don't necessarily need drugs or medical treatment to accomplish this—just friends," says Dr. Kennedy.

And perhaps one of the greatest health benefits of friendship is the youthfulness of extended life—of extra years of enjoyment and satisfaction.

One of the first studies linking social relationships and longevity took place in Alameda County, California. Researchers there found that over a nine-year period, the people with the strongest social and community ties were the least likely to die. Not surprisingly, the most isolated people had the highest death rate.

Three more recent studies duplicated these findings: In each study, people who were isolated were three to five times more likely to die than people who had intimate relationships.

Redford B. Williams, M.D., director of the Behavioral Medicine Research Center and professor of psychiatry at Duke University Medical Center in Durham, North Carolina, sees a definite connection between friendship and longevity. His team studied 1,368 heart disease patients for nine years. They discovered that just being married (even if it was a bad marriage) or having a good friend was a predictor of who lived and who died after a heart attack.

"What we found," says Dr. Williams, "was that those patients with neither a spouse nor a friend were three times more likely to die than those involved in a caring relationship."

As a woman, you'll tend to have more intimate friendships than men do. "Women are more emotional and more willing to express emotional needs. When they feel the need to meet new people or just to talk, they're much more likely to approach someone. It's a good quality," says Michael Cunningham, Ph.D., professor of psychology at the University of Louisville in Kentucky.

But just being willing to express emotions isn't always enough when it comes to making friends. Many women have difficulty developing relationships because they lack certain relationship-building skills. Fortunately, it's never too late to start learning them.

## You Reap What You Sow

Friends don't spring up like wildflowers. They have to be cultivated like roses. And, like roses, they'll keep blooming and growing as long as you nourish them. Here are some tips for growing a garden of friends and reaping the age-erasing benefits of love and friendship.

**Be a friend for life.** Friendships don't happen overnight. They require exchanges of trust and confidence that can only develop over time, says Dr. Cunningham. You have to maintain and nourish your friends by showing genuine and continuing interest in them. Don't just say "How are you?" Say it and really listen to the response. And then tell them how you are doing.

**Try new activities.** Often you attract friends to the extent that you are doing things they are interested in, says Dr. Cunningham. The message: "Be

## Friendly Body Language

In his work with shy people, Arthur Wassmer, Ph.D., a psychologist in private practice in Kirkland, Washington, and author of *Making Contact*, learned that the way you move is just as important as what you say when you're trying to make friends. He offers these six tips for how to present yourself in a social situation. Combine the first letter of each tip to form the word SOFTEN, and you'll find it easy to remember Dr. Wassmer's advice. These tips will make you appear open and inviting to people you meet.

*S*mile
*O*pen posture (don't cross your arms)
*F*orward (lean toward, not away from the person)
*T*ouch (just a light touch on the shoulder or arm)
*E*ye contact
*N*od in agreement

# Your Friend Fido

He has bad breath, leaves hair all over the place and has something of a foot fetish. But at least he's honest. He lets you know right up front that he likes to chew on shoes.

So why do you put up with Fido? Because he's so different from the rest of your life. Relationships are up or down, friends move hither and yon and jobs come and go. But Fido sticks right by your side and loves you—no matter what.

Your dog gives you a whole lot more than fur on the sofa and tooth marks on your best pumps, researchers say. For starters, a pet's companionship lowers your stress level and lowers your blood pressure.

Numerous studies have shown that pets are good for health and longevity. One study of 5,741 people in Melbourne, Australia, showed that pet owners had lower levels of blood pressure and cholesterol than nonowners—even when both groups had the same heart-harming habits, like smoking or a high-fat diet.

In another study, a group of 96 heart attack survivors were observed for a year after they were released from the University of Maryland School of Medicine's coronary care unit in Baltimore. Researchers found that more pet owners were still alive a year later than were those without a pet to go home to. Here, too, the results held firm even after researchers accounted for the patients' individual differences in heart damage and other medical problems.

Another study showed that your dog may play a role in protecting you from heart disease in the first place. Forty-five female dog-lovers were asked to perform a standard experimental stress task at the State

willing to try new activities that will put you in contact with people who might turn out to be good friends," he says.

**Be open and be real.** "Friendship depends on sharing and responding to each other," says Dr. Kennedy. "There's no formula for making friends. The real requirement is just being yourself and showing who you are to someone else."

Many women have the idea that revealing themselves is a tremendous risk, that they might face ridicule, says Arthur Wassmer, Ph.D., a psychologist in private practice in Kirkland, Washington, and author of *Making Contact*. This feeling usually comes from low self-esteem and makes women believe they aren't worthy of sharing their feelings with another person, he says. In reality, he

University of New York at Buffalo. Later, the women took the test again, either alone, with their dogs present in the room or accompanied by a supportive female friend. The results? The women's cardiovascular reactions to stress were milder when their dogs were nearby. The researchers speculate that it is the loving, uncritical presence of pets that lowers physical responses to stress.

Although all sorts of companion animals have been shown to have therapeutic effects, dogs do seem to have an edge, particularly in providing comfort and support to older people. A study at the School of Public Health at the University of California, Los Angeles, showed that recently bereaved elderly people who didn't own pets saw their doctors 16 percent more than pet owners did and 20 percent more than dog owners. Dog owners saw their doctors less partly because they reported greater feelings of attachment to their pets. The researchers think that another factor in dogs' healing companionship is that they often take their owners for health-promoting walks.

How about a feathered friend? A few studies suggest the possibility of some increased risk of lung cancer for those living with a pet bird, possibly due to lung-damaging fungus spores that spread to the air from bird droppings. But other researchers say the connection is not as strong as originally was reported.

So the choice is yours—whether you decide to walk a dog, stroke a cat or talk to a canary, you're getting love, easing stress and bolstering your heart health. So what's a little shedding and tooth marks on your shoes?

adds, you're almost never going to get a bad response from someone when you try to be genuine and open with something personal.

**Ask for what you need.** Just because you tell someone your problems doesn't mean you'll get the emotional support you need, according to Dr. Cunningham. You have to ask for the type of support you need. If you want advice, say so. If you want acceptance and sympathy, let your friend know that too.

**Find a group of sympathetic people.** It's a catch-22, but people who are lonely and needy have the most trouble making friends. Their neediness scares others off. Dr. Cunningham says people develop "social allergies" to needy people and become wary and irritated with them. That's why it helps to look for friends among people who understand what you're going through. If you're a grieving widow or a recovering addict or if you suffer from any number of alienating problems, look into the self-help or 12-step groups in your area. There's bound to be one for you. These groups can help an isolated person deal with her problems and eventually become less needy and thus more attractive to others.

**Have male buddies.** Try having simple nonsexual friendships with men you like. Sometimes women appreciate their men friends because they provide the male point of view, and it can be useful to hear the male angle once in a while. The guy can offer brotherly advice that gives the woman a different perspective than she would get from her female friends.

**Reach out and fax someone.** These days, people are so busy that it can be difficult to find time for friends. But there are always telephones, faxes and old-fashioned letters. You don't have to have constant direct contact to maintain a good friendship.

**Don't put all your eggs in one basket.** It can be dangerous to rely on one person for all of your emotional support, whether it's a friend or your husband. What if your only friend gets tired of listening to you talk about your problems? Or what if you're suddenly widowed and left without anyone to turn to? You'll suddenly be lonely and isolated, and you will probably feel a lot older in a short period of time. It's wiser to spread your emotional needs around to various people.

# GOALS

## *A Road Map to Vitality*

**A**fter your first step, you wanted to run. After your first somersault, you wanted to do a back flip. After you landed your first job, you wanted a better one.

You've had goals all your life. Each time you accomplish a meaningful task you feel a surge of pride and exuberance. Like most women, goals are an essential part of your life. They give you vitality and energy; they keep you going.

"Goals presume there is a future worth living," says Marilee C. Goldberg, Ph.D., a psychotherapist in private practice in Lambertville, New Jersey, who specializes in cognitive and behavior therapy. "They can keep you moving forward, which keeps you optimistic, and having something to look forward to can help you feel younger."

"Goals sustain a woman's sense of well-being and purpose. It's just natural to feel better about yourself and feel worthwhile if you're being productive in some way," says Barry Rovner, M.D., a geriatric psychiatrist at the Thomas Jefferson Medical Center in Philadelphia. "It's this basic: Like your heart needs blood, your mind needs to have a focus or a goal," he says. "People without goals feel lost and adrift."

## They Do a Body Good

All of us have goals, including the mundane ones like paying bills on time. In fact, in any given week the average woman is fulfilling dozens of goals that may include reaching a sales quota at work, getting home in time to see her daughter's soccer game or taking an evening stroll with her husband, says Paul Karoly, Ph.D., professor of psychology at Arizona State University in Tempe.

"We all have the same general desire in life, and that is to get from point A to point B," Dr. Karoly says. "At the core, that means having goals and learning to navigate toward them. Studies indicate that people who have reasonable goals are more satisfied with life and feel better about themselves."

Goals can also help you keep your mind and body in peak condition, says Dennis Gersten, M.D., a psychiatrist in private practice in San Diego and publisher of *Atlantis: The Imagery Newsletter*. "If you don't have goals, what happens? You won't be motivated to maintain your health and keep up your body," he says. "Your life won't have meaning and you won't feel complete. So having goals makes you whole spiritually, physically and emotionally. And being whole can make you healthier and relieve stress."

Goals prevent boredom, and that's important because boredom can put you at higher risk for disease, says Howard Friedman, Ph.D., professor of psychology and community medicine at the University of California, Riverside, and author of *The Self-Healing Personality*.

"Something's going on there, but we really don't know how it all fits together," Dr. Friedman says. "It may be that when you feel challenged by a goal, it triggers a psychophysiological process in the body. Or it could be that people who have goals do other positive things like eat better and exercise more."

In addition, difficult but achievable goals may be more invigorating than goals that are perceived as easy or impossible, Dr. Karoly speculates.

"If you see the task as either easy or impossible, then you have no motivation," Dr. Karoly says. "If you see it as reasonably possible, then it's worth your while to try it. When you do, your heart rate may increase and you may feel more energetic."

## Is Your Goal Really a Dream?

Imagine you want to drive from New York to Los Angeles. But when you get in the car, there's no road map and the highway has no signs. You'd have no way of knowing how far you'd traveled or if you were going in the right direction. That's what it's like to have a dream or vision without goals.

Goals are the road maps, the highway signs, that help you stay on course so you can fulfill your dreams, Dr. Goldberg says. Dreams or visions are often difficult to fulfill simply because they're vague. Goals are specific.

"People get confused about the distinction between goals and visions, and that sets them up for failure," Dr. Goldberg says. "Saying 'I want to be popular' is a vision, not a goal. That statement has no criteria to measure if you're making progress and is impossible to fulfill. A goal would be 'I'm going to phone ten people and ask them to have coffee with me, and I won't stop trying until one of them says yes.' You can measure that. You'll definitely know if you made the phone calls and whether someone said yes."

## Mapping Your Strategy

Your goals don't need to be grandiose or spectacular to energize you, says Dr. Gersten. But whether you're trying to spend more time with your family, organize a yard sale or raise $1 million to build a new community center, the more carefully you shape your goals, the more likely your dreams will be transformed into reality. Here's how.

**Write 'em down.** Committing your goals to paper will make them more tangible to you, says Dr. Friedman. Keep your list in a conspicuous place and check off your goals as you achieve them. Be sure to include a mixture of easy goals that will encourage you, such as reading the newspaper every day, and several more difficult ones that will challenge you, like increasing your productivity at work 10 percent.

**Do first things first.** After you list your goals, decide which ones are most important to you and start working on them. "People often do the least important things first, and the things that are really important to them never get done," Dr. Friedman says.

**Be picky.** Try not to spread yourself too thin. If you have more goals than you can realistically accomplish, you'll drain your energy and feel discouraged and depressed. It's better to have one or two well-defined goals that are meaningful to you than a dozen less important ones, Dr. Friedman says.

**Love your goal.** Choose goals that you feel passionate about, and you'll be more likely to follow through on them, Dr. Gersten says. So if you start collecting silver spoons, but your heart really isn't in it, you're probably not going to stick with it. But if you're a devoted tennis fan, odds are you'll be more successful if you start collecting autographs or other memorabilia.

**Go for the positive.** "Instead of concentrating on what you don't want, create a goal that expresses what you do want," Dr. Gersten says. Positive goals are more pleasurable and more effective than negative ones. If you say, for example, "I won't eat eclairs," you're focusing your attention on a negative goal. That can actually make eclairs more tempting to you. A better goal would be "I'm going to eat a more balanced diet that includes more vegetables, fruits and grains. Then if I want an occasional eclair as a treat, I can have one without feeling guilty."

**Be real.** Goals not only need to be specific, they should be realistic, Dr. Goldberg says. If you say you're never going to watch television again, that's probably not realistic because goals that include absolute words like "always" or "never" seldom are achievable. A more specific and reasonable goal might be to limit your viewing to no more than two hours of television each evening.

**Make it good for you.** A goal that is torturous to achieve or jeopardizes your health isn't worthwhile. "Some women will say 'I'll kill myself to do this thing,'" says Dr. Goldberg. "You have to take your well-being into account no matter what your goal is. So if you want to plant a garden, but you have a sore back, forcing yourself to get down on your knees and do it is a poor idea. If it's really that important to you, ask a friend or pay someone to do it."

**Set deadlines.** Without time lines to nudge us along, many of us would never reach our goals. "Setting a deadline doesn't mean that you're bad if you don't make it," Dr. Goldberg says. "But a deadline does give you a point in time to shoot for. Then if you haven't accomplished everything you'd planned when time is up, forgive yourself, re-evaluate your plan and reset your time line."

**Divide and conquer.** Chopping your goal down into several intermediate steps will make it seem less overwhelming and more achievable, Dr. Goldberg says. If you want to set aside $2,500 over the next two years for a trip to England, you're probably going to have a harder time saving the money if you set your sights on getting the whole amount than if you find ways to save $3.50 a day or $24 a week.

**Involve your friends.** If you tell a friend about your goal or, better yet, get her to help you work on it, you'll be more motivated to stick to it, Dr. Friedman says.

**Find an idol.** If someone you admire has achieved a goal similar to yours, use that person for inspiration, Dr. Gersten says. Put her picture or quotes in a prominent place like on your desk or refrigerator. Take a moment each day to imagine the thrill of achieving what she did.

**But don't compete.** You should learn from the success of others, but you shouldn't set out to outdo them. If you're a songwriter, for example, you should study the works of the great pop artists, but you shouldn't feel like you need to sell more recordings than Madonna to be a success. "You'll be less stressed and more creative if you try to be the best that you can be, rather than try to be the best in the world," Dr. Gersten says.

**Let go of your ego.** Prepare yourself for rejection and criticism. In fact, you should welcome it because criticism can help you focus your goal. "When you begin working on a goal that is important to you, you should put your ego aside and let people chop your work up," Dr. Gersten says. "For example, I'm writing a book, so I gave it to six friends and asked them to tear it apart. Then I paid an editor to do the same thing. As a result, I had to completely reorganize the manuscript. But if you want to successfully reach your goal, you have to open yourself up to criticism like that."

**Forget perfection.** If you think you have to do something perfectly, you'll probably never achieve your goals. Remember, you don't have to do something perfectly. "You want to do your very best, but your goal shouldn't be perfection," Dr. Gersten says.

**Keep your perspective.** Goals are fine, but if they interfere with your family or social life, you could be headed for trouble, according to Brian Little, Ph.D., a professor of psychology at Carleton University in Ottawa, Ontario. "Your goal might be to lose 20 pounds, so you begin jogging for an hour every morning," he says. "But unless you talk to your husband, you might not realize that he enjoys talking to you during that hour because it's the one time of the day that you can be alone together before the kids get up. So your goals not only have to fit your needs, they also have to be timely, fair and take the social needs of others you care about into consideration." In this case, instead of jogging for an hour, perhaps you could compromise and do it for 30 minutes twice a day.

**Envision success.** Imagine that you've already achieved your goal and people are praising your effort. It may motivate you to accomplish the goal and do it well. "I imagine the book that I'm writing is at the top of the *New York Times* best-seller list, and that makes me want to create the best book that I can," Dr. Gersten says.

**Treat yourself.** Give yourself rewards, such as a new compact disk, a manicure or a nonfat frozen yogurt when you complete a goal, no matter how small, Dr. Goldberg suggests. It serves as an incentive to set and accomplish new tasks. And don't forget to give yourself a pat on the back.

**Update your goals.** "It's important to reassess your goals every six months because circumstances may have changed, and some goals may not fit your needs anymore," Dr. Goldberg says. If that's the case, don't hang on to it. Let it fade away and then choose something else that is important to you *now*.

# HONESTY

## *Truth's Healthy Consequences*

It's Monday morning and the boss is boiling. The computer crashed over the weekend and erased the Borkburger files, wiping out six days' worth of work.

Oops. You meant to make backup copies Friday, but got swamped with long-distance calls, last-minute details and spur-of-the-moment planning for a weekend getaway. So what do you say to the boss?

A) "Sorry, Edith. Lots of unexpected things came up Friday. I got really busy and forgot."

B) "Sorry, Edith. Mary over there forgot to do it."

C) "Sorry, Edith. My aunt Jenny is sick, the car overheated, my dog has fleas and . . . gee, that's a really pretty dress you're wearing."

Try "A"—the truth—for your health's sake. Honesty is more than just the best policy. It's a great anti-aging prescription, too, capable of relieving tons of stress and worry, helping you sleep easier at night, strengthening relationships and restoring self-confidence.

"The bottom line about honesty is that it makes you feel better," says psychologist Nathaniel Branden, Ph.D., head of the Branden Institute for Self-Esteem in Beverly Hills and author of *The Six Pillars of Self-Esteem*. "When you tell the truth, you respect yourself and you strengthen your self-esteem."

That doesn't mean you should always blurt out exactly what's on your mind. Such relentless honesty can lead to strained friendships and angry, revenge-minded colleagues, according to Michael W. Mercer, Ph.D., an industrial psychologist, president of the Mercer Group in Chicago and author of *How Winners Do It: High-Impact People Skills for Your Career Success*.

"But once you establish that you are honest, people will respond positively," Dr. Mercer says. "They'll begin to value your opinion, because what you say is what you mean."

# Unraveling the Yarns

Everyone knows someone like Falsehood Fanny Baker, voted Most Likely to be Lying at Any Given Moment by her high school classmates. Through the years you watched Fanny progress from "The dog ate it, Teacher" to "Of course I love you, Sweetheart" to "I would never *think* of going to Aspen without looking up Goldie and Kurt, darling."

Dr. Mercer says some women feel the urge to fudge a little to make their lives seem a little more important. The problem is that once they start, it's tough to stop adding new layers of lies. Pretty soon they're telling one person one thing, the next person something else and their bosses something else again.

The result? Dr. Mercer says these people build giant expectations, promising themselves and others things they're not capable of delivering. They try to be something they simply cannot be: perfect. That disappoints them and their acquaintances; they start feeling lousy about themselves and fret all the time about who's going to find them out.

"It's a whole lot easier on everyone to just tell the truth," Dr. Branden says. "That way you don't ever have to remember what you said the night before or two months before. And other people come to know exactly what you're all about."

# Make a Commitment

It sounds so simple: Just tell the truth. But experts say that honesty takes commitment and a fair amount of courage. If you want to add more honesty to your life, try these truthful tips.

**Take responsibility.** Honesty comes from within. It's an open expression of how you feel and what you think. And Dr. Branden says it's best to express yourself that way.

"Remember: Your opinions and feelings count," he says. Dr. Branden also says it's a good idea to tell people the truth in the first person. Say "I need to tell you about something that's bothering me" or "This is how I feel about what's been happening in our relationship."

These "I" phrases serve two purposes, according to Dr. Branden. First, they're a signal to the other person that you're talking from your heart. It's much more intimate to say "I'm worried about your drinking" than to say "You're making a fool out of yourself by drinking so much."

Second, "I" phrases are a form of self-affirmation. By talking openly about your feelings in the first person, you're telling yourself that your thoughts matter. "It's an excellent way to build self-esteem," Dr. Branden says.

**Make honesty a goal.** "Resolve to tell the truth, starting now," says Dr. Branden. "It may seem scary at first, but the sooner you begin, the better."

Start small if you wish. Let your friend at work know that you think his report could use a little more polish. Tell your husband that you think it's time to retire his favorite T-shirt.

# Truth Doesn't Have to Hurt

Your boyfriend meets you at a restaurant wearing the single most repulsive plaid blazer you have ever seen. "Do you like it?" he asks, strutting to the table. What do you say?

A) "That is the single most repulsive plaid blazer I have ever seen."
B) "That is the single most gorgeous plaid blazer I have ever seen."
C) "I have never seen a blazer quite like that."

Well, "B" is out because it's just untrue. "A" is risky. You might end up eating alone. "C" may seem like a cop-out, but is it really?

"It's important to be honest. But be honest and tactful," suggests Michael W. Mercer, Ph.D., an industrial psychologist and president of the Mercer Group in Chicago.

Remember that honesty is a very powerful tool. People like to feel good about themselves, so spilling the raw truth may lead to hard feelings, Dr. Mercer says.

Some people can handle more bluntness than others. "People who get along in life act a little differently with everyone they meet," Dr. Mercer says. "You need to figure out who you can tell the truth to flat-out and who you have to handle with care."

For more sensitive people, Dr. Mercer suggests opening phrases like "You have a point," "That's quite an idea/report/leotard" and "I've been listening to you, and you may be right." That gives you a little room to dodge, to start a conversation without putting the other person on the defensive.

Once you've shown people respect and won their trust, Dr. Mercer says you can work up to your point more easily. "There's no sense making someone angry for no reason," he says. "You'll never be able to communicate that way, whether you're completely honest or not."

Soon you'll feel better about sharing deeper feelings with friends and lovers—which is why they're friends and lovers in the first place.

**Clear the decks.** Mom thinks you've been going to church every Sunday for the past 13 years. But Pastor Peterson wouldn't know you from Eve herself. Tell Ma the truth. She might be a little hurt at first, but Dr. Branden says it will relieve the pressure of always having to lie to her. Ultimately, he says, it probably will strengthen your relationship.

Dr. Mercer offers a basic rule: If a fib from the past still bothers you, come clean about it. Try an opening line like this: "I told you something in the past that wasn't true. I really value our relationship, so I want to set it straight." Telling someone you care about them first will soften the blow, Dr. Mercer says.

**Know your limits.** Everyone wants to be liked. But sometimes the desire for approval makes you commit to things you can't possibly do. Don't spread yourself too thin trying to please the world, Dr. Mercer says. And never promise to complete a task that you have neither the time nor the expertise to handle.

"If you can't hang wallpaper, you're better off telling your friend to hire a professional," Dr. Mercer says. Otherwise, your friend will end up with crooked wallpaper, and you could end up with one less friend.

**Accentuate the positive.** Remember that honesty is a positive emotion. Being honest doesn't mean only telling people what you dislike about them, Dr. Branden says. Tell them what you like—their hairstyle, their work, their willingness to listen.

**Be a little easier on yourself.** You aren't perfect, but that doesn't mean you're a failure. "Admit that you have strengths as well as weaknesses," Dr. Mercer says. "See yourself in a positive way, and it will become a lot easier to always tell the truth."

# HORMONE REPLACEMENT THERAPY

## A Midlife Option

You've made a lot of health decisions in your lifetime: what type of contraception to use, how and when to exercise, which doctor to go to.

Now with menopause ahead, you face another. And this time, it feels like a real biggie. You keep mulling over the question: "Should I take hormone replacement therapy?"

Millions of women baby boomers are asking themselves the same thing. It's estimated that more women than ever—from 40 to 50 million—will be entering menopause during the next two decades.

We've all heard about the possible difficulties of menopause: hot flashes and night sweats, vaginal dryness and skin changes and increased risk for heart disease and osteoporosis once menopause has passed. We've also heard about hormone replacement therapy as a means to combat these aging effects.

In fact, whether to take hormone replacement therapy is often one of the first questions women have about menopause, says Joan Borton, a licensed mental health counselor in private practice in Rockport, Massachusetts, and author of *Drawing from the Women's Well: Reflections on the Life Passage of Menopause*. "It's still a very difficult decision to make. I see a lot of women being very thoughtful and trying to get as much information as possible," she says.

The choice is difficult, because there are both benefits and risks to taking hormone replacement therapy, or HRT. Women often find themselves trying to weigh the pros—HRT can relieve hot flashes and vaginal dryness, protect against heart disease and osteoporosis and maintain youthful skin and hair—against the cons—women worry that it may increase their risk for breast cancer, uterine cancer and gallstones. HRT also causes women to start having their periods again, which some view as an inconvenience. Most experts agree that the decision is an individual one and depends largely on a woman's health history and her own experience with menopause.

# Understanding Estrogen

HRT is a formulation of hormones designed to replenish a woman's natural hormone levels. In the years preceding menopause, called perimenopause, a woman's natural estrogen levels steadily decline. Then after she stops ovulating and has her last period (when menopause actually begins), her estrogen levels plunge even further. The average age for menopause is 51, but it can occur earlier; about 1 percent of women experience menopause before age 40.

Estrogen plays a vital role in maintaining tissues and organs throughout a woman's body, including her skin, vaginal tissue, breasts and bones. So when estrogen levels dip low during menopause, there can be vaginal dryness, skin wrinkling and deterioration in bone mass and strength. Estrogen also affects a number of bodily functions, such as metabolism and body temperature regulation. So when estrogen levels decline, a woman's cholesterol can rise, placing her at increased risk for heart disease. Her body's internal thermometer can also be thrown off kilter—thus the hot flashes and night sweats.

Years ago, the hormone formulations designed for menopausal women contained just estrogen and were called estrogen replacement therapy, or ERT. But those formulations contained levels of estrogen that proved to be too high; the pills were found to contribute to the formation of blood clots. And giving estrogen alone proved dangerous: Studies showed it promoted uterine cancer.

So researchers redesigned the formulas, lowering the estrogen content and adding a synthetic form of the hormone progesterone called progestin. In addition to regulating estrogen, progesterone prompts the shedding of the uterine lining. The combination of estrogen and progestin is what is known as HRT. The lower doses of estrogen are high enough to replace what's missing and to provide protection for the heart but low enough so as not to promote clots. And the progestin offers protection against uterine cancer because it triggers the uterine lining to slough off, thereby preventing the dangerous buildup that can progress to cancer if unchecked. So today, if a menopausal woman decides she wants to take hormones and she still has her uterus, the recommendation of most doctors is low-dose estrogen plus progestin.

But some women have difficulty tolerating progestin, experts say. It can cause unbearable PMS-like symptoms. These women can receive low-dose estrogen alone, but if they do, they must undergo regular biopsies of the uterus to monitor for cancer. If a woman no longer has her uterus, she's eligible to receive low-dose estrogen alone, but some doctors recommend estrogen and progestin in these cases.

HRT involving both estrogen and progestin can be taken in several different ways. The progestin component of the therapy is available only in a pill, which women can take either in higher doses for 10 to 12 days at the end of their menstrual cycles or in lower doses every day of the month.

Estrogen, however, is available in a number of different forms, including creams, patches and pills, and is taken either every day of the month or for the first three weeks of the menstrual cycle.

Estrogen creams are inserted into the vagina with applicators and have their greatest impact on vaginal tissue; this form of estrogen is most effective for vaginal dryness and urinary tract problems. Estrogen patches are the size of a small bandage and are worn on the abdomen; estrogen is released from the patch in timed sequences and passes directly into the bloodstream. This form is appropriate for women who have medical conditions that prohibit them from taking estrogen orally, such as gallbladder disease or high blood pressure.

Because the estrogen from both creams and patches goes directly into the bloodstream, it does not pass through the digestive tract and the liver, where it would normally have its greatest effect on reducing cholesterol. Cream and patch forms of estrogen are therefore thought to be less effective in protecting against heart disease.

The pill form of estrogen is taken by mouth and is thought to be the best method for fighting heart disease. The most common estrogen pill, called Premarin, is made from natural sources—estrogen from mares—while other pills are made from synthetic sources.

## Immediate Concerns

Hot flashes and vaginal dryness are the two main symptoms that send a woman to her doctor about menopause and HRT, says Brian Walsh, M.D., director of the Menopause Clinic at Brigham and Women's Hospital in Boston.

Hot flashes are estimated to affect 75 to 85 percent of menopausal women. Eighty percent of women who get hot flashes experience them for more than a year, and 25 to 50 percent complain of them for more than five years. Hot flashes can vary from a mild to moderately warm sensation that lasts between 1 and 5 minutes to an extremely hot feeling that lasts up to 12 minutes and involves profuse sweating and flushing.

Hot flashes may occur during the day or at night, when they're known as night sweats. Women may wake up hot and sweating, says Dr. Walsh. They are often so drenched that they must change their nightclothes, further interrupting their sleep and leaving them exhausted and irritable during the day. HRT is highly effective against hot flashes, experts say.

Vaginal dryness also responds to HRT, experts say. The tissue of the vagina has estrogen receptors in it. When estrogen declines with menopause, the lining of the vagina and uterus thins, and vaginal dryness results.

A woman's skin may also have estrogen receptors, so when menopause arrives, skin can begin to wrinkle. HRT is effective in maintaining smooth, youthful-looking skin, experts say.

# Heart Helper

A big concern for women who go through menopause is heart disease, since risk of it increases from one in nine women before age 65 to one in three women after 65, according to the American Heart Association.

The reason a woman's risk goes up is that estrogen helps keep levels of HDL (high-density lipoprotein) cholesterol, the good kind, high and levels of LDL (low-density lipoprotein) cholesterol the bad kind, low. It also helps prevent blood vessel walls from attracting cholesterol. When a woman's natural levels of estrogen decline with menopause, these protections against heart disease are removed.

Will taking HRT restore the protection? Some studies indicate that it may.

The problem with existing studies is that they are based mostly on the older formulations of ERT—those containing just estrogen. The majority of these studies indicate that taking estrogen without progestin will decrease a woman's heart disease risk by 50 percent compared with what her risk would be if she didn't take it, says Cynthia A. Stuenkel, M.D., associate clinical professor in the Department of Medicine and Reproductive Medicine at the University of California, San Diego.

But what about HRT, which uses both estrogen and progestin? Well, less research has been done on those formulations. And there's some question among researchers about whether progestin reduces the protective effect of estrogen.

A study published in the *New England Journal of Medicine*, however, looked at the effects of both HRT and ERT on heart disease. The report analyzed data from the Atherosclerosis Risk in Communities Study, a large study of 15,800 people from four areas of the country. Based on their findings, researchers reported that the levels of good cholesterol were similar for users of estrogen alone and users of estrogen plus progestin. And both groups had higher levels of good cholesterol than women who did not use estrogen. The researchers also estimated that women who took estrogen alone decreased their risk of heart disease by 42 percent compared with nonusers and that women who used estrogen with progestin would have even greater benefit, although just how much more wasn't specified.

# Bone Bonanza

Another concern for menopausal women is osteoporosis, a disease in which the density and strength of bone, particularly in the hips and wrists, declines. Experts say that four in every ten women develop the disease. The consequences can be devastating—an estimated 1.5 million Americans suffer osteoporosis-related fractures each year. After menopause, between 25 percent and 44 percent of women experience hip fractures due to osteoporosis. And by the time they are 90 years of age, women are twice as likely as men to fracture their hips.

Research suggests that using HRT will decrease a woman's risk of suffering osteoporosis-related fractures by 50 percent. And for women who already have osteoporosis, HRT is still thought to be effective and may increase their bone mineral density, a measurement of bone strength, by 5 percent.

How long does a woman need to take HRT in order to protect her bones? In Boston, the Framingham Osteoporosis Study analyzed the bone mineral densities of 670 white women from the Framingham Heart Study. (The Framingham Heart Study began in 1948 and followed study participants through their lives to evaluate risk factors for heart disease.) The Framingham Osteoporosis Study concluded that women needed to take hormone therapy for more than seven years for their bone mineral densities to increase. Women who took it for only three to four years had bone mineral densities similar to women who had never taken it. So according to this study, women may need to stay on HRT for at least seven years for their bone mineral densities to increase significantly.

Researchers also found that when women took HRT for seven to ten years or more and then stopped, the protective effect of HRT against declining bone density lasted only until age 75. After that, any effect of prolonged therapy appeared to be slight. This is important, given that a woman's risk for osteoporosis is greatest in her eighties and nineties.

The findings of this study have prompted discussion in the medical community about how long women need to take HRT to maintain bone density into the last decades of life. Some physicians are tossing around the idea of keeping women on HRT indefinitely—that is, they would start on it after menopause and stay on it through their eighties and nineties. Other doctors are considering the possibility of waiting longer after menopause to start HRT.

# Risks of HRT

There are other health issues and risks for women who take hormones. First, there's the risk of uterine cancer, which affects about 1 in 1,000 women per year, says Dr. Walsh. Taking estrogen alone increases a woman's risk for endometrial cancer about fourfold, says Dr. Walsh. That's why doctors today don't recommend estrogen alone for a woman who still has her uterus. But women who take estrogen and progestin may actually have a lower risk than if they didn't take hormones at all, says Dr. Walsh. Their risk is possibly 30 to 40 percent lower, he says.

Taking HRT places a woman at risk for gallstones, particularly in the first year, says Dr. Walsh. In addition, there are women for whom HRT or ERT is not appropriate. Neither is recommended for women who have known or suspected cancer of the uterus or breast, who have had problems with blood clots called pulmonary embolus or who have active liver disease, says Dr. Walsh.

# The Breast Cancer Question

A major concern for most women considering HRT is whether it will increase their risk for breast cancer. The breast contains estrogen receptors, and the administration of estrogen in animals promotes cancer. So there's some reason to suspect that taking HRT or ERT could promote breast cancer in women.

The relationship between HRT and breast cancer is controversial; various studies on the issue have come to different, often contradictory conclusions. But one study by researchers at the Centers for Disease Control and Prevention in Atlanta compiled the results of a number of different studies and came to the following conclusions: Current users may be at increased risk, but it appears that the risk is relative to how long a woman takes ERT. There does not appear to be an association between ERT use and breast cancer in women who have taken it for less than 5 years, but women who have used it for over 15 years may have about a 30 percent increased risk. Women who used ERT in the past but are not currently taking it do not appear to be at increased risk for breast cancer.

# What You Can Do

So how does a woman decide? It's not easy. But here's what you can do.

**Find the right doctor.** Doctors may vary in their approaches to HRT, so it's important to find one you're comfortable with and who respects your feelings and opinions, says Borton. Don't be afraid to shop around for a doctor, and ask your friends about theirs.

**Know your family history.** In deciding about HRT, it's important to know your family history, says Dr. Walsh. Find out if anyone in your family has a history of heart disease, osteoporosis, breast cancer or endometrial cancer. Tell this to your doctor.

**Weigh your risks.** Deciding on HRT is often a matter of balancing your risk for one disease against your risk for another. One solution is to try "to decide as a woman what you are at risk for and what your risk profile is and to make an intelligent decision about what diseases you ought to be preventing that you are likely to get," says David Felson, M.D., of the Boston University Arthritis Center.

**Keep menstrual records.** When women go on HRT, they often get their periods again, particularly if they are taking progestin with estrogen. Hormone preparations can affect your flow. So record your bleeding pattern, says Dr. Walsh. Take a calendar, mark the days when you bleed and show it to your doctor, so she can determine whether the timing and amount of flow are appropriate, he says.

**Expect time for adjustment.** It may take four to six weeks for the hormones to kick in and for you to feel an effect, says Dr. Walsh. And once you're on them, it may take several months to get your therapy adjusted so that your periods become regular.

**Do those breast exams.** All the questions about the connection between HRT and breast cancer aren't definitively answered. So cover your bases and perform monthly breast self-examinations; they'll enable you to detect breast cancer early if you develop it. One of the most important things a woman can do is perform monthly breast self-examinations, says Dr. Walsh. "Most breast cancers are found by the woman herself, which is why it makes sense for her to examine her breasts once a month," he says. "That's 11 more times than her doctor has a chance to find a breast lump."

**Get your mammogram.** A mammogram is another way to detect breast cancer. Most doctors recommend that women have their first mammograms between the ages of 35 and 40. It's important for women on HRT to get mammograms on a regular basis, says Dr. Walsh. "People argue about how often and starting at what age, but by age 50, women should definitely be having mammograms at least every year," he says. Mammograms "allow the breast cancer to be detected when it's small and it's potentially curable," says Dr. Walsh.

**Have a cancer check.** Another type of follow-up test that women can have is called an endometrial biopsy. This checks the lining of the uterus, or endometrium, for cancer. Some doctors do a baseline biopsy at the start of HRT and then do a biopsy as an annual screening, although not all doctors do this with women who are receiving both estrogen and progestin. The test is more important when a woman is taking just estrogen, because the protective effect of progestin is absent. Ask your doctor about her approach.

**Look for support.** Other women going through menopause can be a tremendous source of support, says Borton. Talk to other women your age—either women you already know or those you meet in a support group—about their thinking, decisions and experiences surrounding HRT, she says. Hearing other women's experiences can often help. Call your local hospital for support groups in your area. Or start one of your own.

# HUMOR

## *It's No Joke—Humor Is Healthy*

"If you never want to see a man again, say 'I love you. I want to marry you. I want to have children.' They leave skid marks."

—*Rita Rudner*

Remember that game of Truth or Dare you played at Sally Winkler's fifth-grade slumber party? You know, the one where Janie Pratt had to kiss Sally's dog on the lips—and the dog kissed back? You laughed so hard that the little rubber bands on your braces popped out of your mouth.

At that tender age you had already stumbled upon one of life's most powerful natural age erasers: humor. In these hurry-up, way-too-serious days of adulthood, you can use a smile and a chuckle to help make yourself feel like a kid again. Humor can relax your body, ease your mind, relieve stress and boost your creativity.

"A sense of humor is not a cure-all or end-all for healthy living," says Joel Goodman, Ed.D., director of the Humor Project in Saratoga Springs, New York. "But it's a great way to beat stress and worry, and it can really make you feel better about life. And the best part of all is that you can do it for yourself."

## Happy Mind, Happy Body

"The bad times I can handle. It's the good times that drive me crazy. When is the other shoe going to drop?"

—*Erma Bombeck*

When something strikes you as funny, you laugh. And when you laugh, your body responds, says psychiatrist William F. Fry, M.D., associate clinical professor emeritus at Stanford University School of Medicine in Palo Alto, California. You flex, then relax, 15 facial muscles plus dozens of others all over your

513

body. Your pulse and respiration increase briefly, oxygenating your blood. And your brain experiences a decrease in pain perception, possibly associated with the production of pain-killing, pleasure-giving endorphins.

There's evidence that laughter can spur your immune system, increasing activity of lymphocytes and other "killer cells" (antibodies) and possibly raising levels of disease-fighting immunoglobulin A in your bloodstream, according to Kathleen Dillon, Ph.D., a psychologist and professor at Western New England College in Springfield, Massachusetts. One study even showed that the Immunoglobulin A may pass through breast milk to children and that humorous moms and happy babies suffer fewer respiratory infections.

By the time you're done giggling, your body is calmer, your brain is clearer and you may even discover that your headache or stiff neck has disappeared. Research shows you also might be more capable of solving problems that seemed impossible a few grumpy minutes before. Not bad for half a minute's work—if you can call laughing work.

## Laughing It Off

> "My ancestors wandered lost in the wilderness for 40 years because even in biblical times, men would not stop to ask for directions."
> —*Elayne Boosler*

The long-term effects of humor are harder to measure. The late author Norman Cousins credited laughter with helping him beat a potentially fatal connective tissue disease. After his diagnosis, Cousins moved into a hotel room, watched funny videos and movies, read funny books and magazines—and staged a stunning recovery.

Despite Cousins's success story, experts say that humor by itself won't cure disease or make you live longer. Still, many doctors have started working humor into treatments for everyone from cancer patients to people undergoing psychotherapy. "When used judiciously, I think it can indeed help with recovery," Dr. Fry says. "If nothing else, it makes the patient feel better for short periods of time."

Even if you're perfectly healthy, a well-honed sense of humor can raise your self-esteem—and maybe even make you more popular. "Humor can help you deal with unpleasant or difficult circumstances," Dr. Goodman says. "If you're able to laugh at yourself or a difficult situation, you're probably going to cope better and feel better in the long run."

Oh, and one other thing: Don't worry about developing laugh lines on your face. You're going to get some wrinkles no matter what you do, be it frowning or squinting or laughing. And specialists like Karen Burke, M.D., Ph.D., a dermatologist in private practice in New York City, say "positive" wrinkles like laugh lines give your face some character—just as frown-faced women can develop creases that make them look perpetually glum.

# Honing Your Funny Bone

"Women should try to increase their size rather than decrease it, because I believe the bigger we are, the more space we'll take up, and the more we'll have to be reckoned with. I think every woman should be fat like me."
—*Roseanne Arnold*

Dear old Mrs. Crabclaws. You remember her—the fourth-grade teacher whose idea of funny was spending a half-hour after school clapping erasers. Well, Dr. Goodman says that even she could have developed a working sense of humor.

"Everyone can laugh, though you might find that hard to believe," Dr. Goodman says. "The trick is to work on your sense of humor, to hone it, so that you can use it to your advantage."

So how do you make your life a little funnier? Experts offer these tips.

**Focus on funny stuff.** Try looking for humor in everyday life. It might help, Dr. Goodman says, to pretend you're Allen Funt of *Candid Camera* for a few minutes each day. "Act like you're carrying around a video camera," he says. "Look for people who are doing funny things, or animals or children or anything that might make you laugh. The more you look for humor, the more you'll find it."

**Take a child's-eye view.** Buried under a pile of paperwork? If it looks high to you, think how towering—and wicked cool—a seven-year-old would find it. Dr. Goodman says you should try picturing what most stressful adult situations would look like to a kid. The barking boss? The whining salesman? Your nagging Aunt Myrtle? They all look a little less threatening when seen with a childlike perspective.

**Check your humor pulse.** When it comes to laughter, it takes different jokes for different folks. Dr. Fry suggests spending a week or so to gauge your own sense of humor. Which comic strips make you laugh? Which movies? Which friends or co-workers? Do you find yourself chuckling at your child's antics? Once you've figured it out, start a laugh library. Clip funny comics and stick them on your refrigerator door. Rent or buy funny movies or stand-up comic routines. Shoot home videos of your wacko dog or your bumbling neighbor Bob.

"It's a simple thing to do," Dr. Fry says. "Still, many women don't think to add a little laughter into their lives. and that's too bad, because it really can make you feel better."

**Meet your laugh quota.** Dr. Goodman suggests trying to get 15 laughs a

# The Laugh Library

Some days it's hard to work up a smile without a little outside help. That's when you need to check out a chuckle from your personal library of laughter.

"Everyone should have a collection," says Patch Adams, M.D., director of the Gesundheit Institute in Arlington, Virginia. "There are times when you can just grab a funny book or movie and change your whole day."

Dr. Adams dispensed with frumpy bedside manners years ago and now visits his patients while dressed like a gorilla, a dead French king or even Santa Claus. The nonprofit Gesundheit Institute has been around since 1971, and in that time Dr. Adams and others have treated more than 15,000 patients with humor therapy–styled medicine, helping them laugh themselves back to health. Dr. Adams has found that a humorous context helps prevent burnout and seems to affect the healing process in a positive way. Dr. Adams is so sold on the idea of humor and healing that he's pushing for construction of a "silly hospital" with hidden passages, slides and chutes and other decidedly unmedical features.

Dr. Adams has more than 12,000 items in his personal collection, including 1,500 cartoon books, scores of funny videos and dozens more comedy albums. Among his favorites:

day, even if you have to look for the humor. "There's no magic in the number," he says. "It just seems about right to me. If you manage to reach your humor quota, you're probably feeling pretty good about life."

Even if you don't particularly feel like laughing, try it once in a while anyway. The reflexes, the smile and the physiological changes your body will undergo just might make you feel better. You may even find yourself beginning to inject humor into tense situations—a great tool everywhere from the boardroom to the bedroom.

**Choose wisely.** Laughter can be contagious, but so can the plague. If you start making racist or ethnic jokes, people will start avoiding you. "Pick subjects that will bring people together in good humor," Dr. Fry says. "And never single someone out. That will make that person with-

• *Being There*, a movie starring the late Peter Sellers. "I honestly can't stop laughing from the opening credits to the end," Dr. Adams says.
• *The Search for Signs of Intelligent Life in the Universe*, a play and best-selling book by Jane Wagner and a movie starring Lily Tomlin.
• Comic strips like "Calvin and Hobbes," "The Far Side," "Pogo" and "The Neighbors."
• Funny books from modern authors like Dave Barry and Lewis Grizzard.
• Any classic video from slapstick artists like the Three Stooges and Jerry Lewis, plus all works by the Marx Brothers (try *Duck Soup*) and Monty Python (try *Monty Python's Life of Brian* or *Monty Python and the Holy Grail*).
• Comedy records from Woody Allen ("a great stand-up guy before he went into movies"), Jonathan Winters ("a true genius"), Lenny Bruce, Sid Caesar and many others.

Starting a comedy collection, especially albums, can even save you some money—if you shop like the experts. Try checking out garage sales, where you're almost certain to encounter at least one 25-cent comedy album in every stack of records.

"And they've only been played three or four times, probably, so there's a lot of life left in them," Dr. Adams says.

draw—and could give her incentive to get back at you when you're most vulnerable," he says.

**Draw the line.** Not everything is funny. And humor won't solve every dilemma. "There are times when you have to take things seriously," Dr. Goodman says. "Laughing at everything can be a form of avoidance. It helps to have a good attitude, sure, but there are certain times that we need to be sensible—like at funerals or in court or at important business meetings—and we need to consider if it will work for or against us."

# IMMUNITY

## A Mighty Defense against Aging

Somewhere in your body, right at this moment, your immune system is choreographing a deadly waltz with viruses, bacteria, fungi and any other unwelcome intruders.

Like a professional dance troupe, a healthy immune system seems to have perfect timing and synchronization. At its best, it is an aggressive age fighter that helps keep you feeling good, looking good and brimming with energy, says Terry Phillips, Ph.D., director of the immunogenetics and immunochemistry laboratories at George Washington University Medical Center in Washington, D.C.

"If the immune system is doing its job, and you have good health, you don't even think about it," Dr. Phillips says. "The best way to keep it that way is to do all the things that are going to keep it naturally strong like exercising, eating right and coping with stress as best you can."

But as we age, our immune system, like an aging dancer, loses some of its dexterity. This incredibly complex defensive system gradually weakens and is less able to pounce on and destroy invading organisms.

"The immune system certainly ages and clearly functions less optimally as we get older. We believe that loss of immune system function is related to the onset of cancer, autoimmune diseases like rheumatoid arthritis and the frequency and severity of infectious diseases. At 27, for example, pneumonia is a nuisance, but at 70 it can be life threatening," says Michael Osband, M.D., adjunct professor at Boston University School of Medicine.

## A Look at the All-Star Cast

The immune system actually consists of millions of cells that have many specialized roles. Some play starring roles, while others are stimulated to act only in specific situations. Among the key performers are B-cells and T-cells, which are types of white blood cells. B-cells hang out in the spleen and lymph nodes waiting for specific invaders, also known as antigens. Once a B-cell identifies an invader, it releases antibodies into the bloodstream. These Y-shaped proteins latch on to the antigen and tag it for destruction by various cells.

T-cells mature in the thymus—a small gland in the throat—and are one of the most important parts of the immune system. They are among the few cells in the body that can distinguish normal cells from foes like cancer cells, viruses, fungi and bacteria, says John Marchalonis, Ph.D., professor and chairman of the Department of Microbiology and Immunology at the University of Arizona College of Medicine in Tucson. How T-cells learn to do that is complicated. But basically, on the surface of each T-cell is a receptor, a chemical molecule that recognizes one of the ten million known antigens. So when a T-cell detects an antigen, not only does it seek out and attempt to destroy that intruder, but it also sends out signals to the other parts of the immune system that determine how aggressively the body will attack the invader.

T-cells, for example, can activate macrophages, amoeba-like cells that literally gobble up the intruder or signal the B-cells to crank up their production of antibodies.

## A Slow Decline

The immune system reaches its prime just about the time that you enter puberty. Then the thymus begins to wither away, and your T-cell production and function drop considerably. Although you may continue to make T-cells throughout your life, these cells don't identify invaders and choreograph the defensive effort of the immune system as well as the ones produced when the thymus was at its peak, Dr. Osband says. Why the thymus shrinks remains a mystery, but some researchers suspect that the hormones that trigger puberty also may turn off the thymus.

"You generally don't make a lot of T-cells after the thymus goes away. The thymus is important because that's where T-cells learn to recognize antigens," Dr. Osband says. "Clearly, that learning process doesn't stop when the thymus goes, but your T-cells are left to learn on their own. It's like trying to educate yourself by reading an encyclopedia instead of going to college."

Genetics and free radicals—chemically unstable oxygen molecules that cause havoc through the body—also contribute to the decline of the immune system, says Marguerite Kay, M.D., professor of microbiology and immunology at the University of Arizona College of Medicine.

In addition, some invaders like HIV (human immunodeficiency virus), the virus that causes AIDS, attack the immune system directly and destroy it.

## Keeping Your Immunity Strong

While some declines in immune power may be a natural part of aging, researchers including Dr. Phillips say that making just a few lifestyle changes can

## Shoot Down the Sniffles

Your immune system is tough, but every year you seem to attract the attention of the latest version of the flu bug. Yet all it takes to protect most people against the illness is a shot. In fact, an annual flu vaccination is probably the best health deal in town, says William H. Adler, M.D., chief of clinical immunology at the National Institute on Aging in Baltimore.

Don't wait to get immunized until everyone around you is hacking and coughing. That may be too late, since it takes at least two weeks for the vaccination to completely kick in. If possible, get your shot by early October. About one-third of the people who are vaccinated will still get the flu, though usually a much milder case than if they weren't protected at all. Expect to pay between $10 and $15. At some doctors' offices, you don't even need an appointment; you can just walk in and a nurse will administer the vaccine on the spot.

---

keep your immunity vigilant long into your life. "In the end," Dr. Phillips says, "it's how well we look after ourselves that decides how well our immune systems look after us." Here are some ways to boost your body's natural defenses.

**Soothe stress.** Researchers have long suspected that stress suppresses the immune system, and emerging evidence supports that theory.

Researchers at Carnegie Mellon University in Pittsburgh, for example, gave cold viruses in the form of nasal drops to 400 volunteers. Placebo drops were given to 26 subjects. The researchers then identified stress levels in both groups and watched for new infections. The highly stressed volunteers ended up being twice as likely to develop colds as the low-stressed volunteers. None of the 26 people who received the placebo got a cold.

Scientists believe that steroids produced by the adrenal glands are released during stress and suppress the activity of immune system cells, Dr. Phillips says.

How you ease stress is an individual choice, but for starters, you could play with your kids or pet, participate in a hobby like gardening or woodworking, do meditation or yoga, watch a funny movie or television program or just read an enjoyable book.

**Get some Zzzs.** "Sleep is the repair shop for the immune system," Dr. Phillips says. During sleep, your brain and body rest but your immune system doesn't. So when you're snoozing, your immune system has less competition for the nutrients needed to strengthen your disease-fighting mechanisms. Without enough rest, your immune system will suffer. In a study of 23 people, for example, researchers at the University of California, San Diego, School of Medicine found a 30 percent decrease in immune response after these people missed three or more hours of sleep in a night.

Try to get at least six to eight hours of sleep a night, Dr. Phillips suggests.

**Stop smoking.** Tobacco smoke contains formaldehyde, a chemical that can paralyze macrophages in the lungs and make you more susceptible to upper respiratory ailments, including colds and flus, Dr. Phillips says. So if you smoke, quit.

**Sweat it out.** Moderate exercise helps prevent bacteria from gathering in the lungs and strengthens the vigilance of the immune system by increasing circulation of antibodies in the blood, says William H. Adler, M.D., chief of clinical immunology at the National Institute on Aging in Baltimore.

After a 15-week study of 18 women in their thirties who were asked to walk 45 minutes a day, five days a week, researchers at Appalachian State University in Boon, North Carolina, found that the walkers had half as many colds and flus as a group of sedentary women.

To keep your immune system at its best, do aerobic exercise like walking, jogging, swimming or bicycling at least 20 minutes a day as often as possible.

# Eat, Drink and Be Immune

"The role of diet in immunity is very direct," says Jeffrey Blumberg, Ph.D., associate director of the U.S. Department of Agriculture Human Nutrition Research Center on Aging at Tufts University in Boston. "Specific nutrients play very particular roles in pushing immunity up and down."

Here's an A-to-zinc guide to some vitamins and minerals that could help keep your immunity in high gear.

**Get on the A list.** Vitamin A fortifies the top layer of skin against cracks through which invaders can enter and fights cancer tumors, possibly by boosting white blood cell activity. But since too much vitamin A can be toxic, it's probably a good idea to get your daily requirements from food rather than high-dose supplements, says Ranjit Chandra, M.D., research professor at Memorial University of Newfoundland in St. John's and director of the World Health Organization Center for Nutritional Immunology. The Recommended Dietary Allowance (RDA) is 800 micrograms retinol equivalents (or 4,000 IU). One medium sweet potato has more than double your daily requirement of vitamin A. Other foods rich in vitamin A are liver, carrots, spinach, broccoli, lettuce, apricots and watermelon.

**Boost your beta-carotene.** An antioxidant, beta-carotene, which is converted to vitamin A in the body, also combats free radicals and may strengthen the immune system's ability to prevent cancer. Like vitamin A, beta-carotene is found in foods such as carrots, spinach, broccoli and lettuce. But, unlike vitamin A, beta-carotene is not toxic and can be taken as a supplement with little danger. Dr. Osband suggests taking six to nine milligrams a day.

**Don't forget B$_6$.** "When older people were fed diets deficient in vitamin B$_6$, their immunity was lowered substantially," Dr. Blumberg says. "When their intake was then increased one step at a time, immunity gradually returned to normal—but only after intake of more than 1.6 milligrams (the RDA) was provided."

You can get the RDA of 1.6 milligrams of vitamin B$_6$ by eating two large bananas. Other good dietary sources are chicken, fish, liver, rice, avocados, walnuts, wheat germ and sunflower seeds. Vitamin B$_6$ can be toxic in very large doses (1,000 to 2,000 milligrams per day), Dr. Blumberg says.

**Supercharge with C.** From keeping viruses from multiplying to stimulating tumor-attacking cells, vitamin C gives almost every part of the immune system a boost, Dr. Blumberg says. Fruits and vegetables like oranges, strawberries, broccoli and red bell peppers are good sources of this nutrient. It appears that optimal dosages range from 500 to 1,000 milligrams a day, says Dr. Blumberg.

**The sun shines on D.** Although scientists know that vitamin D is an immunity booster, they are mystified by its role. They do know that vitamin D is needed for strong bones, which is significant because immune system cells are formed in the bone marrow. Fortunately, most people get their fair share of vitamin D. (The RDA for vitamin D is 5 micrograms or 200 IU a day.) An eight-ounce glass of fortified milk has about 100 IU. It's also abundant in cheeses and oily fish such as herring, tuna and salmon. You can also get vitamin D from sunlight, since ultraviolet radiation triggers a vitamin D–making substance in the skin. In summer, about 10 to 15 minutes of sun a day will give you all the vitamin D you need. Vitamin D is toxic in large amounts, so doctors say it should never be taken in supplements.

**Eat your E.** A real powerhouse, vitamin E can boost your immunity across the board. In particular, it prevents free radical damage to cells, improves white blood cell activity and increases interleukin-2, a substance that promotes the growth of T-cells. It also turns off prostaglandin E$_2$, a naturally occurring substance that suppresses the immune system.

Vitamin E—also considered an antioxidant—can be found in oils, nuts and seeds, but it's difficult to get a health-promoting or immune-boosting dose through food alone, says Dr. Blumberg. Healthy diets generally provide only 20 IU a day. Optimal dosages appear to be between 100 to 400 IU a day, he says.

**Ax the fat.** In animal studies, a diet consisting of 40 percent of calories from fat—the typical American diet—had a detrimental influence on the immune system, says Dr. Chandra. So try to reduce your fat consumption to 25 percent of calories.

To do it, use low-fat or nonfat dairy products, trim skin or visible fat from meats and eat no more than one three-ounce serving (about the size of a deck of cards) of poultry, fish or red meat a day. Be sure to eat at least six servings of grain products like breads, beans and rice and at least five servings of fruits and vegetables like apples, pears, broccoli and spinach daily.

**Pump up your iron.** Iron is a vital catalyst that helps your immune system nab intruders and corral renegade cells like cancer. Most women need about 15 milligrams of iron a day. A dinner of a three-ounce broiled lean steak, a medium-size baked potato and a half-cup of peas provides more than seven milligrams. Other iron-rich foods are clams and oysters, pork, dark chicken meat, dried apricots and green leafy vegetables. But don't depend on iron supplements unless they are prescribed by a doctor. Too much iron can cause health problems such as constipation, skin discoloration, cirrhosis of the liver and diabetes.

**Maximize your magnesium.** Some studies suggest that magnesium deficiency can cause the immune system to run amok, attack normal cells in the body and trigger autoimmune diseases like rheumatoid arthritis, Dr. Phillips says. Taking a magnesium supplement may be a good idea for women on water pills (diuretics) or high blood pressure drugs. Both make you lose this mineral. So does drinking excessive amounts of alcohol. The rest of us can get the RDA of 280 milligrams without supplements by regularly eating leafy vegetables, potatoes, whole grains, milk and seafood.

**Stock up on selenium.** This nutrient, an antioxidant that's a known cancer fighter, may be required to fire up your immune system's infection-fighting team. You should be getting plenty in your normal diet. The RDA of selenium for women is 55 micrograms, and you'll get 138 micrograms from a tuna sandwich alone. All fish, shellfish and whole-grain cereals and breads are selenium rich. Very high doses can impair immune responses, however, so supplements should not exceed 200 micrograms a day. Dr. Chandra says.

**Try zinc, the missing link.** "Of all the minerals, zinc is probably the most important for maintaining immunity," Dr. Phillips says. A shortage can cause a drop in production of the white blood cells that surround and destroy microscopic invaders. Zinc also helps the body process vitamin D, another important nutrient that bolsters immunity. To get the RDA of 12 milligrams from your diet, eat lean red meat, oysters, milk, oats, whole grains, eggs and poultry. Avoid supplements providing more than 40 milligrams, Dr. Blumberg warns. Beyond these levels, zinc can actually slow the immune system down.

# LEARNING

## *Have It Your Way*

**H**igh school algebra? College chemistry? They're history. As an adult you can learn what you want, when you want, any way you want—and with a sense of fulfillment, accomplishment and fun.

"It's one of the great things about being a grown-up," says Ronald Gross, chairman of the University Seminar on Innovation in Education at Columbia University in New York City and author of *Peak Learning: A Master Course in Learning How to Learn*. "When you were in school you were pretty much told what to learn. Now you can pick your own topics and change whenever you feel like it. It gives you a great feeling of freedom."

And a feeling of youthfulness, too. When you were a girl the world seemed a boundless place, full of potential and hope. Learning can bring that feeling back. So read the great philosophers. Program a computer. Learn how to fix your lawn mower. It's like being a child again, discovering why it rains or what makes the sky blue. And your life isn't ruled by final exams, hall passes or pop quizzes.

## Flex Your Brain

Let's start by debunking one of the great myths of aging. Yes, you are losing 50,000 to 100,000 irreplaceable brain cells a day. But it doesn't make a bit of difference because you started with more than 100 billion. By the time you reach the age of 70, you'll still have 99 percent of your original total.

Experts say it's not the number of cells that counts, anyway. It's what you do with them. "The adage 'use it or lose it' applies to the mind as well as the muscles," says Marian Diamond, Ph.D., professor of neurosciences in the Department of Integrated Biology at the University of California, Berkeley. Physical exercise makes muscles grow and mental exercise makes the connections between brain cells grow.

"Studies show that the area in the brain devoted to word understanding is significantly larger in the average college graduate than in the average high school graduate," Dr. Diamond says. "Why? Because college graduates spend more time working with words."

So there's no reason adults can't learn as well as children do. In fact, being an adult often makes learning easier. "You can put things in context," says Gross. "When you're learning something, like philosophy, you have years of experience that will help you see where things fit in. You never had that edge when you were young," he says.

Experts say older women may even handle the rigors of college life better than younger women. A study of 85 women students at the Pennsylvania State University in University Park found that those who were 26 years old and up felt less stress at school than students of typical college age. Past experience with raising families and having careers may buffer against the stress.

# A Primer for Women

The key to learning is overcoming the notion that the whole process is boring—or scary. It doesn't have to be either. "Learning can be life's greatest joy," Gross says. "It's what makes humans human." And the part about being scared? "Why worry when you're doing it for yourself?" Gross asks. "Failing is not an issue. There's not going to be a test. Learn for the sake of learning and you'll see how great you feel."

Ready to get started? Experts offer these tips.

**Follow your heart.** What have you always wanted to learn? Gardening? Spanish? Arc welding? Gross says you should make a list—and don't worry about whether the items seem "important" enough. Remember, you're learning for yourself.

Pick one or two topics, save the rest for later and take it from there.

**Show some style.** In school everyone learned the same way: by being quiet, listening to the teacher, going home and studying. Some people thrived and others didn't.

That's because people learn in different ways. Some do best in large groups. Some like to go off on their own. Others like to interact with one or two good friends, to share ideas.

How about you? Do you like seminars with lots of people or one-on-one sessions? Are you sharpest at night or in the morning? Do you concentrate best with the radio playing softly in the background?

"How you learn plays a large part in what you learn," Gross says. "Figure out your own style and make yourself comfortable."

**Take your time.** It's one thing to learn to play chopsticks. It's another to play Beethoven's Fifth Symphony. And it's yet another to play Beethoven's Fifth while cooking a pear tart à la Julia Child and running a road race like Mary Decker Slaney.

# Are You a Grouper or a Stringer?

What's the best way to learn? Your way. If you like to read the end of a book first, great. If you like to juggle ten topics at once, super. Experts agree that following your own style is key to learning.

To see how you can learn best, take this quiz developed by David Lewis and James Greene of the Mind Potential Study Group in London. Circle either *a* or *b* after each question.

1. When studying one unfamiliar subject, you:
   a. prefer to gather information from diverse topic areas.
   b. prefer to focus on one topic.
2. You would rather:
   a. know a little about a great many subjects.
   b. become an expert on just one subject.
3. When studying from a textbook, you:
   a. skip ahead and read chapters of special interest out of sequence.
   b. work systematically from one chapter to the next, not moving on until you have understood earlier material.
4. When asking people for information about some subject of interest, you:
   a. tend to ask broad questions that call for rather general answers.
   b. tend to ask narrow questions that demand specific answers.
5. When browsing in a library or bookstore, you:
   a. roam around looking at books on many different subjects.
   b. stay more or less in one place looking at books on just a couple of subjects.
6. You are best at remembering:
   a. general principles.
   b. specific facts.
7. When performing some tasks, you:
   a. like to have background information not strictly related to the work.
   b. prefer to concentrate only on strictly relevant information.

In other words, take your time. Otherwise, you may burn out on learning. "Too much stimulation loses its value," Dr. Diamond says. "By all means, enrich your mental life and keep your brain active but allow yourself adequate time to assimilate new information."

8. You think that educators should:
    a. give students exposure to a wide range of subjects in college.
    b. ensure that students mainly acquire in-depth knowledge related to their specialties.
9. When on vacation, you would rather:
    a. spend a short amount of time in several places.
    b. stay in one place the whole time and get to know it well.
10. When learning something, you would rather:
    a. follow general guidelines.
    b. work with a detailed plan of action.
11. Do you agree that, in addition to specialized knowledge, a person should know some math, art, physics, literature, psychology, politics, languages, biology, history and medicine? If you think people should study four or more of these subjects, score an a on this question.

Total the *a* and *b* answers. If you marked six or more of the questions with an *a*, you're a grouper. If you answered six or more with a *b*, you're a stringer.

What does this mean? Groupers are "big picture" people who need to learn in an unstructured fashion, according to Ronald Gross, chairman of the University Seminar on Innovation in Education at Columbia University in New York City and author of *Peak Learning: A Master Course in Learning How to Learn*. You should hop right into a subject, read manuals from back to front if you feel like it and never be afraid to take on several tasks at once. And don't worry about the details at the beginning. You'll pick them up as needed.

Stringers are much more detail-oriented. They like to follow a plan, or a structure that will take them logically through a subject. Gross suggests reading the tables of contents in several good books on your subject of choice. Develop a plan of attack. And make sure you have absorbed material before moving on. You'll enjoy learning more if you develop a sense of mastery along the way.

**Abandon ship!** So you always wanted to learn to sail. And there you are, sailing solo, trimming the jib and gybing the main. But it's just not as much fun as you thought it would be.

Head for the lifeboats and try something else. "There's no sense staying with something that isn't what you really want to do," Gross says. "And there's certainly no shame in it. Just try something else instead."

There's one exception. Before you jump overboard, make sure it's for the right reason. Are you quitting because it's not interesting? Or are you having trouble with it because you're still learning the basics? Mastering a new task means sailing through some rough water. But riding out the storm has its rewards.

**Challenge yourself.** Do you only like crossword puzzles that you can solve? Then you're not challenging yourself. While pushing too hard inhibits learning, not going hard enough can be stifling, too. Gross says you should always leave another bridge for yourself to cross. "Proceed at your own pace, but always proceed," he says. If you reach a goal, bask in the victory. Then set another goal and go after it.

**Don't be afraid to ask.** If you're taking a knitting class and don't know a knit from a purl, drop the needle and raise your hand. If you're not sure how hard to tighten an oil filter, call a garage and ask. Or consult the nearest librarian (a library card is one of the most powerful learning tools around). "Part of learning is knowing when to ask questions," Gross says. "Try to work things out for yourself. But you're not doing yourself any good if you reach a dead end and stay there."

# LEISURE TIME

## *No Woman Can Do without It*

From the moment the alarm rings in the morning, you're on the go. You make coffee, take a quick shower, rouse the kids, fix breakfast, get dressed, dash to work, spend eight intense hours or more on the job, pick up your son after baseball practice, drop your daughters off at soccer, fix dinner, help your children with their homework, get them into bed, iron clothes, make lunches and then do some paperwork you wanted to finish before the meeting tomorrow.

Whew! You need time out here. Leisure isn't a luxury, doctors say. It's a necessity if you want to feel young.

Leisure plays an important role in your overall health and well-being, says Leslie Hartley Gise, M.D., associate professor of psychiatry at Mount Sinai Medical Center in New York City. If you don't get enough of it, you can begin to feel grouchy, fatigued and depressed. Over time, life without leisure can lead to ulcers, migraines, cardiovascular disease, high blood pressure and other physical ailments, she says.

"Leisure activities can certainly help you feel more satisfied with your life. Could that translate into making some people feel younger? My guess would be yes," says Howard Tinsley, Ph.D., professor of psychology at Southern Illinois University at Carbondale. "Some may think of it as literally feeling younger, while others may feel like they just have more zest for life. They may feel more energized and excited to wake up in the morning."

## Adding to Your Reserves

One way to look at the importance of leisure is to imagine that your body is a vast oil field that has two types of energy. Some of the oil, called superficial energy, is like gasoline. It provides the quick bursts of energy we need for day-

529

to-day living. But the other type, called deep energy, is like a slow-burning oil that keeps us going in times of illness and other extensive periods of stress. Its energy is irreplaceable and is intended to last a lifetime, says Walt Schafer, Ph.D., professor of sociology at California State University, Chico, and director of the Pacific Wellness Institute in Chico.

"With adequate sleep, adequate time away from pressure and adequate play, we can replenish those superficial energy reserves," Dr. Schafer says. "But if we don't, then we start tapping into those deep energy reserves, and that accelerates the aging process."

## Learning to Play

Unfortunately, many women simply haven't learned how to create leisure time or use it properly. To them, play is just another chore.

"Some women treat their leisure as if it were a job," Dr. Schafer says. "Their leisure is task-oriented, demand-oriented and packed with pressure to perform well. Instead of experiencing the joy and playfulness of leisure, they're putting themselves at risk of draining their energy reserves even further."

Ironically, the pressure from that approach to fun can create stress—the very thing that leisure is supposed to relieve. And experts suspect that stress siphons youthfulness from your body.

"We all want to feel useful. We all want to feel as if we're contributing. But if that's all you do, then you're short-changing yourself," says Jeanne Murrone, Ph.D., a clinical psychologist at the Center for Mental Health, a clinic affiliated with the Charlotte-Mecklenburg Hospital Authority in Charlotte, North Carolina. "Leisure is the time to renew yourself. Without that renewal time, you're going to burn out. So leisure—that time when you don't have to do something perfectly, but just for the enjoyment of it—is probably just as necessary for us as sleeping, exercising and eating properly."

Here are some ways to create more time for leisure in your life.

**Planning takes knowledge.** Leisure doesn't just happen. It takes effort and planning to work fun activities into your life. Read the newspaper, scan the bulletin boards in your neighborhood supermarkets. Phone your local parks and recreation department and ask about outdoor trips, sports leagues and craft classes, suggests Patsy B. Edwards, a leisure counselor in private practice in Los Angeles. You can also explore your library, community college and church for new activities.

Set aside time each day for a leisure activity you enjoy, even if it is just a ten-minute walk around the block, Dr. Schafer says.

**Find motivation that makes sense.** Find a reason to make room in your life for leisure, says Carol Lassen, Ph.D., clinical professor of psychology at the University of Colorado School of Medicine in Denver. It might be as simple as telling yourself that you want to live longer or have a better relationship with your spouse, kids or friends. But whatever it is, it has be something that is more important to you than work. If it's not, you're less likely to stick with it.

# Where Does the Time Go?

Most of us actually have more free time than we think. How we spend it is the problem, experts say.

On average, women have about 41 hours of free time a week when they're not working, doing household chores or sleeping, says William Danner of Leisure Trends, a Glastonbury, Connecticut, company that analyzes how Americans use their time. But because the number of leisure activities—including sports like wind-surfing, hobbies like jewelry making and entertainment like country music—is expanding rapidly, the amount of time we can devote to any one activity is shrinking.

But one activity—watching television—is gobbling up more of our leisure time than you might suspect. In fact, a Leisure Trends survey of over 5,000 people found that 30 percent of our leisure time—almost one in three of our free-time hours—is spent anchored in front of the tube. In comparison, socializing and reading—the second and third most popular activities—accounted for only 8 and 6 percent, respectively, of the available leisure time each day.

---

## Don't Think about It

By the end of the day your boss wants you to come up with some innovative ways to solve a problem that has been vexing your company for months. But it seems the harder you think about the problem, the tougher it becomes to dream up bedazzling ideas.

So stop trying so hard, says Jeanne Murrone, Ph.D., a clinical psychologist at the Center for Mental Health, a clinic affiliated with the Charlotte-Mecklenburg Hospital Authority in Charlotte, North Carolina. Go for a walk, do a crossword puzzle or some other leisure activity. The miraculous thing about leisure is it not only can keep you youthful, it may also give you a creative edge over your more intense co-workers.

"Some of your most creative times can occur when you're not thinking about work," Dr. Murrone says. "It's like making bread. You can put all the ingredients together, but unless you put it aside for awhile and allow the dough to rise and rest, it's not going to be very good bread. Leisure serves much the same purpose. If you leave some space in your life for leisure, you may find yourself being more productive and creative."

If you want to spend your prime doing better things, experts recommend the following approach.

**Keep a diary.** For a week, write down what you're doing every 30 minutes including things like showering, cooking dinner and working, says Roger Mannell, Ph.D., a psychologist and chair of the Department of Recreation and Leisure Studies at the University of Waterloo in Waterloo, Ontario. At the end of the week take a look at your diary and see how much time you spent working and how much free time you had.

Each day rate your satisfaction with each leisure activity. Was tennis on Tuesday more fun than that party on Friday? If you're filling your time with obligations you don't find rewarding, you should make changes.

**Set limits.** It's important to draw boundaries between your work and home life. For example, avoid taking work home at night. "By doing that, you're letting both your employer and your family know that your leisure time is just as important to you as getting to work on time, meeting your deadlines and whatever else you do on the job," Dr. Murrone says.

**Learn to shift gears.** Create a space at the end of your day—even if it is only 10 to 15 minutes—to be alone with your thoughts so you can make the transition between work and home. Walking, reading the newspaper or listening to music could do it for you. For some people, it's just a matter of changing their clothes, says Dr. Lassen.

**Make your own fun.** What is leisure for one person is work for another. Know yourself and what you think is fun. Make a list of your strengths and weakness, what you like to do and what you detest. Then make your leisure choice based on that list. "Gardening, for example, is fun for some people, but for others it's boring work," Dr. Schafer says. "I do white-water kayaking and I think it's joyful and great fun, but for others it might be terrifying."

**Be imperfect.** Some people avoid doing certain types of leisure activities because they don't feel they can master them. "It's important to recognize that you don't have to do everything well," Dr. Murrone says. "Write a story but don't edit it, draw a picture but don't show it to anyone, so it can be as messy as you want. You don't have to win the golf tournament, you don't have win the race, you don't have to create a painting that is a masterpiece. It's really not a matter of how well you do, but that you enjoy doing it."

# LOW-FAT FOODS

## *Eating Lighter and Liking It*

You've been down the low-fat trail countless times before. You know that the secret to looking good and living long is to clean up your act and get all that grease, lard and oil out of your diet. So you slash fat with a vengeance, blow your grocery budget on some green-colored "health food" and pretend that you're happy.

It doesn't take long before your taste buds start to tingle, your stomach begins to rumble and your imagination runs amok with bizarre images of oversize ice cream sundaes, sizzling steaks and buckets of golden-brown french fries. Before you know it, you're loading your shopping cart with enough chips and Twinkies to fill a warehouse. And another diet attempt bites the dust.

Low-fat eating used to be a lonely, miserable experience—thin on flavor and hardly satisfying. But these days, we don't have to starve, suffer or sacrifice taste to trim the excess fat from our diets. Today, supermarkets offer an array of fresh produce and aisle after aisle of satisfying, good-tasting low- or reduced-fat items that make keeping an eye on fat a piece of cake.

"It's a misconception that cutting back on fat means giving up all the foods we love," says Judy Dodd, R.D., former president of the American Dietetic Association and a food and nutrition adviser. "There are no bad foods, only bad eating habits, which are easy to change if you take things one step at a time." Here's how.

## Do Your Body a Favor

Suppose you've gotten along fine for years with your old favorites. Or you're not particularly overweight. Do you really need to bother changing to a low-fat lifestyle as you get older? The answer is a resounding yes. Most

# A Diet for Longer Life

What if a special kind of low-fat diet would take you farther than you think—even into extra decades? Some scientists say that if you sharply reduce the total number of calories you eat, you may live years or even decades longer. The catch? This diet must be forever—and it calls for loads of self-denial.

The Very Low Calorie Diet (VLCD) is also called a modified fast. Some researchers define VLCDs as diets containing 800 calories or less per day. But others consider a low-fat, nutrient-packed diet of up to 1,800 calories per day for women or men to be a reasonable modified fast.

And it works, says Roy Walford, M.D., professor of pathology at the University of California, Los Angeles, and author of *The 120-Year Diet.* Dr. Walford served as chief medical officer for Biosphere 2—a closed ecosystem in Arizona where for two years the resident scientists experienced an unexpected food shortage. On strict daily rations of 1,800 to 2,200 calories (instead of the normal 2,500 they expected given their high levels of physical activity), they all lost weight and showed marked reductions in blood pressure and cholesterol.

These results are consistent with food restriction in rodents, which increased life span and slowed down almost all age-associated physical changes and diseases, says Edward J. Masoro, Ph.D., a physiologist and director of the Aging Research and Education Center of the University of Texas Health Science Center at San Antonio. But Dr. Masoro feels that a

experts agree that a high-fat diet is a major cause of all kinds of killers, including cardiovascular disease, high blood pressure, diabetes, stroke and some types of cancer.

If a long, disease-free life isn't a good enough reason to go low-fat, here are three you can't ignore: your hips, your thighs and your tummy. "The fat you eat is much more likely to become the fat you carry," says Robert Kushner, M.D., director of the Nutrition and Weight Control Clinic at the University of Chicago. "Fat contains about nine calories per gram, which is about twice as many calories as proteins and carbohydrates. And unlike proteins and carbohydrates, which are easily burned and metabolized by the body, fatty foods burn slowly and are more likely to be stored in the fatty areas of the body."

long-term modified fast is "unchartered" in humans and doubts that many people would adopt such a strict diet for most of their life span.

But if you're a closet Spartan, here's how to do a VLCD safely.

**Ask your doctor to help.** No one should embark on a long-term fasting diet without medical supervision, experts say.

**Know your history.** If you are prone to gallstones, steer clear of VLCDs, says James E. Everhart, M.D., of the Division of Digestive Diseases and Nutrition at the National Institute of Diabetes and Digestive and Kidney Diseases. Studies have shown that up to 25 percent of people on VLCDs develop gallstones, he says.

**Eat no junk.** "A healthy modified fast has to be very high in nutrients, with no junk food," says Dr. Walford. There's simply no room for high-fat food or wasted calories.

**Read Pritikin.** Next to *The 120-Year Diet*, the diet closest to that of the Biosphere team is the Pritikin Longevity Center plan—largely vegetarian, high in fiber and with only ten percent of its calories from fat, says Dr. Walford.

**No alcohol.** The Biosphere results came from an alcohol-free modified fast, Dr. Walford says.

**Take a vitamin and mineral supplement.** "Take a multivitamin with at least the Recommended Dietary Allowance of everything to avoid deficiencies," says Dr. Walford. Additionally, the Biosphere team took 400 IU of vitamin E and 500 milligrams of vitamin C each day.

The problem, says Dr. Kushner, is that our bodies store excess calories as fat cells. If we ate 100 calories of fat, almost all would be stored as fat cells on our waist and hips. But in converting the same amount of carbohydrates or protein to storage fat, your body would actually burn up about 20 percent of that total. In other words, fewer calories are converted to body fat when we eat carbs and proteins than when we eat fat alone.

In fact, a wealth of scientific research indicates that just a little less fat in your diet can lead to a trimmer, slimmer you. According to one study at Cornell University in Ithaca, New York, people on low-fat diets lose weight even when they don't try to restrict their total calories or the amount of food they eat. For eleven weeks, the thirteen participants in this study merely reduced their fat intake to 20 to 25 percent of total calories and, in the process, lost weight at the rate of about one-half pound per week. Best of all, they experienced no hunger pangs, cravings or depression.

Studies also show that a low-fat diet reduces your risk of developing chronic disease. James W. Anderson, M.D., and researchers at the University of Kentucky showed that adults 30 to 50 years old with moderately high levels of serum cholesterol (the artery-clogging substance that produces high blood pressure, heart disease and stroke) can lower their cholesterol levels by as much as 9 percent just by trimming their fat intake to 25 percent of total calories. What's more, when that low-fat diet is coupled with a high intake of soluble fiber (the fat-free substance found in oat bran and whole-grain products), serum cholesterol can be reduced even further: up to 13 percent.

The bottom line: If health and longevity are among your goals, low-fat foods can help take you there.

# Facts on Fat

So this all means that fat is a bad thing, right? Wrong! Actually, it's an essential nutrient that acts as a source of energy for the body and provides vital compounds to our body's cells so they can carry out their daily functions.

It's only when we eat too much fat—which most women do—that fat has the potential to start trouble. "The typical American woman gets as much as 40 percent of her calories from fat, which is far too much," says Diane Grabowski, R.D., nutrition educator at the Pritikin Longevity Center in Santa Monica, California. "That's much, much higher than the diets of other cultures. It's no coincidence that America also has a much higher incidence of heart disease and obesity than other nations in the world."

Most foods contain some fat in one quantity or another. Sometimes it's visible, like on a piece of steak; other times it's carefully hidden. And the make-up of fat can differ from food to food. When you look at it under a microscope, fat actually consists of compounds called fatty acids. Nutritionists have identified three primary fatty acids based on their chemical composition: saturated, monounsaturated and polyunsaturated.

Every fatty food contains these three fatty acids in different combinations. For example, animal fats, butter and tropical oils (like palm and coconut oil) have extremely high concentrations of saturated fats. Margarine, fish and certain cooking oils (like safflower and corn oil) contain mostly polyunsaturated fat. And other oils (like canola and olive oil) as well as avocados and certain nuts, consist mostly of monounsaturated fats.

All three types are equally fattening to our waistlines, so if you're watching your fat intake, it's best to cut back on all three. But experts believe we should place extra emphasis on eating fewer foods that are high in saturated fats. "Saturated fats tend to raise the level of cholesterol in the blood, which raises the risk of heart disease," says Grabowski.

# THE FAT TALLY

This table lists the percentages of saturated and unsaturated fat in commonly used cooking oils and fats. (The percentages may not add up to 100 percent since many of these fats have small amounts of other fatty substances.)

| Oil/Fat | Saturated Fat (%) | Monounsaturated Fat (%) | Polyunsaturated Fat (%) |
|---|---|---|---|
| **11 TERRIFIC COOKING OILS AND FATS . . .** | | | |
| Canola oil | 7 | 60 | 30 |
| Safflower oil | 9 | 13 | 76 |
| Walnut oil | 9 | 23 | 65 |
| Sunflower oil | 11 | 20 | 67 |
| Corn oil | 13 | 25 | 59 |
| Olive oil | 14 | 76 | 9 |
| Soybean oil | 15 | 24 | 59 |
| Peanut oil | 17 | 47 | 32 |
| Rice oil | 19 | 42 | 38 |
| Wheat germ oil | 19 | 15 | 63 |
| Margarine | 20 | 48 | 32 |
| **. . . PLUS 7 TO AVOID** | | | |
| Coconut oil | 89 | 6 | 2 |
| Butter | 64 | 29 | 4 |
| Palm oil | 50 | 36 | 9 |
| Lard | 39 | 45 | 11 |
| Chicken fat | 30 | 45 | 20 |
| Cottonseed oil | 26 | 18 | 53 |
| Vegetable shortening | 25 | 45 | 20 |

Monounsaturated fats, on the other hand, do not seem to produce this rise in blood cholesterol levels, while studies have shown that polyunsaturated fats can actually lower your cholesterol count. That's why if you are going to be using oils in your cooking or eating foods that do contain fat, you are much better off if those foods or oils contain mostly monounsaturated or polyunsaturated fats.

# A LITANY OF LOW-FAT FOODS

This handy guide will give you a good idea of the kinds of foods you should make a part of your low-fat eating program and how many grams of fat each one contains.

| Food | Portion | Fat (g.) |
|------|---------|----------|
| **BREAD AND BREAD PRODUCTS** | | |
| Italian | 1 slice | 0.0 |
| Melba toast | 1 slice | 0.0 |
| Matzo | 1 piece | 0.3 |
| Rice cake | 1 | 0.3 |
| Pita | 1 | 0.6 |
| Cracked wheat | 1 slice | 0.9 |
| Mixed grain | 1 slice | 0.9 |
| Rye | 1 slice | 0.9 |
| White | 1 slice | 1.0 |
| English | 1 | 1.1 |
| Pumpernickel | 1 slice | 1.1 |
| Tortilla, corn | 1 | 1.1 |
| Whole-wheat | 1 slice | 1.1 |
| Oat bran | 1 slice | 1.2 |
| Bagel | 1 | 1.4 |
| French | 1 slice | 1.4 |
| Taco shell | 1 | 2.2 |
| **CEREALS** | | |
| Wheat flakes | 1 cup | 0.0 |
| Cornflakes | 1 cup | 0.1 |
| Corn squares | 1 cup | 0.1 |
| Puffed rice | 1 cup | 0.1 |
| Puffed wheat | 1 cup | 0.1 |
| Farina | 1 cup | 0.2 |
| Shredded wheat | 1 biscuit | 0.3 |
| Bran flakes | 1 cup | 0.7 |
| Wheat germ, toasted | 1 Tbsp. | 0.8 |
| Raisin bran | 1 cup | 1.0 |
| Bran squares | 1 cup | 1.4 |
| Oat rings | 1 cup | 1.5 |
| Oatmeal, instant | 1 package | 1.7 |
| Oatmeal, cooked | ½ cup | 2.4 |

| Food | Portion | Fat (g.) |
|---|---|---|
| **CHEESES** | | |
| Yogurt cheese | 1 oz. | 0.6 |
| Cottage cheese, 1% fat | 1/2 cup | 1.2 |
| Parmesan, grated | 1 Tbsp. | 1.5 |
| Swiss, diet | 1 oz. | 2.0 |
| Mozzarella, skim milk | 1 oz. | 4.5 |
| Cottage cheese, 4% fat | 1/2 cup | 4.7 |
| Ricotta, part skim | 1/4 cup | 4.9 |
| Monterey Jack, light | 1 oz. | 6.0 |
| Feta | 1 oz. | 6.1 |
| Blue cheese | 1 oz. | 8.1 |
| American | 1 oz. | 8.9 |
| **CHICKEN** | | |
| Breast, no skin, roasted | 3½ oz. | 3.5 |
| Thigh, no skin, roasted | 1 small | 5.7 |
| Chicken roll, light meat | 3½ oz. | 7.3 |
| Breast, with skin, roasted | 3½ oz. | 7.8 |
| Leg, no skin, roasted | 3½ oz. | 8.0 |
| Leg, no skin, stewed | 3½ oz. | 8.1 |
| Breast, fried, floured | 3½ oz. | 8.8 |
| Thigh, fried, floured | 1 small | 9.2 |
| **CONDIMENTS** | | |
| Horseradish, prepared | 1 Tbsp. | 0.0 |
| Soy sauce, low-sodium | 1 Tbsp. | 0.0 |
| Teriyaki sauce | 1 Tbsp. | 0.0 |
| Worcestershire sauce | 1 Tbsp. | 0.0 |
| Cranberry sauce | 1/4 cup | 0.1 |
| Ketchup | 1 Tbsp. | 0.1 |
| Sweet relish | 1 Tbsp. | 0.1 |
| Yellow mustard | 1 Tbsp. | 0.3 |
| Brown mustard | 1 Tbsp. | 1.0 |

*(continued)*

# A LITANY OF LOW-FAT FOODS—
## CONTINUED

| Food | Portion | Fat (g.) |
|---|---|---|
| **CRACKERS** | | |
| Rye wafers | 1 | 0.0 |
| Whole-wheat, low-sodium | 1 | 0.0 |
| Rye snacks | 1 | 0.4 |
| Wheat snacks | 1 | 0.4 |
| Graham | 1 | 0.5 |
| | | |
| **DESSERTS** | | |
| Gelatin | ½ cup | 0.0 |
| Angel food cake | 1 slice | 0.1 |
| Vanilla wafer | 1 | 0.6 |
| Fig bar | 1 | 1.0 |
| Fruit-flavored frozen yogurt | ½ cup | 1.0 |
| Vanilla pudding, sugar-free, 2% milk | ½ cup | 1.2 |
| Gingersnap | 1 | 1.6 |
| Chocolate pudding, sugar-free, 2% milk | ½ cup | 1.9 |
| Orange sherbet | ½ cup | 1.9 |
| Chocolate/vanilla sandwich cookie | 1 | 2.3 |
| Chocolate chip cookie | 1 | 2.7 |
| Vanilla, ice milk | ½ cup | 2.8 |
| Cupcake, no icing | 1 | 3.0 |
| Sponge cake | 1 slice | 3.1 |
| Chocolate pudding | ½ cup | 4.0 |
| Tapioca pudding | ½ cup | 4.0 |
| Rice pudding with raisins | ½ cup | 4.1 |
| Macaroon | 1 | 4.5 |
| Apple turnover | 1 oz. | 4.7 |
| Brownie, chocolate icing | 1 | 5.0 |
| Cupcake, chocolate icing | 1 | 5.0 |
| Plain doughnut | 1 | 5.8 |
| Vanilla, ice cream | ½ cup | 7.2 |
| Strawberry shortcake | 1 | 8.9 |

| Food | Portion | Fat (g.) |
|---|---|---|
| **Eggs** | | |
| White only, raw | 1 large | 0.0 |
| Whole, raw | 1 large | 5.0 |
| **Fish** | | |
| Anchovy, fillet, canned | 1 | 0.4 |
| Tuna, light, canned in water | 3$\frac{1}{2}$ oz. | 0.5 |
| Cod, cooked | 3$\frac{1}{2}$ oz. | 0.9 |
| Haddock, cooked | 3$\frac{1}{2}$ oz. | 0.9 |
| Flounder, broiled | 3$\frac{1}{2}$ oz. | 1.5 |
| Sole, broiled | 3$\frac{1}{2}$ oz. | 1.5 |
| Halibut, broiled | 3$\frac{1}{2}$ oz. | 2.9 |
| Rainbow trout, cooked | 3$\frac{1}{2}$ oz. | 4.3 |
| Swordfish, cooked | 3$\frac{1}{2}$ oz. | 5.1 |
| **Fruits** | | |
| Plums | 2 small | 0.0 |
| Grapefruit | $\frac{1}{2}$ medium | 0.1 |
| Peach | 1 medium | 0.1 |
| Casaba melon, cubed | 1 cup | 0.2 |
| Figs | 2 small | 0.2 |
| Honeydew melon, cubed | 1 cup | 0.2 |
| Orange | 1 medium | 0.2 |
| Papaya, sliced | 1 cup | 0.2 |
| Apricot | 2 small | 0.3 |
| Grapes | 12 | 0.3 |
| Kiwifruit | 1 medium | 0.3 |
| Cantaloupe, cubed | 1 cup | 0.4 |
| Dates | $\frac{1}{2}$ cup | 0.4 |
| Prunes | $\frac{1}{2}$ cup | 0.4 |
| Raisins | $\frac{1}{2}$ cup | 0.4 |
| Apple, unpeeled | 1 medium | 0.5 |
| Banana | 1 medium | 0.6 |
| Blueberries | 1 cup | 0.6 |
| Mango | 1 medium | 0.6 |

*(continued)*

# A LITANY OF LOW-FAT FOODS—
## CONTINUED

| Food | Portion | Fat (g.) |
|---|---|---|
| **FRUITS—CONTINUED** | | |
| Nectarine | 1 medium | 0.6 |
| Strawberries | 1 cup | 0.6 |
| Bartlett pear | 1 medium | 0.7 |
| Pineapple chunks | 1 cup | 0.7 |
| Watermelon chunks | 1 cup | 0.7 |
| Cherries, sweet | 12 | 0.8 |
| **GRAVIES AND SAUCES** | | |
| Chili sauce | ¼ cup | 0.0 |
| Tomato sauce, canned | ¼ cup | 0.1 |
| Barbecue sauce | ¼ cup | 1.2 |
| Beef gravy, canned | ¼ cup | 1.2 |
| Turkey gravy, canned | ¼ cup | 1.2 |
| Taco sauce | ¼ cup | 1.4 |
| Mushroom gravy, canned | ¼ cup | 1.6 |
| Marinara sauce, canned | ¼ cup | 2.1 |
| Spaghetti sauce, canned | ¼ cup | 3.0 |
| Chicken gravy, canned | ¼ cup | 3.6 |
| **JUICES** | | |
| Prune | 1 cup | 0.1 |
| Cranberry | 1 cup | 0.1 |
| Grape | 1 cup | 0.2 |
| Apple | 1 cup | 0.3 |
| Orange | 1 cup | 0.5 |
| **LEGUMES AND BEANS** | | |
| Mung beans, sprouted | 1 cup | 0.2 |
| Lima beans, boiled | 1 cup | 0.5 |
| Lentils, boiled | 1 cup | 0.7 |
| Navy beans, cooked | 1 cup | 1.0 |
| Red kidney beans, canned | 1 cup | 1.0 |
| Split peas, dried, cooked | 1 cup | 1.0 |
| Pinto beans, boiled | 1 cup | 1.2 |

| Food | Portion | Fat (g.) |
|---|---|---|
| White beans, boiled | 1 cup | 1.2 |
| Refried beans | 1 cup | 2.7 |
| Garbanzo beans, canned | 1 cup | 4.6 |

## MEATS

| Food | Portion | Fat (g.) |
|---|---|---|
| Canadian bacon | 1 slice | 2.0 |
| Tenderloin pork roast, lean | 3½ oz. | 4.8 |
| Ham, extra lean | 3½ oz. | 5.5 |
| Veal roast, shoulder and arm, lean | 3½ oz. | 5.8 |
| Lamb chop, rib, lean, broiled | 1 | 7.4 |
| Leg of lamb, lean, roasted | 3½ oz. | 7.7 |
| Veal, rib, lean, braised | 3½ oz. | 7.8 |
| Ham roast, lean | 3½ oz. | 8.9 |
| Roast beef, bottom, lean | 3½ oz. | 9.6 |
| Pot roast, arm | 3½ oz. | 9.9 |

## MILK PRODUCTS

| Food | Portion | Fat (g.) |
|---|---|---|
| Evaporated, skim | ½ cup | 0.3 |
| Skim | 1 cup | 0.4 |
| Nondairy creamer | 1 Tbsp. | 1.0 |
| Nondairy whipped topping, frozen | 1 Tbsp. | 1.2 |
| Half-and-half | 1 Tbsp. | 1.7 |
| Buttermilk | 1 cup | 2.2 |
| Low-fat, 1% | 1 cup | 2.6 |
| Sour cream, imitation | 1 Tbsp. | 2.6 |
| Cream, light | 1 Tbsp. | 2.9 |
| Sour cream, cultured | 1 Tbsp. | 3.0 |
| Low-fat, 2% | 1 cup | 4.7 |
| Cream, heavy, whipping | 1 Tbsp. | 5.5 |
| Whole | 1 cup | 8.2 |

## MUFFINS

| Food | Portion | Fat (g.) |
|---|---|---|
| Oat bran with raisins | 1 small | 3.0 |
| Blueberry | 1 small | 4.0 |
| Corn | 1 small | 4.0 |
| Bran | 1 small | 5.1 |

*(continued)*

# A LITANY OF LOW-FAT FOODS—
## CONTINUED

| Food | Portion | Fat (g.) |
|---|---|---|
| **NUTS AND SEEDS** | | |
| Chestnuts, roasted | ½ cup | 0.9 |
| Sesame seeds, roasted | 1 Tbsp. | 4.3 |
| Pumpkin/squash seeds, roasted | ½ cup | 6.2 |
| **OILS AND FATS** | | |
| Low-calorie mayonnaise | 1 tsp. | 1.3 |
| Margarine, diet, corn | 1 tsp. | 1.9 |
| Whipped butter | 1 tsp. | 2.4 |
| Whipped margarine | 1 tsp. | 2.7 |
| Regular mayonnaise | 1 tsp. | 3.7 |
| Regular butter | 1 tsp. | 3.8 |
| Soft margarine, corn or safflower | 1 tsp. | 3.8 |
| Stick margarine, corn | 1 tsp. | 3.8 |
| Olive oil | 1 tsp. | 4.5 |
| Vegetable oil | 1 tsp. | 4.5 |
| **PASTAS AND GRAINS** | | |
| White rice, cooked | 1 cup | 0.0 |
| Bulgur, cooked | 1 cup | 0.4 |
| Macaroni, whole-wheat, cooked | 1 cup | 0.8 |
| Spaghetti, cooked | 1 cup | 1.0 |
| Spinach pasta, cooked | 1 cup | 1.3 |
| Brown rice, cooked | 1 cup | 1.8 |
| Egg noodles, cooked | 1 cup | 2.0 |
| Spanish rice | 1 cup | 4.2 |
| **ROLLS AND BISCUITS** | | |
| Brown 'n' serve roll | 1 | 2.0 |
| Hard roll | 1 | 2.0 |
| Hamburger/hot dog bun | 1 | 2.1 |
| Biscuit | 1 small | 5.1 |
| **SHELLFISH** | | |
| Shrimp, cooked | 3½ oz. | 1.1 |

| Food | Portion | Fat (g.) |
|---|---|---|
| Scallops, steamed | 3½ oz. | 1.4 |
| Clams, cooked | 3½ oz. | 5.8 |
| | | |
| **TURKEY** | | |
| Breast, no skin, roasted | 3½ oz. | 0.7 |
| Turkey loaf, from breast | 3½ oz. | 1.6 |
| Smoked | 3½ oz. | 3.9 |
| Turkey ham, from thigh | 3½ oz. | 5.0 |
| Dark meat, no skin | 3 oz. | 7.2 |
| Turkey pastrami | 3½ oz. | 7.2 |
| Turkey roll, light meat | 3½ oz. | 7.2 |
| | | |
| **VEGETABLES** | | |
| Carrot, raw | 1 medium | 0.1 |
| Celery | 1 stalk | 0.1 |
| Romaine lettuce, shredded | 1 cup | 0.1 |
| Sweet potato, baked | 1 medium | 0.1 |
| Swiss chard, boiled | 1 cup | 0.1 |
| Zucchini, boiled | 1 cup | 0.1 |
| Butternut squash, baked | 1 cup | 0.2 |
| Cauliflower, raw | 1 cup | 0.2 |
| Potato, baked, peeled | 1 medium | 0.2 |
| Spinach, raw, chopped | 1 cup | 0.2 |
| Acorn squash, baked | 1 cup | 0.3 |
| Mushrooms, raw | 1 cup | 0.3 |
| Sweet pepper, raw | 1 small | 0.3 |
| Tomato | 1 medium | 0.3 |
| Broccoli, boiled | 1 cup | 0.4 |
| Cabbage, boiled | 1 cup | 0.4 |
| Green or waxed beans, boiled | 1 cup | 0.4 |
| Asparagus, boiled | 1 cup | 0.6 |
| Summer squash, boiled | 1 cup | 0.6 |
| Brussels sprouts, boiled | 1 cup | 0.8 |
| Corn, fresh, boiled | 1 small ear | 1.0 |
| Onion ring, fried | 1 | 2.7 |
| French fried potatoes, frozen | 10 | 4.4 |

# Low-Fat Superstars

Cutting fat shouldn't be an all-or-nothing affair. In fact, many of the foods you love are already low in fat. And others aren't so bad—as long as you don't eat them every day. Here are some choices that Grabowski recommends that you include on your low-fat menu.

*Potatoes and sweet potatoes.* Spuds—of the baked variety—are a light and filling energy source. Just don't smother them with butter, sour cream or gravy.

*Legumes.* Beans, peas and lentils offer the same essential vitamins, minerals and proteins found in meats, but virtually none of the fat.

*Fruits and vegetables.* While there are a handful of high-fat fruits and vegetables (such as avocados and coconuts), most contain very little or no fat. And what little you find is usually monounsaturated or polyunsaturated. Fruits and veggies are also excellent sources of nutrients such as fiber, vitamins, minerals and carbohydrates.

*Whole-grain breads and cereals, pastas, and brown rice.* These foods are virtually fat-free, unless we overload them with butter and sauces. They're also our best sources for complex carbohydrates—the nutrients that give our bodies the most reliable, long-lasting form of energy—and fiber, which fights disease and aids digestion.

*Fish and fowl.* A low-fat diet doesn't mean you have to go without meat. If you make fish, shellfish and poultry your primary meat sources, you'll get all the protein and minerals of red meats, but not nearly as much fat.

# Lose the Fat, Keep the Flavor

You don't have to go cold turkey to cut back on your fat intake. Some simple, gradual changes to your eating habits are all it takes to make some major reductions. "Look at what you're already eating and how you could eat the same foods with less fat," advises Susan Kayman, R.D., Dr.P.H., a dietitian and consultant with the Kaiser Permanente Medical Group in Oakland, California. Here are some suggestions.

**Don't add fat to a good thing.** A lot of the foods we eat are naturally low in fat until we heap on those extras like butter, dressings and creams. Your fat-reducing program can start by using less condiments and fatty add-ons. For example, using only a tablespoon of jam on your morning toast instead of butter will save you 100 calories of fat. Or try mustard on your sandwiches instead of mayo. "In a year's time, that'll make a big difference," Dr. Kayman says.

**Season to perfection.** Add herbs, spices or tomato or lemon juice to liven up less flavorful foods without adding fat, says Grabowski.

**Choose low-fat cheese.** Cheese is one of the most common fat boosters in a woman's diet, says researcher Wayne Miller, Ph.D., director of the Indiana University Weight Loss Clinic in Bloomington. Most cheeses average about 66 percent of calories from fat, but some shoot well into the 80 percent range. You can generally distinguish high- and low-fat varieties by their color, Dr. Miller says; white cheeses like mozzarella, Swiss, ricotta and Parmesan are lower in fat than yellow cheeses like cheddar and American.

**Minimize milk fat.** Switching from whole milk to 1 percent can substantially cut your fat intake: 1 percent milk gets 23 percent of its calories from fat, while whole milk gets 48 percent. For better results, choose skim milk; it has virtually no fat. If you have trouble getting used to the taste of skim or low-fat milk, Dr. Miller suggests you make the transition slowly, combining it with regular whole milk and gradually increasing the amount of skim or 1 percent in the mix.

**Try low-fat versions of your favorites.** "It's harder to totally swear off ice cream than to simply trade it for low-fat varieties or low-fat frozen yogurt," says Dr. Kayman. These days, with all the special low-fat and nonfat products available, finding healthy alternatives to favorite foods is easier than it's ever been. One study found that substituting fat-free products in just seven categories (cream cheese, sour cream, salad dressing, frozen desserts, processed cheese, baked sweets and cottage cheese) cut fat intake by 14 percent a day.

**Look for leaner meats.** There's room for red meat in a low-fat diet if you make the right choices and eat it only two or three times a week, says Dodd. Best choices include cuts like London broil, eye of round steak and sirloin tip, which get less than 40 percent of their calories from fat. Keep portions to about three or four ounces (the size of a deck of cards), trim all visible fat off before cooking and prepare it by grilling, broiling or baking.

**Forgo frying.** Cutting back on fried foods will cut a load of fat from your diet. Cooking anything in oil, even lean poultry, boosts its fat content considerably, says Dr. Miller. According to the U.S. Department of Agriculture, the average breaded fried chicken sandwich at a fast-food joint has 15 grams more fat than a quarter-pound burger. Go instead for broiled or baked foods, he suggests.

**Skin the bird.** Chicken and turkey are already leaner alternatives to beef and pork, says Grabowski, but you make them even leaner if you peel the skin off before eating.

**Fridge and skim.** Grabowski recommends an easy way to make gravies and broths less fatty: After cooking, just stick them in the refrigerator for several hours. Much of the fat will congeal and rise to the top, and all you'll have to do is skim it off with a spoon or a strainer. When you're ready to serve, just reheat or microwave.

**Fill up when hunger strikes.** If you replace fat with other more filling, nutrient-dense foods, you can actually eat more and still lose pounds or maintain a healthy weight, says Annette Natow, R.D., Ph.D., of N.R.H. Nutrition Consultants in Valley Stream, New York, and co-author of *The Fat Attack Plan*. Count on carbohydrates—pasta, cereals, breads, beans and most fresh vegetables and fruits—to fill you up without the fat. Most of these foods in their whole or unprocessed forms are also full of fiber, which binds with fat and speeds it from your system.

**Lose your sweet tooth.** Many sugary foods are also high in fat. A chocolate bar, for example, gets most of its calories from fat, says Dr. Natow. Sweet cravings are often really fat cravings in disguise. If you want something sweet, try some fresh fruit or a bowl of sugared breakfast cereal with low-fat milk, she says. Or when you're cooking, use cocoa, which has less fat than baking chocolate.

## Managing Your Fat Intake

By following the guidelines above, you should be able to cut your fat intake to about 30 percent of total calories, which is the government's official recommendation.

Still, many experts say the 30 percent goal doesn't go far enough. For example, according to Grabowski, the fat-fighting regimen at the Pritikin Center calls for reducing your intake to 10 percent of total calories.

But unless your doctor specifically recommends that you cut back that much, a more realistic goal is around 20 to 25 percent. To achieve that, you'll need to closely monitor the amount of fat you're eating. "It's not enough to know that chips are bad," says Ron Goor, Ph.D., former coordinator of the National Cholesterol Education Program and co-author of *Choose to Lose Diet: A*

# YOUR PERSONAL GOALS

This chart shows you the maximum number of grams of fat you should be eating each day to both ensure that you're getting no more than 20 percent of your total calories from fat and maintain your current weight. If you're trying to lose weight, aim for the fat limit of your goal weight.

| Your Weight (lb.) | Calorie Intake | Fat Limit (g.) |
|---|---|---|
| 110 | 1,300 | 29 |
| 120 | 1,400 | 31 |
| 130 | 1,600 | 35 |
| 140 | 1,700 | 38 |
| 150 | 1,800 | 40 |
| 160 | 1,900 | 42 |
| 170 | 2,000 | 44 |
| 180 | 2,200 | 48 |

*Food Lover's Guide to Permanent Weight Loss.* "You need to know how bad." Here's what you should do.

**Make a fat budget.** Knowing how much fat you can eat each day is like having a salary, Dr. Goor says. "Once you know what you can afford, you can blow your budget on a double cheeseburger if you want, as long as you eat less fat for the rest of the day." Your budget is based on your total daily calorie intake.

**Keep a food diary.** Get hold of a fat- and calorie-counting guide (available at bookstores and supermarkets) and keep a record of all the food you eat for about three days, says Dr. Goor. This will give you a good idea of how your normal diet shapes up. It will heighten your awareness of what you put in your mouth, making you more likely to consider low-fat alternatives. And months from now, it will give you a way to measure your progress.

**Check labels.** Most packaged foods list their fat content per serving. You'll need to tally these numbers throughout the day and keep a keen eye on portion sizes, which are often unrealistically small, Dr. Goor says. For example, the fat listing on a box of Oreos is for one cookie. If you eat six in a sitting, be sure to multiply accordingly.

# MAKEUP

## *Less Really Can Be More*

Remember the good old days at the drugstore makeup counter? When you and your friends bought up bright orange lipstick, green mascara and frosted eye shadow in four shades of pastel, not to mention sparkly blush, black nail polish and little stars to stick on your face and ears?

Ouch. Did we really do that?

Yeah. But not anymore.

To look young and fresh and full of life—instead of like a worn-out neon sign—use makeup to your advantage. Here's how, starting at the beginning with your foundation.

**Darker may be better.** One of the first signs that time is marching on are the fine lines that show up on our faces. To soften them, try a slightly darker foundation than the one you've been using, says Marina Valmy, a cosmetician at the Christine Valmy Skin Care School in New York City.

"If your hair is graying or you love to wear black, choose a foundation with a slightly pink cast or dust a small amount of pink blush over your cheeks, forehead, nose and chin," says Carole Walderman, a cosmetologist and esthetician and president of Von Lee International School of Aesthetics and Makeup in Baltimore.

The right foundation will also even up your skin tone.

**Do a clean sweep.** Instead of your fingers, use a wooden tongue depressor or orange stick, available at the pharmacy, to scoop foundation from the bottle, says Leila Cohoon, a cosmetologist and esthetician and owner of Leila's Skin Care in Independence, Missouri. This will prevent bacteria from getting into your makeup and either destroying its potency or causing breakouts on your skin.

"Dab foundation with a clean applicator onto a makeup sponge that has been dampened with clean water," says Walderman.

**Use a light touch.** "Apply foundation very lightly, without scrubbing it in," Walderman says. Rubbing hard can tear the delicate tissues under the skin.

Near your eyes, use just your ring finger, which exerts less pressure than a sponge, and apply from the outer corner of the eye in toward the nose with very light strokes, she says.

**Conceal and highlight.** Bring out your best features, like those great cheekbones, and mask little flaws, like those little bags under your eyes, with a touch of concealer blended well, says Walderman. Concealer is available in a wide range of shades, and one slightly lighter than your foundation is best for you, she adds.

To conceal under-eye circles, apply concealer with a small brush into the dark crease only. If you cover the area entirely, in daylight it can make the circles look puffy, says Walderman.

If you have a large problem area to conceal, such as a dark patch of pigmentation, try special makeup, suggests Cohoon. "It's pure pigment, not made with heavy oils or a wax base, and covers very naturally," she says.

**Powder only if you need to.** Use translucent powder as a finisher "very lightly, just to take off shine in oily areas like the nose, forehead and chin, but don't pack it into the face," says Walderman. "That will just accentuate any lines and wrinkles."

And avoid powder colors labeled "pearlized" or "frosted." Why? These contain light-reflecting particles that act as highlighter. If you highlight the hills (your skin surface), the valleys (wrinkles or large pores) look deeper, Walderman says.

**Blend well.** It should not be noticeable where your face ends and your neck begins, so make sure your foundation doesn't end in a line across your jaw.

**Finish with a spritz.** If you like a dewy look, follow your foundation and powder with a light spritz of toner or distilled water, says Walderman. It moistens and sets your makeup without a chalky, pasty look.

# Bring a Blush to Your Cheeks

You may not blush as often as when you were a kid, but it's still nice to add warmth to your complexion with a touch of cheek color.

**Apply it subtly.** Aim for a barely showing, natural blush and don't apply it too close to the nose, which will make your nose look wider, says Walderman. Apply just a trace of blush at a 45-degree angle on the cheek to "lift" the face for a younger look, she says. Never apply blush any lower than the bottom of your nose or any higher up than the outside corner of the eye.

**Do the fade.** Blend cheek color thoroughly with a soft makeup brush, fading it out lightly just past the outer corner of your eyes toward the temple, Walderman says.

**Consult a pro.** If you can't figure out which blush shade is flattering, ask for help at the makeup counter. The makeup specialists can usually tell you which blush colors suit you, says Valmy. Professional color consultants are another option—but you'll have to pay for their service.

## Seven Gimmicks to Avoid

Some makeup techniques you've been using for years may make you appear older than you are. To keep your look young and natural, beware of these habits.

*Blaring blue shadows.* Turquoise eye shadow, or any bright blue, has gone the way of the patent-leather liner look, says Leila Cohoon, a cosmetologist and esthetician and owner of Leila's Skin Care in Independence, Missouri.

*Waxy foundations.* Old-fashioned, wax-based pancake makeup belongs on TV anchors, not anchoring down your skin, says Cohoon.

*Cavernous contouring.* Dark contouring powder along cheeks to create fake hollows is way too obvious, says Carole Walderman, a cosmetologist and esthetician and president of Von Lee International School of Aesthetics and Makeup in Baltimore.

*Clown cheeks.* You'll still see women now and then with hectic little rouge spots on their cheeks. It's neither subtle nor flattering, says Cohoon.

*Red jaws.* Blush belongs high along cheekbones, not down along the jawline, which weighs down the face, says Cohoon.

*Dark, bushy brows.* You don't want to overemphasize eyebrows when you're older, says Walderman. It can be harsh and hard-looking.

*The matte mask.* The experts say, keep it light, light, light! A light touch with makeup can give you a natural, young-looking complexion. Troweling it on layers on years.

## Eye Shadow Secrets

Our eyes may still be the windows to our souls, but the shades may be getting a bit crinkly with wrinkles and lines. Makeup can help conceal the change.

**A little dab'll do ya.** Use less shadow than you've been accustomed to, says Valmy. Heavy doses of eye shadow call attention to folds and lines.

**Correct with color.** If your eyes seem too close together, too far apart, too deep or lacking depth, or you're beginning to notice hooded lids, shadow to the rescue, says Cohoon. "If your eyes are too close together, put darker shadows on the outer portion of the upper lid," she says. "If they are too far apart, apply the dark more toward the center."

Deep-set eyes will appear to come forward with lighter shades of shadow, and you can bring more depth to your eyes with darker eye makeup. Remember to use a light touch, though, she adds.

If hooded lids are a problem, the best solution is a soft blending of three related colors, with the palest just under the brow bone. This diminishes the look of excess skin, Cohoon says. But don't use shadow that's frosted, shiny or too dark.

**Know what flatters.** If you have dark eyes, use soft brown eye shadow with a red base, not a green base, says Valmy. If your eyes are light, use a brown or gray shade with a green base rather than blue. The greener base picks up highlights in light-colored eyes, she explains.

**Don't echo dark circles.** If you find that you often have dark circles under your eyes, avoid shadows with a plum or brown tint. They will accentuate the circles, says Walderman.

**Lift corners for a youthful eye.** Counter the tendency of your eyes to droop at the corners by applying shadow subtly in a 45-degree angle up toward the brow at the outside corner of the eye, Walderman says.

# Eyeliner Artistry

You don't have to give up eyeliner, but you do want a softer, subtler eye definition, says Cohoon.

**Reconsider the color.** Unless you are black, using black liner will look too harsh. Others should choose soft browns, taupes and grays instead, suggests Walderman.

**Go lightly.** Use eyeliner sparingly and as close as possible to your eyelashes to give sparse lashes more fullness, says Valmy.

**Apply softly.** Sharpen your eyeliner pencils freshly for each use, says Walderman. The reason? The sharp point makes it easier for you to stroke on liner without pulling the delicate skin of your lids. If you use liquid liner, never apply it in a straight, flat line. Always smudge your liner for a soft, smoky look, she says. Dip a clean cotton swab under running water and wring it out first before smudging.

**Keep lines apart.** Don't let upper- and lower-lid eyeliner meet at the corners of your eyes. Doing that will only make your eyes look smaller, explains Walderman.

# Tending to Lashes and Brows

Your eyelashes and brows do get sparser with age, but there are several ways to enhance the illusion of silky fullness.

**Use mascara carefully.** Mascara is still an eyelash's best friend. To avoid those irritating blots and raccoon circles beneath your eyes, after you apply mascara, touch face powder very lightly just under the lower lashes with a small brush, says Valmy.

**Flirt with fakes.** These days, very natural looking artificial lashes are available in both strips and individual clusters, says Walderman. You apply the strips just at the base of your own lashes, sticking them into place on the lid. With practice, it will appear as though the lashes are growing out of your own lid, she says.

If you use false strip lashes, though, apply mascara only to your own lashes first and let it dry, or you'll lose lashes when you remove the strip, Valmy says.

A full set of individual lashes can take up to 45 minutes to put on, Walderman says. But they can stay with you up to six weeks until your own lashes complete their growth cycle. They'll stick right through showers and swimming because they're attached with a permanent glue. Individual lashes come in sets of about four lashes per root, and you attach each set onto one of your own lashes. Avoid oil-based cleansers around the eye while you're wearing them, as they will take off the lashes, Walderman says.

**Groom your brows.** A good color guide for brows is that one shade lighter than your hair color tends to look most natural, says Walderman. If your hair is light brown, gray or white, taupe is more flattering, she says.

If your brows are too light, you can use a #2 graphite writing pencil—they're no longer made from lead, so there's no health risk, says Valmy. "You can fill in sparse places, and it will look very nice and natural," she says.

# Liven Your Lips

Your lips are part of your complexion, too, and as you get older, they can bring a lovely touch of color to your face.

**Cruise for corals.** Coral tones are best for older lips, says Walderman. If your skin tones are cool, look for a pinkish coral. If they are warm, an orange-touched tone is fine. But make sure you don't go too far with orange, as it can accentuate the natural yellowing of your teeth as you age.

**Flatten your feathers.** Feathering is the irritating creeping of lip color into fine lines on the upper lip. A lip liner pencil will stop it in its tracks, says Valmy. To make lip color adhere better and last longer, apply lip liner around the edges of your lips. Then apply lipstick, blot it and apply another coat, she says.

**Avoid waxing.** If lip wrinkles and feathering lipstick are a real problem, and you normally wax the downy hair on your upper lip, try bleaching instead, says Walderman. "Down on the lip absorbs moisture that would otherwise melt lipstick and encourage it to enter creases," she says.

**Balance your mouth shape.** Sometimes the upper lip thins a little as we age, says Cohoon. If this is the case, draw your lip line slightly outside the edge of your upper lip and fill in with lipstick.

# MARRIAGE

## *It Could Be for Better*

**G**etting married can be one of the scariest things you'll ever do. But what draws you to that walk down the aisle is the hope that life will be better when you're married than it was when you were single. Will it? Maybe.

If you're happily married, you probably drink less, eat fewer junk foods and exercise more regularly. You may seem more relaxed and upbeat and get sick less often.

"Clearly, a satisfying marriage can help you feel younger and more alive. It's good for your health, and it can help you live a more productive and happier life," says Howard Markman, Ph.D., a University of Denver psychologist and co-author of *We Can Work It Out: Making Sense of Marital Conflict.*

## What's So Good about It

If you ask a dozen scientists if being married will help you live longer, you might get 12 different answers. Researchers at the National Center for Health Statistics, for example, estimate that married women live about ten years longer than single women. Many studies show that single and divorced women are more prone to illness, injury and suicide than happily married women.

In a survey of 47,000 households, the National Center for Health Statistics found that married women were more likely to say their health is good or excellent than single, divorced or widowed women. Married women also were less likely to have chronic illness, reported six fewer sick days per year than divorced women and recovered more quickly from colds, flu and injuries than single or divorced women did. And divorced women reported twice as many injuries.

Other studies indicate that the life span of single and married women is about the same. But there's also research that suggests single women outlive their married friends, says Estelle Ramey, Ph.D., physiologist and professor emeritus at Georgetown University Medical Center in Washington, D.C.

Why such conflicting statistics? Because, say experts, it's not marriage itself but the happiness of the marriage that contributes to a woman's longevity.

"A woman's health seems to follow the health of the relationship," says Robert W. Levenson, Ph.D., a psychologist at the University of California, Berkeley. "If the marriage is satisfying, then their health seems to be good. If they're in an unsatisfying marriage, their health suffers.

It's not the same for men, however, who benefit from any kind of marriage. For men, the quality of married life doesn't seem to matter. Their health seems to improve even if they're in a wretched marriage.

Researchers are puzzled by this difference. Some suspect single women eat better, exercise more and generally take better care of themselves than single men. So when a couple weds—and a married man usually adopts his wife's lifestyle—there are few changes that would have a positive influence on a woman's health. At the same time, she's usually spending more time on household chores and cooking.

Others like Dr. Levenson speculate that as men in bad marriages detach themselves emotionally from the relationship, women work harder and harder to heal the wounds. That effort takes its toll on a woman's health.

"In a bad marriage, there's a lot of anger, recrimination and other emotions flying around, but for some reason it doesn't stick to men the way it does to women. Men walk away from it," says Dr. Levenson. "Women are much less likely to withdraw. They often hang in there trying to solve the problems in the marriage until the bitter end. That can produce a lot of stress that is potentially bad for your health," he says.

## It May Help in a Crisis

Even if a married woman does get a life-threatening ailment, she is more likely to seek treatment earlier and has a better chance of survival than her single sister. In fact, after looking at 27,779 cases of cancer, James Goodwin, M.D., director of the Center on Aging at the University of Texas Medical Branch at Galveston, concluded that married women had survival rates that were comparable to single women who were ten years younger.

"That was a rather striking finding," Dr. Goodwin says. "The treatments for cancer—chemotherapy and radiation—can make you feel very sick. So it just makes sense that having a supportive partner makes it easier for patients to cope."

A happy marriage can help you recover from other serious illnesses, too. In a small preliminary study, women who suffered heart attacks and were able to talk openly and honestly with their husbands about it reported better health and were less likely to have chest pains or be readmitted to the hospital within a year following the attack, according to Vicki Helgeson, Ph.D., a psychologist at Carnegie Mellon University in Pittsburgh.

# The Look of Love

When you look at your husband these days, do you see yourself staring back? It's a good possibility, particularly if you're in a long-lasting relationship.

After closely examining the photographs of 12 couples who had been married for at least 25 years, a panel of observers at the University of Michigan in Ann Arbor concluded that facial features of couples do become more similar after years of living together.

Why? Couples tend to unconsciously mimic each other's facial expressions, says Robert Zajonc, Ph.D., professor of psychology at the University of Michigan in Ann Arbor. Over time, this mimicry reshapes facial muscles and wrinkles so that their faces acquire many of the same features. Couples also tend to adopt the same hand gestures, body posture and gait, Dr. Zajonc says.

Women who are satisfied with their marriages also are less likely to suffer from major depression than women who are in troubled unions, says James Coyne, Ph.D., professor of psychology in the Departments of Family Practice and Psychiatry at the University of Michigan Medical School in Ann Arbor.

In addition, researchers at Ohio State University found that the more put-downs, sarcasm and other hostile words and gestures newlywed couples used when discussing marital conflicts, the more likely they would have higher blood pressure and weakened immune systems. No, a marital argument on Tuesday doesn't mean you'll get a cold on Wednesday. But researchers conclude that couples who often engage in ugly arguments may be more susceptible to infection and disease.

## Keeping Those Bells Ringing

You have your spats, your passion wavers and sometimes boredom suffocates you. Despite all that, you treasure the man in your life. But even the best relationships need occasional tune-ups. Here are some suggestions to keep your marriage ticking.

**Make the moment happen.** If you don't schedule time together, it may never happen. Try to spend at least 20 minutes a day just talking with each other. "You exercise that much each day to keep your body in shape; you need

## Calling It Quits

Your relationship is colder than an ice cube. Your passion has been missing for so long that you've considered calling the search-and-rescue squad. But is it time for you to split up?

"Ending a marriage is the psychological equivalent of cutting off your own arm or leg. It's going to hurt," says John Mirowsky, Ph.D., professor of sociology at Ohio State University in Columbus.

But there are some clear indications that it may be time to end your marriage. And they range from alcohol or drug problems to emotional or physical abuse to the simple inability to communicate anymore.

"My patients always ask me when they should leave. I tell them 'You'll know when it's time,' " says Sherelynn Lehman, a licensed family, marriage and sex therapist in private practice in Cleveland. "It's when your soul dies, when your spirit gets trampled on. I say 'til death do you part' means the death of the spirit. If you're dying inside, then perhaps it's time to move on."

to spend at least that much time keeping your marriage in shape, too," says Sherelynn Lehman, a licensed family, marriage and sex therapist in private practice in Cleveland.

**Listen until you hear him.** If your husband tells you that he feels frustrated because you seem to be tuning him out, stop, acknowledge that he may be right and take time to really listen to him, says Dennis Gersten, M.D., a psychiatrist in private practice in San Diego. Let him know that you heard what he said by repeating his concern back to him: "I know it must be frustrating that I worked late and didn't phone you." If that's not what he's upset about, then ask him to repeat it until you understand. "Say 'I'm really trying to understand your concern, but I don't seem to be getting it. Could you say it in a different way that might make it clearer to me?' " Dr. Gersten suggests.

**Surprise him.** "To keep the spark in the marriage alive, you need to be creative," says Ruth Rice, Ph.D., a psychologist in private practice in Dallas. Arrange occasional surprises like a weekend at a bed-and-breakfast or a moonlit walk around a lake or just slip a romantic card under his pillow.

**Play together, stay together.** Common interests and hobbies relieve boredom and are the glue that holds many good marriages together. "The couple that really enjoys doing things together like traveling, golf or tennis is going to have an advantage as they get into the later years of their marriage and they have more time on their hands," says Martin Goldberg, M.D., a psychiatrist and director of the Marriage Council of Philadelphia, a counseling service.

**Laugh it up.** "Being able to be childlike and laugh together is important because it means that you feel comfortable enough to allow yourselves to be vulnerable with each other," says Arlene Goldman, Ph.D., a psychologist and sex therapist on the faculty of the Family Institute of Philadelphia.

**Focus on your feelings.** The surest way to start a fight, according to Dr. Goldman, is to say things like "You're wrong" or "I think you're being silly."

---

# Retying the Knot

More than half of all marriages end in divorce. You were devastated when your union fell apart. But here you are, thinking about heading for the altar again.

In a sense that's good, because divorced women who remarry probably regain many of the health advantages of happily married women, says Patrick McKenry, Ph.D., a professor of Family Relations and Human Development at Ohio State University in Columbus.

But before you enter the chapel of love, you should ponder a few things that can increase your chances of a happy and lasting marriage this time around.

First, don't rush into a new marriage. "The way a lot of women try to adjust to divorce is to remarry," Dr. McKenry says. He says a woman needs about one to two years before moving on to another serious relationship.

Ask yourself what you expect out of marriage, suggests Joel Kahan, M.D., a psychiatrist at the Medical College of Georgia School of Medicine in Augusta who has studied multiple marriages. "If a woman doesn't want or expect a strong, intimate relationship, then perhaps she shouldn't be married," Dr. Kahan says. "She'll need to work on that issue before she dives into another relationship."

Carefully consider what went wrong in your last marriage and ask yourself if similar problems loom in your new relationship. "A huge number of women remarry men who are very much like their previous spouses. That's one of the most important things to avoid," says Sol Gordon, Ph.D., psychologist, professor emeritus at Syracuse University in New York and author of *Why Love Is Not Enough*. If your new love has any bothersome traits that remind you of your ex-husband, ask yourself if you think you can cope with them better this time. If not, don't get married.

She adds, " 'You' statements are almost always thoughts and are usually hurtful." Instead, try saying "I feel anxious when I don't know where you are. One way you can help me cope with that feeling is to get a message to me so I know where I can get in touch with you." That's much less challenging than "You're always late."

**Look at yourself first.** Focus on your own faults rather than your partner's, Dr. Markman suggests. You have more control over your own behavior than your partner's actions, and often when one person in a relationship starts making changes, the other will follow.

**Small changes make a difference.** "Making big changes in a relationship is really the result of making a series of small changes," Dr. Markman says. "If you can say just one less critical thing to your spouse each day, you could be on your way to significant change."

**Stop the sting.** A sharp-tongued put-down in the middle of an argument may feel good, but the hurt of that one zinger will erase your last 20 acts of kindness from your husband's memory, Dr. Markman says. It's better to bite your tongue than to needlessly open a new wound.

**No finger-pointing.** Blaming your husband rather than acknowledging that

## Coping with a Cheatin' Heart

Your best friend is the talk of the office now that her love affair has destroyed her marriage. Fortunately, nothing like that could ever happen to your relationship, right?

"You can never be 100 percent certain that your marriage will be immune from affairs," says Sherelynn Lehman, a licensed family, marriage and sex therapist in private practice in Cleveland and author of *Love Me, Love Me Not: How to Survive Infidelity.* "You must woo your mate every day. You can't let down your guard." Out there, she says, is someone who thinks your husband is a really good catch.

Women and men are often attracted to affairs out of boredom or loneliness, Lehman says. Maintaining good communication and keeping zest in your sex life are among the keys to preventing an affair. But an affair doesn't mean all is lost.

"A marriage rocked by an affair is like an egg that cracks. Although the crack will always be there, you can work around it. The marriage doesn't have to shatter, but counseling is essential," Lehman says.

you share some of the responsibility for a problem in your relationship increases the likelihood you'll end up in divorce court, Dr. Markman says. To break out of that pattern, try telling your husband "I know we've been caught up in this pattern of criticizing each other at the drop of a hat lately, so I'm going to work on being less critical of you and try to see you in a more positive light."

**Divide housework fairly.** If you or your husband is doing more than your share of the housework, that can cause resentment, Dr. Rice says. List everything you need to accomplish: cleaning, laundry, shopping, yard work, bill paying, home repairs. Then negotiate a fair division that includes an equal number of things that each of you enjoys doing and things you consider to be drudgery. If your budget allows it, consider hiring people to help you.

**Let gadgets do it.** If television is important to one of you but not the other, watching it may rob you of quality time together, Dr. Rice says. Get a VCR, tape the show and watch it later. If the telephone is constantly ringing, get an answering machine and screen your messages so you can spend time with your spouse.

# MASSAGE

## Much-Kneaded Relief

**Y**ou've been waiting all week for this hour of ecstasy. Anxiety at work—rub, rub. Tension at home—stroke, stroke. Those aching muscles and joints—tappity-tappity-tap. They're all melting away with each pass of your massage therapist's hands.

After 45 minutes, that age-erasing magic has worked again. No sore back. No stiff neck. You rise refreshed and relaxed, leaving what feels like 20 years of pain and worries there on the massage table.

"Nothing makes you feel more rejuvenated than a massage," says Madeline P. Rudy, a licensed massage therapist with Massage Therapy in West Reading, Pennsylvania. "If you're looking for a way to put yourself back in sync and feel younger, there isn't a better thing out there."

### Studies in Relaxation

Any woman will tell you that a massage feels great. Yet medical science still doesn't know exactly why.

"There's not a lot of research out there yet," says Tiffany Field, Ph.D., director of the Touch Research Institute at the University of Miami School of Medicine. The institute is the first organization in the country dedicated to studying massage's medical benefits.

Dr. Field says we have gained a few insights into the way massage works, however. For one thing, it seems to restrict the body's release of cortisol, a hormone that plays a big role in triggering stress reactions. The less cortisol you produce, the less stress you may feel, Dr. Field says. Massage also has been shown to improve the deep, resting phase of sleep. And it may boost your production of serotonin, a hormone linked to positive mood changes and improved immunity, Dr. Field says.

In a Touch Research Institute study of medical faculty and staff, 15 minutes of daily massage appeared to lessen anxiety, make people more alert and increase the speed with which they could complete math problems. "The key to a better work force," Dr. Field says, "could be regular massage."

The institute is working on a series of 34 studies, with hundreds of participants, that looks at massage therapy's effects on everything from depression and pregnancy to high blood pressure and migraine headaches. The studies also look at how massage therapy could help males who test positive for HIV (human immunodeficiency virus, the virus that causes AIDS) improve their immune function.

For now, some doctors say they need to know more about what massage can do before they start prescribing it as therapy.

"No one is willing to accept any nebulous explanation that involves the metaphors of energy, toxins, good vibes or any other poetic verse," says Larry Dossey, M.D., co-chairman of the panel on Mind/Body Interventions, Office of Alternative Medicine at the National Institutes of Health in Bethesda, Maryland, and former chief of staff at Medical City Dallas Hospital.

But that attitude may be changing. Many insurance companies now cover massage if a doctor orders it. And some massage therapists note that some of their best, most loyal clients are physicians.

## Some Hands-On Advice

If you're thinking about trying massage therapy, Rudy says you should be prepared to spend anywhere from $25 to $65 per session, with a typical session lasting about 50 to 55 minutes. Go as often as you like or as often as you can afford. For more guidance, try these tips.

**Shop carefully.** The last place you want to end up in is a massage "parlor," with its creepy clientele and sometimes questionable practices. To find a reputable, qualified massage therapist, ask questions before you go. "Look in the phone book," Rudy says. "Make sure they're a member of the American Massage Therapy Association (AMTA). Ask if they went to accredited schools to learn massage. And always avoid places that offer 'discreet billing.' That's a sign that they may not be on the up-and-up."

The AMTA has a customer referral service that will help you find a registered massage therapist in your area. Write the group at 820 Davis Street, Suite 100, Evanston, IL 60201.

**Pick your pleasure.** When it comes to massage, there really are different strokes for different folks. Swedish massage—with its kneading, rubbing and use of oils—is the method most people think of. But there's also shiatsu, or oriental massage, in which a therapist works pressure points along nerve pathways to relieve pain and stress (Rudy says some people may experience some discomfort with this method). There's specialized sports massage, which focuses

*(continued on page 566)*

# You Can Do It Yourself

Sometimes that Friday afternoon massage seems weeks away. You know you'll feel good when you go, but what about now?

Try self-massage. These little pick-me-ups can do wonders for you. And they require nothing except a couple of tennis balls, a quiet corner and your own two hands.

## Head

Pressure points in your skull can relax your whole body.

"There are two very significant acupressure points at the base of the skull on what's called the occipital ridge," says Robert DeIulio, Ed.D., a licensed psychologist and muscle therapist in private practice in Wellesley Hills, Massachusetts. "If you apply consistent pressure there, you can achieve total relaxation."

How do you do it? Put two tennis balls in a sock and tie the end. Lie on your back on the floor and place the sock behind the upper neck, so that the two balls each touch the skull ridge that's right above the hollow spot. Stay like that for 20 minutes. Listen to soothing music, if you like. "Those acupressure points send messages down the spinal column to relax all the muscles," says Dr. DeIulio.

## Face

Just touch your face. There's no need to knead it. With a very light touch, cup your cheeks and temples with your hands using no more pressure than the weight of a nickel. Hold your hands there for a minute. "The warmth of the hands relaxes the muscles and connective tissue, bringing on an overall sense of relief," Dr. DeIulio says.

## Jaw

Pull the sides of your ears gently straight outward, then straight up, then straight down. Or, with your index finger, press the tender spot next to your earlobe where it attaches to your head. Press and release, alternating ears, 10 to 15 times.

## Torso

Get a quick boost by rubbing the area above your kidneys. That's at waist level where the tissue is still soft. Rub briskly with your fists in a circular motion. "It's a nice way of energizing the body," says Dr. DeIulio.

## Feet

Few things on this Earth feel as good as a foot massage. Here are a few winning techniques. After you try them out on one foot, switch feet and repeat.

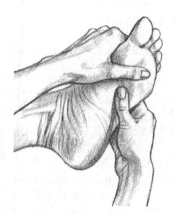

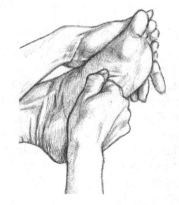

*Make a fist and press your knuckles into the bottom of your foot, moving from your heel to your toes. Repeat five times.*

*Sit on a chair and place one foot on the opposite thigh. Rub some massage oil or lotion onto your foot if you like. Apply pressure with your thumbs to the sole of your foot, working from the bottom of your arch to the top near your big toe. Repeat five times.*

*Massage each toe by holding it firmly and moving it from side to side. Extend each toe gently out and away from the ball of your foot. Then apply pressure to the areas between your toes.*

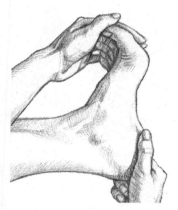

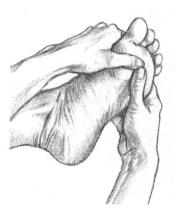

*Hold your toes in one hand and bend them backward, holding them there for five to ten seconds. Then bend them in the opposite direction and hold for five to ten seconds. Repeat three times.*

*Press and roll your thumbs between the bones of the ball of your foot.*

on soothing overworked muscles and joints. And there's a grab bag of techniques and sub-techniques like Rolfing, Feldenkrais, Trager, Alexander and Aston-Patterning, which promote everything from body-lengthening to spine realignments to posture improvements.

"The key is to talk to therapists first," Rudy says. "You want to find someone whose specialty matches your needs. And you want to make sure they're legitimate."

**Respect your limits.** Massage is about relaxation. And let's face it: Some women just aren't comfortable disrobing for a Swedish massage.

"Only go as far as what feels right," Rudy says. "Maybe you'll have to work your way up to it. This is your special time. Enjoy it."

Therapists should be conscious of your feelings. They should cover parts of the body they're not working on and should not touch your breasts or genital areas. They shouldn't ask you for intimate details of your life or give details of theirs. They're supposed to respect your wishes. If they don't, find another massage therapist.

"The whole thing," Rudy says, "is about health and well-being and feeling better. If there's tension or pressure in a relationship, go somewhere else."

**Know when to say no.** Massage isn't for everyone. AMTA guidelines say that people with phlebitis or other circulatory ailments, some forms of cancer or heart disease, infections or fevers should not use massage therapy. In most cases, avoid massage for about three days after suffering a fracture or serious sprain. If you have any doubts, ask your physician.

# MEDICAL CHECKUPS

## Well Worth Penciling In

Nobody's particularly wild about lying down half-naked on a cold table to have their bodies examined by a near-stranger. Yet we do it, because we know that medical checkups are good for us.

In fact, each year American women make roughly 130 million more visits to the doctor's office than men do. And we also live an average of seven years longer than men. Some experts say that these two statistics are by no means unconnected.

By getting a regular checkup, you and your doctor can keep an eye out for developing problems and perhaps put a stop to them. Just as important, meeting with your doctor can give you both a chance to discuss certain lifestyle factors that can make the difference between a long and vigorous life or a short one plagued with problems you shouldn't have until you're 85.

## Choosing Dr. Right

Getting a checkup seems simple enough, but where it can quickly start to resemble the quest for the Holy Grail is when you start looking for a doctor. Who's qualified? What should you, as a smart consumer, be looking for?

"Basically, anyone who holds himself out by training and practice as a primary care physician should be fully qualified to take care of checkups for normal, healthy adults," says Douglas Kamerow, M.D., director of the Clinical Preventive Services Staff for the Office of Disease Prevention and Health Promotion in the U.S. Public Health Service. "But, in my opinion, there are really only two groups that are qualified by their training to do so: general internists and family physicians."

Some experts in women's health, however, would narrow the list even further and add a few provisos. "My number-one choice would be a general internist,"

# How Often Should You Go?

The annual physical. When most people think of a checkup, they tend to picture a yearly barrage of pokes, prods and needle pricks that are done like clockwork whether they're needed or not. This has a lot to do with tradition.

Back in 1922 the American Medical Association (AMA) first endorsed the annual examination of healthy people, and for many years after it was standard practice. "It was only in 1983 that the AMA withdrew support for this concept," says Douglas Kamerow, M.D., director of the Clinical Preventive Services Staff for the Office of Disease Prevention and Health Promotion in the U.S. Public Health Service.

In this brave new world of checkups, the current medical wisdom is that for healthy people, a more tailored program of preventive services can be effective. In layman's terms, this means fewer checkups will do just as well as the time-honored annual physical.

If you have no serious ailments that need monitoring, most experts advise that you touch base with your primary care physician every three to five years from age 30 to 39, every two to three years from age 40 to 49 and, past 50, every year.

But, adds Dr. Kamerow, a pap smear is still recommended annually regardless of your age if you have shown any potential signs of trouble in the cervix or if you have multiple sex partners.

says Lila Wallis, M.D., clinical professor of medicine at Cornell University Medical College, former president of the American Medical Women's Association and founder of the National Council of Women's Health in New York City. "And not just any general internist, but one who has had special training in office gynecology and the psychological needs of female patients."

According to Dr. Wallis, a family practitioner would do if a general internist was not available. "The only reason he or she wouldn't be my first choice is that the family practitioner has to learn so much more about children that it could dilute the amount of time spent keeping abreast of women's health developments."

And gynecologists, who many women make their first choice, actually come in third. "While general internists and family practitioners already have a firm knowledge of the rest of the body, gynecologists specialize specifically in women's sexual organs and reproductive tract," notes Dr. Wallis. "This gives them far more to learn than the other two to become a primary care physician."

Specialization is not something you want to overlook, adds Dr. Wallis. "Many internists have areas of specialization such as cardiology or hematology. But you want to be careful that they aren't neglecting continuing education courses in women's health issues to the advantage of their other interest."

# Preparing for Your Checkup

Miss Marple may have been able to get to the truth based on the merest of clues, but your doctor needs solid information. You can best provide that information by doing a bit of homework before your visit.

**Keep a food log.** When it comes to health habits, the murkiest information tends to surround diet. How often do you really notice what you eat throughout the day: that mid-morning candy bar, a bag of chips in the car. It all adds up, but it's easily forgettable when making a report on your eating habits to your doctor. And what in reality is not the healthiest of eating habits suddenly becomes squeaky clean in the doctor's office.

"If you know you're going in for a checkup and plan on discussing diet, it's not a bad idea to keep a precise food log for a week beforehand," suggests Dr. Kamerow. "Don't change your eating habits, just keep track of them. It's the little forgettable things like snacks that add up to a lot of dietary fat, and it's these things that you'll need to focus on when talking to your doctor."

**Climb your family tree.** Coming up with a complete family history of illnesses will also require a little attention and, depending on what you discover, may affect the types of tests you'll need. "People with a family history of certain health problems may be at greater risk of developing them, and it's reasonable to screen these people more regularly or earlier for these diseases," says Dr. Kamerow.

While there may well be hundreds of diseases that can be passed along genetically, there are, in fact, only a few that you really need to be concerned with. "Breast cancer is a primary concern," says Dr. Kamerow. "The U.S. Preventive Services Task Force does not recommend mammograms before the age of 50. But one may want to make an exception for women who are at high risk by evidence that their mother or sister had it, especially if the cancer was pre-menopausal."

Osteoporosis is another concern for women. "A family history of osteoporosis might predispose me to suggest a bone mineral density study at menopause, which I might not normally use routinely," says Dr. Wallis. A family history of heart disease or any cancer including ovarian, colon, breast, uterine and pancreatic should also be discussed with your doctor.

**Prepare your files.** You'll want to make sure your doctor has records from any other physicians you may have visited. You'll also want to inform her of any medications you are taking and any problems that you feel you may be experiencing because of them. You may also want to prepare a list of current health complaints complete with symptoms and dates if possible.

# Getting the Most from It

You've picked the doc, done your homework and now you're cooling your heels in the waiting room listening to a Muzak version of "Eleanor Rigby." What lies in wait for you beyond the smiling nurse? Or, more to the point, what should happen in the examination room to make for a perfect checkup?

"One of the most important components of the physical is a breast examination," says JoAnn E. Manson, M.D., co-principal investigator of the cardiovascular component of the Nurses' Health Study, associate professor of medicine at Harvard Medical School and co-director of women's health at Brigham and Women's Hospital, both in Boston. "After that and, of course, a pelvic exam and pap smear, there is a whole list of options that can be performed, some more important than others."

Dr. Manson strongly suggests that your doctor perform the following:

- Measure your blood pressure, weight and height.
- Inspect your tongue and gums for any signs of oral cancer or need for dental care.
- Check the artery in your neck for pulse and listen for bruits—abnormal sounds that can indicate a clogged artery.
- Inspect the neck area for thyroid size and nodules for possible cancer.
- Examine your skin, especially in sun-exposed areas, for any signs of skin cancer.
- Listen to your chest for heart sounds and lung congestion, crackles or wheezes.

"In some people, especially those who are young and healthy, it may be less important to check the liver, kidneys, spleen and reflexes and test for signs of nerve damage," says Dr. Manson. "The need for many of these tests depends on age, prior medical history and risk factors. So not all women should expect to have all these tests performed at every checkup."

What else might you expect?

"It's also not a bad idea to do a nonfasting total blood cholesterol screening, and this is especially needed if there is a history of heart disease in the family," says Dr. Kamerow.

Pap smears are also standard issue. Most of the experts recommend an annual Pap smear. Regular Pap smears are especially important for sexually active women outside of a monogamous relationship, because many physicians feel that the human papilloma virus, a sexually transmitted disease, is a major cause of cervical cancer. If your sexual activity is not directed toward only one person, Dr. Kamerow suggests that you get routine screenings for other sexually transmitted diseases, such as chlamydia, as well.

When it comes to the more exotic blood and urine tests, electrocardiograms and x-rays, the U.S. Preventive Services Task Force does not routinely recommend them for the healthy patient.

# After Menopause

As we reach menopause, one test might be added to our routine checkup. "There is no better way of determining how a woman's bones will fare later than a bone mineral density study at menopause," says Dr. Wallis. "If the patient exhibits any risk factors, such as a family history of osteoporosis, a pale complexion, red or blonde hair, a northern European origin, lack of exposure to sun, lack of exercise or a lack of calcium intake, I would definitely suggest she undergo it."

Taking anywhere from five minutes to a half-hour (depending on the technology used), a bone mineral density study is a painless, noninvasive scan performed by machines that use low-dose radiation to measure bone mass.

The other change in checkup routine happens at 40. At that age, most doctors recommend regular mammograms for women. "Some would also recommend a fecal occult blood test and a sigmoidoscopy to screen for colorectal cancer," says Dr. Kamerow.

Of the three tests, the fecal occult blood test offers the least amount of patient discomfort, only requiring a stool sample to be brought from home so that the physician can check for blood as a possible symptom of colorectal cancer. Mammograms, while nothing more than low-dose breast x-rays, may cause some discomfort when the breast is firmly compressed between two plates. Finally, the sigmoidoscopy. It's not pleasant. A thin, hollow, lighted tube is inserted into the rectum and lower part of the colon to look for precancerous polyps.

# Taking the Doctor's Advice Home

Take a deep breath and relax. The poking and prodding are behind you. Now it's time to direct the hard light of science onto your lifestyle. "Outside of the few tests and shots you should get, the most important thing that can be done at a checkup is to team up with your doctor and take stock of your health habits," states Dr. Kamerow. The big four topics of discussion should be exercise, diet, sexual practices and vices such as smoking and drinking, he says. "Poor habits in these areas contribute mightily to the leading causes of disease and death in this country, and yet they are the very things we cannot test or fix with medicine."

If you smoke, talk to your doctor about ways to quit. The same goes for "recreational" drugs, excessive use of medications, such as sedatives and diet pills, and alcohol abuse. If you are prone to adventurous sex, have a sobering conversation on safe sex as well as the potential dangers involved in bed hopping. Diet? Haul out that food diary and go over it in detail. As for exercise, ask your doctor for tips to incorporate more physical activity into your life.

Don't worry about taking up too much of your doctor's time. "The most important thing that goes on at a checkup is the counseling and the activity that the patient then does because of that counseling," says Dr. Kamerow. "Doctors are beginning to realize that the most healing thing they can do is provide information and motivation."

# OPTIMISM

## A Proven Power for Health

You sometimes wonder whether that cheerful woman in the office down the hall is missing a few marbles. Even when she goes through hard times, she always seems to find a positive spin on things. You ask yourself, "Doesn't she ever feel down like the rest of us? Are optimists oblivious to the dark side of life?"

Not at all. Optimism is not about ignoring what's real, but becoming aware of your thoughts about why things happen, says Martin Seligman, Ph.D., professor of psychology and director of clinical training at the University of Pennsylvania in Philadelphia and author of *Learned Optimism*. "And there's a good chance that optimism may keep you healthier during the course of middle age and old age."

What's really at the heart of optimism, Dr. Seligman says, is how you explain negative experiences to yourself. When something bad happens to a pessimist, she's likely to get into a sort of dark and hopeless mental muttering that has her thinking things like "It's all my fault, it's permanent and everything is ruined."

The optimist's explanation? It was bad luck, it will pass and I'll handle it differently next time because I learn from my experiences. With this kind of reasoning, an optimist feels a greater sense of control over her future—and her health.

## Comeback Power

Optimism can give you real resilience as you get older. "Research has shown that optimistic attitudes and beliefs are associated with fewer illnesses and quicker recovery from illness," says Christopher Peterson, Ph.D., professor of psychology at the University of Michigan in Ann Arbor and author of *Health and Optimism*.

"You're not going to find an 85-year-old with a smiley button who looks 20," Dr. Peterson says. But since optimists are more likely to feel that they can take charge of their health and not just passively slide into old age, they tend to take better care of themselves. "They sleep better, don't drink or smoke as much, exercise regularly and are more free from depression," he says.

So who's likely to live longer and age more gently? If you're fatalistic and believe there's nothing you can do to slow down aging, you may be less motivated to stay away from age-accelerating habits, Dr. Peterson says. But optimists tend to make healthier choices.

"And when optimists do fall ill," Dr. Peterson says, "they go to the doctor and shut down and rest, believing this will make a difference. They stay home, drink fluids and follow the doctor's advice. They allow themselves to heal."

## Attitude Is Everything

Optimism's negative sibling—pessimism—may lower your resistance to illness, increase your chances of heart disease and even shorten your life, researchers say.

Pessimism may weaken the immune system. That's the finding of researchers from Yale University, the University of Pennsylvania and the Prince of Wales Hospital in Sydney, Australia. They interviewed 26 women and men to find out what kind of explanations they gave for their health problems and then tested their immune cell activity. The researchers found that the pessimists had higher levels of T-suppressor cells, which interfere with the action of cells that boost immunity. The researchers don't know the exact mechanics of how pessimism inhibits immunity, but they do think it might be an important risk factor in immune-related diseases.

Your immune system isn't the only part of the body that's suppressed by pessimism. Dr. Seligman described pessimism as a kind of depression—and one study shows that a heavy heart is more prone to heart disease—in men, at any rate. Researchers at the Centers for Disease Control and Prevention in Atlanta tracked the health and attitudes of 2,832 adults for 12 years. They found that those with the most negative and hopeless attitudes were at greater risk of developing heart disease. Although the study included only men, depressed women may be more vulnerable, too, Dr. Seligman says.

Many studies have indicated that women are diagnosed with depression more often than men. The reasons given vary widely—from genetic differences, stress levels and unequal salaries to women's greater willingness to recognize their depression and seek help for it.

But psychologist Susan Nolen-Hoeksema, Ph.D., of Stanford University in California has reviewed hundreds of studies on depression and gender and concludes that most of these reasons are not supported by convincing evidence. Instead, she offers another explanation for why more women are depressed than men.

An important clue may lie in the different ways women and men respond to depressing thoughts and situations, Dr. Nolen-Hoeksema suggests. Studies have also shown that men tend to take action to distract themselves when they are depressed. But women more often analyze and brood over their state—a ruminating process that may deepen pessimistic feelings.

And there's a lot to be said for cultivating optimistic attitudes now, before the challenges of old age arrive. Some researchers speculate that pessimism begins to have a negative effect on health in middle age, around ages 35 to 50. And other studies show that if you're feeling grim, you might even expect an early visit from the grim reaper.

Researchers at the Center for Gerontology and Health Care Research at Brown University in Providence, Rhode Island, studied the responses of 1,390 older women and men to questions about their daily lives and the problems of aging. Those who believed their problems were the inevitable result of aging had a 16 percent higher death rate over the next four years than those who believed their problems were due to a specific, treatable condition.

"People who are saying their problems are just due to age are saying 'I have something that's not really treatable,' " says William Rakowski, Ph.D., the gerontologist who co-authored the study at Brown. "Whereas, the optimists—people who say it's a specific, treatable condition—are saying 'I can do something about it.' "

# Learning How to Hope

What if grubbing in the garden of gloom has been your lifelong habit? You can learn to cultivate a more upbeat attitude, and it's never too late to start, says Dr. Seligman. "I'm a born pessimist myself, so I've had to learn these techniques, and I use them every day," he says.

**Notice how your friends feel.** Look at your friends' attitudes, says Dr. Peterson. "Optimism and pessimism are both contagious states," he says. "So to 'catch' optimism, associate as much as possible with positive people."

**Negotiate with negative types.** Likewise, you can't be the only optimist in a family of pessimists, Dr. Peterson says. You're likely to cave in, go numb under the onslaught and become a pessimist yourself. So if it's a family member who spouts negativity all day long, try saying "It really drives me crazy when you talk like this. Can we be negative once a week instead?"

**Savor your successes.** We're trained to be modest, says Dr. Peterson, but there's no need to belittle your own triumphs with "I was just lucky." Instead, you can say to yourself "I worked really hard, I did a good job and I'm proud of myself," he says. That's the optimistic way of thinking about good events that you brought about by your own efforts.

**Face facts, but never give up.** Optimism doesn't mean you're not in touch with hard facts, says Dr. Rakowski. "Be realistic about what's happened in your life: 'Yes, I've had it tough'; 'I was a victim of circumstance there'; 'That

---

# When Pessimism Pays Off

Although extreme pessimism never does anybody any good, some jobs call for a steady dose of realism. And in these fields, moderate pessimism may spell success, says Martin Seligman, Ph.D., professor of psychology and director of clinical training at the University of Pennsylvania in Philadelphia and author of *Learned Optimism*.

According to Dr. Seligman, moderate pessimists do well in these areas:

- Design and safety engineering
- Technical and cost estimating
- Contract negotiation
- Financial control and accounting
- Law (but not litigation)
- Business administration
- Statistics
- Technical writing
- Quality control
- Personnel and industrial relations management

When do you need to be a die-hard optimist? In sales, brokering, public relations, acting, fund-raising, creative jobs, highly competitive jobs and high-burnout jobs, an optimistic outlook is a must, he says.

---

was my fault'; 'That wasn't'; 'I did this well.' " And then use optimism to resolve that, in spite of it all. Tell yourself "With effort, initiative and good luck, I will still have good things to look forward to," he says.

**Make the best of hard times.** Some people face a great deal of adversity and still call themselves optimists, Dr. Rakowski says. Why? "When you're optimistic, you're also believing 'I can make the most of what I've got,' " he says. "Sometimes you need to redefine your objectives and let go of an initial expectation. Then your basic objective is still to make the most of what you have."

**Distance yourself from your beliefs.** It is essential to realize that your beliefs are just that—beliefs, not facts, Dr. Seligman says. If a jealous rival at work said to you "You're a terrible manager and you'll never make it in this business," you'd know to ignore her insults. But what about the spiteful things we say to ourselves? ("I can't balance the checkbook. I'm so stupid.") They can be just as baseless as jealous insults, only it's bad thinking—a mental reflex you don't have to find convincing. "Check out the accuracy of your reflexive beliefs and argue with yourself," he says.

**Learn your optimism A-B-C.** Three things happen when you face a tough situation, and A-B-C is a good way to remember the pattern, says Dr. Seligman. You respond to *a*dversity with a *b*elief, which determines the *c*onsequence. For example, you're on the phone trying to make a sale, and your first caller hangs up on you—adversity. When you respond with an optimistic belief—"Oh well, that's one no out of the way. It brings me closer to the yes,"—then the likely consequence is that you'll feel relaxed and energetic. Compare that with a knee-jerk negative belief—"I'll never get any better at this"—which produces an equally negative consequence—you feel lousy about yourself.

**Derail negative thoughts.** When you become aware of your negative thoughts, you can learn to stop pessimistic thinking. When a persistent negative thought runs repeatedly through your mind, try techniques like these: Smack your palm hard on your desk and say—loudly—"Stop!" Or put a rubber band around your wrist and snap it every time you have the thought. (One wag says this helps you "snap out of it.") Or write down the thought and set aside a time to think it over later. These techniques can stop a bout of pessimism before it starts.

**Give a little.** If painful circumstances have made you unhappy, doing what you can to help others may give you a more optimistic view, says Dr. Rakowski. Whether you do volunteer work or simply offer to listen to a friend's troubles, you can find a way to give, he says. There's a real sense of fulfillment in giving that can lift you out of your pain, he says.

**Get help for depression.** "If you're a real pessimist, odds are you're fairly depressed," says Dr. Peterson. "It's a good bet that undergoing therapy for depression will make you healthier and improve your life." Cognitive behavioral therapy, during which you learn to challenge defeatist ways of thinking, is particularly helpful in turning depression around, he says. Chronically unhappy people do a running negative commentary on their lives that they're often not aware of, he says. A therapist can teach you ways to divert yourself when you get in these moods. These techniques won't reduce the frequency of episodes of depression you have, but will shorten them, he says. And in some cases, a prescription for antidepressant medication may help.

# RELAXATION

## *Mother Nature's Secret Life Enhancer*

In your dreams, you lie in a lounge chair on a balmy beach next to a serene, turquoise sea. In reality, you can't remember the last time you've been to the beach or just had a moment when you didn't need to be anywhere or do anything.

But relaxation is something that you cannot afford to forgo until your next vacation, whenever that will be. In fact, taking a few minutes each day to relax and let life's strains roll off isn't a luxury; it's a necessity if you want to stay vigorous, productive and healthy.

"There are three main things you can do to prolong your life. One is to exercise, one is to maintain proper nutrition and the other is to relax. Relaxation can definitely help you age better. It's important for preventing a wide variety of disorders and for increasing your effectiveness and efficiency in life," says Frank J. McGuigan, Ph.D., director of the Institute for Stress Management at United States International University in San Diego. "I don't think there's any question that relaxation can have a positive effect on phobias, depression, anxiety, high blood pressure, ulcers, colitis, headaches and lower back pain."

## Slow Down, You Move Too Fast

For many of us, relaxing means shopping, talking with a friend or playing an enjoyable round of golf.

But while those activities can be stress relieving, they also can trigger competition and frustration, two things that actually make it harder to relax, says Richard Friedman, Ph.D., associate professor of psychology at the State University of New York at Stony Brook.

"We know from carefully conducted experiments that most people don't really get into a relaxed physiological state when they're doing things that society generally considers relaxing, like reading a newspaper, playing sports or watching television," Dr. Friedman says. "The true way to get into a relaxed physiological state is essentially to let your mind go into neutral."

Popping your brain out of gear momentarily frees your mind so you're not judging anything or pondering weighty decisions. For a few seconds or minutes, you're not thinking about what you could have done yesterday or what might happen tomorrow. Taking several of these mental rest stops each day lessens anxiety and helps you let go of stress and tension, Dr. Friedman says. This physiological state, called the relaxation response, has been shown to lower heart rate, metabolism, blood pressure and breath rate, slow brain waves and elicit feelings of peace and tranquillity, says Herbert Benson, M.D., associate professor of medicine at Harvard Medical School, chief of the Behavioral Medicine Division at the New England Deaconess Hospital, both in Boston, and author of *The Relaxation Response*.

Sometimes relaxation or a feeling of ease and well-being arises naturally, like after a long, enjoyable run or an intimate conversation with a close friend. But if you've ever had anyone tell you to "relax" when you've felt stressed, besides making you more frustrated or upset, you know how difficult it is to consciously allow yourself to regain a sense of stability and calm.

"To relax, you really can't try too hard. This is similar to trying to fall asleep. Often the effort involved in attempting to make yourself go to sleep will probably keep you awake all night," says Saki Santorelli, Ed.D., associate director of the Stress Reduction Clinic at the University of Massachusetts Medical Center in Worcester.

To truly unwind, Dr. Santorelli says, you actually need to concentrate or focus your attention on your breath or some other sensation that will allow your mind to settle into an inherent sense of stillness. There are plenty of ways to unwind, but before we talk about them, let's find out a bit more about the physical and psychological benefits of relaxation.

# Mellow Out for Better Health

When you're stuck in traffic, struggling to meet a deadline or facing any other stressful situation, your muscles tense, you breathe faster and deeper, your heart beats more rapidly, blood vessels constrict and blood pressure rises, the digestive tract shuts down and perspiration increases. Over time, constant stress elevates blood pressure, total blood cholesterol and blood platelet counts, all of which can lead to atherosclerosis (hardening of the arteries) and heart attacks. Add to that the other hazards of a modern lifestyle, such as a high-fat diet and too little exercise, and you're a disaster waiting to happen.

In a study of monkeys, whose cardiovascular systems are similar to ours, researchers at Bowman Gray School of Medicine of Wake Forest University in

Winston-Salem, North Carolina, found that emotional stress (caused by the disruption of the animals' social bonds) significantly increased coronary blockages. And these blockages occurred regardless of diet and blood cholesterol levels—two of the major risk factors for heart disease. When the monkeys were fed a typical high-fat diet, emotional stress magnified the process of atherosclerosis 30 times.

Stress is also linked to ulcers and colitis and can trigger backaches, headaches, leg pain, chronic fatigue, depression, anxiety and insomnia. It also can aggravate arthritis and diabetes, Dr. McGuigan says.

In fact, eight of ten people seen by primary care physicians have some stress-related symptoms, says Robert S. Eliot, M.D., director of the Institute of Stress Medicine in Jackson Hole, Wyoming, and author of *From Stress to Strength: How to Lighten Your Load and Save Your Life*.

Fortunately, practicing relaxation techniques can relieve or prevent almost all of the harmful effects of chronic stress, Dr. Benson says.

Relaxation training, for instance, is a core element in a successful program to clear clogged arteries and reverse heart disease without surgery pioneered by Dean Ornish, M.D., president and director of the Preventive Medicine Research Institute in Sausalito, California. While Dr. Ornish believes that all of the components of his program are important—including regular exercise and a nearly fat-free vegetarian diet—he says that relaxation training is probably one of its most powerful components.

"We have shown, using PET scans and angiograms, that people who practice some form of relaxation like yoga or meditation and who meet regularly with a support group experience a greater degree of heart disease reversal than if they only attack the problem at the physical level, say just with diet or cholesterol-lowering drugs," Dr. Ornish says. A PET scan is positron emission tomography, a three-dimensional imaging technique that measures heart blood flow.

Studies by Dr. Benson and other researchers have also consistently shown that relaxation techniques significantly relieve high blood pressure, another risk factor for heart disease.

In addition, relaxation techniques can relieve even the most severe symptoms of premenstrual syndrome (PMS), according to Harvard Medical School researchers. In a five-month study of 46 women, the researchers found that women who meditated for 15 to 20 minutes twice a day reduced their symptoms of PMS by 58 percent. That was more than twice the improvement perceived by women who read twice a day and nearly 3½ times better than women who merely kept a diary of their symptoms.

Relaxation can also short-circuit low back pain and headaches. Muscle relaxation, for example, helped 21 people whose severe chronic tension headaches weren't relieved by drugs reduce the number and severity of their headaches by 42 percent, according to researchers from the Center for Stress and Anxiety Disorders at State University of New York at Albany. Another group of people who simply tracked their headache activity showed no improvement at all.

# Getting Down to Basics

You probably first experienced fight or flight, the two basic responses to stress, at a young age—particularly if you were ever caught wearing your sister's favorite dress without permission. But Dr. Eliot suggests we might be better off if we learned another approach.

"When you can't fight and you can't flee, then flow," he says.

While learning to be more relaxed and at ease takes time and attention, it can be done. "I look at relaxation as being comfortable in your own skin," Dr. Santorelli says. "That's tough for all of us at times, but it's possible to begin cultivating that capacity at any age."

Here are a few basics to help you mellow out.

**Snuff out the smokes.** "Our studies show that smoking causes blood vessels to clamp down and restrict blood flow," Dr. Eliot says. "That's like trying to drive with your foot pressed down on the brake. If there's a single thing that people can do to feel less stressed and more relaxed, it's kicking the habit."

**Whittle your weight.** "It's hard to feel relaxed if you're carrying around extra weight," Dr. Eliot says. "Your clothes don't feel comfortable and your body image suffers." Being overweight also contributes to high blood pressure, heart disease and diabetes. Ask your doctor if losing weight could help you.

**Team up with carbs.** "Protein seems to raise energy levels and keep you alert," Dr. Eliot says. "So if you have a hamburger late at night, you'll probably be rehashing yesterday's sales meeting until dawn." Carbohydrates, on the other hand, trigger the release of hormones that will relax you. So if you want to unwind at night, eat a plate of spaghetti, baked beans or other complex carbohydrates for dinner.

**Write it down.** Over a dozen studies have shown that if you write about your problems you can help relieve stress, improve your immunity, make fewer visits to the doctor and have a more optimistic view of life, says James Pennebaker, Ph.D., professor of psychology at Southern Methodist University in Dallas. Spend 20 minutes a day writing about your deepest thoughts and feelings, Dr. Pennebaker suggests. Don't worry about grammar or style; just write how you feel about things that are really upsetting you. Then when you're done, throw the paper away. You may feel a sense of relief when you're done.

**Time is on your side.** "Every time after you look at a clock or your watch during a day, take a deep breath while consciously raising and lowering your shoulders or dropping your jaw," Dr. Santorelli says. "That probably takes ten seconds and will serve as a reminder to you that you can be at ease while going about your daily schedule."

**Laugh it off.** Humor is a powerful relaxation technique, Dr. Eliot says. Laughter triggers the release of endorphins, chemicals in the brain that produce feelings of euphoria. It also suppresses the production of cortisol, a hormone released when you're under stress that indirectly raises blood pressure by causing the body to retain salt. So share a good laugh with a friend or keep a handy file of humorous anecdotes and drawings in a drawer that you can quickly pull out.

**Make time for others.** "Take a moment to practice basic kindness," Dr. Santorelli says. "Smile and say hello to a co-worker, play with a pet or talk to a close friend. If you do, you might feel better and more relaxed and possibly be more productive."

**Snooze away.** Get plenty of uninterrupted sleep, Dr. Eliot advises. If you get less sleep than you need, you might wake feeling tense and incapable of coping with life's basic hassles. Try to get at least six to eight hours of sleep each night. Avoid alcohol or sleeping pills. Although they can help put you to sleep, they can also interfere with your natural sleeping patterns and actually cause you to have a less restful night, Dr. Eliot says.

# Going with the Flow

There are many methods available for the development of calmness and stability. No single method is right for everyone. The key is finding one that feels comfortable to you. "I feel that it is important to set aside a block of time each day to practice these methods and then incorporate them into your daily life. Often these can be so unobtrusive that most people won't know that you're doing anything special," says Dr. Santorelli. Here are some ideas.

**Pay attention to your breath.** Paying attention to your own breathing is a simple form of meditation that can be very calming, Dr. Santorelli says. Sit in a comfortable chair or on the floor so that your back, neck and head are straight but not rigid. Exhaling deeply, allow the inhalation to come naturally. Simply pay attention to the gentle rising and falling of your abdomen, the movement of your ribs or the sensation of the breath moving through your nostrils. There is no need to try "relaxing." Just focus your mind on your breathing. If your mind starts to wander, gently escort your mind back to your breathing.

As an alternative, lie on the floor, put a book on your abdomen and take several slow, deep breaths, Dr. Eliot suggests. Focus on the book moving up and down on your belly. As you breathe in, think to yourself "Cool, clear mind." Then as you blow out, think "Calm, relaxed body."

**Take a slice of life.** Another way of cultivating moment-to-moment awareness is to focus your attention on a food, Dr. Santorelli says. Take a single slice of orange or apple, or an almond or raisin or some other food you like. Look at it carefully. Roll it around in your fingers. Focus your mind on its color, texture or fragrance. Then after a few moments, consciously decide to take one small bite. Chew it slowly, paying attention to its taste and what happens to it in your mouth. Feel your tongue engulf it. Then slowly and consciously swallow it.

As an alternative, try focusing intently on an everyday activity like showering or washing dishes. "Some people say that they feel much more at ease after practicing in this way," Dr. Santorelli says.

**Climb every mountain.** Visualizations and imagery can encourage the development of calmness and well-being, Dr. Santorelli says. Closing your eyes, once again become aware of your breath and bring to mind a favorite mountain in your life. It could be one you've climbed or yearned to visit. Allow your body to become the stable foundation, sloping sides and summit. Feel yourself steady, solid, grounded. As your sense of stability and steadiness grows, allow the weather to vary—some days the mountain will be covered in sunlight, other times with rain, snow, sleet or hail. Although the weather changes, notice that the mountain remains steady and dignified. "This image helps you realize that you can feel stable and secure and endure any storm that life has in store for you, like being stuck in a traffic jam, facing a deadline or living with the death of a loved one," Dr. Santorelli says.

**Move that body.** Exercise triggers the release of endorphins, but exercising the mind and body simultaneously may produce even better results, according to researchers at the University of Massachusetts Medical Center in Worcester. They asked 40 sedentary people to begin walking 35 to 40 minutes a day, three times a week, while listening to relaxation tapes. The tapes guided the walkers through a meditation that helped them focus on the one-two rhythm of their steps. The researchers concluded that this routine provoked more feelings of euphoria and reduced anxiety than in a matched group who exercised at the same intensity but didn't listen to the tapes.

"If you focus your mind on an unchanging, repetitive rhythm like exercise, the mind tends to go blank. That blankness is what you're shooting for," Dr. Friedman says. "It gives the brain a chance to restore itself and calm down."

To try it, pick an exercise (such as walking, running, swimming, climbing stairs or jumping rope) that has a natural rhythm. Focus your attention on that rhythm—even to the point of repeating the words "one, two" in your head in cadence with the exercise. Try to stay in that rhythm. As with breathing or other types of meditation, your mind may start to wander after a couple of minutes. If it does, refocus your attention on the repetitive movement of the exercise, Dr. Benson says.

Try doing this 20 minutes a day, three times a week, Dr. Benson suggests.

**Unleash those muscles.** There are about 1,030 skeletal muscles in the body. When you feel under stress, these muscles naturally contract and create tension, Dr. McGuigan says. One way to counteract that is progressive relaxation. By systematically flexing and releasing muscles, progressive relaxation can whisk that tension right out of your body.

"It's a good technique for beginners because it's practical and doesn't depend on imagination," says Martha Davis, Ph.D., a psychologist at Kaiser Permanente Medical Center in Santa Clara, California, and co-author of *The Relaxation and Stress Reduction Workbook*. "It works because it exaggerates the tension in the muscle so that you become more aware of what tension feels like. Secondly, you fatigue the muscle so that when you let go, the muscle is more than ready to relax," she says.

Although there are many variations, Dr. Davis suggests this approach: Clench your right fist as tightly as you can. Keep it clenched for about ten seconds, then release. Feel the looseness in your right hand and notice how much more relaxed it feels than when you tensed it. Do the same thing with your left hand, then clench both fists at the same time. Bend your elbows and tense your arms. Release and let your arms hang at your sides. Continue this process by tensing then relaxing your shoulders and neck and wrinkling then relaxing your forehead and brows. Then squeeze your eyes and clench your jaw before moving on to tense then relax your stomach, lower back, thighs, buttocks, calves and feet. It should take about ten minutes to complete the entire sequence. Try to do these exercises twice a day.

**Stretch them, too.** Unlike progressive relaxation, which contracts muscles, gentle stretching allows muscles to stretch and relax. That's better for some people, particularly those with chronic muscle pain, says Charles Carlson, Ph.D., professor of psychology at the University of Kentucky in Lexington.

"If you tense a muscle that is already in pain, you'll likely just create more pain. That doesn't help you relax," Dr. Carlson says. "Gentle stretching does two things. First, if you gently stretch a muscle and release it, it will generally relax. But secondly, when you focus your attention on doing the stretch, it also helps the mind relax. Muscle stretching should always be done slowly and without pain. There should be no overstretching or bouncing of muscles."

As an example of stretch-based relaxation, begin by pushing your eyebrows up with your index fingers and pushing down on your cheeks with your thumbs. (While doing any of these stretching exercises, note what the tension feels like so you'll learn to monitor your muscle tension, Dr. Carlson advises). Hold that position for about ten seconds, then release and let the muscles around your eyes relax. After a minute of relaxing your muscles, let your head slowly sag toward your right shoulder for about ten seconds, then slowly sag your head toward the left shoulder for another ten seconds.

Next, at chest height, place your hands together as if you were praying. Then, keeping your fingertips and palms together, spread your fingers as if you were creating a fan. Move your thumbs down along the midline of your body until you feel a light stretch in the lower arms. Hold that position for ten seconds. Then relax.

Next, interlock your fingers and raise your hands over your head. Straighten your elbows and rotate your palms outward. Let your arms fall back over your head until you feel resistance. Hold that position for ten seconds, then quickly release and let your arms rest at your sides for one minute.

Do these exercises at least once a day or whenever you feel tense.

# RELIGION
# AND SPIRITUALITY

## *The Strength of an Ageless Soul*

When the spirit whispers, we all hear different things.

Many women hear the sound of the sacred in a holy book or favorite hymn. Others find their spirits lifted in meditation. Some find their spirituality in communion with the natural world. Some, in a new theology that avoids exclusively masculine terms. The sources of our faith and belief—and ways of manifesting them—are as varied as we are. But the benefits are the same, says Mark Gerzon, author of *Coming Into Our Own: Understanding the Adult Metamorphosis.*

Private and public expressions of spirituality—from meditation and prayer to attending religious services—increase emotional fulfillment while helping to relieve stress and depression. They also decrease your risk of heart disease and cancer. Researchers say they may even help prevent alcoholism, drug use and suicide.

What matters most in gaining these benefits is to experience your own spirituality in your own way, Gerzon says. "The key thing about spirituality in the second half of life is that we've lived enough and seen enough people pass from this earth to feel an urgency," he says. "We begin to listen to our inner voices. And when we do, where they lead us is not predictable. They may lead us back to the church of our childhood, but they may also lead us to other places we never expected," he says.

"So we need to broaden our view of what spiritual means. For some it could be tending flowers in the garden and for others, saying Hail Marys at morning mass," says Gerzon.

Perhaps your sense of the sacred has more to do with nature walks or loving relationships than participating publicly in religious rites. Many people draw meaning and strength from such a private spirituality, says Gerzon.

One way of searching for a sense of wholeness is through meditation or prayer, which have been shown to decrease heart rate and blood pressure and to help you cope better with stress.

# The Healing Power of Community

Most scientific conclusions about religion and health have been drawn from organized religion because religious organizations provide researchers with measurable groups of subjects involved in specific behaviors, such as attending worship services or participating together in community service. But perhaps there is something about religious community itself—aside from a shared belief system—that makes you healthier.

When you join in a religious community's social life, you become part of a caring network that will be there for you in hard times, says Dave Larson, M.D., adjunct associate professor of psychiatry at Duke University Medical Center in Durham, North Carolina, president of the National Institute for Healthcare Research in Rockville, Maryland, and former senior research psychiatrist at the National Institutes of Health Office of Alternative Medicine.

And women are particularly good at creating these networks of friendship and support, Dr. Larson says, because they are raised to value communication and nurturing and to work together.

Other researchers have also recognized the healing benefits of a spiritual community. "When people get sick they visit each other, bringing food; they notify relatives and take each other to the doctor," says Lawrence Calhoun, Ph.D., a psychologist at the University of North Carolina at Charlotte. "When you're a meaningful part of a community like that, it can soften the sting of getting older."

Health experts have known for years that stress contributes to many physical problems including nausea, diarrhea, constipation, high blood pressure and heart rhythm abnormalities.

Studies have shown that strong religious beliefs go a long way to relieve stress—even if you simply hold your beliefs privately. But the stress-relieving effects of faith are most powerful, experts say, when you are regularly involved with a religious community.

Researchers at Ben Gurion University of the Negev and Soroka Medical Center in Beersheba, Israel, studied how 230 members of a religious kibbutz community coped with stressful life events. People within the community found that their individual faith and coping skills were strengthened by the support the community offered. And that resulted in quicker recovery from stress—including the stresses associated with getting older.

# Living a Fuller—and Longer—Life

Another study highlights the broad-ranging health benefits of attendance at religious services and active participation in a congregation's social life. Psychol-

# Meditation the Easy Way

For busy, over-stressed women, moments of tranquility and stillness are precious and rare. But there is a way to maximize the benefits of prayer and contemplation, says Herbert Benson, M.D., associate professor of medicine at Harvard Medical School, chief of the Behavioral Medicine Division at the New England Deaconess Hospital, both in Boston, and author of *The Relaxation Response*.

Dr. Benson conducted some of the first scientific studies into the effects of prayer and faith on stress reduction. To help patients learn how to relax, he taught the simplest meditation method: Sit quietly in a comfortable position and silently repeat a word or phrase while passively disregarding other thoughts.

When patients were offered the choice of a word, sound or phrase to repeat, 80 percent of them chose a word or prayer from their faith. And that led to a discovery, Dr. Benson says. People who used words from their own religion rather than neutral words (like "one" or "be calm") stuck with the program better. And their health improved as a result of the "relaxation response," which is characterized by decreased heart rate and blood pressure and feelings of tranquillity.

The words may vary, Dr. Benson says, but the benefits don't. "In all the different religious contexts, there seems to be a similar potential for health-enhancing effects," he says. Here's how to bring those benefits into your life every day.

Choose a word or short phrase that's easy to pronounce and short enough to say silently as you exhale. When thoughts arise, as they inevitably will, gently return to the focus word. Practice this kind of meditation for 20 minutes twice a day.

ogists Stanislav Kasl of Yale University and Ellen Idler of Rutgers University studied 2,812 elderly women and men in New Haven, Connecticut. They found that outwardly religious Catholics, Protestants and Jews were less likely to become medically disabled than those who considered attending church or synagogue unimportant. These people also remained more physically independent as they got older, largely because of their public religious environment.

Hanukkah, Easter, Christmas and other religious holidays may mean even more to you as the years go by. The New Haven study also found that very religious people are much less likely to die during the months before and after major religious holidays. But one particular finding may inspire you to take a more active role in the important celebrations of your faith. Although death rates for both Jewish men and women dipped during Passover, the women were less protected. The researchers believe this is probably because women are excluded from any role in the most important aspects of the Passover ritual.

Religion in your life can also be potent protection against cancer. This may be because some groups of believers such as Mormons and Jehovah's Witnesses encourage healthy lifestyle choices, like eating a vegetarian diet or avoiding smoking. Analysts from the University of Florida's Center for Health Policy Research in Gainesville reviewed data on cancer deaths across the United States and found that counties with the highest number of religious people also have the lowest rates of cancer.

Even faiths that do not recommend specific dietary or health habits still have a protective effect, the researchers believe, simply because they encourage moderation—cautioning their members against unhealthy excesses of any kind.

## Healing the Heart

Spirituality offers particularly strong protection against a major killer: heart disease, says Dr. Larson.

A study of 85 women and 454 men in Jerusalem found that people who define themselves as "secular" (nonreligious) have a greater risk of heart disease than those who follow the path of Orthodox Judaism. Even after the researchers accounted for smoking habits and cholesterol and blood pressure levels, a strong association between lowered heart disease risk and religious practice remained for both sexes.

Although the researchers are unsure which aspects of belief are responsible, they speculate that the strong social support system of traditional Orthodox communities, like those present in many other types of congregations, plays a heart-protecting role, probably by reducing isolation and stress.

In another study of religion and the heart, Dr. Larson and his colleagues studied data on blood pressure in more than 400 men in Evans County, Georgia. They found that either a personal belief in God or attendance at religious services (even without belief) tended to lower blood pressure, but people who both believed and attended had the lowest readings.

## Like a Bridge over Troubled Water

Not only does an active spiritual or religious life keep many forms of stress and disease at bay, but it also helps shield you from mental and emotional illness.

Dr. Larson and his research team reviewed more than 200 studies on religious commitment and mental health. They found that people who are religious have lower rates of depression, alcoholism, suicide and drug use than less religious people do. Young people who are religious do better in school and are less likely to be delinquent and sexually active. Married people who attend church regularly report greater marital happiness, are more satisfied with their sexual lives and experience lower rates of divorce.

The studies also showed that religious faith is directly connected to a higher sense of satisfaction with life in general and a greater ability to cope with life's stresses and problems, Dr. Larson says. The researchers examined specific "real life" behaviors, such as attending services, rather than attempting to measure attitudes or beliefs.

# Embrace the Spirit

You may feel a growing yearning for a deeper sense of meaning in your life. Here's how to re-connect with your spiritual side.

**Begin at the beginning.** Before you re-commit to your childhood religion or embrace another faith, examine it, says Alan Berger, Ph.D., director of Jewish studies in the Department of Religion at Syracuse University in New York. "Ask yourself 'What is it that my tradition teaches?' " he says. "Don't feel you have to accept it, but do know it."

**Go beyond the don'ts.** If religion seems only like a series of rules or thou-shalt-nots, Dr. Berger says, "You need to un-skew your view. Go find yourself a better teacher, a new community. Read the texts yourself or with a partner and uncover the various levels of meaning. Understand that life is a fluid and dynamic experience that people need help with. Religion is the attempt to search for meaning in an otherwise chaotic universe."

**Accept yourself.** "It's fine to say 'I don't really know what I am, spiritually,' " says Brother Guerric Plante, a monk at the Abbey of Gethsemane in New Haven, Kentucky. "Honesty has everything to do with spiritual growth." Once you're open with yourself about any confusion you feel, the way will become more clear.

**Search with others.** Read the religion and support group announcements in your newspaper to find a group or organization that may offer help for your spiritual search, Brother Plante says. "Faith can come through others—their example, their talk, their interest in others. Group therapy, religious services or even a 12-step group for addiction can rekindle a spiritual life if you're sincerely searching."

**Meditate or pray.** Clear time from your schedule to sit in quiet contemplation and listen to the stillness within you, says Gerzon. "If we derive meaning and purpose in life only from doing, we're in trouble," he says. "We need to find it from being, and meditation is a good way to start learning about how to simply be."

**Broaden your view.** Sometimes just encouraging your sense of curiosity and wondering about life will lead you to spiritual truths. When you ponder some of the age-old questions such as "Why am I here?" or "What is the meaning of life?" you encourage your spiritual insight to unfold, says Gerzon. "It's possible to find the spiritual dimension in answers, but we're more likely to find it in the questions themselves," he says. "When we're really moved by the spirit of life, it's because we're touching what we don't know, not what we know."

**Go against your grain.** You're more likely to grow spiritually if you seek out activities that are different from what you usually do all day, says John Buehrens, a minister for over 20 years and president of the Unitarian Universalist Association in Boston. If you spend your day locked away from others in a corporate office, then serving a meal to the needy might be just what you need. But if you're a lawyer at a free clinic or a social worker, you may benefit more from a religious discussion group, he says.

Buehrens's own spiritual discipline? "I'm a pointy-headed, pear-shaped intellectual," he says. "So one of my spiritual disciplines is getting some regular exercise. It really is a time of meditation and prayer for me."

**Care about others.** You need to get out of yourself to feel spiritually healthy, Buehrens says. "That's why community is so important to real spiritual growth, because we're drawn out of ourselves. We'll never find peace along religious, racial and ethnic lines unless we do this." His advice for isolated seekers? "Go help in a soup kitchen, go visit a nursing home and get your nose out of your navel," he says.

**Keep a spiritual journal.** Writing in a daily journal about your spiritual questions, doubts, beliefs and experiences can illuminate the meaning and value in your life, says Buehrens. "You may find that your unconscious is trying to get through to you with more life-enhancing and creatively responsible methods."

**Don't be afraid to question.** "All spiritual traditions try to teach an enhanced awareness of being, greater spiritual vitality and deeper compassion for other people," Buehrens says. But any spiritual community that doesn't respect questioning or the importance of your individual conscience may be an unhealthy one, he says. His advice? Follow your own conscience to the spiritual path that's right for you.

# RESISTANCE TRAINING

## Give Your Life a Lift

You've watched your grandmother struggle through the simplest tasks. It takes all the energy she can muster just to get out of a chair. And a walk down the hallway takes forever. She's managing to get by on her own, but just barely.

You swear you're never going to let yourself get like that.

So you get plenty of aerobic exercise, eat right and try to get enough sleep. The prescription right off the Geritol ads.

But aren't you forgetting something?

It's called resistance training, otherwise known as weight lifting. And it can help you maintain, if not improve, your quality of life.

Resistance training improves muscle strength and endurance—qualities that will enable you to do the activities you love well into old age. It can also help improve your cholesterol level, enhance your bone strength, maintain or lose weight and improve your body image and self-esteem.

"If people stay with it, continue to be active and continue to do activities that stress the muscles, they can fight off some of the effects of aging," says Alan Mikesky, Ph.D., an exercise physiologist and professor at Indiana University School of Physical Education in Indianapolis. "People can continue to do things they enjoy in life longer. And not only that, but also maintain their performance in what they're doing," says Dr. Mikesky.

## Good and Strong

One of the major—and most obvious—benefits of resistance training is its effect on muscle strength. Maintaining or increasing muscle strength is crucial to maintaining independence as we age, says Miriam E. Nelson, Ph.D., a research scientist and exercise physiologist at the U.S. Department of Agriculture's Human Nutrition Research Center on Aging at Tufts University in Boston. Adequate muscle strength is what enables you to do things like carry your own luggage, climb stairs and get in and out of bed.

Resistance training increases muscle strength by putting more strain on a muscle than it's used to. This increased load stimulates the growth of small proteins inside each muscle cell that play a central role in the ability to generate force. "When you lift weights, you stress or challenge the muscle cells, and they adapt by making more force-generating proteins," says Dr. Mikesky.

Weight training also helps improve muscle endurance, says Dr. Mikesky. So in addition to giving you the strength you need to lift a suitcase, it will give you the endurance you need to carry that suitcase for a longer period of time.

It doesn't take long to improve muscle strength, says Dr. Mikesky. "You can increase strength very quickly, in as little as 2 to 3 weeks," he says. Noticeable increases in muscle size take longer—about 6 to 8 weeks. Some studies have shown strength increases of 100 percent or more in 12 weeks, he says. The bad news is that you can lose strength gains just as quickly. "If you miss a week of workouts and go back and put the same weight on, it's harder," explains Dr. Mikesky.

There are several different methods for resistance training, including free weights, weight machines, calisthenics and resistance tubing. Free weights involve the use of dumbbells and bars stacked with weight plates; the lifter is responsible for both lifting the weight and determining and controlling body position through the range of motion. Weight machines, on the other hand, allow you to lift plates, but the machine dictates the movement that you perform. Calisthenics, such as chin-ups, push-ups and sit-ups, utilize your own body weight as the resistance force. Resistance tubing involves the use of an elastic band that provides resistance to active muscles. In one study at Indiana University–Purdue University at Indianapolis, 62 older adults were put on a 12-week training program with elastic tubing. The participants showed an average increase in strength of 82 percent, as measured by the increase in the tubing's level of resistance.

"The difference between free weights and machines is that machines are more user-friendly," says Mark Taranta, a physical therapist and director of the Physical Therapy Practice in Philadelphia. Training with machines doesn't require a lot of skill or coordination. "With free weights, more balance is required and there are more learning techniques required," he says.

There are different theories on the best type of resistance training program to follow. A lot of it depends on your individual goals. In general, lifting a heavy weight in three sets of 8 to 12 repetitions is the best way to build strength. And lifting a lighter weight for more repetitions helps to build endurance and tone.

# Heft for the Heart

Weight training can also give your cardiovascular health a lift, experts say. Studies on the effect of weight training on cholesterol profiles are controversial, says Dr. Mikesky, but some studies suggest an improvement in cholesterol levels that's similar to that of endurance training, he says.

In one study, six men and eight women used resistance training three days a week for 45 to 60 minutes each session. They showed significant changes in their cholesterol levels as a result. For the women, the ratio of total cholesterol to good, or HDL (high-density lipoprotein), cholesterol dropped 14.3 percent. This measurement is the best predictor of heart disease because it helps estimate how much bad, or LDL (low-density lipoprotein), cholesterol you have.

In the men, the ratio of total cholesterol to HDL was reduced by 21.6 percent. Ideally, you want your total cholesterol-to-HDL ratio to be low; a ratio of less than 3.5 is desirable. A ratio between 3.5 and 6.9 indicates moderate risk and a ratio over 7.0 indicates high risk.

In another study of 88 healthy, white pre-menopausal women, 46 women were put on a resistance training program that included weight-lifting exercises for the major muscle groups in the arms, legs, trunk and lower back, and the remaining women made up a control group. The resistance training group lifted 70 percent of their maximum weight in three sets of eight repetitions three days per week. Five months of resistance training led to significant decreases in total cholesterol and LDL cholesterol. No significant effect on HDL or triglycerides was observed.

There's some indication that higher-volume weight training—the kind that involves lifting a lighter weight for more repetitions—may have more of an effect on cholesterol levels than weight training that involves lifting heavier weights for fewer repetitions, according to Janet Walberg-Rankin, Ph.D., associate professor in the Exercise Science Program in the Division of Health and Physical Education at Virginia Polytechnic Institute and State University in Blacksburg.

While researchers don't fully understand how weight training lowers cholesterol, one means might be its effect on body composition and weight, says Dr. Walberg-Rankin. Weight training sometimes leads to weight loss and the reduction of body fat, and that can cause cholesterol to drop, she says.

# A Good Way to Bone Up

Resistance training can certainly have an effect on your body composition. Muscles burn more calories than fat, so by increasing muscle mass, you increase your metabolic rate and can burn calories and reduce fat tissue.

One study of women whose calorie input was restricted modestly found that when women used weight training in addition to dieting, there was an increase in lean body mass even though they were losing weight.

Resistance training puts stress on bone as well as muscle and thereby helps increase bone mineral mass and prevent osteoporosis, experts say. While aerobic weight-bearing exercise like walking and running helps maintain bone strength in the legs and hips, it's less effective on the spine and upper body. Resistance training helps maintain bone strength in those areas, says Dr. Walberg-Rankin.

One study of 40 menstruating women ages 17 to 38 conducted at the University of Arizona in Tucson found that weight lifting provided greater stimulus for increasing bone density than endurance exercise did. Women who lifted weights had greater bone density in their wrists, spine and hips.

## Boost Your Body Image

Resistance training is a good way to feel better about the way you look. One study of 60 sedentary women ages 35 to 49 conducted at Brigham Young University in Provo, Utah, found that women who resistance trained improved their body images 2.4 times that of women who participated in a walking program. Body image improved most in women who trained hard and consistently, the researchers found.

One reason weight training may be so effective in boosting self-esteem is that feedback is immediate. In addition to being able to see muscle growth and improved muscle tone, progress is easy to detect. "You know in two weeks when you can lift more weights on a machine," says Dr. Walberg-Rankin. That's a little easier to detect than an improvement in your aerobic fitness, she says.

## How to Get to It

Why wait when you can be lifting weights? Here are some tips for getting started.

**Check it out.** Your physical health, that is. If you are going to start a resistance-training program, you should see your doctor for a physical first, says Dr. Walberg-Rankin. Your doctor will do a physical exam and take a health history. If you have a history of osteoporosis, heart disease or high blood pressure, be sure to mention it.

**Don't go it alone.** If you're going to start resistance training, you must get instruction from an experienced person, says Dr. Walberg-Rankin. If you belong to a health club, get a qualified instructor to help you. Look for certification from the American College of Sports Medicine or the National Strength and Conditioning Association. Your instructor can help you decide on the best resistance training method for you and get you started on a program. If you are doing a home program with a gym machine or dumbbell weights, consult a video on proper weight-lifting techniques, she says. If you're interested in using resistance tubing, consult a physical therapist or exercise physiologist.

**Be sure to breathe.** While you're lifting, do not hold your breath, says Dr. Walberg-Rankin. Breathe in or out while lifting, she says. It doesn't really matter when you breathe in or out, she says; just be sure to do it throughout the exercise. Holding your breath can cause your blood pressure to skyrocket, which can be very dangerous.

**Start out light.** "Start low and progress slowly," says Dr. Mikesky. That means start with a lighter weight that you can lift 10 to 15 times and then progress slowly over the weeks to lifting heavier weights.

**Keep at it.** If you're persistent and consistent about lifting, your strength should gradually increase over a number of months. You may reach a point where you plateau, says Taranta, but it's important to keep lifting even at that plateau level to maintain strength.

**Do lifts you like.** There are many different exercises for each muscle group. "If you don't like an exercise, don't stay with it. Find one you like," says Dr. Mikesky.

**Lower slowly.** Focus on lowering the weight slowly. That half of the movement, called a negative, or eccentric, contraction, actually stimulates more muscle growth, says Dr. Nelson. One method is to take a longer time lowering the weight than raising it. Try lifting the weight to the count of three and lowering it to the count of four.

**Get started.** It's never too late to start weight training, says Dr. Mikesky. Muscle can adapt and increase in strength well into your older years, he says. Research at Tufts University has shown strength gains between 100 and 200 percent in individuals well into their nineties.

# SEX

## *It Does a Body Good*

You and your friends have wondered for years about the "glow" a woman supposedly gets after having good sex. But how many of you have actually seen it?

Next time you're feeling good after sex, get up and look at yourself in the mirror: You're beautiful, confident, energetic and alive. See? There really *is* a glow.

You know why you feel so good. But that glow is more than a feeling. Scientists attribute it to endorphins—chemicals that are released in the brain after sex. These chemicals create a sense of euphoria and ease your stress, says Helen S. Kaplan, M.D., Ph.D., director of the Human Sexuality Teaching Program at New York Hospital–Cornell Medical Center in New York City.

Medical researchers say regular doses of sex can also soothe chronic aches and pains, spur creativity, rev up energy and make you feel youthful.

"Anything that makes you feel good, alive and physically excited will make you feel more youthful. All of those things are associated with sex," says Lonnie Barbach, Ph.D., a sex therapist and psychologist in San Francisco and writer of the video *Sex after Fifty*.

Intimacy can also bolster your immune system and protect you against disease, Dr. Kaplan says.

For instance, sex has helped women cope with the pain of such chronic diseases as arthritis, says Sanford Roth, M.D., a rheumatologist and director of the Arthritis Center in Phoenix. Endorphins relieve the pain, but Dr. Roth believes sex has a vital psychological impact, too.

"Many times when patients come to me, pain isn't their number-one issue. They're more concerned about how the disease is affecting the quality of their lives, and sexuality is an important part of that," Dr. Roth says. "So maintaining sexual function in the face of disease helps people feel better about themselves and their lives."

Sex also might put an end to the pain that spawned the age-old excuse "Not tonight, dear, I have a headache." While sex isn't a sure cure, researchers have found it actually can relieve some headaches. In one small study, 47 percent of people with migraines said sex relieved their pain, according to George H. Sands, M.D., assistant professor of neurology at the Mount Sinai School of Medicine in New York City. One possible reason is that orgasms short-circuit the nervous system activity that's causing the pain. (On the other hand, sex can sometimes *cause* headaches. If it does, discuss it with your doctor.)

## Sex Can Be Forever

You probably were sexually stimulated in the womb before you were born, and you can remain sexually active until you die, says William Masters, M.D., of the Masters and Johnson Institute in St. Louis. In fact, seven out of ten women older than 70 who have partners have sex at least once a week.

"Sex is a natural function throughout your life if you have an interesting partner and remain healthy. It's not going to go away," Dr. Kaplan says. "It's abnormal for sex to disappear. The normal person has sex until the end of her life."

Sex can also be self-affirming. "Sex can help make you feel competent. It's a way of connecting with someone else. It can help you feel in charge of your own destiny," says Marty Klein, Ph.D., a licensed marriage counselor and sex therapist in Palo Alto, California, and author of *Ask Me Anything: A Sex Therapist Answers the Most Important Questions for the '90s.* "Sex is a place where you can go and not be bound by the ordinary rules of life."

"Sex often becomes more—not less—important as we age," Dr. Kaplan says. "It's one of the last processes to be affected by aging. First, the skin and your vision goes, then you get arthritis and heart disease. But you can still have sex. It's one of the enduring pleasures of life."

## Making Great Sex Better

For good sex, keep your body healthy by avoiding smoke and fatty foods, which can clog blood vessels and make arousal and orgasm difficult. Here are some other tips to add zing to your sex life.

**Get physical.** Aerobic exercise three times a week, 20 to 30 minutes a session, can improve your sex drive and performance, says Roger Crenshaw, M.D., a psychiatrist and sex therapist in private practice in La Jolla, California. Researchers at Bentley College in Waltham, Massachusetts, found, for example, that women in their forties who swam regularly had sex about seven times a month and enjoyed it more than their sedentary peers, who only had sex three times a month. In other words, the swimmers were as sexually active as women 10 to 20 years younger.

**Talk it over.** Talking with your partner helps both of you explain what you want sexually. If you don't tell him what you really want, then don't expect him to please you, says Shirley Zussman, Ed.D., a sex and marital therapist and co-director of the Association for Male Sexual Dysfunction in New York City. Avoid saying negative things like "That doesn't feel good" or "You know I don't like that." Instead, keep it positive: "I enjoy sex with you, but I have some ideas about making it even better."

**It's show time.** While talking helps, often showing your partner what pleases you is just as useful. If he's grabbing your breasts or rubbing you too hard, for example, gently take his hand and show him how you prefer to be stroked, Dr. Klein suggests.

# Picking the Right Contraceptive

While no birth control method has a 100 percent success rate, a contraceptive may be a powerful safeguard against pregnancy and sexually transmitted diseases (STDs) if used properly, says Michael Brodman, M.D., professor of obstetrics and gynecology at the Mount Sinai School of Medicine of the City University of New York.

There are many types of birth control available to women including the Pill, intrauterine devices (IUDs), diaphragms, female condoms, sponges, spermicides, hormonal injections and a surgically implanted conception rod that works for up to five years.

Choosing the birth control method that's right for you might require advice from your doctor. But a few general guidelines will help you make your choice, Dr. Brodman says.

First, if you're using contraception to avoid STDs, use a barrier contraceptive such as the female condom, sponge or diaphragm or have your partner wear a condom. A spermicide containing nonoxynol 9 should be used with both the diaphragm and the male condom because it is effective against the virus that causes AIDS.

If you're using contraceptives for birth control and you absolutely cannot take any chances, use the Pill, an implant or hormonal injections because they have the highest success rates, Dr. Brodman suggests.

If the male condom is your choice, you must use a spermicide because condoms are only 80 percent effective in preventing pregnancy when used alone. Spermicides must also be used with the diaphragm, which may shift during intercourse and allow sperm to enter the uterus, increasing the likelihood of pregnancy.

# What Men Really Want from Women

You want to talk, he wants sex. You want to snuggle, he wants sex. You want commitment, he says oops, it's time to go. Perplexed? Join the club.

"Men are often more able to separate sex from the emotional relationship. Unlike most women, they can have relationships that are purely physical," says Lonnie Barbach, Ph.D., a sex therapist and psychologist in San Francisco. "A lot of men have difficulty getting into intimacy. Sex is a way they can do that. So they often start their relationships with sex and bring the feelings in later."

"Men are toxic to too much closeness," agrees Anthony Pietropinto, M.D., a psychiatrist in New York City and author of *Not Tonight, Dear: How to Reawaken Your Sexual Desire.* "Many men don't like women who want you to talk about your deepest emotions."

Men like novelty in their sexual lives, Dr. Pietropinto says. They're more likely to suggest that you wear provocative clothing or seek exotic places to have sex.

When you do make love, a man is probably more concerned about his performance than you are. "A woman wants to know if the guy likes being close to her and finds her attractive. The guy is interested in finding out how he did," Dr. Pietropinto says.

On the bright side, many of these traits fade as a man ages and his sex drive declines. After about age 45, men need more psychological stimulation and as a result often become more sensitive, caring and receptive to a woman's emotional needs, says Helen S. Kaplan, M.D., Ph.D., director of the Human Sexuality Teaching Program at New York Hospital–Cornell Medical Center in New York City.

**Broaden your horizons.** "Intercourse is overemphasized as a sexual activity," Dr. Klein says. "Most couples would benefit from seeing sex as a much broader set of experiences." So take time to kiss, hug, caress, hold hands, talk or do other sexually pleasing activities such as mutual masturbation that make you feel close to your partner, he suggests.

**Make time for whoopee.** "I know it sounds comical, but some couples say they just don't have time for sex," says Carol Lassen, Ph.D., a psychologist and clinical professor of psychology at the University of Colorado School of Medicine in Denver. "Why? Everything else comes first. They can't have sex be-

# The Joy of Celibacy

"Marriage has many pains, but celibacy has no pleasures," according to Samuel Johnson, an eighteenth-century wit. But that assessment is way off target, experts say. Many couples and more than a few single women find celibacy gratifying and say that it actually bolsters their relationships and self-esteem.

About one in ten married couples abstain from sex, according to Michael S. Broder, Ph.D., a clinical psychologist in Philadelphia and author of *The Art of Staying Together*. Some people are celibate because of religious convictions, medication side effects or chronic illnesses. But a growing number of couples are actually celibate because they want to strengthen their bond in other ways.

Many singles choose abstinence in part to protect themselves from AIDS and other sexually transmitted diseases or even to finish their M.B.A., says Shirley Zussman, Ed.D., a sex and marital therapist and co-director of the Association for Male Sexual Dysfunction in New York City. Some single women say that they are simply waiting for someone really special.

"One big advantage of choosing to be celibate for some period of your life is that it gives you an opportunity to fully understand the place of sex in your life or relationship," says Harrison Voigt, Ph.D., a clinical psychologist, sex therapist and professor at the California Institute of Integral Studies in San Francisco. "It offers you a chance to see how well you can really relate to others outside of the sexual sphere."

Here are some guidelines for choosing celibacy.

- Realize that you'll continue to have sexual urges but you don't have to act on them.
- Consider your celibacy a vacation—a time to rest or try new experiences. Instead of thinking of it as a deprivation, consider it a choice. See it as an opportunity to find deeper meaning in your life.
- Remember, it doesn't have to be forever. You can stop being celibate anytime you choose. When you do, sex may be even more exciting and rewarding than ever.

cause they have to do the laundry or watch a football game or just get some sleep. They have very little time left for each other."

Rather than letting sex get lost in the daily grind, schedule time for it, says Michael Seiler, Ph.D., author of *Inhibited Sexual Desire* and assistant director of the Phoenix Institute in Chicago. "You'd make reservations in a fancy restaurant for 7:00 Saturday night. Why not say you'll meet in the bedroom at 9:00 P.M. Tuesday?" he says. "How do you know you'll be in the mood? You don't. But you don't know if you'll be hungry on Saturday night, either."

**Check your hang-ups at the door.** "Leave work, religion and your performance expectations outside the bedroom door," Dr. Barbach suggests. "Simply go into the bedroom with your body and your feelings. Focus on the emotional connection you have with your partner and the pleasure your body has in store."

**Keep it fun.** "Do you know what the Eskimos call sex? Laughing time," Dr. Zussman says. "Sex can be fun, frivolous and relaxing. We are so far from that in our society. We feel like we have to have fantastic sex each and every time." Forget performance, Dr. Zussman says. Just concentrate on having a good time with your partner and sex will be much more like laughing time than working overtime.

**Get back to basics.** "Couples stop doing the very things that brought them together in the first place," Dr. Seiler says. "They don't write each other little notes or send flowers. They don't give each other back rubs or go out on dates. You really have to work to keep the fun and play in the relationship. Without it, there won't be any fun and play in the bedroom."

So prepare a romantic candlelight dinner or ask him to take an evening walk around the block. Hold hands. You might be pleased with where it leads.

**Get a good sexual cookbook.** If your sex life, like stale soda, has lost most of its fizz, try browsing through sex manuals or watching erotic videos together for new ideas, says Domeena Renshaw, M.D., director of the Sexual Dysfunction Clinic at Loyola University of Chicago Stritch School of Medicine in Maywood.

**Keep an eye on him.** "Sustained eye contact during sex breeds intimacy. Often, it's more intimate than kissing or holding hands," says Harrison Voigt, Ph.D., clinical psychologist, sex therapist and professor at the California Institute of Integral Studies in San Francisco. "It's a way to get people in touch with a powerful form of union that isn't physical."

**Create a ritual.** Lighting a candle, massaging each other's feet or collaborating on the exchange of some special intimacies can become a part of a unique ritual that can help some couples connect emotionally before sex, Dr. Voigt says. "A ritual is basically a mutual agreement that sex should be something unique for the couple. It doesn't have to be complex, but it should change the context of sex into something that is special rather than just rolling over in bed and saying 'Hey, let's do it.' "

**Don't keep score.** If you had sex four times last week and had an orgasm each time, but had sex only once this week and did not have an orgasm, don't push to keep pace. "Frequency isn't as important as truly enjoying the sex that you do have," Dr. Zussman says.

**The bedroom isn't a workplace.** Your bedroom should be a place where you and your partner can retreat for intimate interludes. If it's cluttered with computers, the television, a typewriter and filing cabinets, it's more like an office. "There's something about disorder that distracts from romance. The bedroom should have a certain tranquillity," Dr. Zussman says.

---

# What Your Dream Lovers Are Telling You

You dream that you're naked at a elegant party. Embarrassed, you try to hide behind your husband, but Tom Cruise spots you from across the room, walks up and asks you to dance.

What does it mean? Nothing except that you're probably a typical woman.

"For women, sexual dreams usually are romantic and, more often than not, about a man she knows or someone like a boyfriend, movie star or rock musician who is emotionally significant to her," says Robert Van de Castle, Ph.D., professor emeritus of behavioral medicine at the University of Virginia Medical Center and past president of the Association for the Study of Dreams.

Women who have sexual dreams probably have better sex lives than those who don't dream about sex that much, he says. That's because women who are comfortable with their sexuality in the real world are more likely to dream about it.

If you have a sexual problem, it can show up in your dreams. "If a woman can't reach orgasm, she might dream that she is made of snow, symbolizing that she feels cold and frigid," Dr. Van de Castle says.

But some sex dreams might not be about sex at all, says Gayle Delaney, Ph.D., a San Francisco psychologist and author of *Sexual Dreams*. "For example, if you dream about having sex with a co-worker, it rarely means you have an unrecognized desire to have sex with that person," she says. "If that co-worker is incredibly selfish, your dream may represent some selfish aspect of your own character or the character of someone you are intimate with."

You can't even escape aging in your dreams. "Generally, we tend to dream about sexual partners who are our own age," Dr. Van de Castle says. "The vast majority of the people you see in your dreams are within 20 years of your own age."

# SKIN CARE

## Easy as Pie and Worth the Effort

**Y**our life is so busy you barely have time to sleep or eat or go to the grocery store. You definitely don't have time for skin care—or do you?

The truth is, safeguarding your skin doesn't have to take much time at all. And, despite the hype that surrounds big-name products and mind-boggling multi-step beauty routines, it really doesn't have to be complicated or expensive.

It just has to cleanse, moisturize and protect your skin from photoaging—the wrinkling, crinkling, blotch effects of too much time in the sun.

If you use daily sun protection, doctors say you'll find that after a while your skin will repair some of the damage itself, leaving you looking younger and fresher and feeling good about it.

Some products, such as Neutrogena Moisturizer, that combine moisturizers with sunscreens and tints will save you time.

So let's look at a realistic routine that will leave your skin looking its youthful best, but won't detonate your day planner.

### Go Gently into That Good Day

No matter if your skin is normal, oily, dry or sun-damaged, the watchword for cleansing is "gentle," dermatologists say. Gentle cleansers and gentle handling. Why? Every time you rub, pull, scrub or otherwise yank your skin around, you may loosen the tiny fibers beneath the surface that promote firmness and a youthful look.

"Everything you do to your face adds a little age damage," says Albert M. Kligman, M.D., a professor of dermatology at the University of Pennsylvania School of Medicine in Philadelphia.

**Choose gentle products.** Forget harsh cleansers and astringents, advises Seth L. Matarasso, M.D., assistant professor of dermatology at the University of California, San Francisco, School of Medicine. Inexpensive mild soaps like Purpose, Basis, Neutrogena and Dove are all you need.

If your skin's particularly dry, even a thorough morning rinse with a soap substitute such as Cetaphil or no soap at all is fine, Dr. Matarasso says. Just experiment to see what feels best to you.

**Nuts to the nut scrubs.** Washing with those ground-up nut scrubs and abrasive sponges is like taking kitchen cleansers to your skin, says Carole Walderman, a cosmetologist and esthetician and president of Von Lee International School of Aesthetics and Makeup in Baltimore. The tiny scratches they leave behind inflame your skin and gather bacteria, so they can promote breakouts when you thought you'd left acne behind for good.

**Keep water temperature moderate.** Use warm, not hot, water to rinse off your cleanser, says Leila Cohoon, a cosmetologist and esthetician and owner of Leila's Skin Care in Independence, Missouri. And don't bother with a cold-water splash to "close your pores" afterward. Pores do not open and close as commonly thought.

**Pat yourself dry.** Pat your face not-quite dry with a soft towel as gently as a toddler's touch, says Dr. Matarasso. "Leave just a damp film on your skin, like a dew."

**Try mild toners.** For an optional extra-clean feeling, use a soothing flower-water, such as Rosewater, and toner after you cleanse and rinse, says Walderman. "In our thirties our pores can start to look larger, because gravity is pulling down around the hair follicles, making them look deeper," she says. "Toners will temporarily close pores, maybe for around 45 minutes, leaving a nice background for applying makeup." Apply toner with a cotton pad that has first been saturated with water and then squeezed out, using gentle upward strokes.

# The Beauty of Moisturizers

Moisturizers do not add moisture to the skin, no matter what the ad writers say. They do help retain the water you've left on your face and body after washing, though, which plumps up fine wrinkles and smooths the surface, says Dr. Matarasso. If you towel 'til you're bone-dry, any moisturizer—no matter how expensive—will just sit on top and feel greasy. But if you leave a damp film after you rinse, the moisturizer will help water get into the pores and sink deeper into your skin. If your skin is oily, you may not need a moisturizer; it may aggravate acne.

Here's what else you need to know about moisturizing.

**Ask about AHAs.** Alpha hydroxy acids (AHAs) are derived from food sources such as red wine, sour milk and fruit. Some studies show that these acids can increase cell turnover in sun-damaged skin, smoothing and firming its

# Fast Home Facials

If you have a package of dry red beans, a food processor and a few simple ingredients, you can easily treat yourself to a luxurious home facial now and then. Marina Valmy, a cosmetician at the Christine Valmy Skin Care School in New York City, offers these recipes to use twice a week to refresh your skin.

For normal to dry skin:

*Start with a cleansing mask.* Put 2 cups of dry red beans in your food processor and grind to a powder. Then mix about ½ cup with a little water to form a paste and spread all over your face (except for your eye area) as a mask. Leave the mask on for about five minutes, then rinse thoroughly with water. Save the rest of the bean powder in a tightly closed jar for another time.

*Follow with a hydration mask.* Mix 1 teaspoon honey, 1 egg yolk, ½ teaspoon olive oil and ½ teaspoon half-and-half or heavy cream. Apply to your face, including the eye area, and leave on for 15 to 20 minutes while you relax. Then rinse with water.

For oily skin:

*Cleanse with the red-bean mask (above), then follow with a toning mask.* Mix 1 teaspoon plain low-fat yogurt, ½ egg white, ¼ teaspoon avocado oil and 1 teaspoon mashed fresh parsley. Leave on for 15 to 20 minutes and rinse with water.

texture. Though they're hot topics in beauty magazines, researchers differ on whether the AHAs in many new moisturizers actually reduce fine wrinkling.

The problem may be the low concentrations found in commercial products, says Dr. Matarasso. Most cosmetic moisturizers use very small amounts of AHAs, he says. If you'd like to see what AHAs can do for you, your best bet is to discuss high-concentration AHA moisturizers with your dermatologist.

**Choose non-clogging lotions.** If you just want a good everyday moisturizer, but have a tendency to break out now and then, choose a moisturizer labeled "noncomedogenic," says Thomas Griffin, M.D., a dermatologist with Graduate Hospital and clinical assistant professor of dermatology at the University of Pennsylvania School of Medicine, both in Philadelphia. These products won't clog pores.

**Check the pH.** If your skin is sensitive, use a product that is the same acid balance (pH) as normal skin, which is in the range of pH 4.5 to 5.5, says Cohoon. "Many labels say 'pH-balanced,' but that means nothing," she says. "It might mean pH-balanced acid, or pH-balanced alkaline, which is not good for your skin. You want it to be pH-balanced acid for skin care."

How to be sure? "Buy pH papers (such as pHydrion) from your skin-care salon and dip them in the product," Cohoon says. "The paper will change color, and you compare it to an enclosed color chart, which will show you what pH the moisturizer is."

**Go lightly on the eye area.** Use just a lightweight eye cream on the eye area during the day, says Walderman. Some women use heavy eye creams, which tend to make makeup appear thick and pasty.

# Saving Your Face and Body

Any way you wear it, sunscreen is the single most important age-erasing step in skin care. Even if you've been slapdash in the past, using a sunscreen right now will pay youthful dividends for decades to come.

**Make it simple.** Unless you enjoy applying layer after layer of potions and lotions, the easiest way to add sunscreen to your routine is to use a lotion or cream-based sunscreen as your moisturizer, says Dr. Matarasso.

**Be sure it's real protection.** Choose a sunscreen or moisturizer-sunscreen combination with a sun protection factor (SPF) of at least 15, says Dr. Kligman. And sunscreens that block both the UVA and UVB forms of light (often called full-spectrum suncreens) will offer you the best protection against both surface burning and the deeper tissue damage that causes wrinkles and sags, he says. Many cosmetic moisturizers trumpet their sun protection capabilities, but most contain very low SPF sunscreens.

# As You Sleep

At night you cleanse again. Add an overnight moisturizer if your skin tends toward dryness, or perhaps tretinoin (Retin-A) if you're actively battling sun damage. Then, sweet sleep, which in its own way brings you younger-looking skin by removing stress and strain from your complexion.

Try adding these tips to your nightly cleansing routine.

**Remove makeup.** It's true what they say: You should never sleep with it on. For a very thorough job, use a cleanser with petrolatum for removing makeup, says Marina Valmy, a cosmetician at the Christine Valmy Skin Care School in New York City. But only at night; petrolatum is too heavy for daytime cleansing or moisturizing, she says. Your favorite gentle soap is an option, too; just clean and rinse thoroughly.

**Try a deep-pore cleanser.** Three times a week, use a deep-pore cleanser and a soft facial brush for deep-cleaning your skin, says Walderman.

**Sleep with a wrinkle-fighter.** If sun damage has etched your skin with fine lines, ask your doctor about a prescription for Retin-A cream, says Jonathan Weiss, M.D., assistant clinical professor of dermatology at Emory University School of Medicine in Atlanta. "Retin-A is a wonderful product for sun damage," he says. "It can improve the yellowed appearance of the skin and make it more pink. But its greatest improvement is on wrinkles and age spots." Dr. Weiss points out that the Food and Drug Administration has not yet approved Retin-A for the treatment of sun-damaged and wrinkled skin, though the cream does seem effective.

With your dermatologist's help, you can customize the concentration of Retin-A that best suits your skin. "After you cleanse with a mild soap, let your skin dry completely for 10 to 20 minutes," says Dr. Matarasso. "Then apply a pea-sized amount of Retin-A everywhere—around your eyes (leaving about a half-inch bare under your eyes), mouth, chest, forearms and back of hands. If you use Retin-A, you won't need a moisturizer at night unless the Retin-A causes a little redness and flaking. If that happens, use a moisturizer that night and alternate with Retin-A." You can also use petroleum jelly around your eye area. (For more on Retin-A, see Wrinkles, page 384.)

**Moisturize if you like.** If you like the feeling of moisturizer at night and your skin has gotten a little drier over time, apply a rich night cream, suggests Walderman. And this is the time to use heavier eye creams on the skin all around your eyes. Too heavy for daytime use or under makeup, these products are good for holding in natural moisture while you sleep, she says.

**Don't forget lips.** Put petroleum jelly on your lips at night, says Valmy. Because lip skin is very thin, the blood circulation is very near the surface and can encourage lips to dry out. The jelly won't allow the moisture to evaporate, and it prevents you from waking up with chapped lips.

# SLEEP

## *The Pause That Refreshes*

What would you do if you were told that you could look and feel younger as well as boost your energy level without spending a single cent or even having to leave home?

For most of us, the reply would be simple: What do I have to do?

The answer? Get some sleep.

It's no exaggeration that sleep's benefits can add volumes to the quality of your life. But sleep is often the first thing to go when we get overworked or overwrought and stay up just another hour or two or three to finish a project, do the ironing, read a report, scrub the bathroom floor . . .

"You can't cheat sleep without somehow cheating yourself," says Mark Mahowald, M.D., director of the Minnesota Regional Sleep Disorders Center at the Hennepin County Medical Center in Minneapolis.

## The Secret Youth Enhancer

We all know a sleep-deprived person when we see one: droopy eyes with dark circles; a dazed, gloomy, spaced-out expression; poor posture; slow-walking; slow-talking. Not exactly the picture of youth. But what if we start exercising good sleep habits on a regular basis? Can we actually add vitality and reverse some of these signs of aging?

Unless there are other medical problems, the answer is yes. "Sleep is a part of a constellation of behaviors that maximizes the quality of our lives," Michael Vitiello, Ph.D., associate director of the Sleep and Aging Research Program at the University of Washington in Seattle. "When you sleep better, you feel better. You're more likely to perform at optimal levels and to maintain healthy lifestyle behaviors like exercise and healthy eating. Combine sleep with these

# To Nap or Not to Nap?

"Many individuals who don't get all the sleep they need at night benefit from a short siesta in the afternoon," says Timothy Monk, Ph.D., director of the Human Chronobiology Research Program at the University of Pittsburgh School of Medicine. "There is a natural dip in alertness in the mid-afternoon, part of our circadian rhythms. Many of those who are sleep-deprived or who have very strong napping instincts are often revitalized by a 30-minute nap in this period."

But not everyone has the time for a nap, and napping is not for everyone. "If you have insomnia, you may have a strong desire to nap in the afternoon, but that can worsen your sleeplessness at night," says Karl Doghramji, M.D., director of the Sleep Disorders Center at Thomas Jefferson University Hospital in Philadelphia. "In addition, many people are poor nappers. They actually feel worse after a nap due to what we call sleep inertia—the groggy feeling that can linger for hours."

What should you do? Dr. Monk and Dr. Doghramji say to experiment. If napping makes you feel good the rest of the day, if it doesn't interfere with your evening sleep and if your schedule permits, by all means take a siesta when you feel that afternoon slump. About 20 to 45 minutes just after lunch is usually best.

other behaviors and all those things we associate with youth—appearance, energy and attitude—will ultimately improve."

## Body and Mind Together

Scientists know that the body releases its greatest concentration of growth hormone—the substance that helps our bodies repair damaged tissue—during sleep. Sleep-deprived lab animals suffer a complete breakdown in their vital functions. And recent studies have shown that sleep-deprived individuals seem to experience a decrease in the activity of natural killer cells and other immune system good guys that keep the body infection-free.

Most sleep specialists believe the mind benefits equally from a good night's sleep.

"Sleep deprivation makes us moody and irritable," says Dr. Mahowald. It also limits our ability to concentrate, make judgments and perform mental tasks. As a result, it can affect our job performance or, even worse, lead to industrial or traffic fatalities."

Sleep, it turns out, is really a highly active state made up of a series of regular cycles. There are stages to each cycle: Stages one to three occur during light sleep and stage four (also called delta sleep) represents our deepest sleep. A fifth stage of sleep (called rapid eye movement or REM) occurs when we dream. Adequate delta and REM sleep, experts believe, are essential. Without either, we feel lousy and our abilities to learn, memorize and reason are sharply impaired.

## Your Changing Sleep Patterns

Do you expect to run as fast or play tennis as well in your forties, fifties or sixties as you did in your teens, twenties and thirties? Of course not. But how about sleep? You probably think it will take no effort at all or even be easier. But for most of us, a good night's sleep could become harder to get.

Beginning in middle age and continuing into our golden years, it will take many of us longer to fall asleep. We'll experience frequent awakenings and spend less time in the valuable delta and REM stages. We'll spend less time sleeping, period.

"As we age, our internal clocks are much more easily disturbed," says Timothy Monk, Ph.D., director of the Human Chronobiology Research Program at the University of Pittsburgh School of Medicine. "The main effect can be that we don't sleep as well and we enter a state of malaise and depression—like a chronic case of jet lag."

## Getting What You Need

How much sleep do you need? It depends on the individual. Some of us can function perfectly on only four hours of sleep per night; others require as many as ten to feel refreshed. For most women, seven to eight hours does the job, but only you can answer the question for yourself. "There is no magic number. You should get as much sleep as you need to feel rested and able to function at your maximum the next day," says Dr. Mahowald.

How can you maximize the quality and quantity of your sleep? Here's help.

**Stay on a regular schedule.** Going to bed and waking up at the same time every day (including weekends) helps maintain a consistent circadian rhythm—your body's natural clock, says Dr. Monk. This will condition your internal clock so that you will fall asleep easier, sleep more soundly and wake feeling refreshed.

**Eat three regular meals at regular times.** "Our daily rhythms can become easily disrupted by external factors," says Dr. Monk. "You need certain external cues to keep your body clock running right. Keeping consistent meal times will help."

**Take time to unwind.** You can't expect to leap from the rat race directly into the sack. Give yourself two hours before bedtime to relax and turn off the world by reading, watching television, listening to music or any other activity you find restful. Take care of business, bills and other stress makers during the day or early evening.

**Establish a routine.** Many people can't sleep well because their lifestyles are too chaotic before they go to bed. If you can develop a regular pattern of activities and behaviors every night just before bedtime, sleeping can be a kinder experience. For example, suppose each evening you took the dog for a walk, read the newspaper, showered, brushed your teeth and went to bed? You'd be relaxed and you would get yourself into a good presleep rhythm.

**Maintain a proper environment.** Improving your surroundings can make sleep a better experience. Most people find light and noise disruptive, so turn off your radio and draw the shades. Also, check the thermostat; most people sleep better with a temperature on the cooler side of normal.

**Go only when you're tired.** Don't stay in bed trying to make sleep happen, says Dr. Vitiello. You'll only condition yourself not to fall asleep while you're there. Instead, get up and read a book or do something constructive until you feel tired.

**Don't stockpile sleep.** If you have an early morning or an active day ahead of you, going to bed earlier probably won't help you, says Dr. Vitiello. Most people just spend that extra time in bed awake, only to have trouble falling asleep later. "While it's easy to accumulate a sleep debt, it's not possible to save up on your sleep," he says.

**Avoid late meals and snacks.** A small snack before bed is okay, but don't eat a full meal, spicy foods or a Dagwood sandwich less than three hours before bedtime, says Karl Doghramji, M.D., director of the Sleep Disorders Center at Thomas Jefferson University Hospital in Philadelphia. Your rumbling stomach may keep you up for hours or may make your sleep less refreshing.

**Cut the caffeine.** Save your coffee, tea, colas, chocolates and other foods containing caffeine for the morning or early afternoons, says Dr. Doghramji. Caffeine is a powerful sleep inhibitor that stays in the bloodstream for up to six hours.

**Limit your liquids after 8:00 P.M.** For obvious reasons: Frequent trips to the bathroom can keep you up all night.

**Forget the nightcap.** We all know alcohol will make you drowsy at the drop of a hat. But it also makes you toss and turn in your sleep and changes the pattern of REM and non-REM sleep. You are also more likely to experience frequent brief awakenings throughout the night. Even if you spend many hours asleep, they probably won't be good hours, and you'll feel rotten in the morning.

**Avoid medications.** Sleeping pills and other sedatives, although often helpful, can also upset your sleep patterns, says Dr. Doghramji. In addition, it's easy to get hooked, especially if you use them improperly. Your best bet is to try to fall asleep without any chemical assistance. If you must take sleeping pills, do so only under a doctor's watchful eye.

**For sleep and sex only.** The bed was designed for two purposes only, says Dr. Vitiello. "If you introduce activities like paying bills, eating pizza and watching television, the body gets confused and may not want to go to sleep in bed."

**Make love ... or don't.** Some women find that sex before sleep is relaxing; others feel that it keeps them up for hours afterward, says Dr. Mahowald. If making love knocks you out, go for it. If not, save your passion for another time of the day.

**Shift your shift.** "We were built to work during the day and sleep at night," says Dr. Monk. "The aging shift worker should seriously consider switching to a position or work schedule that doesn't require odd hours rather than fight the body's natural inclinations."

**Be wise with exercise.** It's a myth that heavy exercise will wear you out and make you sleepy, says Dr. Mahowald. But people who are physically fit and active will be better sleepers, so make exercise a part of your daily regimen. A mild walk before bedtime is okay if it relaxes you, but save your heavy workouts for earlier in the day; they'll keep you awake for quite a while.

**Set aside worry time.** "You'll never sleep well if you lie in bed obsessing over your worries," says Dr. Vitiello. "Set aside 30 minutes or so away from the bedroom before bedtime as worry time and get your troubles out of your system. Don't use the bed as a setting for anxiety."

# STRETCHING

## Get Loose, Feel Good

Every once in a while, you find the time to stretch. When you do, you love the way it makes you feel—loose, limber, relaxed. But those days are few and far between.

Usually you spend your time in overdrive, running from one activity to the next, with barely the time to sit and catch your breath, let alone stretch. You manage to squeeze in some walking or an aerobics class about three times a week, but that's about all you can usually manage. And stretching isn't really all that important anyway, right?

Wrong.

A general warm-up followed by regular stretching raises the temperature within our muscles and enables us to move smoothly and with a full range of motion—like we did when we were younger. In addition to relieving stress and tension, it improves flexibility, enhances performance and helps prevent injuries.

## Oh, Those Aging Muscles

As we get older, our muscles and joints tend to become tighter, says John Skowron, physical therapist at Raleigh Community Sports Medicine and Physical Therapy in North Carolina. That's because as we age, connective muscle tissues shorten. That makes it harder to do the activities we're used to, whether on the playing field or around the house, because our muscles just aren't ready.

Here's what happens: Anytime you do an activity, whether it's reaching up to paint a wall, carrying something downstairs or going for a run, your muscles move. Certain muscles contract, or shorten, with movement, while the opposing muscles relax, or lengthen. When the muscles and surrounding elastic tissue that need to lengthen are too tight, they can't move the way we want them to and we lose what health experts call our full range of motion; that is, our movement becomes restricted.

# Advanced-Placement Stretching

If you're a beginner, the type of stretching described in this chapter—static stretching—is probably the best way to get started. But if you're already into static stretching and are looking for other possibly more effective methods, here are some suggestions.

*Passive stretching.* Passive stretching is similar to static stretching, only a gentle force is applied by a partner to increase flexibility. For example, to stretch the hamstrings in your right leg, lie on your back with your left leg bent and the sole of your left foot flat on the floor. Raise your right leg, slightly bent, upward until you feel a stretch. Then have a partner apply a gentle force to push the stretch a little farther.

*PNF Stretching.* Proprioceptive Neuromuscular Facilitation, or PNF, stretching is a technique that stimulates certain reflex centers and nerves. It generally requires a partner, who provides resistance so that the muscle being stretched can be contracted against resistance before the stretch is continued. For example, begin the right hamstring stretch. While in the same position described above, have a partner raise your right leg until you feel a stretch. Then, as a partner provides resistance against your push (she can do this by placing a shoulder against the back of your thigh), contract, or tighten, your hamstring without moving it and hold the contraction for 3 to 6 seconds. Then relax, have your partner move you into the stretch farther and hold it for another 20 to 30 seconds.

*AI Stretching.* AI stretching is a completely different approach advocated and practiced by Aaron Mattes, Ph.D., a kinesiologist in southern Florida and author of *Flexibility: Active and Assisted Stretching.* Through his work with both professional athletes and the elderly, Dr. Mattes says he has observed some remarkable results from what he calls AI stretching, or active isolated stretching. In contrast to static stretching, AI stretching involves performing each stretch for 1½ to 2 seconds, relaxing, then stretching again. It also involves contracting the muscle opposite the one you are stretching and using a rope or towel to move the limb to the point where the stretch is felt.

For example, to stretch your right hamstring, lie on your back with your left leg bent and foot flat on the floor. Then, with a rope or towel wrapped around your right foot and your right leg extended, lift your right leg up, contracting your right quadriceps while you gently use the rope to assist the leg into the stretch. Hold the stretch for 1½ to 2 seconds, return your leg to the starting position, relax and repeat.

This can cause all kinds of trouble. Sometimes it prohibits us from participating in activities at all. Other times we can participate, but our performance is compromised. Then there are the times when it leads to injury. When our body realizes it can't use a certain muscle group fully, it often tries to compensate by asking another muscle group to work harder than usual, a demand that can sometimes cause that part of the body to break down. And sometimes the muscles themselves are damaged—their tissues can tear, which is what happens when someone "pulls" a muscle.

Part of the reason we get tighter after age 30 has to do with our lifestyles, says Michael Kaplan, M.D., Ph.D., director of the Rehabilitation Team, a sports medicine and physical therapy clinic in Catonsville, Maryland. "Before they're 30, people tend not to have as many responsibilities. They often don't have the job that they have to do plus the house that they have to support, the kids they have to do things for," he says. Eventually. any of these responsibilities takes up most of their time; folks become less active and, as a result, less mobile and less flexible.

"There's no reason why people in their thirties and forties and even older can't have just as much flexibility as when they were younger—or even more flexibility," says Dr. Kaplan. "A 60-year-old can have more flexibility than a 20-year-old," if she works at it and stretches, he says.

## Improving Flexibility

Here's how it works. When you stretch a muscle, say the hamstring muscle at the back of your leg, you place tension on it and the muscle begins to lengthen. Initially, a stretch reflex inside the muscle tries to protect it from lengthening and asks the muscle to contract. But if the stretch is held long enough, then a structure located where tendons adjoin to muscles, called the Golgi tendon organ, sends a message that triggers the muscle to relax farther and lengthening continues.

That's what happens when you do the type of slow and steady stretching—called static stretching—that has generally been accepted as the right way to stretch these days. The idea is to move into the stretch slowly and gradually, hold it for 20 to 30 seconds, relax and repeat. Research conducted at the Institute for Sports Medicine at Lenox Hill Hospital in New York City showed that the majority of muscle relaxation occurs within 20 seconds of stretching.

## How It Can Help

In addition to improving performance and helping to prevent injuries, stretching can help improve strength, says Mark Taranta, a physical therapist and director of the Physical Therapy Practice in Philadelphia. "People have to realize that strength will increase as flexibility increases," he says. "If you're flexible, you're able to generate more force," because the muscle is in a lengthened position.

And if you're feeling stressed out, stretching can provide some relief. "Stretching reduces tension," says William L. Cornelius, Ph.D., associate professor of physical education in the Department of Kinesiology, Health Promotion and Recreation at the University of North Texas in Denton. One way researchers have assessed this is by measuring the electrical activity elicited by muscles with a technique called electromyography, or EMG. Studies have shown that stretching helps reduce the amount of electrical activity passing through muscles, a sign that tension has been reduced, says Dr. Cornelius.

## How to Do It Right

You too can reap the benefits of stretching if you pay attention to your stretching technique. Here's what to keep in mind.

**Warm up first.** "You should warm up the muscle before you stretch it," says Lucille Smith, Ph.D., assistant professor at the Human Performance Laboratory at East Carolina University in Greenville, North Carolina. The general guideline is to warm up until you break a sweat. For activities involving the entire body, warm up with a brisk walk or light jog. If you're going to be exercising only one area of your body, concentrate on that area. Warming up raises the temperature of the muscle and makes it less susceptible to injury. "When the muscle is heated up, it's more pliable," says Taranta.

**Go slow and steady.** When you stretch, make it a slow and steady one, says Dr. Cornelius. Don't bounce. Move into each stretch gradually until you feel tension in the muscle and connective tissue, he says. Hold that position for 20 to 30 seconds, relax and do it again.

**Be sure to breathe.** "You really have to concentrate on your breathing," says Taranta. If you hold your breath, that can contribute to tensing of your muscles, whereas breathing helps relax them, he says.

**Know every little bit helps.** You don't have to have 20 to 30 minutes to devote to stretching, says Dr. Kaplan. If you stretch your neck, shoulders, back, hips and legs for 2 minutes each at 30-second intervals, that makes for a 10-minute stretching workout.

**Get into a routine.** It's important to be consistent about stretching, says Taranta. If you don't stretch regularly, it won't have much effect, he says. Aim to stretch three times a week to start. Once you're in the habit, aim for every day.

**Pay attention to the temperature.** When it's cold out, you may need to spend a little extra time stretching to get your muscles warm; when it's hot, a little less, says Taranta.

**Do more in the morning.** If you exercise in the morning, or have to do physical labor first thing, take the time to warm up and stretch a little longer than usual. "Core temperature and body temperature probably would be lower, and you'd probably be stiffer first thing in the morning versus later in the day, when you've already been moving around," says Dr. Smith.

**Get in a group.** Join or form a group of people interested in stretching together, says Dr. Kaplan. Yoga classes are one option. Or, if you are part of a soft-ball or volleyball team, make stretching together part of your practices and games, he says. "By yourself, you may lose incentive."

# Go for the Basics

There are lots of stretching options. Here are a few basic stretches for each body area to get you started.

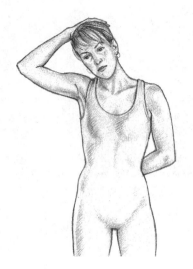

*If your neck is feeling sore or tight, stretching can do wonders. While standing or sitting, hold your left arm behind your back. Then tilt your head as if you were trying to touch your right ear to your right shoulder. Use your right hand to pull gently on your head if you need more of a stretch. Hold the stretch for 10 to 20 seconds, relax and repeat. Try this three or four times for the left side of your neck, then reverse and do the same for the right side.*

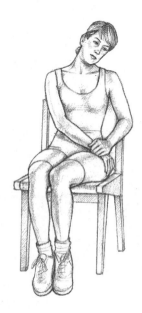

*Here's another stretch to keep your neck from tightening up. Sit on a chair and cross your right arm across your body so that your right wrist rests on your left hip. Grasp your right wrist with your left hand. Tilt your head as if you were trying to touch your left ear to your left shoulder. At the same time, pull gently on your right arm with your left hand. You'll feel the stretch on the right side of your neck. Reverse the directions to do the same exercise for the left side of your neck.*

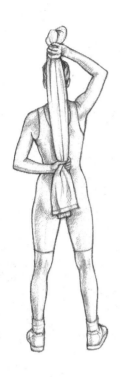

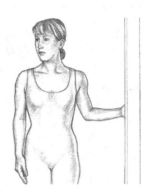

*Standing in a doorway, let your right arm hang down by your side. Bend your left arm to 90 degrees and place the palm of your left hand against the door frame. Slowly turn your body to the right until you feel a gentle stretch in your left shoulder. Hold it for 20 to 30 seconds, relax and repeat. Reverse the instructions to stretch your right shoulder.*

*The shoulders are another area where stress and tension can take their toll. While standing with feet hip-width apart, grasp a towel in your right hand. Flip the towel up and over your head, as shown. Reach behind your back with your left hand and grasp the end of the towel. Stretch your left shoulder by pulling upward on the towel with your right hand. Hold the stretch for 20 to 30 seconds, relax and repeat several times. Reverse the instructions to stretch your right shoulder.*

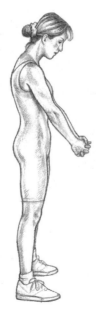

*Standing with your feet hip-width apart, clasp your hands together in front of your body, keeping your arms straight. Raise your arms a couple of inches away from your body. Bend your head forward and gently pull your shoulder blades apart. Hold the stretch for 20 to 30 seconds, relax and repeat several times.*

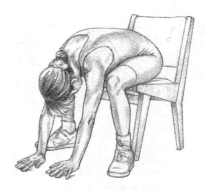

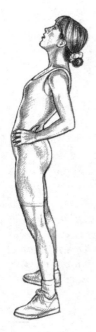

*Sit on a chair with your knees apart. Bend forward and try to touch your hands to the floor. You should feel a gentle stretch in your lower back. Hold the stretch for 20 to 30 seconds, relax and repeat.*

*And then there's that achy-breaky back. To get some relief, try this stretch. Stand up straight with your feet hip-width apart. Place both hands on your hips and arch gently backward. Hold the stretch for 20 to 30 seconds, relax and repeat.*

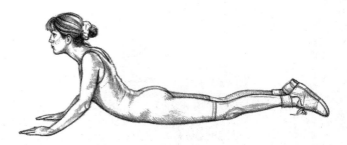

*Lie on your stomach on the floor and place the palms of your hands on the floor by your chest. Press your upper body upward, keeping your hips on the floor. Remember to keep your lower back and buttocks relaxed. Hold the stretch for 20 to 30 seconds, relax and repeat several times.*

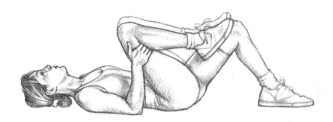

*Lying on your back, bend both knees while keeping your feet flat on the floor. Then pull your right knee toward your chest and, grasping the back of your thigh, pull your knee toward your chest until you feel a gentle stretch in your lower back. Repeat with the opposite knee. You can also perform this stretch by pulling both knees toward your chest simultaneously.*

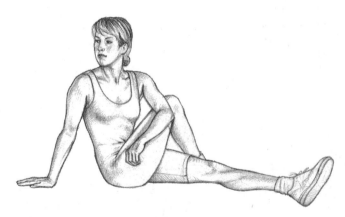

*Sit on the floor with both legs extended straight in front of you. Bend your right leg and cross it over your left leg so that the sole of your right foot is flat on the floor. Slowly twist your upper body to the right and place your left elbow over the outside of your right knee. Gently push on the bent knee with your elbow until you feel a stretch in your right buttock. Hold the stretch for 20 to 30 seconds, relax and repeat several times. Do the same for the opposite side.*

To stretch your quadriceps, or thigh muscles, stand on your right leg, bend your left leg up behind you and grasp your left foot in your left hand. Pull your left heel toward your buttocks until you feel a stretch in the front of your thigh. Hold for 20 to 30 seconds, relax and repeat several times. Do the same for your right leg.

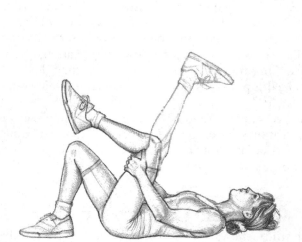

Here's a stretch for your hamstrings, the muscles at the back of your thigh. Lie on your back and bend both knees so that the soles of your feet are flat on the floor. Grasp the back of your left thigh with both hands. Holding your left thigh, slowly straighten your left leg until a gradual stretch is felt in your hamstrings. Hold the stretch for 20 to 30 seconds, relax and repeat several times. Repeat the stretch for your right leg.

# VEGETARIANISM

## Why Beans Beat Beef

Let's cut right to the meat of the matter here: If you're a typical American woman, you're eating too much fat. And you're getting most of it from foods like meat loaf, burgers and pepperoni pizza.

The result can be an age-erasing disaster. Diets heavy with added fat can lead to elevated cholesterol levels, high blood pressure and digestive tract problems. And then there are other problems like flabby thighs and growing hips that you didn't have to worry about just a few short years ago.

If you're searching for a way to regain a little vigor, lose weight and help ward off serious health problems down the road, you might want to take a look at a meatless lifestyle.

"Very simply, vegetarians tend to be healthier people," says Reed Mangels, R.D., Ph.D., a nutrition adviser to the Vegetarian Resource Group in Baltimore. "You get much of your fat through animal products, and the fewer animal products you eat, the better you're probably going to feel."

## Leaner, Lighter, Livelier

Study after study shows that vegetarians are better off than their meat-eating sisters. Researchers in Germany, for instance, found that a group of 1,904 vegetarians had about half the overall mortality rate of meat eaters over an 11-year period.

The German study showed that vegetarian women suffered about 25 percent fewer cases of digestive tract cancer than would have been expected in people eating normal diets. They also had less than half the expected amount of heart disease.

Other studies conducted on Buddhists, Seventh-Day Adventists, people in the developing world and Westerners show that vegetarians generally have lower blood pressure than meat eaters. Vegetarians also may have less risk of developing diabetes.

Vegetarians also report less trouble with constipation and gallstones. And people who switch to vegetarian diets say they just plain feel better—with more energy and vigor—after dropping meat from their diets.

What's behind all these magic results? For one thing, vegetarians tend to weigh less—partly because they eat less fat, Dr. Mangels says, and partly because they tend to lead more active lifestyles.

Vegetarians also smoke less. "Many of them have made a serious long-term commitment to their health," says Dr. Mangels. "It's reflected in their lifestyles, not just in the food they eat."

Most vegetarians eat diets that are much lower in fat than the typical American diet. On average, Americans eat 36 percent of their calories in the form of fat.

Less fat, less weight, more exercise and fewer cigarettes can have a ripple effect on your health, according to Dr. Mangels. "It all goes hand in hand," she says. "You eat better, you feel better, your heart may be stronger, so you feel like doing more. The end result is better overall health."

There's even some evidence that vegetarian diets can help fight arthritis pain. Symptoms of the most common form of arthritis, osteoarthritis, may be relieved because people who weigh less don't put so much stress on joints like their knees, Dr. Mangels says.

And people with rheumatoid arthritis may get relief from a vegetarian diet tailored to their needs, researchers in Norway report. They put 27 people with rheumatoid arthritis on a fast, then introduced vegetarian foods slowly to their diets, rejecting the foods that resulted in pain flare-ups. After a year, those in the study said they felt less tenderness in their joints, less morning stiffness and greater strength in their grips.

## Steering Away from Red Meat

Sounds good, huh? But give up meat? Forever?

Maybe not entirely. You don't have to cut out meat completely to reap most of the health benefits of vegetarianism. "If you can keep your meat intake to a small portion, like a side dish, you're probably all right," says Suzanne Havala, R.D., a nutrition adviser for the Vegetarian Resource Group and a dietitian who co-wrote the American Dietetic Association's position paper on vegetarianism.

Besides, Havala says, by the time you discover what variety vegetarian meals can offer, you may start missing meat less and less. "From my experience, people find vegetarian meals so delightful that they would just as soon forget about the meat altogether."

Here are some tips to get you started.

# A World without Meat

When you were a kid, you learned all about the four basic food groups: meat, dairy, vegetables and bread.

As you grew up, you switched to new groups: steaks, shakes, chips and cheesecake.

It may be time to regroup.

"You don't need to eat meat to be healthy," says Suzanne Havala, R.D., a nutrition adviser for the Vegetarian Resource Group in Baltimore and a dietitian who co-wrote the American Dietetic Association's position paper on vegetarianism.

Here's a quick vegetarian primer, courtesy of Havala. And those food groups are:

*Breads, cereals and pasta.* Eight or more servings a day. Examples of serving sizes include one slice of whole-grain bread, half of a bun or bagel, one-half cup cooked cereal, rice or pasta and one ounce of dry cereal.

*Vegetables.* Four or more servings a day. Serving sizes are one-half cup cooked vegetables or one cup raw. Be sure to include one raw serving that's rich in beta-carotene, such as carrots.

*Legumes and meat substitutes.* Two to three servings a day. Examples of serving sizes include one-half cup cooked beans, four ounces of tofu and two tablespoons of nuts or seeds.

*Fruit.* Three or more servings a day. Serving sizes are one piece of fresh fruit, three-quarters cup of juice and one-half cup cooked or canned fruit.

*Dairy or alternatives.* Optional, two to three servings a day. Examples of serving sizes are one cup low-fat or skim milk, one cup low-fat or nonfat yogurt, 1½ ounces low-fat cheese and one cup calcium-fortified soy milk.

*Eggs.* Optional, three to four yolks a week. This includes eggs in baked foods. Note: Strict vegetarians, or vegans, do not eat eggs. Egg substitutes work fine in most recipes.

**Lower the steaks.** You don't have to eliminate red meat all at once, Havala says. "It's easier that way for some people. But lots of people like to taper off until they're not eating any meat after a few weeks or months," she says.

Try starting with one meatless day a week. How hard is that? As hard,

Havala says, as eating cereal and a piece of fruit for breakfast, a peanut butter and jelly sandwich with a piece of fruit for lunch and pasta tossed with steamed veggies and a salad for supper.

Work your way up to two, then three or more meatless days per week. At that point, you can easily make the jump to full vegetarianism, if you want.

**Fake it.** Health food stores and some supermarkets sell products called meat analogs. You've probably heard of them—tofu burgers and meatless hot dogs are the most common. "Some people need to see something that looks like a meat dish at first," Dr. Mangels says. "Try them for a while. They might help you make the transition."

**Don't fixate.** People used to think that vegetarians had to plan their meals right down to the last gram to get adequate nutrition. "If you just make sure to get enough calories to meet your energy needs by eating a variety of fruits, vegetables, grains and legumes, you should be fine," says Havala.

Something to avoid: picking a favorite food and eating it five times a day. "Balance is the key," Dr. Mangels says. "Don't eat only grapefruit for two weeks straight, then switch to baked potatoes for half a month."

**B careful.** Vegans—strict vegetarians who eat no animal products, including eggs or milk—must make sure they get enough $B_{12}$, a vitamin that aids in nervous system function. The vitamin is found mainly in animal products and in supplements. The Recommended Dietary Allowance is two micrograms.

If you drink low-fat milk, eat low-fat cheese or cook yourself an omelet, you're all set. But if you don't, try a whole-grain breakfast cereal or soy milk.

**Junk the junk.** No diet, meatless or otherwise, needs to include lots of junk food. "To reap the most benefits from a vegetarian diet, limit or eliminate sugar and fat-filled foods," Havala says.

**Ferret out the fat.** Meat is loaded with fat. But it's not the only place you'll find those nasty mono- and polyunsaturated and saturated fiends. To lower your fat intake, Dr. Mangels suggests steaming foods, sautéing them in water, broth, juice or wine and going easy on the cheese and mayo. "Low-fat salad dressings aren't a bad idea, either," she says.

**Power up the proteins.** Meat isn't the only food that's packed with protein. You'll get more than enough with a balanced vegetarian diet. "There's plenty of protein in grains, vegetables and legumes. Common meatless dishes such as bean burritos, vegetarian chili and stir-fried vegetables with rice are packed with protein," Havala says.

**C your way to enough iron.** Again, a balanced vegetarian diet provides plenty of iron. But the best source of absorbable iron is still found in meat. You can increase the absorption of the iron found in vegetables by taking vitamin C. Havala suggests eating a vitamin C source at every meal. Foods high in vitamin C include tomatoes, broccoli, melons, peppers and citrus fruits and juices.

**Don't have a cow over calcium.** You'll get plenty of calcium in a balanced vegetarian diet, Dr. Mangels says. If you drink milk and eat low-fat cheeses, you're in good shape. Calcium also can be found in collard greens, seeds and nuts, kale and broccoli.

**Hit the road.** "You don't have to be a stay-home eater just because you're a vegetarian," Dr. Mangels says. "You can eat out all you want. Just find a place with a good salad bar and you're set." Most restaurants will give you a plate of steamed vegetables on request, too.

"Or try a Chinese restaurant. You can eat meal after meal there and never even think about missing meat," adds Dr. Mangels.

# VITAMINS AND MINERALS

## Life's Bare Necessities

$A$h, the usual breakfast. Half a dry bagel and a cup of coffee with artificial sweetener, hold the milk. Lunch? No time for anything but a diet soda. Oh well, you're trying to lose weight anyway.

When you finally arrive home, the kids are in a hurry to go to Little League, and you and your mate are ravenous. So you pull out the chips and he pulls out the frozen pizza. A few hours later your body is begging for sustenance. You respond with a pint of butter pecan ice cream.

This is no way to live—literally. Your body needs reinforcements, the right raw materials to keep it young, healthy and vital.

Those raw materials are vitamins and minerals, the tools your body must have to meet its daily work and activity demands. These microscopic marvels rejuvenate and energize your cells and make every single process in the body possible.

When they're present, everything is smooth sailing. But when they're not, you're in for a crash landing. Taken to extremes, deficiencies in vitamins and minerals can lead to ugly diseases like scurvy, pellagra and rickets—dreaded illnesses that cause loose teeth and bloody gums, weak and brittle bones, unhealthy skin and hair and even death.

Thankfully, American women have a diet decent enough to keep these diseases at bay—partially due to the fact that many of the foods we eat, such as cereals, breads and milk, are fortified with vitamins and minerals. But it is still possible that you're not getting all the vitamins you need, especially if, like many women, you're trying to drop a few pounds or are too busy to do anything but eat on the run.

*(continued on page 630)*

627

# THE 13 ESSENTIAL VITAMINS

Here's a table of vitamin requirements for women ages 25 to 50.

| Vitamin | Daily Intake |
|---|---|
| **Vitamin A** | 800 mcg. RE or 4,000 IU (1,300 mcg. RE or 6,500 IU if pregnant or nursing) |
| **B Vitamins** | |
| Thiamin | 1.1 mg. (1.5 mg. if pregnant; 1.6 mg. if nursing) |
| Riboflavin | 1.3 mg. (1.6 mg. if pregnant; 1.8 mg. if nursing) |
| Niacin | 15 mg. (17 mg. if pregnant; 20 mg. if nursing) |
| Vitamin $B_6$ | 1.6 mg. (2.2 mg. if pregnant; 2.1 mg. if nursing) |
| Folate | 180 mcg. (400 mcg. if pregnant; 280 mcg. if nursing) |
| Vitamin $B_{12}$ | 2 mcg. (2.2 mcg. if pregnant; 2.6 mcg. if nursing) |
| Biotin | 30 to 100 mcg.* |
| Pantothenic acid | 4 to 7 mg.* |
| **Vitamin C** | 60 mg. (70 mg. if pregnant; 95 mg. if nursing) |
| **Vitamin D** | 200 IU or 5 mcg. (10 mcg. if pregnant or nursing) |
| **Vitamin E** | 12 IU or 8 mg. alpha-TE (15 IU or 10 mg. alpha-TE if pregnant; 18 IU or 12 mg. alpha-TE if nursing) |
| **Vitamin K** | 65 mcg. |

NOTE: Daily intake values are Recommended Dietary Allowances (RDAs) unless otherwise noted.
*Value is the Estimated Safe and Adequate Daily Intake. There is no RDA for this vitamin.

| Age-Erasing Benefit | Food Sources |
| --- | --- |
| Needed for normal vision in dim light; maintains normal structure and functions of mucous membranes; aids growth of bones, teeth and skin | Yellow-orange fruits and vegetables; dark green leafy vegetables; fortified milk; eggs |
| Carbohydrate metabolism; maintains healthy nervous system | Pork; whole- and enriched-grain products; beans; nuts |
| Fat, protein and carbohydrate metabolism; healthy skin | Dairy products; whole- and enriched-grain products |
| Fat, protein and carbohydrate metabolism; nervous system function; needed for oxygen use by cells | Meats; poultry; milk; eggs; whole- and enriched-grain products |
| Protein metabolism; needed for normal growth | Meats; poultry; fish; beans; grains; dark green leafy vegetables |
| Red blood cell development; tissue growth and repair | Green leafy vegetables; oranges; beans |
| Needed for new tissue growth, red blood cells, nervous system and skin | Meat; poultry; fish; dairy products |
| Fat, protein and carbohydrate metabolism | Found in small amounts in many foods |
| Fat, protein and carbohydrate metabolism | Whole- and enriched-grain products; vegetables; meats |
| Builds collagen; maintains healthy gums, teeth and blood vessels | Citrus fruits; peppers; cabbage; strawberries; tomatoes |
| Calcium absorption; bone and tooth growth | Sunlight; fortified milk; eggs; fish |
| Protects cells from damage | Vegetable oils; green leafy vegetables; wheat germ; whole-grain products |
| Clotting of blood | Cabbage; green leafy vegetables |

"As we age, our requirements for certain vitamins and minerals actually increase," says Jeffrey Blumberg, Ph.D., associate director of the U.S. Department of Agriculture Human Nutrition Research Center on Aging at Tufts University in Boston. "We tend to eat less food overall on a daily basis. So if your diet is already lacking a little in certain nutrients, as you get older, you stand a greater chance of widening that deficiency, and in some way your body will pay the price for it."

Low vitamin and mineral levels can lead to increased susceptibility to infection, slow healing, decreased mental capacity and chronic fatigue, nutritionists say. The bottom line is obvious: To look, feel and perform at your best, you can't make a habit of skimping on your vitamins and minerals.

## Vitamins Are Vital

Inside our bodies, hundreds of biochemical reactions are taking place 24 hours a day. And just like chemical reactions in a laboratory, these internal chemical reactions need catalysts to facilitate and regulate them. Vitamins are organic chemical compounds that act as catalysts. Each has a specific function—from helping bone growth to maintaining healthy skin to assisting the cells in processing energy. Fall short in just one vitamin, and any number of vital functions that depend on that vitamin can be compromised.

Nutritionists divide the 13 essential vitamins into two groups based on their behavior in the body. Water-soluble vitamins—vitamin C and the eight B vitamins (thiamin, riboflavin, niacin, $B_6$, pantothenic acid, $B_{12}$, biotin and folate)—are short-lived, fast-acting compounds that are stored in the watery parts of body cells. But not for long. The body quickly puts these vitamins to work assisting cells in chemical reactions and energy processing, and usually excretes any excess.

Fat soluble vitamins—A, D, E and K—are found in the fatty parts of cells and regulate a wide variety of metabolic processes. They tend to be put in long-term storage and are then drawn upon as the body needs them.

While many studies have acknowledged vitamin intake as a factor in lowering the risk of chronic disease, several vitamins have been singled out for their ability to slow down or even prevent the onset of age-related diseases, like heart disease and cancer, and potentially slow the aging process itself. These vitamins—C, E and beta-carotene (a substance that the body converts to vitamin A)—are known as antioxidants for their ability to neutralize destructive oxygen-derived particles believed to initiate many disease processes.

## Minerals Are Musts

From the earth we originally came, and from the earth we draw a variety of nutrients to keep ourselves in good working order.

Like vitamins, minerals help keep the body functioning. But unlike vitamins, they are inorganic and not metabolized by the body. Instead, they act more like building blocks, providing structure to bones and teeth, serving as major components in blood, skin and tissue and keeping our bodily fluids in balance.

There are two categories of minerals. The major minerals—calcium, chloride, magnesium, phosphorus, potassium and sodium—are found in large quantities in the body and are abundant in food sources. We require large amounts of these minerals.

The trace minerals—chromium, copper, fluoride, iodine, iron, manganese, molybdenum, selenium and zinc—are found in much smaller amounts in our bodies and in our food, and as such, our daily requirements are lower.

Some minerals are stored in the body, on reserve to replace those we lose in our urine and sweat. If we don't replenish our mineral stores as rapidly as they are being depleted, we run the risk of developing such diseases as iron deficiency anemia and osteoporosis, two serious health problems that afflict millions of women.

# A Woman's Nutritional Needs

Getting the right amount of these essential nutrients takes planning, and to make that task easier, the National Research Council's Food and Nutrition Board has established guidelines for vitamin and mineral consumption. They're called Recommended Dietary Allowances (RDAs).

RDAs are the amount of a nutrient judged to be adequate for the average healthy person. "Because the levels exceed the actual needs of most people, you can actually be below the RDAs for a nutrient but still be well above the deficiency level," says Paul R. Thomas, R.D., Ed.D., staff scientist with the Food and Nutrition Board of the National Academy of Sciences in Washington, D.C. "Falling short of the RDAs usually isn't dangerous, but if your vitamin and mineral intake is routinely some 20 to 30 percent below the RDAs, deficiency problems could develop over time."

That's great for the woman who wants to avoid anemia. But what if you want superior health? "A growing body of evidence indicates a direct link between increased longevity and improved overall health when certain vitamin and mineral intakes exceed the RDAs," says Dr. Blumberg. "This suggests that perhaps the RDAs are inadequate for the changing needs of the aging adult."

But even too much of a good thing can be bad. "Taken in extremely high doses, many vitamins and minerals can be toxic," cautions Diane Grabowski, R.D., nutrition educator at the Pritikin Longevity Center in Santa Monica, California. "They can interfere with the functioning of vital organs like the heart, liver or kidneys. Or they can produce any number of harmless but aggravating side effects such as heartburn, nausea or frequent urination."

(continued on page 634)

# THE 15 ESSENTIAL MINERALS

Here's a handy table of the major and trace mineral requirements for women ages 25 to 50.

| Mineral | Daily Intake |
|---|---|
| Calcium | 800 mg. (1,200 mg. if pregnant or nursing) |
| Chloride | 750 mg.* |
| Chromium | 50 to 200 mcg.† |
| Copper | 1.5 to 3.0 mg.† |
| Fluoride | 1.5 to 4.0 mg.† |
| Iodine | 150 mcg. (175 mcg. if pregnant; 200 mcg. if nursing) |
| Iron | 15 mg. (30 mg. if pregnant; 15 mg. if nursing) |
| Magnesium | 280 mg. (300 mg. if pregnant; 355 mg. if nursing) |
| Manganese | 2.0 to 5.0 mg.† |
| Molybdenum | 75 to 250 mcg.† |
| Phosphorus | 800 mg. (1,200 mg. if pregnant or nursing) |
| Potassium | 2,000 mg.* |
| Selenium | 55 mcg. (65 mcg. if pregnant; 75 mcg. if nursing) |
| Sodium | 500 mg.* |
| Zinc | 12 mg. (15 mg. if pregnant; 19 mg. if nursing) |

NOTE: Daily intake values are Recommended Dietary Allowances (RDAs) unless otherwise noted.

| Age-Erasing Benefit | Food Sources |
| --- | --- |
| Strong bones and teeth; muscle and nerve function; blood clotting | Dairy products; green leafy vegetables; sardines with bones; tofu |
| Aids digestion; works with sodium to maintain fluid balance | Foods with salt |
| Carbohydrate metabolism | Vegetables; whole grains; brewer's yeast |
| Blood cell and connective tissue formation | Grains; legumes; shellfish |
| Strengthens tooth enamel | Fluoridated water; fish; tea |
| Maintaining proper thyroid functioning | Milk; grains; iodized salt |
| Carries oxygen in blood; energy metabolism | Red meat; fish; poultry; whole grains; dark green leafy vegetables; legumes |
| Aids nerve and muscle function; strong bones | Beans; nuts; cocoa; grains; green vegetables |
| Bone and connective tissue formation; fat and carbohydrate metabolism | Spinach; nuts; pumpkin; tea; legumes |
| Nitrogen metabolism | Unprocessed grains and vegetables |
| Energy metabolism; teams up with calcium for strong bones and teeth | Meat; poultry; fish; milk; beans |
| Controls acid balance in the body; works with sodium to maintain fluid balance | Vegetables; fruits; meats; milk |
| Helps vitamin E protect cells and body tissue | Grains; meat; fish; poultry |
| Fluid balance; nervous system function | Salt; processed foods; soy sauce; seasonings |
| Wound healing; growth; appetite | Seafood; meats; nuts; legumes |

*Value is the Estimated Minimum Requirement. There is no RDA for this mineral.
†Value is the Estimated Safe and Adequate Daily Intake. There is no RDA for this mineral.

Research is in the works to determine the exact levels of each vitamin and mineral needed for optimal health. Until such results are found, doctors say that your goal at the very least should be to shoot for 100 percent of the RDAs for every essential vitamin and mineral, especially if you lead an active life.

# Food: Our Best Source

With the range of fresh and healthful foods available these days, most women shouldn't have that much trouble hitting 100% of their RDAs. "A well-balanced diet consisting of a variety of nutrient-rich foods will easily supply all the vitamins and minerals you need, probably even more," says Grabowski.

Here are some tips for getting the maximum vitamin and mineral content from the foods you eat—and for the least amount of calories.

**Go for the basics.** "Concentrate on eating from the five basic food groups—fruits, vegetables, lean meats and legumes, grains and cereals and low-fat or nonfat dairy products," says Grabowski. "If you eat a lot of snacks that are nutritionally inferior or junk food, you're just giving your body empty calories that are devoid of vitamins and minerals."

**Focus on fruits and veggies.** "You should eat a minimum of five good-size servings of fruits and vegetables every day," says Grabowski. "In most cases, the darkest or most vibrantly colored fruits and vegetables have the richest vitamin and mineral content." Color your diet with such perennial favorites as cantaloupe, oranges, peaches, tomatoes, spinach, yams and carrots. Also ask your greengrocer about some of the more exotic fruits and vegetables to add variety. Most tropical fruits are rich in vitamins.

**Eat 'em raw or just-cooked.** Cooking food draws out or destroys many vitamins and minerals, so whenever you can, try to eat fruits, vegetables and grains in their natural raw or unprocessed state or minimally cooked.

**Don't boil.** Boiling tends to leach out more minerals and vitamins from foods than other cooking methods, says Grabowski. "The less time spent in the oven, on the stove or surrounded by hot water, the better." She recommends steaming or microwaving.

**Trap nutrients.** Exposure to air can rob vitamins and minerals from food. So can sunlight when it penetrates glass bottles or cellophane wrap. Grabowski recommends using airtight, opaque containers. For long-term storage of foods or juices, try freezing. It keeps nutrients intact for a long time.

**Watch out for medications.** Certain drugs and over-the-counter medications can interfere with the body's vitamin and mineral stores. Aspirin, laxatives, diuretics, antibiotics, antidepressants and antacids can accelerate the excretion of some vitamins and minerals or impede their absorption. If you are taking any of these medications, consult your doctor before quitting or trying alternatives.

# The Skinny on Supplements

If you think you might be falling short in your RDAs, seek out a health or nutrition professional who can evaluate your diet and tell you which nutrients you might need more of. But don't expect supplements to completely make up for poor eating habits—they won't. If you try supplements, taking levels in excess of the RDAs should be done only in consultation with a physician.

Here are some guidelines for selecting and using supplements.

**Go multi.** A safe and beneficial supplement would be a once-a-day-type multivitamin with minerals, says Grabowski. Such a supplement should contain a mixture of all or most of the essential vitamins and minerals and contain approximately 100% of the RDAs for each.

**Take care with single supplements.** In most cases, you probably don't need extra doses of specific vitamins and minerals if you are taking a multivitamin and eating right. Exceptions would be if you are under a doctor's treatment for a deficiency or if you are seeking antioxidant protection by taking extra vitamin C, vitamin E and beta-carotene. Otherwise, avoid single supplements—especially vitamin A, vitamin D and iron, says Dr. Thomas. These nutrients are toxic in high doses and can result in such side effects as vomiting, hair loss, bone abnormalities, anemia, cardiovascular damage and liver and kidney failure.

**Don't forget your calcium.** Calcium is vital for bone strength and for staving off osteoporosis—the bone-thinning disease that creeps up on many women after menopause. But studies show that most women don't get enough—the recommended 800 milligrams a day before menopause and 1,000 milligrams a day thereafter. That's why calcium supplements are recommended for women as added protection against bone loss.

The most easily absorbed calcium supplements are those made with calcium citrate, says Margo Denke, M.D., assistant professor of medicine at the University of Texas Southwestern Medical Center at Dallas Center for Human Nutrition and a member of the nutrition committee of the American Heart Association. They are more easily absorbed by the body than supplements made with calcium carbonate, she says. Calcium citrate can be found in some over-the-counter supplements or in calcium-fortified orange juices. Just check the labels.

But you may prefer to get your calcium from inexpensive over-the-counter antacid tablets made from calcium carbonate. It's best to take these with meals, says Clifford Rosen, M.D., director of the Maine Center for Osteoporosis Research and Education in Bangor. The acid your body produces when you eat will break down the calcium carbonate and allow it to be absorbed, he says.

Some antacid brands, such as Gelusil, Maalox and Mylanta, are not recommended for use as regular supplements, however, because they also contain aluminum. Your best choices are Tums or Rolaids—both aluminum-free.

**Look into generics.** Generic and store brands are typically comparable in quality to big-name brands, says Dr. Thomas. In fact, generics are often produced by the same manufacturers as the big-name brands but cost a lot less. Your pharmacist should be able to tell you if a generic is worthwhile.

**Forget "super-supplements."** You may see "high potency" or "extra strength" labels. These products typically contain levels of vitamins and minerals that greatly exceed the RDAs and may be hazardous, says Dr. Thomas. Or you may just end up excreting the excess, in which case you're wasting your money.

**Say no to gimmicks.** Phrases like "anti-stress formula" are bogus, says Dr. Thomas, and although "time-released" and "effervescent" are legitimate descriptors, in some supplements these qualities may not matter. For example, effervescence in calcium may be helpful but it is not needed in vitamin C. Check with your physician or nutritional professional.

**A vitamin is a vitamin.** Also ignore claims about natural or organic ingredients, says Dr. Thomas. There is no standard definition of *natural*. Some "natural" supplements, in fact, may contain mostly synthetic nutrients.

**Avoid multiple dosages.** If the label tells you to take more than one a day, check the total amount to see how it compares with the RDA. If it's way over, this may be a ploy to get you to shell out more money, Dr. Thomas says.

**Pop 'em with a meal.** As a general rule, supplements will be absorbed more efficiently by the body if they are taken during a meal rather than on an empty stomach, says Dr. Thomas. They will also break down better if they're taken with water or some other beverage.

**Check the expiration date.** When shopping for supplements, make sure an expiration date is on the label. If the date has passed or is just around the corner, find a bottle with a longer shelf life.

**Keep 'em in a cool, dry place.** Light, heat and moisture can rob supplements of their potency. Because of this, a kitchen cabinet, away from the heat of the stove, is probably a better place to keep your supplements than on the windowsill or in a bathroom medicine chest. The refrigerator is another good storage place. Try to use a non-transparent container. And always secure the cap tightly.

# YOGA

## Finding Peace in the Chaos

You're looking for an oasis, a tranquil place where you can pull yourself together after a day of impossible deadlines, impossible people and impossible dreams.

For lots of women, the answer is yoga. If you're looking for something that will leave you feeling relaxed, limber, self-confident and youthful, it may be a perfect fit for you, too.

"So many things you do in life are energy users." says Alice Christensen, founder and executive director of the American Yoga Association in Sarasota, Florida. "But yoga provides a constant source of energy. When you practice yoga, you actually have more vitality and vigor. In that way, I really think it can help to make you feel younger."

## New Health from an Ancient Art

Yoga has been around for thousands of years. Literally translated, it means "union." Yoga advocates believe that mind, spirit and body are inseparable. And they believe that exercises called asanas, or poses, can aid in flexibility, relaxation, increased strength and inner peace.

Though there are as many as eight different branches of yoga, most western women focus on hatha yoga. This yoga stresses relaxation through asanas and breathing techniques and is often taught in classes at local YM/YWCAs or fitness clubs.

Hatha yoga is not aerobic exercise. But studies show it can help soothe your body and mind in a number of ways.

The most obvious benefits appear to come in stress reduction and mood enhancement. A study of 170 college students showed that those taking beginner yoga classes had less tension, depression, anger, fatigue and confusion after class

637

# Scan Away Your Stress

It's one of those days. Everything—from the car to the job to the trip to the grocery store—has gone wrong. Now you have a tension headache, a throbbing neck and shooting pains in your back and shoulders.

All is not lost. An effective meditative method for dealing with pain is a yogalike exercise called the body scan. It can help you focus on those aches and slowly work them out of your body. Taught to patients at the University of Massachusetts Medical Center, the body scan is a great way to identify and beat your own stress hot spots.

Here's how to do it.

Lie on your back, close your eyes and simply breathe. After a few minutes start concentrating on the toes of your left foot. Note the sensations: Are they warm, cold, tired or cramped? After a minute or so imagine releasing the weight of your toes, feeling them melt right into the floor.

Now concentrate on your left leg, practicing the same routine on your foot, ankle, calf, knee, thigh and hip. Then do the same for your right leg. Move up your torso pausing at your pelvis, lower back, belly, upper back, chest and shoulders. On your arms, move on to the fingers of both hands, the back of the hands, the palms, the wrists, the forearms, the elbows, the upper arms and the shoulders. Finally, move on to your neck, then your head, paying attention to your chin, mouth, nose, eyes and eyebrows, forehead, ears and scalp.

The American Yoga Association in Sarasota, Florida, advocates a similar complete relaxation exercise that is introduced just before meditation, though its plan works from the head down and then up the back of your body.

"The subtle benefit of practicing this type of exercise is that you'll become more aware of your body on a daily basis," says Alice Christensen, founder and executive director of the American Yoga Association. "Then, even when you're sitting at your desk at work, you'll notice 'Oh, my stomach's tense' or 'I'm clenching my teeth.' "

"The simple act of bringing awareness to the tense area will help you to release the tension."

than they did before. The students' reported feelings were similar to others who had started more strenuous activities like swimming. The study reported that the students began to notice stress reduction after taking their first class.

Yogic breathing techniques also may help people with asthma. A British study of 18 patients showed yoga breathing could reduce symptoms of asthma, though it did not eliminate them. Some doctors are now prescribing yoga as part of therapy to help their asthma patients gain more self-control over their breathing difficulties.

Christensen says yoga also can be tremendously helpful to people with back pain, as long as they follow the yoga principles of stretching slowly and only as far as the body wants to go. And she says it may help people with arthritis as well. Though there are few studies linking yoga and arthritis, Christensen says many of her students with common age-related arthritis report feeling more flexible and in less pain after starting a yoga class. Christensen warns, though, that people with bone-crippling rheumatoid arthritis should not attempt yoga exercise when their joints are swollen and painful.

In addition to the physical advantages of yoga, there's a meditative side that's impossible to measure with a stethoscope. "Yoga quiets the constant talk that's in your mind," Christensen says. "You deal constantly with scattered thoughts, other people's voices, emotions, desires. And you don't even notice it after a while."

Yoga can help clear that from your mind. "It helps improve your concentration and allows you to become more observant of your thoughts, feelings and reactions," says Christensen. "Much of the time we move through the world like the steel ball in a pinball machine, bouncing off one thing after another. Yoga meditation increases awareness so you can make more conscious choices in your life."

# Getting Started

Sounds good, doesn't it? Here are some tips to help you reap yoga's considerable benefits.

**Take a deep breath.** Yoga begins with breathing, something we rarely think about. Most of us inhale from our chests taking quick, shallow breaths. Yoga practitioners, however, breathe from their diaphragms—the large, dome-shaped muscle that arches across the base of the lungs. When a person inhales deeply, the diaphragm expands, allowing more air into the lung's lower lobes.

To get started, sit comfortably on the floor, supporting your hips by sitting on a firm cushion. Or you can sit on the edge of a chair. Place your hands on your belly, a little below your navel. This is the area—not your chest—that should expand when you inhale. Remember to always breathe in and out through your nose. When you inhale, feel your hands rise. When you exhale, contract your belly. Breathe smoothly and evenly. After a few breaths, place your hands on your legs and continue breathing with your eyes closed, concentrating on the sound of the breath.

Ideally, you should breathe from your diaphragm all the time—at work, at home, in the car, wherever. Christensen says this helps you get more oxygen

*(continued on page 642)*

# Yoga for Beginners

If you're interested in trying yoga, these four poses are a good place to start. Remember: Go at your own pace and don't stretch past the point of comfort.

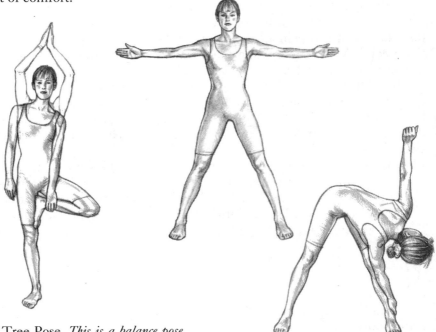

The Tree Pose. *This is a balance pose that improves poise, posture and concentration. Stand with your feet parallel. Shift weight to your right leg and place the heel of your left foot against your right ankle. Hold on to a wall or chair for support if you need to. Slowly raise the left foot higher, assisting with your free hand, until the foot reaches your right inner thigh. Place your arms at your sides, then slowly bring them over your head as straight as possible with your palms together. Relax your stomach and your breath. Stare at one spot for balance. Hold for several seconds or as long as you can comfortably. Then slowly lower and repeat on the opposite side.*

The Twisting Triangle. *This exercise limbers the back, hips and legs and may help to relieve depression. Stand with your feet pointed straight ahead, as wide apart as you can stand comfortably. Breathe in and raise your arms out to the sides, then breathe out and twist to the left. Grasp the outside of your left ankle with your right hand, extend your left arm straight up with fingers slightly curled and look up at your left thumb. Hold for just a moment, then breathe in and return to a standing position with your arms outstretched. Breathe out and repeat to the right leg. Stretch three times to each leg.*

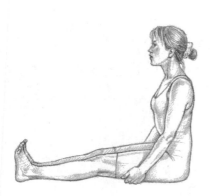

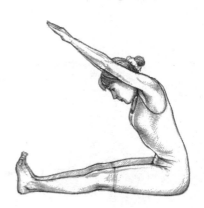

Seated Sun Pose. *This exercise limbers the back and legs, massages the internal organs and improves circulation. Sit on the floor with your legs outstretched and your toes pulled back toward your face (above). Breathe in and raise your arms to the sides and overhead. Stretch and look up (below).*

*Then tuck your head, start to breathe out and slowly bend forward as far as you can without straining (above). Get a good grip on your legs wherever you can reach, bend your elbows and gently pull your upper body down toward your legs (below). Use your arms to pull, not your back muscles. Hold for a few seconds. Breathe in and raise your arms back up overhead. Then breathe out and lower your arms to your sides. Repeat twice more.*

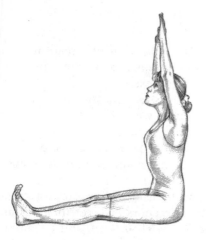

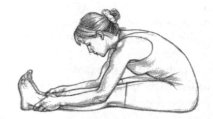

## Yoga for Beginners—Continued

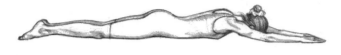

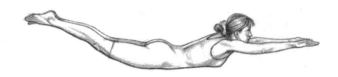

The Boat Pose. *This is an excellent exercise to strengthen the back and improve posture. Lie on your stomach with your arms outstretched in front and your forehead on the floor (above). Breathe out completely, then breathe in as you raise your legs, arms and head all at once, looking up (below). Breathe out and lower your body. Repeat twice more.*

into your system, making you more alert. You'll also find yourself breathing at a more relaxing pace of maybe 10 or 14 times per minute instead of the typical 16 to 18 times. Remember, always breathe through your nose.

**Find a good class.** Lots of places offer yoga classes, but not every class is the same. Christensen suggests looking for a teacher who practices yoga every day and sees her own yoga teacher on a regular basis. Ask the teacher for references. Take a trial class before you invest long-term time or money. And if you have specific problems, like a bad back or arthritis, make sure you find a teacher who will individualize instruction for you.

**Go for mail order.** If you're having problems locating a class, the American Yoga Association has a correspondence course. The course packet includes an instruction book *(The American Yoga Association Beginner's Manual)* and an audiocassette on relaxation and meditation. The course can be helpful when you're practicing at home, even if you're enrolled in a class. The association also offers a videotape and other instructional materials. A catalog is available on request. For more information write to the American Yoga Association, 513 South Orange Avenue, Sarasota, FL 34236.

**Set your own pace.** Yoga isn't a contest. You're not there to out-stretch or out-meditate or out-breathe your friends who practice yoga or the other people in the class.

"At the very least, you need to know that you should not compete," says Martin Pierce, director of the Pierce Program, a yoga studio in Atlanta. "If you are looking around at others thinking you must do as well as they do, you are going to create more stress for yourself." Direct your attention inward, Christensen says. "Pay attention to your own experiences and you will achieve the most lasting results."

**Strike that pose.** Lots of yoga stretches, or asanas, are easy for beginners, Christensen says.

Remember: Don't push your body. Stretch slowly and evenly. Don't bounce. And push only as far as your body lets you. "Going too far will injure you. Be a friend to your body," Christensen says.

Always check with your doctor before you start practicing yoga or any exercise program.

**Stick with it.** You may start feeling better after just one yoga session, but don't stop there. "People can't expect to benefit greatly from yoga without making a commitment to it," says Jon Kabat-Zinn, Ph.D., director of the Stress Reduction Clinic at the University of Massachusetts Medical Center in Worcester.

"Yoga practice should be regular—daily, if possible," Christensen says. "At the very least, if you want results, it demands three exercises and a few minutes of breathing and meditation. This can take as little as 15 minutes. If you find yourself wanting to practice more, an hour a day is plenty. The important thing is to enjoy what you do."

**Keep working out.** Beginner yoga is not aerobic exercise. Christensen recommends that you continue with bicycling, walking, running or some other activity that gives your heart a workout. "Think of yoga as an added dimension to your fitness program," she says. "It is never boring because besides offering the physical benefits of limberness, health and strength, it adds meaning to life."

# SOURCES AND CREDITS

"How Long Will You Live?" on page 12 is adapted from *Health Risks* by Elliot J. Howard, M.D. Copyright © 1986 by Elliot J. Howard, M.D., and Susan A. Roth. Reprinted by permission.

"What Do You See in the Mirror?" on page 67 is adapted from *The Body Image Trap* by Marion Crook, published by International Self-Counsel Press Ltd. Reprinted by permission of the publisher.

"Are You Burning Out?" on page 74 is adapted from *Burnout: The High Cost of High Achievement* by Herbert J. Freudenberger. Copyright © 1980 by Herbert J. Freudenberger and Geraldine Richelson. Used by permission of Doubleday, a division of Bantam Doubleday Dell Publishing Group, Inc. (Foreign distribution or foreign language reprints by permission of Herbert J. Freudenberger, Ph.D.)

"Are You in Alcohol's Grip?" on page 138 is adapted from the *American Journal of Psychiatry*, vol. 127, no. 12, 1655, June 1971. Copyright © 1971 the American Psychiatric Association. Reprinted by permission.

The table in "What's a Healthy Weight, Anyway?" on page 278 is from the U.S. Department of Agriculture and U.S. Department of Health and Human Services.

"Is Stress Adding Up?" on page 330 is adapted from *Is It Worth Dying For?* by Robert S. Eliot, M.D., and Dennis L. Breo. Copyright © 1984 by Robert S. Eliot, M.D., and Dennis L. Breo. Used by permission of Bantam Books, a division of Bantam Doubleday Dell Publishing Group, Inc.

"Is Work Wearing You Out?" on page 332 is from the American Institute of Stress. For more information, write to 124 Park Avenue, Yonkers, NY 10703.

# INDEX

Note: <u>Underscored</u> page references indicate boxed text. **Boldface** references indicate illustrations. Prescription drug names are denoted with the symbol Rx.